Role Development for the Nurse Practitioner

Edited by
Susan M. DeNisco, DNP, APRN, FNP-BC, FAANP

Professor and Director, Family Nurse Practitioner
and Doctor of Nursing Practice Program
Sacred Heart University
Fairfield, Connecticut

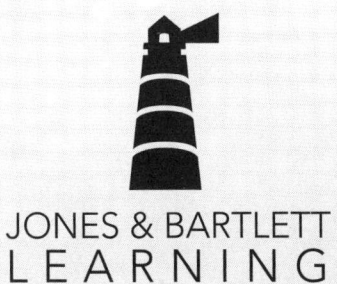

JONES & BARTLETT
LEARNING

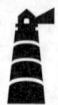

World Headquarters
Jones & Bartlett Learning
25 Mall Road
Burlington, MA 01803
978-443-5000
info@jblearning.com
www.jblearning.com

Jones & Bartlett Learning books and products are available through most bookstores and online booksellers. To contact Jones & Bartlett Learning directly, call 800-832-0034, fax 978-443-8000, or visit our website, www.jblearning.com.

Substantial discounts on bulk quantities of Jones & Bartlett Learning publications are available to corporations, professional associations, and other qualified organizations. For details and specific discount information, contact the special sales department at Jones & Bartlett Learning via the above contact information or send an email to specialsales@jblearning.com.

Copyright © 2023 by Jones & Bartlett Learning, LLC, an Ascend Learning Company

All rights reserved. No part of the material protected by this copyright may be reproduced or utilized in any form, electronic or mechanical, including photocopying, recording, or by any information storage and retrieval system, without written permission from the copyright owner.

The content, statements, views, and opinions herein are the sole expression of the respective authors and not that of Jones & Bartlett Learning, LLC. Reference herein to any specific commercial product, process, or service by trade name, trademark, manufacturer, or otherwise does not constitute or imply its endorsement or recommendation by Jones & Bartlett Learning, LLC and such reference shall not be used for advertising or product endorsement purposes. All trademarks displayed are the trademarks of the parties noted herein. *Role Development for the Nurse Practitioner, Third Edition* is an independent publication and has not been authorized, sponsored, or otherwise approved by the owners of the trademarks or service marks referenced in this product.

There may be images in this book that feature models; these models do not necessarily endorse, represent, or participate in the activities represented in the images. Any screenshots in this product are for educational and instructive purposes only. Any individuals and scenarios featured in the case studies throughout this product may be real or fictitious but are used for instructional purposes only.

The authors, editor, and publisher have made every effort to provide accurate information. However, they are not responsible for errors, omissions, or for any outcomes related to the use of the contents of this book and take no responsibility for the use of the products and procedures described. Treatments and side effects described in this book may not be applicable to all people; likewise, some people may require a dose or experience a side effect that is not described herein. Drugs and medical devices are discussed that may have limited availability controlled by the Food and Drug Administration (FDA) for use only in a research study or clinical trial. Research, clinical practice, and government regulations often change the accepted standard in this field. When consideration is being given to use of any drug in the clinical setting, the health care provider or reader is responsible for determining FDA status of the drug, reading the package insert, and reviewing prescribing information for the most up-to-date recommendations on dose, precautions, and contraindications, and determining the appropriate usage for the product. This is especially important in the case of drugs that are new or seldom used.

23430-5

Production Credits
VP, Content Strategy & Implementation:
    Christine Emerton
Director, Product Management: Matthew Kane
Product Manager: Tina Chen
Manager, Content Strategy: Carolyn Pershouse
Project Manager: Kristen Rogers
Project Specialist: Janet Vail
Digital Project Specialist: Rachel DiMaggio
Senior Marketing Manager: Jennifer Scherzay
Content Services Manager: Colleen Lamy

Product Fulfillment Manager: Wendy Kilborn
Composition: S4Carlisle Publishing Services
Project Management: S4Carlisle Publishing Services
Cover Design: Michael O'Donnell
Rights & Permissions Manager: John Rusk
Senior Media Development Editor: Troy Liston
Rights Specialist: Benjamin Roy
Cover Image, Part Opener, Chapter Opener:
    @ Tomertu/Shutterstock
Printing and Binding: CJK Group Inc.

Library of Congress Cataloging-in-Publication Data
Names: DeNisco, Susan M. author.
Title: Role development for the nurse practitioner / [edited by] Susan M.
    DeNisco.
Description: Third edition. | Burlington, MA : Jones & Bartlett Learning,
    [2023] | Includes bibliographical references and index.
Identifiers: LCCN 2021026306 | ISBN 9781284234305 (paperback)
Subjects: MESH: Nurse Practitioners | Nurse's Role | BISAC: MEDICAL /
    Nursing / General
Classification: LCC RT82.8 | NLM WY 128 | DDC 610.7306/92--dc23
LC record available at https://lccn.loc.gov/2021026306

6048

Printed in the United States of America
25 24 23 22 21   10 9 8 7 6 5 4 3 2 1

This book is dedicated to my late friend and colleague, Dr. Julie G. Stewart. I was most fortunate to have Julie in my life. She was a passionate nurse educator always helping "the underdog," a nurse practitioner working with the poor, and a visionary nurse leader whom I called "the triple threat." Her passion for life, sense of humor, and vision for the future of nursing still helps me carry on. She will always be the Lucy to my Ethel. Rest in peace my dear friend—you have left a legacy behind.

Susan M. DeNisco

Brief Contents

Foreword — xv
Preface — xvi
Contributors — xvii

PART 1 Scientific Underpinning of the Nurse Practitioner Role — 1

CHAPTER 1 Historical Perspectives: The Art and Science of Nurse Practitionering and Advanced Practice Nursing 3

CHAPTER 2 Evidence-Based Practice and Dissemination Strategies 33

PART 2 The Nurse Practitioner–Patient Relationship — 69

CHAPTER 3 Family-Focused Clinical Practice: Considerations for the Nurse Practitioner 71

CHAPTER 4 Vulnerable Populations 99

CHAPTER 5 Mental Health and Primary Care: A Critical Intersection 131

CHAPTER 6 Cultural Sensitivity and Global Health 155

CHAPTER 7 Chronic Disease Management Models, Pain Management, and Palliative Care 187

Brief Contents v

PART 3 Clinical Education for the Nurse Practitioner 213

CHAPTER 8	Quality, Safety, and Prescriptive Authority 215
CHAPTER 9	Clinical Education: The Role of the Student, Faculty, and Preceptor 237
CHAPTER 10	Case Presentation, Consultation, and Collaboration in Primary Care 255
CHAPTER 11	Clinical Prevention/ Community and Population Health 277
CHAPTER 12	Electronic Health Record and Impact on Healthcare Outcomes 305
CHAPTER 13	Telehealth: Increasing Access to Health Care 327

PART 4 The Professional Nurse Practitioner 349

CHAPTER 14	Concepts and Challenges of the Professional Nurse Practitioner 351
CHAPTER 15	Health Policy and the Nurse Practitioner 367
CHAPTER 16	Mentoring and Lifelong Learning 389
CHAPTER 17	Reimbursement for Nurse Practitioner Services............. 403
CHAPTER 18	Professional Employment: Preparing for Licensure, Certification, and Credentialing... 431

| CHAPTER 19 | Nurse Practitioner as a Business Owner: Entrepreneurship and Practice Management........449 |

Index   **461**

Contents

Foreword xv
Preface xvi
Contributors xvii

PART 1 Scientific Underpinning of the Nurse Practitioner Role — 1

CHAPTER 1 Historical Perspectives: The Art and Science of Nurse Practitionering and Advanced Practice Nursing ... 3
Susan M. DeNisco and Julie G. Stewart

Advanced Practice Nursing 4
The Role of the NP: A Historical Perspective 4
Nurse Practitioner Education and Title Clarification 5
The Role of the NP Today 6
Educational Foundation for the Advanced Practice Nurse 6
The Essentials: Core Competencies for Professional
  Nursing Education 6
Core Nursing Concepts, Major Domains, and Competencies 8
Nurse Practitioner Core Competencies 13
Doctor of Nursing Program (DNP) 16
Nurse Practitioners' Approach to Patient Care 18
Nurse Practitioners' Unique Role 21
Seminar Discussion Questions 28
References 29

CHAPTER 2 Evidence-Based Practice and Dissemination Strategies ... 33
Kerry Milner

The History of Evidence-Based Practice 33
Nursing and EBP 34
Evidence-Based Competencies for Advanced Practice Nurses 37

viii Contents

How to Translate EBP into Practice 38
Searching for Evidence 38
Searching Databases for Best Current Evidence 40
What Counts as Evidence? 45
Critical Appraisal of Evidence 48
Evidence Synthesis and Recommendations 53
Outcomes of the EBP Process 59
Shared Decision Making: An Important Often Missed
    Part of EBP 59
Disseminating EBP 62
Barriers to EBP 62
Chapter Summary Points 63
Seminar Discussion Questions 64
References 65

PART 2 The Nurse Practitioner-Patient Relationship   69

CHAPTER 3 Family-Focused Clinical Practice: Considerations for the Nurse Practitioner 71
Susan M. DeNisco

Family Theory 71
Family Resilience and Capacity Models 74
Family Structure, Function, and Roles 80
Family Development 81
Divorced Families 82
Nontraditional Families 82
Structural Assessment and Family Interviews 85
Family Problem List 92
Seminar Discussion Questions 95
References 95
Additional Resources 98

CHAPTER 4 Vulnerable Populations 99
Susan M. DeNisco

Section One: Overview of Vulnerabilities and Disparities 99
Section Two: Overview of Select Special Populations,
    Direct Care, and Access 103
Section Three: Developing Population-Based Programs
    for the Vulnerable 124

Chapter Summary ... 125
Seminar Discussion Questions ... 126
References ... 126

CHAPTER 5 Mental Health and Primary Care: A Critical Intersection ... 131
Anna Goddard and Sara Ann Jakub

NP Role in Holistic Care ... 132
Health Disparities ... 132
What Is Mental Health? ... 135
Management, Treatment, and Referrals Considerations ... 142
Trauma Informed Care ... 146
Importance of Self-Care ... 148
Understanding Scope of Practice ... 149
Seminar Discussion Questions ... 150
References ... 151

CHAPTER 6 Cultural Sensitivity and Global Health ... 155
Michelle A. Cole and Christina B. Gunther

Introduction ... 155
Global Diversity ... 156
Cultural Competency and Clinical Education ... 157
Cultural Awareness ... 160
Environmental Control ... 161
Cultural Humility ... 163
Cultural Competence and the Clinician ... 165
Cultural Immersion Experiences ... 170
Demystifying the Cultural Competence Puzzle ... 171
Language and Communication ... 174
Seminar Discussion Questions ... 180
References ... 181

CHAPTER 7 Chronic Disease Management Models, Pain Management, and Palliative Care ... 187
Mary Lou Siefert, Sylvie Rosenbloom, Elizabeth Ercolano, and Jean Boucher

Introduction ... 187
Palliative Care Definition and Background ... 187
Goals of Care ... 189

Contents

Care Transitions 189
Quality of Life 189
National Organizations 191
Nurses and Palliative Care 192
Conclusion 203
Seminar Discussion Questions 204
References 207

PART 3 Clinical Education for the Nurse Practitioner 213

CHAPTER 8 Quality, Safety, and Prescriptive Authority 215
Sylvie Rosenbloom, Linda S. Morrow, and Tammy A. Testut

An Introduction to Quality 215
Quality in Doctoral Education 216
U.S. Healthcare System 216
Institute of Medicine Quality Reports 218
Professional Accountability and Teamwork 219
Quality and Safety Education for Nurses 220
Patient-Centered Care 223
Communication and Care Coordination 224
Quality Improvement Planning 225
Safety 227
Informatics 229
TeamSTEPPS 229
Prescriptive Authority 229
Chapter Summary 234
Seminar Discussion Questions 234
References 234

CHAPTER 9 Clinical Education: The Role of the Student, Faculty, and Preceptor 237
Susan M. DeNisco

Daily Reflective Questions 239
The Role of Faculty 239
The Role of the Student 241
The Role of the Preceptor 244
Evaluation and Clinical Time Documentation 246

Pathways to the DNP...247
Final Project..248
Current Trends in NP Clinical Education.............................249
The Future of NP Clinical Education 249
The Pandemic's Impact on Clinical Education 250
Seminar Discussion Questions.......................................250
References..251

CHAPTER 10 Case Presentation, Consultation, and Collaboration in Primary Care 255
Susan M. DeNisco and Sylvie Rosenbloom

Introduction to the Case Presentation...............................255
Organizing the Oral Case Study Presentation.........................256
Collaboration, Consultation, and Referral in Primary Care 263
Interprofessional Collaboration 268
Collaborative Health Management Model...............................271
Barriers and Benefits to Effective Interprofessional
    Collaboration 273
Seminar Discussion Questions.......................................273
References..274

CHAPTER 11 Clinical Prevention/Community and Population Health.....................................277
Anna Goddard and Dorothea Esposito

Principles of Epidemiology...277
Prevention Levels..283
HIV and Prevention Levels..286
COVID-19 and Prevention Levels 288
Population Health and *Healthy People 2030*........................293
Emergency Preparedness and the Nurse Practitioner..................297
Seminar Discussion Questions.......................................301
References..302

CHAPTER 12 Electronic Health Record and Impact on Healthcare Outcomes 305
Stephen C. Burrows

Moving to Electronic Documentation/Electronic Health
    Record: Reasons for Doing So...................................305
Influencing Forces...307
Meaningful Use 308

Contents

The Electronic Health Record 310
Converting to Electronic Health Record 314
Electronic Health Records Features and Functionality 318
Technical Considerations 319
Seminar Discussion Questions 321
References 322

CHAPTER 13 Telehealth: Increasing Access to Health Care ... 327
Donna F. McHaney and Nicole Kroll

Introduction to Telehealth 327
Difference between Telehealth and Telemedicine 327
The History of Telehealth 328
Telehealth Modalities 329
Guidelines for the Entry-Level Primary Provider 331
The Role of the Advanced Practice Nurse Practitioner
   in Telehealth 332
Telehealth Regulations 336
Privacy and Protective Health Information Requirements
   Relevant to Telehealth 336
Integration of Telehealth into Clinical Practice 337
Evaluation of Telehealth Systems 343
The Future of Telehealth 344
Seminar Discussion Questions 345
References 345

PART 4 The Professional Nurse Practitioner   349

CHAPTER 14 Concepts and Challenges of the Professional Nurse Practitioner 351
Constance H. Glenn and Geraldine Budd

Professionalism 351
Autonomy 355
Ethics 357
Service/Altruism 359
Leadership 361
Barriers 362
Seminar Discussion Questions 363

Contents   xiii

References 363
Additional Resources 365

CHAPTER 15 Health Policy and the Nurse Practitioner 367
Julie A. Koch and Linda Washington-Brown

History of the NP and Related Health Policy 368
Formal Health Policy Education for NPs 369
Advancing NP Practice Through Health Policy 371
Current Health Policy Issues 375
Getting Involved 380
Nurse Practitioner Health Policy Exemplars 382
Exemplar 1 382
Exemplar 2 384
Seminar Discussion Questions 385
References 385

CHAPTER 16 Mentoring and Lifelong Learning 389
Susan M. DeNisco and Dori Taylor-Sullivan

Preceptor 389
Role Model 390
Coach 391
Mentor 391
Seminar Discussion Questions 399
References 400

CHAPTER 17 Reimbursement for Nurse Practitioner Services 403
Lynn Rapsilber

Introduction 403
Important Steps in Reimbursement Eligibility 403
Coding and Billing Resources 405
Medical Record Documentation 406
Payment for Services 412
Evaluation and Management Documentation Guidelines 413
General Coding Guidelines 413
Key Components of Reimbursement 415
How to Bill for a Visit 425
Coding Conundrums 425

xiv Contents

Value-Based Reimbursement................................. 427
Seminar Discussion Questions................................ 428
References.. 430

CHAPTER 18 Professional Employment: Preparing for Licensure, Certification, and Credentialing 431
Susan M. DeNisco

Nurse Practitioner Certification 431
Nurse Practitioner Licensure for Prescription Privileges 433
Malpractice Insurance.. 434
Résumé vs. Curriculum Vitae Development for Nurse Practitioners... 435
Job Satisfaction 436
Collaboration 437
Empowerment 438
Interviewing Skills 438
Negotiating an Employment Contract 439
Credentialing 441
Collaborative Agreements.................................... 441
The Consensus Model—Stay Tuned! 445
Seminar Discussion Questions................................ 445
References.. 445

CHAPTER 19 Nurse Practitioner as a Business Owner: Entrepreneurship and Practice Management 449
Kimberly Testo and Tiffany Teixeira

Introduction 449
Practice Start-up 450
The Legal Aspects of Owning a Practice 452
Practice Management.. 457
References.. 460

Index **461**

Foreword

The first edition of this unique and timely book was inspired and developed by two doctor of nursing practice (DNP) alumni from one of the most prestigious DNP programs in the country. Collectively, with more than seven decades as nurse practitioners in primary care practice and education, the authors took on the task of summarizing the key aspects of their roles, including preparing for NP certification and licensure, as well as often overlooked areas, such as consultation, collaboration, billing, and reimbursement. Critically important clinical information on the cultural aspects of practice, the intersection of primary and mental health care, and the NP–patient relationship is also highlighted. Chapters on mentoring and professionalism, the hallmark activities of any high-level occupation, are included. This *Third Edition* informs the reader of current trends in health care, including new chapters on telehealth and NPs as entrepreneurs.

Throughout the text, case vignettes and interviews with nurse practitioners are used to highlight key information and inspire critical thinking. The information outlined in this publication will provide the foundation needed to practice at the highest level of NP preparation in order to meet societal needs for quality, cost-effective, and outcome-driven health care. This book will serve as a resource for the NP at a variety of stages, from student to expert clinician.

Margaret A. Fitzgerald, DNP, FNP-BC, NP-C, FAANP, CSP, FAAN, DCC

President, Fitzgerald Health Education Associates, Inc.

Preface

As a new graduate nurse, I was very interested in working with medically underserved populations and was influenced by the work of Mary Breckenridge, a nurse–midwife who founded the Frontier Nursing Service. Off I went to my first professional nursing role as a surgical nurse in a small country hospital in eastern Kentucky. On weekends, I and a physician friend of mine traded the "horse" for a "Jeep" and visited many families that had few resources and no transportation out of the "hollers" to obtain medical care. Following the 2 years spent in Appalachia, I solidified my interest in primary care by working for the U.S. Public Health Service on the western slope of Colorado where I set up clinics for migrant Mexican farm workers. I was then hooked and decided that I could make the largest impact on vulnerable populations by becoming a family nurse practitioner. My 35 years as a primary care provider has afforded me the opportunity to provide direct patient care to both rural and urban populations in a wide variety of settings. Each patient I have been honored to care for has taught me so much and helped fuel my passion for "nurse practitionering." A large part of my career has been spent on passing on my knowledge to the next generation of NPs. I have precepted many NP students over the years and enjoy seeing them blossom from neophyte, entry-level nurse practitioners to those that practice with competence and compassion. I have been fortunate to share my love of educating nurse practitioner students with my late colleague and dear friend, Dr. Julie Stewart. She sits on my shoulder and I often ask myself "What would Julie do?" and then I have a good laugh!

In the words of Khalil Gibran, "Generosity is giving more than you can, and pride is taking less than you need."

Susan M. DeNisco

Contributors

Jean Boucher, PhD, RN, ANP-BC
Associate Professor of Nursing & Medicine
UMass Medical School
Graduate School of Nursing
Worcester, MA

Geraldine Budd, PhD, APRN, FNP-BC, FAANP
Clinical Associate Professor, Family Nurse Practitioner/Doctor of Nursing Practice Program
Davis and Henley College of Nursing
Sacred Heart University
Fairfield, CT

Stephen C. Burrows, DPM, MBA, CPHIMS, FHIMSS
Program Director, Healthcare Informatics
College of Health Professions
Sacred Heart University
Fairfield, CT

Michelle A. Cole, DNP, MSN, RN, CPN
Clinical Associate Professor
University of Connecticut
School of Nursing
Storrs, CT

Elizabeth Ercolano, DNSc, MSN, RN
Associate Research Scientist
Yale School of Nursing
Yale University
Orange, CT

Dorothea Esposito, DNP, MSN, APRN, FNP-BC, NP-C
Clinical Assistant Professor, Doctor of Nursing Practice/Family Nurse Practitioner Program
Davis and Henley College of Nursing
Sacred Heart University
Fairfield, CT

Constance Glenn, DNP, APRN, FNP-BC, CNE
Clinical Assistant Professor, Doctor of Nursing Practice/Family Nurse Practitioner Program
Davis and Henley College of Nursing
Sacred Heart University
Fairfield, CT

Anna Goddard, PhD, APRN, CPNP-PC
Vice President of Quality, Research, & Evaluation
School-Based Health Alliance
Washington, DC

Christina B. Gunther, PhD, MA
Director, Global Health Programs & Health Science Program
Assistant Professor
College of Health Professions
Sacred Heart University
Fairfield, CT

Sara Ann M. Jakub, MA, SYC, LPC
Child and Family Agency of Southeastern Connecticut
New London, CT

Contributors

Julie A. Koch, DNP, APRN, FNP-BC, FAANP
Assistant Dean of Graduate Nursing and DNP Program Director
Valparaiso University
Valparaiso, IN

Nicole Peters Kroll, PhD, APRN, ANP-C, FNP-BC
Clinical Assistant Professor FNP/MSN Program
Davis and Henley College of Nursing
Sacred Heart University
Fairfield, CT
Family Nurse Practitioner
University Occupational Health Partners
College Station, TX

Donna Faye McHaney, DNP, MIS, APRN, FNP-C
Clinical Associate Professor
Director, FNP & DNP Online Programs
Sacred Heart University
Davis and Henley College of Nursing
Fairfield, CT

Kerry Milner, DNSc, RN
Associate Professor
Davis and Henley College of Nursing
Sacred Heart University
Fairfield, CT

Linda S. Morrow, DNP, MSN, MBA, CNOR, CPHQ
Assistant Professor and Program Director Patient Care Services Administration
Davis and Henley College of Nursing
Sacred Heart University
Fairfield, CT

Lynn Rapsilber, DNP, APRN, ANP-BC, FAANP
Owner, NP Business Consultants and NP Wellness Care
Torrington, CT

Sylvie Rosenbloom, DNP, APRN, FNP-BC, CDCES
Clinical Assistant Professor
Sacred Heart University
Davis and Henley College of Nursing
Sacred Heart University
Fairfield, CT

Mary Lou Siefert, DNSc, MBA, RN, AOCN®
Associate Clinical Professor & Director, Doctor of Nursing Practice Program
School of Nursing
Bouvé College of Health Sciences
Northeastern University
Boston, MA

Dori Taylor Sullivan, PhD, RN, CPHQ-Ret., FAAN
Leadership/Education/Quality Consulting
Hobe Sound, FL

Tiffany Teixeira, MSN, APRN, A-GNP-C
New Solutions Pain Management Clinic LLC
Milford, CT

Kimberly M. Testo, MSN, APRN, FNP-C
Owner and Chief Medical Officer
New Solutions Pain Management Clinic LLC
Milford, CT

Tammy A. Testut, PhD, MSN, RN, NEA-BC
Clinical Assistant Professor
Davis and Henley College of Nursing
Sacred Heart University
Fairfield, CT

Linda Washington-Brown, PhD, EJD, PNP, ANP-C, FNP, FAANP, FAAN
Retired Founding Associate Dean, Broward College BSN Program
Clinical Coordinator, Miami Rescue Mission Clinic
Miami, FL

PART 1

Scientific Underpinning of the Nurse Practitioner Role

CHAPTER 1	Historical Perspectives: The Art and Science of Nurse Practitionering and Advanced Practice Nursing. 3
CHAPTER 2	Evidence-Based Practice and Dissemination Strategies 33

CHAPTER 1

Historical Perspectives: The Art and Science of Nurse Practitionering and Advanced Practice Nursing

Susan M. DeNisco and Julie G. Stewart

U.S. News and World Report (2021) lists nurse practitioner (NP) as the second top health care occupation for 2021. According to the American Association of Nurse Practitioners in the 2018 national sample survey, it was estimated 270,000 nurse practitioners were licensed to practice in the U.S. (AANP, 2019). Today, that number has increased to 290,000 NPs (AANP, 2020). By 2029, the Bureau of Labor Statistics projects that the NP role will have grown by 52% percent, compared to 10% for physicians (U.S. Bureau of Labor Statistics, 2021). In 2010, the Institute of Medicine (IOM) released a report that identified the need for nurses to be placed at the forefront of health care. The report strongly recommended that advanced practice registered nurses—including nurse practitioners—be allowed to practice to the full scope of their abilities and that barriers be removed to enable moving forward. We have come a long way since 2010, but there are still milestones to reach and barriers to break.

Nurse practitioners have reached a tipping point as a profession (Buerhaus, 2010). Malcolm Gladwell states that the "tipping point is that magic moment when an idea, trend, or social behavior crosses a threshold, tips, and spreads like wildfire" (Gladwell, 2000, p. 12). Nurse practitioners have been given the opportunity to shine and to experience growth professionally, and they provide a solution to some of the issues affecting health care in America today. The need for NPs is growing as we consider the IOM's recommendation and the large population of aging baby boomers, which is anticipated to increase use of the healthcare system (Van Leuven, 2012). In addition, the Patient Protection and Affordable Care Act signed in 2010 instituted comprehensive health insurance reform and expanded healthcare insurance coverage to 32 million Americans (USDHHS, 2021).

Researchers have validated the cost, quality, and competence of NPs' role in providing primary care with outcomes that are similar to primary care physicians (Hamric, Spross, & Hanson, 2009; Laurant et al., 2005; Mundinger et al., 2000; Wilson et al., 2005). Medical economist and health futurist Jeffrey C. Bauer (2010) reviewed evidence-based data in an article to illustrate how NPs functioning independently can meet the cost-effective needs of healthcare reform while providing high-quality care for patients in multiple settings. Indeed, more than 1 billion patients visit NPs for health care annually (AANP, 2020).

At least 89% of NPs are educated to provide primary care, and 65% are educated as family NPs (AANP, 2020); however, in some states, many NPs are not working in primary care possibly because of the state's restrictions on requiring collaborators and written agreements with physicians. Many states have recognized this barrier and have removed those requirements, and many insurance companies are including NPs in their provider networks. So, will we meet the near future needs for healthcare providers? Today, nurse practitioners are the largest group of advanced practice nurses. As previously mentioned, there are 290,000 NPs who are licensed and practicing with some level of prescriptive authority in all 50 states and the District of Columbia (American Association of Nurse Practitioners, 2020).

Clearly, there is a need to fully understand the role of the NP in order to advance professionalism and unity of the NP workforce. Seminar discussions regarding pertinent issues must be part of the education of student NPs and be included in discussion among those already in practice.

Advanced Practice Nursing

There is still confusion and debate regarding the terminology *advanced nursing practice, advanced practice nursing,* and *advanced practice registered* nurse (DeNisco & Barker, 2021). Based on the definition given by the American Association of Colleges of Nursing (AACN) and other widely accepted usages, the term *advanced practice registered nurse (APRN)* has been used to indicate master's- or doctorally prepared nurses who provide direct clinical care. This term encompasses the roles of nurse practitioner (NP), certified nurse-midwife (CNM), certified registered nurse anesthetist (CRNA), and clinical nurse specialist (CNS). The first three roles require a license beyond the basic registered nurse (RN) license. The role of the clinical nurse specialist requires a master's degree but does not require separate licensing unless the CNS is applying for prescriptive authority. While the focus of this textbook is to educate NP students to provide primary care services, it is not to diminish the important roles the CNM, CRNA, and CNS play in providing access to health care for all. Those roles will be briefly described later in this chapter.

The Role of the NP: A Historical Perspective

The role of the nurse practitioner was developed as a way to provide primary care for the underserved. The role is typically described as having emerged during the

1960s, yet Lillian Wald's nurses of the late 1800s bear a striking resemblance to NPs of today. The nurses of Wald's Henry Street Settlement House in New York City provided primary care for poverty-stricken immigrants, and treated common illnesses and emergencies that did not require referral (Hamric et al., 2009). In 1965, the role of nurse practitioner was formally developed by Loretta Ford, EdD (nurse educator), and Henry Silver, MD (professor of medicine), both of whom were teaching at the University of Colorado (Sullivan-Marx, McGivern, Fairman, & Greenberg, 2010). This nurse practitioner program was developed not only to advance the nursing profession; it was also developed in response to the need for providers in rural, underserved areas. The program was initially funded by a $7,000 grant from the School of Medicine at the University of Colorado (Bruner, 2005; Weiland, 2008). The first program was a pediatric NP program based on the nursing model, yet the program advanced the clinical practice of these students by teaching them how to provide primary care and how to make medical diagnoses.

These early NP pioneers were focused on having a positive effect on advancing the profession, "making a difference," and gaining autonomy (Weiland, 2008, p. 346). However, due to the socioeconomic and political climate of the times, the NP was viewed to be a cost-effective way to provide healthcare providers for the underserved. During the 1970s, federal funding helped to establish many NP programs to address a shortage of primary care physicians, particularly in underserved areas. Idaho was the first state to endorse nurse practitioners' scope of practice to include diagnosis and treatment in 1971. NP programs doubled between 1992 and 1997. By the year 2000, there were 321 institutions that offered either a master's level or a postmaster's-level NP program (Health Resources and Services Administration [HRSA], 2004). By 2002, more than 30% of NPs were working with vulnerable populations, including the homeless, indigent, chronically ill, and elderly (Jenning, 2002). Today, in the United States there are more than 400 nurse practitioners and 290,000 licensed nurse practitioners (AANP, 2019).

Nurse Practitioner Education and Title Clarification

In the 1960s, the role of the NP was not warmly welcomed by nurse educators; therefore, many educational programs to train nurses in the NP role were more often continuing education programs rather than university-housed programs (Pulcini, 2013). In the 1980s and 1990s, NP education moved into the university setting as master's-level programs, although confusion arose when there were efforts to interchange the clinical nurse specialist (CNS) and NP roles. Today, there are well over 400 graduate-level NP programs, and many have gone on to offer a clinical doctorate—the doctor of nursing practice (DNP)—for NP education in response to the American Association of Colleges of Nursing's (AACN's) recommendation that advanced practice nurses be educated at that level by 2015.

In 2008, the *Consensus Model for APRN Regulation: Licensure, Accreditation, Certification & Education* was finalized through the collaborative efforts of the APRN Consensus Work Group and the National Council of State Boards of Nursing APRN Advisory Committee. To clarify who is an advanced practice registered nurse, the document included the following definition (APRN Consensus Work Group, National Council of State Boards of Nursing APRN Advisory Committee, 2008).

An advanced practice registered nurse (APRN) is a nurse:

1. Who has completed an accredited graduate-level education program preparing him or her for one of the four recognized APRN roles;
2. Who has passed a national certification examination that measures APRN, role and population-focused competencies, and who maintains continued competence as evidenced by recertification in the role and population through the national certification program;
3. Who has acquired advanced clinical knowledge and skills preparing him or her to provide direct care to patients, as well as a component of indirect care; however, the defining factor for *all* APRNs is that a significant component of the education and practice focuses on direct care of individuals;
4. Whose practice builds on the competencies of registered nurses (RNs) by demonstrating a greater depth and breadth of knowledge, a greater synthesis of data, increased complexity of skills and interventions, and greater role autonomy;
5. Who is educationally prepared to assume responsibility and accountability for health promotion and maintenance as well as the assessment, diagnosis, and management of patient problems, which includes the use and prescription of pharmacologic and nonpharmacologic interventions;
6. Who has clinical experience of sufficient depth and breadth to reflect the intended license; *and*
7. Who has obtained a license to practice as an APRN in one of the four APRN roles: certified registered nurse anesthetist (CRNA), certified nurse-midwife (CNM), clinical nurse specialist (CNS), or certified nurse practitioner (CNP).[1]

Clearly, NPs are one of the four roles that fall under the umbrella definition for APRN; however, using the title "APRN" does not clearly define which role and educational background the professional has. Each APRN role differs from the others, and state regulatory agencies vary in requirements for licensing in each state, and in many cases, for each APRN role.

The Role of the NP Today

Nurse practitioners are board certified in a variety of specialty areas, including pediatrics, family, adult-gerontology, women's health, and acute care, to name a few. See **Table 1-1** for an overview of all specialty areas, practice settings, and clinical focus.

Educational Foundation for the Advanced Practice Nurse
The Essentials: Core Competencies for Professional Nursing Education

Given changes in higher education, student expectations, and the rapidly changing healthcare system outlined in AACN's Vision for Academic Nursing (2019), new methods to deliver nursing education were recognized as necessary to prepare the

---

1 APRN Consensus Work Group and the National Council of State Boards of Nursing APRN Advisory Committee (2008). Consensus model for APRN regulation: Licensure, accreditation, certification & education. APRN Joint Dialogue Group Report, July 7, 2008.

Table 1-1 Distribution, Top Practice Setting, and Clinical Focus Area by Area of NP Certification

Population*	Percent of NPs	Top Practice Setting	Top Clinical Foci
Acute Care	5.5	Hospital Inpatient (33.0%)	Surgical (16.1%)
Adult^	12.6	Hospital Outpatient Clinic (15.2%)	Primary Care (32.4%)
Adult-Gerontology Acute Care	3.4	Hospital Inpatient (43.3%)	Surgical (13.3%)
Adult-Gerontology Primary Care^	7.8	Hospital Outpatient Clinic (18.7%)	Primary Care (46.6%)
Family^	65	Private Group Practice (12.7%)	Primary Care (46.2%)
Gerontology^	1.7	Long-Term Care Facility (16.6%)	Primary Care (46.2%)
Neonatal	1.3	Hospital Inpatient Clinic (69.1%)	Neonatal (57.8%)
Pediatric – Primary Care^	5.5	Hospital Outpatient Clinic (18.7%)	Primary Care (55.6%)
Psychiatric/Mental Health – Adult	1.8	Psych/Mental Health Facility (23.0%)	Psychiatric (93.6%)
Psychiatric/Mental Health – Family	1.8	Psych/Mental Health Facility (25.8%)	Psychiatric (91.6%)
Women's Health^	2.8	Hospital Outpatient Clinic (15.7%)	OB/GYN (64.1%)

* NPs may be certified in more than one area.
^ Primary care focus
Data from 2017 AANP National Nurse Practitioner Sample Survey; 2018 AANP NP Facts: The Voice of the Nurse Practitioner

nursing workforce of the future. On April 6, 2021, AACN-affiliated academic deans across the country endorsed *The Essentials: Core Competencies for Professional Nursing Education,* which delineates competency expectations for graduates of baccalaureate and graduate nursing programs. This historic and courageous move will transform how nurses are educated for entry-level and advanced roles (AACN, 2021a).

These "New" Essentials are built on the strong foundation of nursing as a discipline, the foundation of a liberal education, and principles of competency-based education. Competency-based education is a process whereby students are held accountable to the mastery of competencies deemed critical for an area of study (AACN, 2021b). Competency-based education allows students to be at the center of the learning experience, progressing through a defined program of study at their own pace with faculty offering feedback and guidance along the way. This approach offers a personalized learning experience, in which students can accelerate through content that can easily be mastered and devote more time on subject matter requiring intense study. Students are consistently assessing their own performance, reflecting on their own progress toward the attainment of competencies required for nursing practice.

Core Nursing Concepts, Major Domains, and Competencies

The Essentials clearly delineates 8 core nursing concepts and 10 major domains and competencies that represent the essence of professional nursing practice. These can be found in **Table 1-2**. The core concepts, domains, and competencies exemplify the uniqueness of nursing as a profession and reflect the diversity of practice settings yet share common language that is understandable across healthcare professions and by employers, students, faculty, and the public (AACN, 2021b). Four spheres of care (disease prevention/promotion of health and well-being, chronic disease care, regenerative or restorative care, and hospice/palliative/supportive care), were used to design the competencies that reach across the lifespan, and include diverse patient populations. While the domains and competencies are identical for both entry and advanced levels of education, the sub-competencies build from entry into professional nursing practice to advanced levels of knowledge and practice.

Advanced-level nursing education programs provide rich and varied opportunities for practice experiences (both direct and indirect care experiences) to prepare graduates with the Level 2 sub-competencies, as well as applicable advanced nursing practice specialty/advanced nursing practice role competencies and requirements. **Table 1-3** shows a comparison of The Essentials Major Domains, Select Nursing Education Competencies, Select Advanced Nursing Practice Sub-competencies, and NONPF Competencies.

Table 1-2 The Essentials: Core Concepts and Major Domains

8 Concepts for Nursing Practice	10 Major Domains
■ Clinical Judgment ■ Communication ■ Compassionate Care ■ Diversity, Equity, and Inclusion ■ Ethics ■ EBP ■ Health Policy ■ Social Determinants of Health	■ Knowledge for Nursing Practice ■ Person-Centered Care ■ Population Health ■ Scholarship for Nursing Practice ■ Quality and Safety Descriptor ■ Interprofessional Partnerships ■ Systems-Based Practice ■ Information and Healthcare Technologies ■ Professionalism ■ Personal, Professional, and Leadership Development

Data from American Association of Colleges for Nursing. (2021). The Essentials. Retrieved from https://www.aacnnursing.org/Education-Resources/AACN-Essentials

Table 1-3 Comparison of The Essentials Major Domains, Select Nursing Education Competencies, Select Advanced Nursing Practice Sub-competencies, and NONPF Competencies

Domain 1: Knowledge for Nursing Practice

Nursing Education Competencies	Select Advanced Nursing Education Sub-competencies	NONPF Competencies
1.2 Apply theory and research-based knowledge from nursing, the arts, humanities, and other sciences.		*Independent Practice*
	1.2f Synthesize knowledge from nursing and other disciplines to inform education, practice, and research.	Integrates knowledge from the humanities and sciences within the context of nursing science.
1.3 Demonstrate clinical judgment founded on a broad knowledge base.		
	1.3d Integrate foundational and advanced specialty knowledge into clinical reasoning.	Develops new practice approaches based on the integration of research, theory, and practice knowledge.

Domain 2: Person-Centered Care

Nursing Education Competencies	Select Advanced-Level Nursing Education Sub-competencies	NONPF Independent Practice
2.2 Communicate effectively with individuals.	2.2j Facilitate difficult conversations and disclosure of sensitive information.	Creates a climate of patient-centered care to include confidentiality, privacy, comfort, emotional support, mutual trust, and respect.
2.7 Evaluate outcomes of care.		
	2.7d Analyze data to identify gaps and inequities in care and monitor trends in outcomes.	Evaluates the relationships among access, cost, quality, and safety and their influence on health care.

Domain 3: Population Health

Nursing Education Competencies	Advanced-Level Nursing Education Sub-competencies	NONPF
3.1 Manage population health.		

(continues)

Table 1-3 Comparison of The Essentials Major Domains, Select Nursing Education Competencies, Select Advanced Nursing Practice Sub-competencies, and NONPF Competencies *(continued)*

	3.1m Develop a collaborative approach with relevant stakeholders to address population healthcare needs, including evaluation methods.	Facilitates the development of healthcare systems that address the needs of culturally diverse populations, providers, and other stakeholders.
3.3 Consider the socioeconomic impact of the delivery of health care.		
	3.3c Analyze cost-benefits of selected population-based interventions.	Evaluates the relationships among access, cost, quality, and safety and their influence on health care.

Domain 4: Scholarship for the Nursing Discipline

Nursing Education Competencies	Advanced-Level Nursing Education Sub-competencies	NONPF Practice Inquiry
4.1 Advance the scholarship of nursing.		
	4.1l Disseminate one's scholarship to diverse audiences using a variety of approaches or modalities.	Disseminates evidence from inquiry to diverse audiences using multiple modalities.
4.2 Integrate best evidence into nursing practice.		
	4.2g Lead the translation of evidence into practice.	Leads practice inquiry, individually or in partnership with others.

Domain 5: Quality and Safety

Nursing Education Competency	Advanced-Level Nursing Education Sub-competency	NONPF Quality
5.1 Apply quality improvement principles in care delivery.		
	5.1i Establish and incorporate data-driven benchmarks to monitor system performance.	Anticipates variations in practice and is proactive in implementing interventions to ensure quality.
	5.1n Advocate for change related to financial policies that impact the relationship between economics and quality care delivery.	Evaluates the relationships among access, cost, quality, and safety and their influence on health care.

Core Nursing Concepts, Major Domains, and Competencies

5.2 Contribute to a culture of patient safety.		
	5.2i Design evidence-based interventions to mitigate risk.	Uses best available evidence to continuously improve quality of clinical practice.

Domain 6: Interprofessional Partnerships

Nursing Education Competency	Advanced-Level Nursing Education	NONPF
6.1 Communicate in a manner that facilitates a partnership approach to quality care delivery.		
	6.1h Facilitate improvements in interprofessional communications of individual information (e.g., EHR).	Contributes to the design of clinical information systems that promote safe, high-quality, and cost-effective care.
6.4 Work with other professions to maintain a climate of mutual learning, respect, and shared values.		
	6.4g Integrate diversity, equity, and inclusion into team practices.	Develops strategies to prevent one's own personal biases from interfering with delivery of quality care.

Domain 7: Systems-Based Practice

Nursing Education Competency	Advanced-Level Nursing Education Sub-competencies	NONPF
7.1 Apply knowledge of systems to work effectively across the continuum of care.		
	7.1h Design policies to impact health equity and structural racism within systems, communities, and populations.	Facilitates the development of healthcare systems that address the needs of culturally diverse populations, providers, and other stakeholders.
7.3 Optimize system effectiveness through application of innovation and evidence-based practice.		
	7.3e Apply innovative and evidence-based strategies focusing on system preparedness and capabilities.	Applies knowledge of organizational practices and complex systems to improve healthcare delivery.

(continues)

Table 1-3 Comparison of The Essentials Major Domains, Select Nursing Education Competencies, Select Advanced Nursing Practice Sub-competencies, and NONPF Competencies *(continued)*

Domain 8: Informatics and Healthcare Technologies

Nursing Education Competency	Advanced-Level Nursing Education Sub-competency	NONPF
8.2 Use information and communication technology to gather data, create information, and generate knowledge.		
	8.2h Use standardized data to evaluate decision-making and outcomes across all systems levels.	Uses technology systems that capture data on variables for the evaluation of nursing care.
8.3 Use information and communication technologies and informatics processes to deliver safe nursing care to diverse populations in a variety of settings.		
	8.3g Evaluate the use of information and communication technology to address needs, gaps, and inefficiencies in care.	Translates technical and scientific health information appropriate for various users' needs.
	8.3k Pose strategies to reduce inequities in digital access to data and information.	Assesses the patient's and caregiver's educational needs to provide effective, personalized health care.

Domain 9: Professionalism

Nursing Education Competency	Advanced-Level Nursing Education Sub-competency	NONPF
9.1 Demonstrate an ethical comportment in one's practice reflective of nursing's mission to society.		
	9.1j Suggest solutions when unethical behaviors are observed.	Applies ethically sound solutions to complex issues related to individuals, populations, and systems of care.
9.3 Demonstrate accountability to the individual, society, and the profession.		
	9.3j Demonstrate leadership skills when participating in professional activities and/or organizations.	Participates in professional organizations and activities that influence advanced practice nursing and/or health outcomes of a population focus.

Domain 10: Personal, Professional, and Leadership Development		
Nursing Education Competency	Advanced-Level Nursing Education Sub-competency	NONPF
10.2 Demonstrate a spirit of inquiry that fosters flexibility and professional maturity.		
	10.2h Mentor others in the development of their professional growth and accountability.	Collaborates with both professional and other caregivers to achieve optimal care outcomes.
10.3 Develop capacity for leadership.		
	10.3j Provide leadership to advance the nursing profession.	Assumes complex and advanced leadership roles to initiate and guide change.

Data from 2017 AANP National Nurse Practitioner Sample Survey; 2018 AANP NP Facts: The Voice of the Nurse Practitioner.

Nurse Practitioner Core Competencies

In addition to the AACN, which strives to advance the education of nurses in general, the National Organization for Nurse Practitioner Faculties (NONPF) sets the standards for nurse practitioner programs. NONPF has stated there are core competencies for nurse practitioners in all tracks and specialties. **Box 1-1** gives an overview of the broad competencies, so the NP student can review and understand how coursework reflects these competencies (NONPF, 2017). The comprehensive components of the competencies that must be met for role development are necessary and useful for developing curricula and for evaluating the NP student during the educational training period, as well as containing standards to which the practicing NP can be held accountable.

For a full description of competencies and curriculum recommendations, please access the NONPF website at https://cdn.ymaws.com/www.nonpf.org/resource/resmgr/competencies/2017_NPCoreComps_with_Curric.pdf.

Beyond the NP: Advanced Practice Nursing Foci

Nurse-Midwives

The first nurse-midwifery school was established in 1925 by Mary Breckenridge, who founded the Frontier Nursing Service (FNS) in Hyden, Kentucky, in response to the high maternal and child death rates in rural eastern Kentucky, an area isolated by geography and poverty (DeNisco & Barker, 2021). The midwives were educated to provide family health services, as well as childbearing and delivery care, at nursing centers in the Appalachian Mountains. As reported by the FNS (2014), by the

> **Box 1-1** Nurse Practitioner Core Competencies
>
> - Scientific Foundation
> - Leadership
> - Quality
> - Practice Inquiry
> - Technology and Information Literacy
> - Policy
> - Health Delivery System
> - Ethics
> - Independent Practice
>
> Data from NONPF. (2017). Nurse Practitioner Core Competencies. https://cdn.ymaws.com/www.nonpf.org/resource/resmgr/competencies/2017_NPCoreComps_with_Curric.pdf

late 1950s the FNS nurse-midwives had attended more than 10,000 births, and maternal and infant outcome statistics in rural Kentucky were better than those for the whole country during the nurse-midwives first three decades of service. The most significant differences were in maternal mortality rates (9.1 per 10,000 births for FNS compared with 34 per 10,000 births for the United States as a whole) and low birth weights (3.8% for FNS compared with 7.6% for the country).

Today, all nurse-midwifery programs are housed in colleges and universities. There are multiple entry paths to midwifery education, but most nurse-midwives graduate at the master's degree level, and several programs culminate in the DNP degree. These programs must be accredited by the American College of Nurse-Midwives (ACNM) for graduates to be eligible to take the national certification examination offered by the American Midwifery Certification Board (AMCB). Midwifery practice as conducted by certified nurse-midwives (CNMs) and certified midwives (CMs) is the autonomous primary care management of women's health, focusing on pregnancy, childbirth, the postpartum period, care of the newborn, family planning, and gynecologic needs of women.

CNMs are licensed, independent healthcare providers who have prescriptive authority in all 50 states, the District of Columbia, American Samoa, Guam, and Puerto Rico. CNMs are defined as primary care providers under federal law. Although midwives are well-known for attending births, 53.3% of CNMs identify reproductive care and 33.1% identify primary care as their main responsibilities in their full-time positions (Schuiling et al, 2010). Examples include performing annual exams; writing prescriptions; providing basic nutrition counseling, parenting education, and patient education; and conducting reproductive health visits. According to the American Midwifery Certification Board, there are 11,826 CNMs and 101 CMs in practice in the United States. Since 1991, the number of midwife-attended births in the United States has nearly doubled. In 2014, CNMs or CMs attended 332,107 births—a slight increase despite a decrease in total U.S. births compared with births in 2011 (ACNM, 2019).

In 2014, CNMs or CMs attended 94.2% of all midwife-attended births, 12.1% of all vaginal births, and 8.3% of total U.S. births (Hamilton et al., 2014). Whereas the majority of midwife-attended births occurs in hospitals, some occur at home and in freestanding birth centers. See **Figure 1-1**.

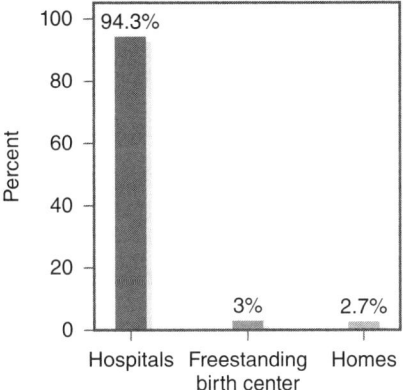

Figure 1-1 Site of Births Attended by Certified Nurse-Midwives and Certified Midwives, 2014

Data from Hamilton B., Martin, J., Osterman, M., Curtin, S., and Mathews, T.: Births: Final Data for 2014. National Vital Statistics Reports; Vol 64, No 12. Hyattsville, MD: National Center for Health Statistics. 2015. Retrieved from http://www.midwife.org/acnm/files/ccLibraryFiles/Filename/000000005950/CNM-CM-AttendedBirths-2014-031416FINAL.pdf

Allowing CNMs to have hospital privileges, as full, active members of the medical staff would promote continuity of care, and birth certificate data would more accurately reflect provider type and outcomes (Buppert, 2021). Medicaid reimbursement for midwifery care is mandatory in all states and is 100% of the physician fee schedule under the Medicare Part B fee schedule. The majority of states also mandates private insurance reimbursement for midwifery services. It is clear that nurse-midwives have improved primary healthcare services for women in rural and inner-city areas. It is imperative that nurse-midwives be given a larger role in delivering women's health care for the greater good of society.

Nurse Anesthetists

According to the American Association of Nurse Anesthetists (AANA), nurses have been providing anesthesia services to patients in the United States for more than 150 years. The first anesthesia administered to patients was chloroform, used for the treatment of wounded soldiers during the American Civil War. The shortages of physicians qualified to administer anesthesia during wartimes continued, and nurse anesthetists were the main providers of anesthesia care for U.S. military personnel on the front lines for World War I, World War II, the Korean War, and the Vietnam War. Nurse anesthetists also provide care in current conflicts in the Middle East (Keeling, 2009).

Historically, nurse anesthetists have been the primary providers of anesthesia care in rural America, enabling healthcare facilities in medically underserved areas to offer obstetrical, surgical, pain management, and trauma stabilization services. In some states, CRNAs are the sole providers in nearly 100% of rural hospitals. According to the U.S. Bureau of Labor Statistics (2021), there are 39,860 employed CRNAs in the United States, with the highest employment rates in the states of Texas, Ohio,

North Carolina, Pennsylvania, and Florida, respectively. Nurse anesthetists enjoy a higher median annual wage than their nurse practitioner and nurse midwife counterparts of $183,580 versus $111,680 (NPs) versus $111,130 (CNMs) (U.S. Bureau of Labor Statistics, 2021)

The credential CRNA came into existence in 1952 when the American Association of Nurse Anesthetists (AANA) established an accreditation program to monitor the quality and consistency of nurse anesthetist education (Keeling, 2009). Today, CRNAs safely administer *45 million anesthetics* to patients each year in the United States, according to the AANA 2020 Member Profile Survey. The scope and standards of practice for CRNAs are similar to those for other advanced practice registered nurses. Nurse anesthetists are licensed as independent practitioners, and they provide care autonomously and in collaboration with surgeons, dentists, podiatrists, and anesthesiologists, among other healthcare professionals. CRNAs provide evidence-based anesthesia and pain care services to patients at all acuity levels in a variety of settings for procedures, including, but not limited to, surgical, obstetrical, diagnostic, therapeutic, and pain management (AANA, 2021). Currently, CRNAs are qualified and have the legal authority to administer anesthesia without anesthesiologist supervision in all 50 states, the District of Columbia, Puerto Rico, and the Virgin Islands; however, some states have put into place restrictions and supervisory requirements in some settings (Joel, 2013).

Doctor of Nursing Program (DNP)

In response to the confusion arising from the variety of doctoral degrees that nurses seeking to advance their education were obtaining, the AACN developed a task force to address the issue in 1999 (Zaccagnini & White, 2011). Until this point, nurses had obtained doctorates in education (EdD), PhDs in nursing or other disciplines, doctorates in nursing science (DNS/DNSc), and doctorates in nursing (ND). In 2004, the AACN formally approved the doctor of nursing practice (DNP) degree, which is focused on clinical practice in contrast to the research-focused doctoral degree obtained with a PhD. This degree is not only for NPs, but offers a clinical doctorate for all nurses who seek to improve healthcare delivery systems and patient outcomes. Although an original goal was to have the DNP as entry level for the NP by 2015, the complexities associated with the endeavor, particularly at the state licensure level, makes this unlikely to enforce in such a short time. However, AACN endorses the DNP as a goal for all APRNs (AACN, 2013). The DNP is recognized as the terminal practice degree (AACN, 2006).

Why is there a need for a DNP when numerous studies have validated the excellent and cost-effective care provided by MSN-level NPs (AANP, 2010a, 2010b)? Owing to the ever-increasing complexity of health care and healthcare delivery systems, it is optimal to have clinicians who are well educated in the areas of health policy, quality improvement, evidence-based practice, and outcomes evaluation. Currently, MSN-level programs for NPs require 42–50 credits—much more than other MSN tracks that typically need approximately 30 credits for completion. In addition, most NP programs require at least 500–600 clinical hours to graduate and take certification examinations. The DNP offers the NP student additional education and preparation to meet the needs of the complex healthcare system of the near future. In addition, NPs work collaboratively with numerous other doctorally prepared clinicians whose doctorate is clinically focused, including pharmacists (PharmD), physical therapists (DPT), physicians (MD), doctors of osteopathy (DO), naturopaths (ND), and others. To achieve educational parity, the clinical doctorate (DNP) is recommended for nurse practitioners.

There are currently 357 DNP programs enrolling students in the United States and at least another 106 new post-baccalaureate and post-master's DNP programs in the planning stages (AACN, 2020). More than 36,000 nurses were enrolled in a DNP program in 2018–2019 (AACN, 2020). At this time, there are differences in the existing programs, particularly as they relate to the scholarship of the terminal project, the title of which in itself has sparked numerous passionate debates among leaders in doctoral-level nursing education. The AACN published *The Essentials of Doctoral Education for Advanced Nursing Practice* (2006) to shape the education for the DNP to meet quality indicator criteria. These essentials were developed to build upon the baccalaureate and master's essentials and are aligned with recommendations from the Institute of Medicine's (IOM) multiple reports emphasizing quality in education, evidence-based practice, and nurses practicing to the full extent of their scope of practice (Zaccagnini & White, 2011).

With this year's introduction of the new *Essentials for Nursing Education*, like the former DNP *Essentials* it contains language that reflects the need for the 3 Ps and the expertise required for APNs, which is detailed in the following for ease of access during seminar discussions.

AACN published a White Paper—*The Doctor of Nurse Practice: Current Issues and Clarifying Recommendations* (2015)—which describes and clarifies the "characteristics of DNP graduate scholarship, the DNP project, efficient use of resources, program length, curriculum considerations, practice experiences, and collaborative partnership guidelines" (AACN, 2015, para. 4). Of particular interest to the DNP educator and student are the components required for the DNP Scholarly Project, which must:

a. Focus on a change that impacts healthcare outcomes either through direct or indirect care.
b. Have a systems (micro-, meso-, or macro-level) or population/aggregate focus.
c. Demonstrate implementation in the appropriate arena or area of practice.
d. Include a plan for sustainability (e.g., financial, systems or political realities, not only theoretical abstractions).
e. Include an evaluation of processes and/or outcomes (formative or summative). DNP Projects should be designed so that processes and/or outcomes will be evaluated to guide practice and policy. Clinical significance is as important in guiding practice as statistical significance is in evaluating research.
f. Provide a foundation for future practice scholarship. (AACN, 2015, p. 4)

The DNP graduate prepared for an advanced practice role must demonstrate practice expertise, specialized knowledge, and expanded responsibility and accountability in the care and management of individuals and families. By virtue of this direct care focus, advanced practice nurses (APNs) develop additional competencies in direct practice and in the guidance and coaching of individuals and families through developmental, health–illness, and situational transitions (Tracy & O'Grady, 2018). The direct practice of APNs is characterized by the use of a holistic perspective; the formation of therapeutic partnerships to facilitate informed decision making, positive lifestyle change, and appropriate self-care; advanced practice thinking, judgment, and skillful performance; and use of diverse, evidence-based interventions in health and illness management (Brown, 2005).

APNs assess, manage, and evaluate patients at the most independent level of clinical nursing practice. They are expected to use advanced, highly refined assessment skills and employ a thorough understanding of pathophysiology and pharmacotherapeutics in making diagnostic and practice management decisions. **To ensure sufficient depth and focus, it is mandatory that a separate course be required for each of these three content areas: advanced health/physical assessment, advanced physiology/pathophysiology, and advanced pharmacology.** In addition to direct care, DNP graduates emphasizing care of individuals should be able to use their understanding of the practice context to document practice trends, identify potential systemic changes, and make improvements in the care of their particular patient populations in the systems within which they practice (AACN, 2006, p. 18).

The National Organization of Nurse Practitioner Faculties provides further clarification related to competencies for the NP educated to the MSN and DNP level (NONPF, 2017a). These areas include independent practice, scientific foundations, leadership, quality, practice inquiry, technology & information literacy, policy, ethics, and health delivery systems. In addition, NONPF (2017b) further delineates eight common APRN Doctoral Competencies and progression indicators for the following domains:

- Patient Care
- Knowledge of Practice
- Practice-Based Learning and Improvement
- Interpersonal and Communication Skills
- Professionalism
- Systems-Based Care
- Interprofessional Collaboration
- Personal and Professional Development

Nurse Practitioners' Approach to Patient Care

Sometimes nurse practitioners may be asked why they didn't become a physician instead of an NP. The best response is that becoming a nurse practitioner provides us with the best of both worlds: nursing and medicine. Nursing continues to be the top trusted profession in the United States at 89%, with physicians in second place at 77% (Gallop Politics, 2020). According to a recent national survey, NPs received extremely high patient satisfaction scores when compared to their physician colleagues (Kippenbrock et al., 2019). Nurse practitioners have a unique approach to health care. This is not to say that there are no physicians who are amazing—because I personally have worked with and been under the care of fantastic physicians—but a common theme I hear from my patient population is that "nurses listen to what I have to say." One study found that only 50% of the patients seen by physicians reported that they felt that the physician "always" listened carefully, compared to more than 80% of NP patients (Creech et al., 2011). In a study of more than 1.5 million veterans, satisfaction levels were highest in primary care clinics when the healthcare provider was an NP (Budzi et al., 2010). The authors state that the interpersonal skills of NPs in patient teaching, counseling, and patient-centered care contribute to positive health outcomes and patient satisfaction. Encouragement to hire more NPs to increase access to cost-effective quality care for the largest healthcare system in the United States was a conclusion reached by these researchers.

Of course, it is important to review and analyze quantitative research regarding the cost-effectiveness and improved health outcomes when NPs are providing primary care, but it is also as important (in many cases, more important) to listen to what patients have to say about their experiences with NPs as healthcare providers.

What Nurse Practitioners Do

In an effort to articulate what a nurse practitioner actually does, it is easy to discuss the tasks involved with the daily work of the NP. These tasks involve reviewing laboratory tests, performing physical examinations, charting, writing prescriptions, and ordering radiological procedures, yet this approach describes the profession or duties of the NP, and not the actual art of nurse practitionering. Dr. Loretta Ford described *holistically oriented goals for self-care* as what sets NPs apart from physicians in primary care (Weiland, 2008).

Nurse practitionering (as a unique verb) incorporates the vital elements of nursing and philosophical theories, communication skills, diagnostic skills, coaching and educating, and most importantly, developing reciprocal relationships with patients. It is the foundation of nursing that forms the basis for taking a holistic approach to the interview, assessment, diagnosis, and mutually agreed upon goals for patient care, which help NPs to engage patients as full partners in aspects of their health care.

Florence Nightingale recognized the main difference between nursing and medicine by writing that while medicine focuses on disease, nursing focuses on illness and suffering, with the goal(s) being to ease suffering and promote disease prevention (Nightingale, 2009). Physicians are trained in a different framework than NPs. In an interesting article, "The Total Package: A Skillful, Compassionate Doctor," the theme was stated thusly:

> Traditionally, medical school curricula have focused on the pathophysiology of disease while neglecting the very real impact of disease on the patient's social and psychological experience, that is, their illness experience. It is in this intersection that humanism plays a profound role. (Indiana University, 2009)

NPs, with their comprehensive, humanistic nursing background, formulate nurse practitionering in that intersection.

The role of the nurse practitioner has the foundation of nursing and has integrated segments of the medical model to become the unique profession of nurse practitioner; therefore, differences in the role and practice of nurses and nurse practitioners exist (Haugsdal & Scherb, 2003; Kleinman, 2004; Nicoteri & Andrews, 2003; Roberts et al., 1997). However, there remains confusion among the public and other members of the healthcare team, as well as among some NP students, as to what NP practice truly means.

It is not surprising that defining nurse practitionering is difficult when one considers that it has historically been difficult to define nursing (Chitty & Black, 2007). Certainly, today we have comprehensive definitions of nursing developed by the American Nurses Association, the Royal College of Nursing, and the International Council of Nurses; however, it seems that Florence Nightingale wrote the first definition of a holistic approach to patient-centered care:

> I use the word *nursing* for want of a better. It has been limited to signify little more than the administration of medicines and the application of poultices. It ought to signify the proper use of fresh air, light, warmth, cleanliness, quiet, and the proper selection and administration of diet—all at the least expense of vital power to the patient. (Nightingale, 2009)

Nursing Theories for Nurse Practitioners

Many nursing philosophies, theories, and models exist today, and NPs can and should build upon these for their professional practice. For example, Henderson (1991) identified 14 basic needs of the patient which are common needs to all humankind.

Jean Watson's 10 Carative Processes exemplify the changing relationship between patient and nurse attending to the unification of body, mind, and soul to achieve optimal health. Watson has spent many years as director of the Center for Human Caring at the University of Colorado in Denver. Watson's Theory of Human Caring meets the criteria for Carper's four fundamental ways of knowing, and Watson defines the metaparadigm of person, environment, nursing, and health in her theoretical base (Watson, 2021).

Hildegard Peplau (1952) focused on the relationship between patient and nurse, during which the nurse takes on the role of counselor, resource, teacher, technical expert, surrogate, and leader, as needed. Whether one is practicing professionally in the United States or elsewhere in our global arena, to be successful in clinical practice, the NP must use transcultural nursing theory, which was founded by Leininger (1995). The NP must use culturally sensitive and aware skills to develop relationships and to assess, diagnose, and treat patients.

King's framework (1981) uses personal, interpersonal, and social interacting systems to form a theory for nursing. Interestingly, when one reviews the Calgary Cambridge guide to the medical interview for physicians in training (Kurtz, Silverman, & Draper, 1998), many of the concepts are the same. The focus is on the concerns of the patient for both of these methods for interacting with patients. King's framework gives the NP the ability to see the patient holistically by including the family and community aspects. Both King's framework and the Calgary Cambridge guide focus on mutual goal setting—taking the time during each step of the interview, assessment, and planning stages to truly understand the patient's issues and perspectives. By frequently eliciting the patient's input, it is easier to develop mutual understanding and develop interventions and goals to reach a state of optimal health.

In the development of a middle range theory, Swanson (1991) defined caring as, "a nurturing way of relating to a valued other, toward whom one feels a personal sense of commitment and responsibility" (p. 163). Swanson stated that five processes characterize caring: knowing, being with, doing for, enabling, and maintaining belief. NPs practice knowing (empathy), being with (presence), doing for (evidence-based practice), enabling (empowerment), and maintaining belief (instilling hope).

In a survey of 200 Illinois NPs to explore their perspectives of their own caring behaviors, researchers used a revised Wolf's Caring Behaviors Inventory instrument and modified it for use with NPs (Brunton & Beaman, 2000). The findings showed the top caring behaviors were: (1) appreciating the patient as a human being; (2) showing respect and being sensitive to the patient; (3) talking to, listening to, and being honest with the patient; (4) maintaining confidentiality; and (5) encouraging patients to call if problems arose. NPs who had worked for a longer period of time in their role expressed more positive connectedness with patients than NPs with less practice experience.

The idea of forming a partnership with the patient is hardly new. Whitlock, Orleans, Pender, and Allan (2002) wrote about this concept in a U.S. Preventative Services Task Force recommendation, "Evaluating Primary Care Behavioral Counseling Interventions: An Evidence-Based Approach." Developing mutually respectful relationships with patients is more likely to prevent patients' resistance to advice on healthy living and behavior change suggestions by healthcare providers. Also detailed in this recommendation is an approach the National Cancer Institute developed to guide physician intervention in smoking cessation known as the "5 As": assess, advise, agree, assist, and arrange.

- **Assess:** Behavioral health risk factors affecting choice of personal choices and behavior change goals.
- **Advise:** Provide individualized behavior change advice, includinformation about the risks and benefits of personal health choices.
- **Agree:** Negotiate appropriate treatment goals based on the patient's interest in and willingness to change the behavior.
- **Assist:** Using behavior change techniques such as self-help and cognitive behavioral therapy to instill confidence and support for the patient in achieving goals; the inclusion of supplemental medical treatments when appropriate (e.g., nicotine patches for tobacco dependence, contraceptive drugs/devices).
- **Arrange:** Schedule follow-up communication in office, by telephone or via telehealth to provide continuity of care and support to adjust the treatment plan as needed, inreferral to specialized treatment (Whitlock et al., 2002).

All of the approaches mentioned in this chapter focus on the need for the healthcare provider to be open to patients' needs, to hear what they really have to say, to understand what they really believe is wrong or right, and to let them work with you to develop goals. The ability to be culturally sensitive—and to be flexible and willing to collaborate and compromise when needed and appropriate—will help to form the framework for a successful patient–NP relationship, and most importantly, assist patients to reach a state of optimum health. This is not to say that becoming expert in these skills is easy or that it can be accomplished in one course; however, the student NP should start practicing these skills as soon as the educational program begins.

Nurse Practitioners' Unique Role

In a survey seeking to identify barriers for nurse practitioners to use standardized nursing language (SNL) for documenting nursing practice, the researchers found that NP survey participants identified that their role was a blending of the nursing and medical models, and most were not aware of what SNL consisted of (Conrad, Hanson, Hasenau, & Stocker-Schneider, 2012). Jacqueline Fawcett (in Cody, 2013) exhorts us to sever our "romance" with medical science and non-nursing professions, and in particular, with NPs being compared to physicians providing primary care. Instead, she advises we integrate nursing science as nurse scholars. With this in mind while clarifying the professional practice of nurse practitioners, it is important to distinguish the profession from that of physicians and physician assistants.

Nicoteri and Andrews (2003) sought to uncover any theory that was unique to NPs and associated attributes. This integrative review of the literature found that the role of the NP is influenced by many disciplines, especially medicine. The authors posited that an emergence of theory that is unique to NPs and grounded in nursing, medicine, and social science was discovered. The authors suggested developing the concept of "nurse practitionering" (p. 500). The concept of nurse practitionering as a unique phenomenon has been written about in only a few journal articles. The term itself is not one used in typical conversation between healthcare providers and patients, nor within the nursing community; thus, there may be confusion with the term. The goal for this endeavor is not to elevate or denigrate one profession or another, but to better understand the components of nurse practitionering.

Hagedorn (2004) posits that the difference between nurse practitioners and "biomedical practitioners" is related to nurse practitioners' humanistic approach to patient care. According to many theorists, such as Jean Watson, Patricia Benner, and Boykin and Schoenhofer, nursing's essence is that of caring (Zaccagnini & White, 2011). The interpersonal focus of nursing within a caring and nurturing framework is the building block of all nursing theories (Brunton & Beaman, 2000; Chinn & Kramer, 1999; Green, 2004; Nicoteri & Andrews, 2003; Visintainer, 1986). If one accepts this as a core element of being a nurse, it would be difficult to imagine one losing this essence when acquiring advanced education that contains skills and competencies associated with the practice of medicine. In fact, NPs should be familiarizing themselves with nursing theories in order to use nursing theory to guide their practice. By doing so, one is practicing beyond the medical model, offering a unique approach to the relationship, assessment, and treatment plan.

In an effort to expand upon the concept of nurse practitionering, the late Dr. Julie Stewart sent an online survey and interviewed ninety NPs in Connecticut about "nurse practitionering" and what they believed it encompassed. Fifty-nine (65.6%) respondents stated that nurse practitionering is a unique term that describes what they do, which is different than solely the practice of nursing or medicine. Because many activities of practice overlap and are subjective, participants were not given definitions of nursing activities versus medical activities. Regarding how much time they perceived is spent in solely nursing activities, 36.7% of participants felt it was low, between 0% and 25%. In contrast, 34.4% of NP participants felt that the amount of time spent performing medical activities was greater, between 36% and 50%. These results are included in **Table 1-4**.

The respondents were requested to enter key terms and phrases that described all that's involved in providing care to patients as a nurse practitioner. Participants were not given terms or phrases from which to choose; rather, this portion of the survey was open-ended. Similar terms were grouped together where deemed appropriate. The most frequent key phrases in order of the number of times mentioned

Table 1-4 Percentage of Clinical Practice Time in Nursing and Medical Activities (N = 90)

Percent of Time	Nursing Activities	Medical Activities
0–25%	**36.7% (n = 33)***	13.3% (n = 12)
26–50%	30.0% (n = 27)	**34.4% (n = 31)***
51–75%	25.6% (n = 23)	32.2% (n = 29)
75–100%	7.8% (n = 7)	20.0% (n = 18)

*Bold denotes highest value.

were nurture/care/empathy ($f = 31$), educate ($f = 30$), assess/diagnose/treat/prescribe ($f = 30$), holistic ($f = 22$), listener ($f = 17$), collaborate ($f = 13$), advocate ($f = 11$), and coach ($f = 5$). The majority of the key phrases and terms in this pilot study confirm that the core of nurse practitionering is based on the nursing model. Key phrases and terms relating to medical practice included *diagnosing* and *treating/prescribing*, which were as frequent as the *caring* (nursing) category, but the nursing elements were mentioned most often.

In an effort to expand upon the key phrases, invitations to participate in interviews to share their perceptions of "nurse practitionering" were sent to 150 NPs in Connecticut. A total of 14 individual interviews were held with a convenience sample of experienced NPs willing to participate and share their perceptions. The 14 participants of the interviews were all female, between the ages of 31 and 70 years, and currently practicing as nurse practitioners.

Authentic Listening

The NPs in this study were exemplars for authentic listening. According to Bryant (2009), listening well involves being present, being interested, spending time, and showing respect. One NP explained:

> I think the biggest reason why people like to come here is they say, "You listen. The docs don't listen to me." It is probably what I do the most and, one of the nurses got very frustrated with me and said, "You nurse practitioners, when a patient comes in to see the doctor and their finger is the problem, the doctor just looks at the finger and the patient is out. You go and you guys talk about everything. You have to talk about everything!"

Another NP described the time she spends teaching patients:

> I prescribed the medications, I go out, I get the inhaler, you know, the sample inhaler and the sample spacer, and I go right back in and I tell the patient, "This is what I am ordering, and this is how you use it," versus the pediatrician or the pulmonologist who says, "Here are your medications. I'll have the nurse come in to teach you how to use it."

Empathy

Empathy is the ability to relate to the patient's thoughts and feelings and develop an understanding of what the patient is experiencing (Baillie, 1996). The NPs in this study are genuinely concerned about the patient's psychosocial well-being, family matters, and future goals and aspirations, as they demonstrate in the following examples from the interviews:

> This woman this morning has lots of what I perceive as small complaints. She's a relatively healthy 28-year-old woman, and I asked her, "Tiffany, are you working?"
> She said, "No."
> I said, "When was the last time you worked?"
> She said, "Oh, 9 years ago, before my daughter was born." Then she said, "It's really hard to get a job."
> I asked, "Do you have your high school diploma?"
> She said, "No."
> So I recommended to her a local learning center program. I encouraged her, and that's where I think the nurse practitioner is different. It was me listening first, caring about what she was telling me, and then offering her something and trying to be an advocate for her.

Empathy enabled another NP to gain a deep understanding of what motivated the patient:

> She has a disabled child at home that needs total care. That's something that I know about her and her situation. That's an example of, I guess, advocating and coordinating and knowing that a lot of people don't have transportation. Like if I want to send them to radiology, I'll ask them, "What time of the day is good for you?" because a lot of these people are grandmothers raising grandkids, and they need to arrange their life. Some of them are pretty capable of making appointments for themselves, but others are not. They are scared to or they don't think that they're going to do it right. Maybe we are enabling them by doing it for them, but we will take the extra time and, you know, ask "What's the best day for you to go for that ultrasound? Morning or afternoon?"

Negotiating

Authentic listening and empathy enabled the NPs in this study to communicate more effectively and negotiate with patients when formulating treatment plans. An integrated literature review on communication styles of NPs and the impact on patients (Charlton, Dearing, Berry, & Johnson, 2008) found that NPs who are trained to use a patient-centered communication style are most likely to have patients with a better understanding of their health and treatment options and who are more likely to follow the treatment plan, thereby achieving better health outcomes. In this study, this occurred with NPs who involved patients in the decision-making process and actively negotiated with the patients:

> One of the things here that we do well, I think, is negotiate with the patients. Part of when I see people [is that] I'm not going to be paternalistic

and tell them you have to do this, this, and that. I have a woman I saw this morning; she came in for follow-up of her labs. She has hypertension, and the first time she had a hemoglobin A1C of 6, and she has a family history of diabetes, so we talked. She's not a dummy; she is a registered nurse. She just became a registered nurse, just got out of school, and I said "Let's talk about this new thing that's coming up. Do you have diabetes? Or are you prediabetic? Let's discuss it." So we negotiated what she was going to do next. I didn't want to say to her, "You have to start on more meds today." Her fasting sugars have been normal, the A1C was 6, and she is a woman that takes care of herself, pretty much. Now she may go on metformin in 3 months, but I know she doesn't like to take pills. She cares about a healthy lifestyle, so we negotiated: try lifestyle changes for 3 months and check the A1C in 3 months; if it goes up, then we'll talk about starting medication.

Going Above and Beyond

NPs describe going beyond what is expected or required of the role of primary care provider. The NPs in our study were motivated to do more for their patients and ensure that patients were satisfied with their care:

> My patient that came in this morning was status posthospitalization. When she was in the hospital, they did a big cardiac and neuro workup. I had sent her out by ambulance the week before, and they kept her for 4 days because they did a really good workup on her, but they didn't do a stress test, so she needed to have that done. And so, I coordinated today for her to have a stress test, and I picked a Spanish-speaking cardiologist for her because I thought she would be more comfortable with that. And then they also recommended that she see a therapist because she's on an antidepressant, so we talked about that today, and I coordinated that for her.

Another NP describes her ability to take on a difficult patient and help to gain his trust, thereby improving his adherence to the treatment plan, and reducing costs for overusing the emergency room:

> Treating marginalized patients with multiple comorbidities is challenging. This challenge is amplified by mental illness and substance abuse, combined with mistrust of the healthcare system. An example of this begins with the discharge of a difficult patient from a clinic for threatening front desk staff and a few nurses. He was belligerent, and when he felt he was not being respected, he threatened staff members, including his physician. He had been followed in the medical resident clinic for his chronic medical illnesses but was not addressing his anger management, cocaine abuse, obsessive compulsive disorder, and depression, and ultimately he was not adherent to medications or medical appointments either. The patient had been fired by multiple agencies in the town he lives in for the same behaviors, and at this point was about to be fired from the only medical provider left within walking distance. He does not own a car and could not afford to travel by bus. Final discharge from the clinic and care would render this man with no primary care locally, except the emergency room.

A final attempt was made to have the patient receive his care with a nurse practitioner, as she could at least provide continuity, if he showed up for the appointment, and she was not afraid. But really, the NP provided more than the same face in the clinic each visit. The NP provided this man with a milieu of empathy and teamwork between patient and care provider. Her approach to practice sparked a level of trust of the practitioner. The patient recognized the NP's genuine interest in providing him individualized care and respect. She built upon this practitioner–patient relationship. The NP helped the patient realize his control of his healthcare commitment and his role in his health outcome. This empowerment and trust lead to successful engagement in following through for his routinely scheduled medical visits, as well as medication adherence. When the patient was ready to address his mental health and addiction, he asked the NP to be his advocate.

The NP's commitment to holistic patient-centered care led to reinstatement of his mental health services. And today, this patient is significantly healthier, drug-free, treating his medical and mental illness, and is one less person sitting in the emergency room.

Another NP describes the impact one can have when going the extra step for a patient:

While at a precollege arts experience, a teen came to the clinic to ask for help with a sore throat. While assessing her I began discussing her comfort with being away from home for the first time. She mentioned that she was really surprised that having three meals a day made her feel so comfortable. (Students eat in the college cafeteria during the program.) Further questioning revealed that she rarely ate except at school as she qualified for free lunch because, "There is an empty refrigerator in my house." When asked if her school had a breakfast program, she said that they did but her mom, "was too busy to apply—says it is too complicated." Her strep culture was positive, so I prescribed antibiotics and had the resident assistant pick them up from the pharmacy. Meanwhile, I asked the young lady if she would like to speak to the nurse practitioner at her school to contact social services for assistance with not only the breakfast program but also what else the assessment would allow. At that point I learned that her mom was in rehab and unable to be reached—that this student had been assigned a foster care person—whom I contacted regarding care and treatment for the strep throat and confirmed the rest of the story. Activation of social services through contact with the NP at the school-based health center started the process in motion. Additional contact with her throughout the 5 weeks proved to positively impact this child's life.

The NPs in this study expressed how much they love being nurse practitioners. They believe in the added value and unique contributions of the NP to health care and get a lot of gratification from putting in extra time and effort. This is supported by a similar study that showed NPs feel that their lives are enhanced and cite internal rewards and gratification from their interactions with patients:

I think the most gratifying thing is when I sit down with them and explain their disease and really spend the time with them that they need. I feel like they really understand the necessity for the treatment plan that I recommend, and I really feel like if I spend the time with them that they are so grateful because they feel like you've really invested in them.... I think that most nurse practitioners will probably say something to this effect, but when they sit down with their patients, they try to treat them like they would want one of their family members treated. And so when people really see that that you're really doing that for them, and distinguish it from the way that they feel like they've been treated by other providers in the past or when they really recognize the amount of energy and the amount of giving—when they really see that—there's nothing more gratifying than that. (Kleinman, 2004)

The preceding studies validate similar components uncovered by Kleinman (2004) regarding nurse practitioners and their relationships with patients. Essential meanings in her phenomenological study included "openness, connection, concern, respect, reciprocity, competence, time, and professional identity" (p. 264).

Based on research and formal and informal interviews, a concept map depicting nurse practitionering was developed (**Figure 1-2**). From that, the Stewart Model of Nurse Practitionering was developed to depict this model of nurse practitioner practice (**Figure 1-3**). This model has as its core the nursing model—the foundation of NP practice. As the NP student evolves through the educational program, scientific knowledge and attributes of the medical model are incorporated in order to provide accurate assessment, medical diagnoses, and appropriate evidence-based treatment modalities to patients needing health care. The circles within the larger circle represent unity and wholeness.

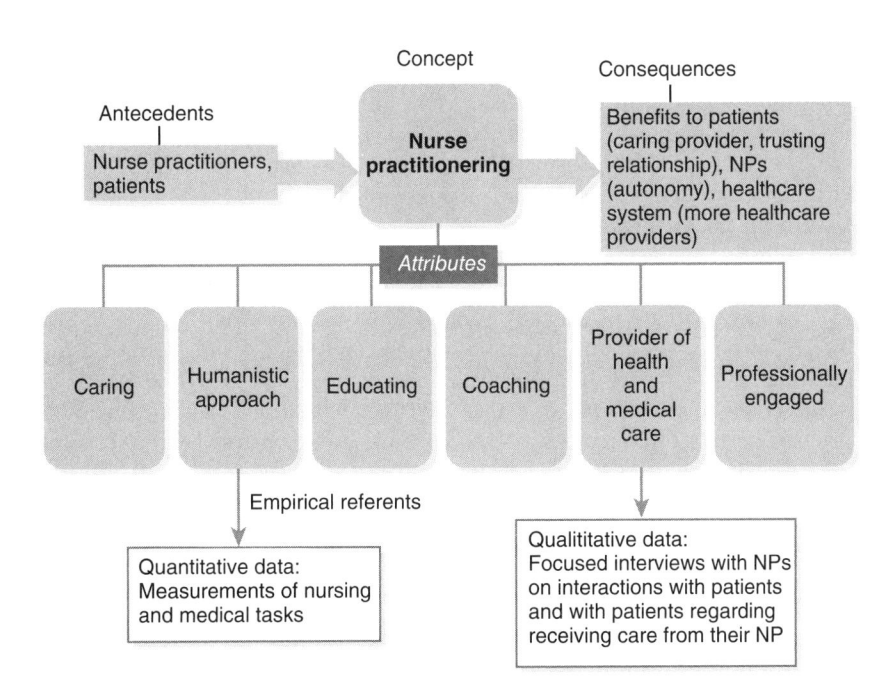

Figure 1-2 Model of Nurse Practitioner Practice

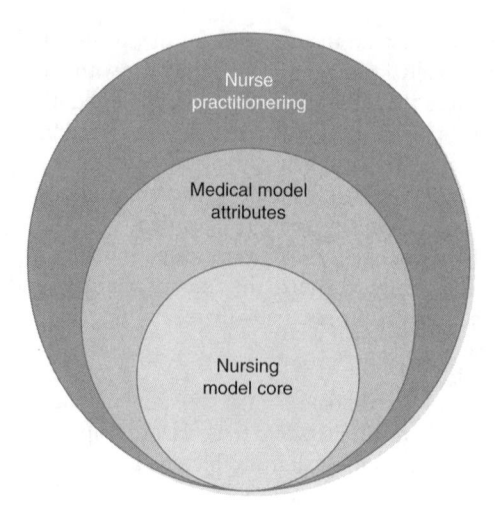

Figure 1-3 The Stewart Model of Nurse Practitionering

It is evident that in order to function successfully within this model, the NP must retain the crucial interpersonal skills required to provide education surrounding health promotion and disease management. Brykczynski (2012), in an article discussing qualitative research that looked at how NP faculty keep the nurse in the NP student, suggests that holistically focused healthcare providers consider thinking of "patient diagnoses" instead of either medical versus nursing diagnoses (p. 558). Nurse practitioner students and novice NPs need to beware of minimizing the importance of nursing as the core foundation from which excellence in practice develops. Rather, all NPs should emphasize the art and science of nursing philosophies and theories as the building blocks for providing health care to patients. It is these very qualities that make NPs unique—what it is that instills trust and confidence, as well as positive patient–NP relationships—which is the circle labeled in Figure 1-2 as "nurse practitionering." In an opinion article in *The New York Times* (Rosenberg, 2012), it is clearly noted that nurse practitioners approach patient care differently than physicians do and that research has proven that it is as effective and "might be particularly useful for treating chronic disease, where so much depends on the patients' behavioral choices" (para. 5). Sullivan-Marx et al. (2010) posit that the NP encompasses both the holistic nursing caring model and more than the physician's curing model—that NPs have a paradigm flexible enough to be able to move between the two. Who better than NP/DNPs to tackle the inequities in health that have been tied to variations in socioeconomic status, racial and ethnic discrimination, and stressors, as well as policies relating to social and economical justice?

Seminar Discussion Questions

1. What was the purpose for the initial role of the nurse practitioner, and does it differ from the role of the nurse practitioner in today's healthcare system?
2. Who are advanced practice registered nurses (APRNs)?
3. What are *The Essentials: Core Competencies for Professional Nursing Education* and what are they used for?

4. Describe the NP core competencies as identified by NONPF, and discuss how students can attain basic mastery of those competencies.
5. What are elements of role transition from RN to NP, and what are you currently experiencing in this process?
6. The concept of "nurse practitionering" has been introduced in this chapter. Comment on your responses to this idea.

References

American Association of Colleges of Nursing. (2006). *The essentials of doctoral education for advanced nursing practice*. Washington, DC: Author.

American Association of Colleges of Nursing. (2011). *The essentials of master's education in nursing*. Washington, DC: Author.

American Association of Colleges of Nursing. (2013). *DNP fact sheet*. Washington, DC: Author.

American Association of Colleges of Nursing. (2015). White Paper: *The doctor of nursing practice: Current issues and clarifying recommendations*. Washington, DC: Author.

American Association of Colleges of Nursing. (2017). *DNP fact sheet*. Washington, DC: Author. Retrieved from http://www.aacnnursing.org/Portals/42/News/Factsheets/DNP-Factsheet-2017.pdf

American Association Colleges of Nursing. (2020). *DNP fact sheet*. Retrieved from https://www.aacnnursing.org/News-Information/Fact-Sheets/DNP-Fact-Sheet

American Association of Colleges of Nursing. (2021a). *Bold action taken to transform nursing education and strengthen the nation's healthcare workforce*. Retrieved from https://www.aacnnursing.org/News-Information/Press-Releases/View/ArticleId/24807/AACN-Approves-New-Essentials

American Association of Colleges of Nursing. (2021b). *The essentials*. Retrieved from https://www.aacnnursing.org/Education-Resources/AACN-Essentials

American Association of Nurse Anesthetists (AANA). (2020). *Professional practice documents: Scope of nurse anesthesia practice*. Retrieved from http://www.aana.com/resources2/professionalpractice/Pages/Scope-of-Nurse-Anesthesia-Practice.aspx

American Association of Nurse Anesthetists (AANA). (2021). *CRNAs and the AANA fact sheet for patients*. Retrieved from https://www.aana.com/membership/become-a-crna/crna-fact-sheet

American Academy of Nurse Practitioners. (2010a). *Quality of nurse practitioner practice*. Austin, TX: Author.

American Academy of Nurse Practitioners. (2010b). *Nurse practitioner cost-effectiveness*. Austin, TX: Author.

American Association of Nurse Practitioners. (2017). *Press release: More than 234,000 licensed nurse practitioners in the United States*. Retrieved from Https://www.aanp.org/press-room/press-releases/173-press-room/2017-press-releases/2098-more-than-234-000-licensed-nurse-practitioners-in-the-united-states

American Association of Nurse Practitioners. (2019). *Nurse practitioner role grows to more than 270,000*. Retrieved from https://www.aanp.org/news-feed/nurse-practitioner-role-continues-to-grow-to-meet-primary-care-provider-shortages-and-patient-demands

American Association of Nurse Practitioners. (2020). *NP fact sheet*. Retrieved from https://www.aanp.org/about/all-about-nps/np-fact-sheet

American Association of Nurse Practitioners. (2021). *Planning your nurse practitioner (np) education: Begin your journey to become patients' partner in health*. Retrieved from https://www.aanp.org/student-resources/planning-your-np-education#:~:text=There%20are%20approximately%20400%20academic,adult%2C%20family%20or%20pediatrics

American College of Nurse Midwives. (2019). *Fact sheet: Essential facts about midwives*. Retrieved from https://www.midwife.org/acnm/files/cclibraryfiles/filename/000000007531/EssentialFactsAboutMidwives-UPDATED.pdf

APRN Consensus Work Group and the National Council of State Boards of Nursing APRN Advisory Committee. (2008). *Consensus model for APRN regulation: Licensure, accreditation, certification & education.* APRN Joint Dialogue Group Report, July 7, 2008.

Auerbach, D. I. (2012). Will the NP workforce grow in the future? New forecasts and implications for healthcare delivery. *Medical Care, 50*(7), 606–610.

Baillie, L. (1996). A phenomenological study of the nature of empathy. *Journal of Advanced Nursing, 24*(6), 1300–1308.

Bauer, J. (2010). Nurse practitioners as an underutilized resource for health reform: Evidence-based demonstrations of cost-effectiveness. *Journal of the American Academy of Nurse Practitioners, 22*, 228–231.

Brown, S. J. (2005). Direct clinical practice. In A. B. Hamric, J. A. Spross, & C. M. Hanson (Eds.), *Advanced practice nursing: An integrative approach* (3rd ed., pp. 143–185). Philadelphia, PA: Elsevier Saunders.

Bruner, K. (2005). *Nurse practitioners' program to celebrate 40th anniversary.* Retrieved from http://www.uchsc.edu/news/bridge/2005/may/NP_anniversary.html

Brunton, B., & Beaman, M. (2000). Nurse practitioners' perceptions of their caring behaviors. *Journal of the American Academy of Nurse Practitioners, 12*, 451–456.

Bryant, L. (2009). The art of active listening. *Practice Nurse, 37*(6), 49.

Brykczynski, K. (2012). Clarifying, affirming, and preserving the nurse in nurse practitioner education and practice. *Journal of the American Academy of Nurse Practitioners, 24*, 554–564.

Budzi, D., Lurie, S., Singh, K., & Hooker, R. (2010). Veterans' perceptions of care by nurse practitioners, physician assistants and physicians: A comparison from satisfaction surveys. *Journal of the American Academy of Nurse Practitioners, 22*(3), 170–176. doi:10.1111/j.1745-7599.2010.00489.x

Buerhaus, P. (2010). Have nurse practitioners reached a tipping point? Interview of a panel of NP thought leaders. *Nursing Economics, 28*(5), 346–349.

Buppert, C. (2021). Hospital privileges. In C. Buppert (7th ed.), *Nurse practitioner's business practice and legal guide.* Burlington, MA: Jones & Bartlett.

Bureau of Labor Statistics, U.S. Department of Labor. (2021). *Occupational outlook handbook, nurse anesthetists, nurse midwives, and nurse practitioners.* Retrieved from https://www.bls.gov/ooh/healthcare/nurse-anesthetists-nurse-midwives-and-nurse-practitioners.htm

Carryer, J., Gardner, G., Dunn, S., & Gardner, A. (2007). The core role of the nurse practitioner: Practice, professionalism and clinical leadership. *Journal of Clinical Nursing, 16*(10), 1818–1825. doi: 10.1111/j.1365-2702.2006.01823.x

Charlton, C. R., Dearing, K. S., Berry, J. A., & Johnson, M. J. (2008). Nurse practitioners' communication styles and their impact on patient outcomes: An integrated literature review. *Journal of the American Academy of Nurse Practitioners, 20*, 382–388. doi:10.1111/j.1745-7599.2008.00336.x

Chinn, P. L., & Kramer, M. K. (1999). *Theory and nursing: Integrated knowledge development* (5th ed.). St. Louis, MO: Mosby.

Chitty, K., & Black, B. (2007). *Professional nursing: Concepts and challenges.* St. Louis, MO: Saunders.

Cody, W. (Ed.). (2013). *Philosophical and theoretical perspectives for advanced practice nursing* (5th ed.). Burlington, MA: Jones & Bartlett Learning.

Conrad, D., Hanson, P., Hasenau, S., & Stocker-Schneider, J. (2012). Identifying the barriers to use of standardized nursing language in the electronic health record by the ambulatory care nurse practitioner. *Journal of the American Academy of Nurse Practitioners, 24*(7), 443–451.

Creech, C., Filter, M., & Bowman, S. (2011). *Comparing patient satisfaction with nurse practitioner and physician delivered care.* Poster presented at the 26th Annual American Academy of Nurse Practitioners Conference, Las Vegas, Nevada.

DeNisco, S., & Barker, A. (2020). *Advanced practice nursing: Evolving roles for the transformation of the profession.* Sudbury, MA: Jones and Bartlett Publisher.

Gallop Politics. (2020). *US ethic ratings rise for medical workers and teachers.* Retrieved from https://news.gallup.com/poll/328136/ethics-ratings-rise-medical-workers-teachers.aspx

Gladwell, M. (2000). *The tipping point: How little things can make a big difference.* New York, NY: Little, Brown & Company.

Green, A. (2004). Caring behaviors as perceived by nurse practitioners. *Journal of the American Academy of Nurse Practitioners, 16*, 283–290.

Hagedorn, M. (2004). Caring practices in the 21st century: The emerging role of nurse practitioners. *Topics in Advanced Practice Nursing eJournal*, 4. Retrieved June 11, 2006, from http://www.medscape.com/viewarticle/496372

Hamilton B., Martin, J., Osterman, M., Curtin, S., and Mathews, T. (2014). Births: Final Data for 2014. National Vital Statistics Reports; Vol 64, No 12. Hyattsville, MD: National Center for Health Statistics. 2015. Retrieved from http://www.midwife.org/acnm/files/ccLibraryFiles/Filename/000000005950/CNM-CM-AttendedBirths-2014-031416FINAL.pdf

Hamric, A., Spross, J., & Hanson, C. (2009). *Advanced practice nursing* (4th ed.). Philadelphia, PA: W. B. Saunders.

Haugsdal, C., & Scherb, C. (2003). Using the nursing interventions classification to describe the work of the nurse practitioner. *Journal of the American Academy of Nurse Practitioners, 15*, 87–94.

Health Resources and Services Administration (HRSA), Bureau of Health Professions. (2004). *A comparison of changes in the professional practice of nurse practitioners, physician assistants, and certified midwives: 1992 and 2000*. Retrieved from http://bhpr.hrsa.gov/healthworkforce/reports/comparechange19922000.pdf

Indiana University. (2009). The total package: A skillful, compassionate doctor. *Indiana University News Room*. Retrieved from http://newsinfo.iu.edu/web/page/normal/9704.html

Jenning, C. (2002). *Testimony: American Academy of Nurse Practitioners before the National Committee on Vital and Health Statistics*. Retrieved from http://www.ncvhs.hhs.gov/021029p3.html

Joel, L. (2013). *Advance practice nursing: Essentials of role development* (3rd ed.). Philadelphia, PA: F. A. Davis.

Keeling, A. W. (2009). A brief history of advance nursing practice in the United States. In A. B. Hamric, J. A. Spross, & C. M. Hanson (Eds.), *Advanced practice nursing: An integrative approach* (4th ed., pp. 3–32). St. Louis, MO: Elsevier.

King, I. (1981). *A theory for nursing: Systems, concepts, process*. New York, NY: Wiley.

Kippenbrock, T., Emory, J., Lee, P., Odell, E., Buron, B., & Morrison, B. (2019). A national survey of nurse practitioners' patient satisfaction outcomes. *Nurs Outlook*, Nov–Dec., 67(6), 707–712. doi: 10.1016/j.outlook.2019.04.010. Epub 2019 May 4. PMID: 31607371.

Kleinman, S. (2004). What is the nature of nurse practitioners' lived experiences interacting with patients? *Journal of the American Academy of Nurse Practitioners, 16*(6), 263–269.

Kurtz, S., Silverman, J., & Draper, J. (1998). *Teaching and learning communication skills in medicine*. Oxford: Radcliffe Medical Press.

Laurant, M., Reeves, D., Hermens, R., Braspenning, J., Grol, R., & Sibbald, B. (2005). Substitution of doctors by nurses in primary care. *Cochrane Database of Systematic Reviews, 2*, CD001271.

Leininger, M. (1995). Culture care theory, research and practice. *Nursing Science Quarterly, 9*, 71–78.

Mundinger, M. O., Kane, R. L., Lenz, E. R., Totten, A. M., Tsai, W. Y., Cleary, P. D., Shelanski, M. L., et al. (2000). Primary care outcomes in patients treated by nurse practitioners or physicians: A randomized trial. *Journal of the American Medical Association, 283*(1), 59–68.

National Organization of Nurse Practitioner Faculties. (2017a). *National Organization of Nurse Practitioner core competencies content*. Washington, DC, Author. Retrieved from https://cdn.ymaws.com/www.nonpf.org/resource/resmgr/competencies/2017_NPCoreComps_with_Curric.pdf

National Organization of Nurse Practitioner Faculties. (2017b). *Common advanced practice registered nurse doctoral level competencies*. Washington, DC, Author. Retrieved from https://cdn.ymaws.com/www.nonpf.org/resource/resmgr/competencies/common-aprn-doctoral-compete.pdf

Nicoteri, J. A., & Andrews, C. (2003). The discovery of unique nurse practitioner theory in the literature: Seeking evidence using an integrative review approach. *Journal of the American Academy of Nurse Practitioners, 15*, 494–500.

Nightingale, F. (2009). *Florence Nightingale: Notes on nursing*. New York, NY: Fall River Press.

Ortiz, J., Wan, T. T., Meemon, N., Paek, S. C., & Agiro, A. (2010). Contextual correlates of rural health clinics' efficiency: Analysis of nurse practitioners' contributions. *Nursing Economics, 28*(4), 237–244.

Peplau, H. (1952). *Interpersonal relations in nursing*. New York, NY: Putnam.

Pulcini, J. (2013). Advanced practice nursing: Moving beyond the basics. In S. DeNisco & A. M. Barker, *Advanced practice nursing: Evolving roles for the transformation of the profession* (2nd ed., pp. 19–26). Burlington, MA: Jones & Bartlett Learning.

Roberts, S. J., Tabloski, P., & Bova, C. (1997). Epigenesis of the nurse practitioner role revisited. *Journal of Nursing Education, 36*, 67–73.

Rosenberg, T. (2012). The nurse as family doctor. *The New York Times.* Retrieved from http://opinionator.blogs.nytimes.com/2012/10/24/the-family-doctor-minus-the-m-d

Schuiling, K. D., Sipe, T. A., & Fullerton J. (2010). Findings from the analysis of the American College of Nurse-Midwives' membership surveys: 2006-2008. *J Midwifery Womens Health, 55*(4), 299-307.

Sullivan-Marx, E., McGivern, D., Fairman, S., & Greenberg, S. (Eds.) (2010). *Nurse practitioners: The evolution and future of advanced practice* (5th ed.). New York, NY: Springer.

Swanson, K. M. (1991). Empirical development of a middle range theory of caring. *Nursing Research, 40*, 161–166.

Tracy, M. F., & O'Grady, E. T. (2018). *Hamric & Hanson's advanced practice nursing: An integrative approach* (6th ed.). Philadelphia, PA: W. B. Saunders.

U.S. Bureau of Labor Statistics. (2021). *Occupational handbook outlook nurse anesthetists, nurse midwives, and nurse practitioners.* Retrieved from https://www.bls.gov/ooh/healthcare/nurse-anesthetists-nurse-midwives-and-nurse-practitioners.htm

U.S. Department of Health and Human Services. (2021). *What is the affordable care act?* Retrieved from https://www.hhs.gov/answers/affordable-care-act/what-is-the-affordable-care-act/index.html

U.S. News and World Report. (2021). *U.S. News & World Report unveils the 2021 best jobs.* Retrieved from https://www.usnews.com/info/blogs/press-room/articles/2021-01-12/us-news-unveils-the-2021-best-jobs

Van Leuven, K. (2012). Population aging: Implications for nurse practitioners. *Journal for Nurse Practitioners, 8*(7), 554–559.

Visintainer, M. (1986). The nature of knowledge and theory in nursing. *Image: Journal of Nursing Scholarship, 18*, 32–38.

Watson, J. (2021). *Caring Science and Human Caring Theory.* Retrieved from https://www.watsoncaringscience.org/jean-bio/caring-science-theory/

Weiland, S. (2008). Reflections on independence in nurse practitioner practice. *Journal of the American Academy of Nurse Practitioners, 20*(7), 345–352. doi:10.111/j.1745-7599.2008.00330.x

Whitlock, E., Orleans, T., Pender, N., & Allan, J. (2002). Evaluating primary care behavioral counseling interventions: An evidence-based approach. *American Journal of Preventative Medicine, 22*(4), 267–284.

Wilson, I. B., Landon, B. E., Hirschhorn, L. R., McInnes, K., Ding, L., Marsden, P. V., & Cleary, P. D. (2005). Quality of HIV care provided by nurse practitioners, physician assistants, and physicians. *Annals of Internal Medicine, 143*(10), 729–736.

Zaccagnini, M., & White, K. (2011). *The doctor of nursing practice essentials: A new model for advanced nursing practice.* Sudbury, MA: Jones and Bartlett.

CHAPTER 2

Evidence-Based Practice and Dissemination Strategies

Kerry Milner

The History of Evidence-Based Practice

The concept of evidence-based practice (EBP) originated in medicine and was first introduced to U.S. healthcare providers in the published literature in a 1992 *Journal of the American Medical Association* article (Ragan & Quincy, 2012). In this article, evidence-based medicine (EBM) was described as de-emphasizing tradition, unsystematic clinical experience, and pathology as sufficient grounds for practice decisions, and it was suggested that critical examination of evidence from practice-based studies should underlie clinical decision making (Evidence-Based Medicine Working Group, 1992). The EBM movement called for physicians to learn the skills of efficient literature searching and the use of formal rules to critically evaluate evidence from the clinical literature.

In the early published definitions of EBM, the areas of foci included identifying, critically appraising, and summarizing best current evidence. However, it became clear that evidence alone was not sufficient to make clinical decisions, so in 2000 the Evidence-Based Medicine Working Group presented the second fundamental principle of EBM. This principle specified that clinical decisions, recommendations, and practice guidelines must not only focus on the best available evidence, they also must include the values and preferences of the informed patient. Values and preferences refer not only to the patients' perspectives, beliefs, expectations, and goals for life and health, but also to the practices individuals use to consider the available options and the relative benefits, harms, costs, and inconveniences of those options (Guyatt et al., 2000).

A similar definition by Canadian medical doctor David Sackett, who is credited with pioneering EBM, emerged around the same time. His definition follows:

> The practice of evidence-based medicine means integrating individual clinical expertise with the best available external clinical evidence from systematic research. By individual clinical expertise we mean the proficiency and judgment that individual clinicians acquire through clinical experience and clinical practice. Increased expertise is reflected in many ways, but especially in more effective and efficient diagnosis and in the more thoughtful identification and compassionate use of individual patients' predicaments, rights, and preferences in making clinical decisions about their care. (Sackett et al., 1996, p. 71)

While EBM was being written about in U.S. scientific literature, Archie Cochrane, a British epidemiologist and physician, had been vocal about the lack of systematic reviews upon which to base medical practice, so he published a systematic review on care during pregnancy and childbirth. It was so well received that he was granted government funding for the Cochrane Center in 1992. The central mission of the Cochrane Collaboration is to promote healthcare decision-making throughout the world that is informed by high-quality, timely research evidence ("Our mission," n.d.). Today the Cochrane Collaboration is an international network of members and supporters from over 130 countries helping healthcare providers, policy makers, patients, their advocates, and caregivers make well-informed decisions about health care by preparing, updating, and promoting the accessibility of systematic reviews.

While the United States, Canada, and England were implementing EBM, in Australia, in response to the growing trend of evidence-based health care, the Joanna Briggs Institute was created at the Royal Adelaide Hospital in 1996 to facilitate evidence-based health care globally (Jordan et al., 2006). The institute's original focus was on nursing, and later it changed to incorporating medicine and allied health practitioners. The institute's definition of evidence-based health care is consistent with early definitions of EBM, stating that clinical decisions should be based on the best available scientific evidence while recognizing patient preferences, the context of health care, and the judgment of the clinician (Jordan, Munn, Aromataris, & Lockwood, 2015).

Nursing and EBP

Concern about overlooking the patient's values and preferences in the early definition of EBM by Evidence-Based Medicine Working Group (1992) prompted nursing to adopt a definition similar to those written by Sackett et al. (1996) and the Joanna Briggs Institute. In 2000, Ingersoll articulated the following definition of EBP for nursing:

> Evidence-based nursing practice is the conscientious, explicit, and judicious use of theory-derived, research-based information in making decisions about care delivery to individuals or groups of patients and in consideration of individual needs and preferences. (Ingersoll, 2000, p. 154)

Unique to this EBP definition was the inclusion of the use of theory as well as evidence when making clinical practice decisions. Leaders in nursing believed that theory and clinical research should be the basis for evidence-based nursing instead of ritual, isolated, and unsystematic clinical experiences, ungrounded opinion, and tradition (Fain, 2014; Ingersoll, 2000). The goal of EBP is to promote effective nursing practice, efficient care, and improved outcomes for patients, and to provide the best available evidence for clinical, administrative, and educational decision making (Newhouse, Dearholt, Poe, Pugh, & White, 2007). Key assumptions of EBP in nursing practice include:

1. Nursing is both a science and an applied profession.
2. Knowledge is important to professional practice, and there are limits to knowledge that must be identified.
3. Not all evidence is created equal, and there is a need to use the best available evidence.
4. Evidence-based practice contributes to improved outcomes.

Two nurse practitioners (NPs), who are educators and researchers in nursing (Melnyk & Fineout-Overholt, 2014), define EBP using Sackett's definition as a platform and identify seven steps in the EBP process. The EBP process, per this definition, starts with an organizational culture that supports EBP and encourages nurses at all levels to wonder "Are we doing the best thing?" Nurses turn a clinical question into a searchable format using an established method (e.g., PICO) and use this focused question to search for the most relevant evidence. Step 3 involves critically appraising the evidence found in step 2, summarizing the strength and quality of the best relevant evidence, and formulating recommendations. The evidence is integrated with a nurses' clinical expertise and patients' values and goals when making a decision or practice change. The next step is to evaluate the outcomes of the EBP decision or practice change. The last step is to disseminate the outcomes of the decision or change locally (e.g., grand rounds) or through traditional methods (e.g., poster or podium presentation, publishable manuscript).

Evidence-based practice for nursing is not EBM, because it is imperative that many sources of evidence are critically appraised when making practice decisions. While randomized controlled trials or systematic reviews may provide the most rigorous scientific evidence for EBM, that evidence may not be applicable to nursing and patient care, which requires a holistic approach and a broad range of methodologies as the basis for care (Houser & Oman, 2010). No one research design is better than another when evaluating evidence on effective nursing practices, and appropriate clinical decision making can only be achieved by using several sources of evidence (DiCenso, Cullum, & Ciliska, 1998; Rycroft-Malone et al., 2004).

Non-research evidence is useful for answering some types of clinical questions. For example, practice-based evidence includes "evidence concerning the contexts, experiences, and practices of healthcare providers working in real-world practice settings" (Leeman & Sandelowski, 2012, p. 171), and the use of qualitative methodologies play an essential role in creating more practice-based evidence in the evidence base for nursing practice used for problem solving and clinical decision making.

Missing from the earlier definitions of EBM and EBP is clinical decision making related to available resources. The reality is that there is a limited amount of healthcare dollars. Therefore, when making evidence-based clinical decisions, nurses and other healthcare professionals must also weigh the cost of benefit, cost of harm, and cost to the system when providing evidence-based care (Hopp & Rittenmeyer, 2012). Nurses, especially at the advanced practice level, must be able to articulate the business case and expected return on investment for EBP (Tucker, 2014).

NPs are actively championing the advancement of EBP in health care and academia. The Helene Fuld Health Trust National Institute for Evidence-based Practice in Nursing and Healthcare Center [formerly the Center for Transdisciplinary Evidence-based Practice (CTEP)] is a world-renowned hub, based at The Ohio State University College of Nursing, that serves as a leader and resource to health professionals, healthcare systems, and academic institutions for implementing best practices through an EBP approach to decision making and sustaining a culture of EBP for the ultimate purpose of improving the quality of health care and its outcomes for all ("About Fuld Institute for EBP," n.d.). The founders are NPs whose mission is to:

- Improve EBP knowledge, skills, and attitudes in clinicians from all disciplines
- Facilitate EBP across the care continuum and healthcare systems
- Assist with creating sustainable EBP culture in healthcare systems
- Synthesize and disseminate evidence to advance evidence-based care
- Influence health policy by advocating for EBP
- Assist clinicians and healthcare organizations with expediting the process of translation of evidence into practice
- Disseminate findings of EBP implementation and research
- Conduct ongoing research on many aspects of EBP

It is clear from the inception of EBM and evidence-based nursing that all healthcare disciplines should be making decisions based on the best available evidence, clinical expertise, patient values and preferences, and available resources. Moreover, leaders in nursing are calling for EBP to be the foundation for everything healthcare providers do (Melnyk, 2016b).

Why Should NPs Use EBP?

If you were diagnosed with breast cancer and were faced with the decision of whether to have a lumpectomy versus mastectomy, and chemotherapy versus radiation, would you want your NP to give you the best and latest information on treatment options and the risks and benefits associated with each treatment from systematic reviews or randomized control trials (RCT) including patients with the same diagnosis and similar personal characteristics? Would you want to know about how others with your type of cancer coped with the treatment based on evidence from well-designed descriptive or qualitative studies?

There are many reasons why NPs should base their practice on the EBP process. First and foremost is, care that is not evidence-based is likely unethical and incompetent (Vincent, Hastings-Tolsma, Gephart, & Alfonzo, 2015). Thus, as the basis of patient care, NPs should integrate research evidence with clinical evidence and patient values while considering available resources in order to provide the best care. NPs should use the EBP paradigm to promote optimal patient outcomes, stimulate innovation in clinical practice, and promote the value of the nursing profession in the healthcare system (Melnyk, 2014). In today's complex and dynamic patient-care environment, nursing practice informed by the best evidence is vital to realizing healthcare improvements and cost savings (Dearholt & Dang, 2017). The role of the NP has expanded over the years to include a wider scope of practice in many states, thus prompting the need for all NPs to acquire EBP skills and use the best current evidence for clinical decision making (Facchiano & Snyder, 2012a). NPs need to practice using the EBP process because studies have shown that patient care outcomes are substantially improved when health care is based on well-designed studies rather than relying on tradition and clinical expertise alone (Houser & Oman, 2010; Melnyk, 2016a).

Existing practices based on tradition or clinical expertise may be harming patients. It is unethical to continue using untested interventions. NPs need to use and understand the EBP process so they can take a lead role in facilitating the evaluation of evidence to develop EBP guidelines, form EBP teams, identify practices and systems that need study, and collaborate with nurse scientists to initiate research (Melnyk, 2016b).

Evidence-Based Competencies for Advanced Practice Nurses

The Doctor of Nursing Practice (DNP) is a practice-focused doctorate that prepares advanced practices nurses for clinical, faculty, and leadership roles; to improve practice and patient outcomes; and to strengthen practice and healthcare delivery ("AACN Position Statement on the Practice Doctorate in Nursing," 2004). The AACN and the DNP essentials are clear that DNP-prepared nurses are the leaders and experts in EBP (Melnyk, 2016b). The following EBP competencies have been developed for NPs working in health systems and should be a part of NP performance evaluations (Melnyk, Gallagher-Ford, Long, & Fineout-Overholt, 2014).

1. Questions clinical practice in order to improve healthcare outcomes.
2. Uses internal evidence (e.g., data from clinical setting) to describe clinical problems.
3. Develops clinical questions in a searchable format (e.g., PICO = Patient population; Intervention; Comparison intervention; Outcome).
4. Conducts systematic, exhaustive searches for external evidence (e.g., evidence from research studies) to answer clinical questions in PICO format.
5. Critically appraises all different evidence types (e.g., clinical practice guidelines, systematic reviews, research studies, evidence reviews; manufacturer guidelines).
6. Synthesizes a body of evidence to determine its strength and worth to clinical practice.
7. Collects data from practice (e.g., patient, system, or quality/performance improvement data) to inform clinical decision making.
8. Plans and implements evidence-based practice changes using internal and external evidence, clinical expertise, and patient preferences to improve healthcare processes and outcomes.
9. Evaluates evidence-based decisions and practice changes for individuals, populations, and systems to determine best practices.

10. Develops evidence-based policies and procedures.
11. Participates in research studies with other healthcare professionals.
12. Is an EBP mentor.
13. Disseminates evidence-based best practices that improve healthcare outcomes.
14. Implements strategies to sustain an EBP culture.
15. Shares best evidence with individuals, colleagues, and policy makers.[1]

Incorporating these competencies into the standards of practice for NPs working in health systems should facilitate higher quality, efficient care, and improved healthcare outcomes (Melnyk et al., 2014).

How to Translate EBP into Practice

Many EBP models exist that help to guide healthcare systems and their clinicians with implementing EBP policies, protocols, and guidelines. It is important for organizations or healthcare systems to have EBP models that assist clinicians with translating research evidence into the practice setting. A central goal of these EBP models is to speed up the transfer of new knowledge into practice, because in the past this has taken years. Use of a model provides an organized approach to EBP implementation and can maximize use of nursing time and resources (Gawlinski & Rutledge, 2008). There are several EBP models that help with translating research into practice. Common aspects of these models include the EBP process that identifies problems and practice questions and reviews the latest evidence, existing clinical practices and practice guidelines, and other data specific to quality indicators in that setting. No one model of EBP exists that meets the needs of all nursing environments. For the purposes of this chapter, some of the more popular models are described in **Table 2-1**.

The ACE Star model, ARCC, PARIHS, EBP Model for Change, and Trinity EBP model are all models or frameworks for systematically putting the EBP process into operation within a healthcare system. The Johns Hopkins Nursing EBP Model and the Iowa Model of Evidence-Based Practice to Promote Quality Care are geared toward clinical decision making at the bedside. The goal of the Transdisciplinary Model of EBP is to accelerate the translation of the EBP process across disciplines within an organization. In summary, there are many models and frameworks that nurse leaders can choose to help guide and integrate EBP into their healthcare system.

Searching for Evidence

Before you can find the best current evidence for clinical decision making, you must identify a clinical problem and translate it into a searchable, answerable question. The PICOT method is a widely accepted format for creating clinical questions.

---

1 Data from Melnyk, B. M., Gallagher-Ford, L., Long, L. E., & Fineout-Overholt, E. (2014). The Establishment of Evidence-Based Practice Competencies for Practicing Registered Nurses and Advanced Practice Nurses in Real-World Clinical Settings: Proficiencies to Improve Healthcare Quality, Reliability, Patient Outcomes, and Costs.

Table 2-1 Evidence-Based Practice Models

Model	Description	Processes
ACE Star (Stevens, 2004)	EBP framework for systematically putting EBP processes into operation	1. Knowledge discovery 2. Evidence summary 3. Translation into practice recommendations 4. Integration into practice 5. Evaluation
Advancing Research and Clinical Practice through Close Collaboration Model (ARCC Model) (Melnyk & Fineout-Overholt, 2014)	Provides healthcare systems with a guide for implementation and sustainability of EBP to achieve quality outcomes	1. Assessment of organizational culture and readiness for EBP 2. Identification of strengths and major barriers 3. Development and use of EBP mentors 4. EBP implementation
Johns Hopkins Nursing Evidence-Based Practice Model (Dearholt & Dang, 2017)	Assists nurses at the bedside in translating evidence to clinical, administrative, and educational practice	1. Practice question 2. Evidence 3. Translation
Iowa Model of Evidence-Based Practice to Promote Quality Care (Titler et al., 2001)	A guide for nurses and clinicians in making decisions about day-to-day practices that affect patient outcomes	1. Identify type of organizational trigger: problem or knowledge focused 2. Form a team 3. Gather and critically appraise evidence 4. Assess if sufficient evidence 5. Pilot practice change or conduct research 6. Evaluate pilot practice change 7. Institute practice change
Promoting Action on Research Implementation in Health Services Framework (PARIHS framework) (Kitson, Harvey, & McCormack, 1998)	Provides healthcare systems a framework for how research findings can be successfully implemented into practice with equal recognition of level of evidence, the context into which the evidence is being implemented, and the method of facilitating the change	1. Critical appraisal of evidence 2. Gain understanding of practice area where change will happen 3. Create a strategic plan for practice change 4. Successful implementation is a function of evidence, context, and facilitation

(continues)

Table 2-1 Evidence-Based Practice Models (continued)

Model	Description	Processes
Model for EBP Change (Rosswurm & Larabee, 1999)	Model for translating EBP into healthcare organization	1. Assess the need for change in practice 2. Locate the best evidence 3. Critically analyze the evidence 4. Design practice change 5. Implement and evaluate change in practice 6. Integrate and maintain change in practice
Transdisciplinary Model of EBP (Newhouse & Spring, 2010)	Interdisciplinary EBP model to accelerate the translation of EBP across disciplines	1. Primary researcher 2. Systematic reviewer 3. Practitioner
Trinity Evidence-Based Practice Model (Vratney & Shriver, 2007)	A conceptual model for EBP that addresses how to overcome barriers to implementation; a guide for growing EBP in your organization while weeding out barriers	1. Breaking ground 2. Planting seeds 3. Sprouting up 4. Showering of education 5. Heating things up 6. Branching out 7. Bearing fruit

Melnyk and Fineout-Overholt (2014) have developed question templates for asking PICOT questions in nursing based on the type of clinical problem (e.g., intervention/therapy, prevention, diagnosis) (see **Figure 2-1**). Examples of intervention and prognosis/prediction PICOT questions are displayed in **Figure 2-2**.

Searching Databases for Best Current Evidence

Successful searching for the best current evidence after developing a PICOT question is the next step in the EBP process. Melnyk and Fineout-Overholt (2014) identified eight steps for an efficient search:

1. Begin with a PICOT question and the P, I, C, O, T should be used as the key words (e.g., P = veteran with diabetes, I = shared medical appointment, C = routine office visit, O = clinical outcomes, T = 1 year) that will be used for the search.
2. Establish inclusion and exclusion criteria before searching (e.g., studies published in the last 5 years).
3. Use controlled vocabulary headings when available (e.g., MeSH).
4. Expand the search using the explode option.
5. Use tools to limit the search so the topic of interest is the main point of the article.
6. Combine searches generated from PICOT key words.

Template for Asking PICOT Questions & Short Definition of Question Type
1. **INTERVENTION** In _____(P), how does _____ (I) compared to _____(C) affect _____(O) within _____(T)?   Questions addressing the treatment of an illness or disability.
2. **THERAPY** In _____(P), what is the effect of _____(I) compared to _____(C) on _____(O within _____(T)?   Questions addressing the treatment of an illness or disability
3. **PROGNOSIS/PREDICTION** In _____(P), how does _____ (I) compared to _____(C) influence _____(O) over _____(T)?   Questions addressing the prediction of the course of a disease or diagnosis
4. **DIAGNOSIS OR DIAGNOSTIC TEST** In _____(P) are/is _____(I) compared with _____(C) more accurate in diagnosing _____(O)?   Questions addressing the act or process of identifying or determining the nature and cause of a disease or injury through evaluation
5. **ETIOLOGY** Are_____ (P), who have _____ (I) compared with those without _____(C) at _____ risk for/of _____(O) over _____(T)?   Questions addressing the causes or origins of disease (i.e., factors that produce or predispose toward a certain disease or disorder)
6. **MEANING** How do _____(P) with _____ (I) perceive _____ (O) during _____(T)?   Questions addressing how one experiences a phenomenon.

Figure 2-1 PICOT Definitions and Questions

Data from Melnyk, B., & Fineout-Overholt, E. (2010). Evidence-based practice in nursing & healthcare. New York, NY: Lippincott Williams & Wilkins, p. 26.

7. Limit final search results with meaningful limits, such as year, type of study, age, gender, and language.
8. Organize studies in a meaningful way using evidence summary tools (e.g., Johns Hopkins Nursing Evidence Based Practice [JHNEBP] Individual Evidence Summary Tool).

Bibliographic databases commonly used for searches by NPs include the Cochrane Library, Cumulative Index to Nursing and Allied Health Literature (CINAHL), Medical Literature Online (MEDLINE), PubMed. Several of these databases require a subscription fee. **Table 2-2** includes a variety of sources for finding evidence to aid clinical decision making; a description of the evidence for each source; the website addresses; and if a fee is needed to access them. In the following paragraphs, some of the more popular databases are described in more detail.

The Cochrane Library is a collection of seven databases that may be used to find the best current evidence in health care. The most popular database is the Cochrane

PICOT QUESTION USING INTERVENTION TEMPLATE

Clinical scenario: You are an extremely busy NP in the primary care division of a Veterans Administration Health System. It has been challenging to meet the complex care needs of veterans with diabetes in the traditional 20-minute clinic visit. You wonder what other care delivery models (e.g., shared medical appointment) may lead to improved clinical outcomes, patient satisfaction, and provider efficiency.

Population: Veterans with diabetes
Intervention: Shared medical appointments
Comparison: Routine clinic visit
Outcome: Improved clinical outcomes
Time: 1-year period

In veterans with diabetes, how does shared medical appointment compared to standard care (routine clinic visit) improve clinical outcomes over 1 year?

PICOT QUESTION USING PROGNOSIS/PREDICTION TEMPLATE

Clinical scenario: A 65-year-old male comes to the cardiology clinic for his regularly scheduled physical examination. He shares that he has seen advertisements for anticoagulant medicine that does not require frequent laboratory testing. He is apprehensive about switching to one of these newer anticoagulant medicines (e.g., dabigatran etexilate) because he has also seen news reports for increased complications related to these newer medicines. The PICOT question would be: Are adult patients who have dabigatran etexilate prescribed compared to warfarin at increased risk for complications? In this scenario, you do not need "T."

Figure 2-2 Examples of Intervention and Prognosis/Prediction PICOT Questions

Table 2-2 Sources of Evidence

Name of Source	Type of Evidence	Access	Fee
ACP PIER (American College of Physicians—Physicians Information & Education Resource)	Includes guidelines and recommendations based on all levels of medical evidence including RCTs, cohort and observational studies, case reports, and expert opinions	https://www.acponline.org/clinical-information	ACP member/fee
Agency for Healthcare Research and Quality (AHRQ)	Clinical Information Effectiveness: ■ Evidence-based practice ■ Outcomes and effectiveness ■ Technology assessments ■ Guidelines: • Preventive services • Clinical practice guidelines • National Guideline Clearinghouse	http://www.ahrq.gov	Free

Name of Source	Type of Evidence	Access	Fee
Campbell Collaboration	Systematic reviews and other evidence synthesis for evidence-based social policy and practice Emphasis on reviews of research evidence on the effectiveness of social and behavioral interventions	https://campbellcollaboration.org/	Free
Center for Evidence-Based Medicine (Oxford)	Conferences, workshops, and EBM tools for how to access, appraise, and use evidence	https://www.cebm.net/	Some free, some fee to access
Clinical Evidence	Database of best available evidence on common clinical interventions	https://www.bmj.com/specialties/clinical-evidence	Subscription
CINAHL Plus with Full Text	Comprehensive nursing and allied health research database, providing full text for more than 770 journals Evidence-based care sheets	https://www.ebsco.com/products/research-databases/cinahl-database	Subscription
Cochrane Collaboration	Cochrane Reviews	https://www.cochrane.org/	Free abstract Subscription for full text
Joanna Briggs Institute	Reliable evidence for health professionals to use to inform their clinical decision making; tools for how to access, appraise, and use evidence	http://joannabriggs.org/	Subscription
NICE: National Institutes of Health and Clinical Excellence	NICE develops evidence-based clinical guidelines on the most effective ways to diagnose, treat, and prevent disease and ill health; also have patient-friendly versions of guidelines to help educate and empower patients, caregivers, and the public to take an active role in managing their conditions	https://www.nice.org.uk/	Free

(continues)

Chapter 2 Evidence-Based Practice and Dissemination Strategies

Table 2-2 Sources of Evidence *(continued)*

Name of Source	Type of Evidence	Access	Fee
Prospero	Protocol details for systematic reviews relevant to health and social care, welfare, public health, education, crime, justice, and international development, where there is a health-related outcome	https://www.crd.york.ac.uk/prospero/	Free
PubMed/MEDLINE/NLM	Provides free access to Medline and the NLM database of indexed citations and original abstracts in medicine, nursing, and health care; search tutorials; evidence-based medical reviews (EBMR)	https://pubmed.ncbi.nlm.nih.gov/	Free abstracts Some free articles Subscription for full text
RePort	Access to reports, data, and analyses of NIH research activities and the results of NIH-supported research	https://report.nih.gov/	Free
Turning Research into Practice Database (TRIP) Database: For Evidence-Based Medicine	Meta-search engine for evidence-based healthcare topics; searches hundreds of EBM and EBN websites that contain synopses, clinical answers, textbook information, clinical calculators, systematic reviews, and guidelines	https://www.tripdatabase.com/	Free
UpToDate	Clinical decision support system that combines the most recent evidence with the experience of expert clinicians	https://www.uptodate.com/home	Subscription

Database of Systematic Reviews. This database contains systematic reviews of primary research in human health care and health policy. This database is maintained by the Cochrane Working Group, and their reviews are held to the highest scientific standards. Abstracts of reviews are available free of charge from the Cochrane website; however, full reviews are available by subscription. The Cochrane Database of Systematic Reviews is found online at https://www.cochrane.org/evidence.

The CINAHL database produced by EBSCO Information Systems has more than 2.6 million records and provides indexing to more than 3,000 journals from nursing and allied health fields. In addition to journals, this database has publications from the National League for Nursing, American Nurses Association, references to healthcare books, nursing dissertations, legal cases, clinical innovations, critical paths, drug records, evidence-based care sheets, research instruments, and clinical trials. To access this database, you need a subscription.

The MEDLINE database is provided by the National Library of Medicine and is widely known as the premier source for bibliographic and abstract coverage of biomedical literature. It has indices that reference more than 5,000 journals and includes at least 300 journals specific to nursing. PubMed is the National Library of Medicine's web interface, through which MEDLINE can be accessed for free. PubMed has free tutorials on how to conduct searches. Abstracts are free, as well as some full text articles; otherwise, a fee is charged to retrieve full text articles. A guide of MEDLINE and PubMed resources can be found at https://www.nlm.nih.gov/bsd/pmresources.html.

The Joanna Briggs Institute is an international collaboration involving nursing, medical, and allied health researchers, clinicians, academics, and quality managers across 40 countries in every continent. The Joanna Briggs Institute connects healthcare professionals with the best available international evidence at the point of care. They offer systematic reviews, best practice information sheets, and critical appraisal tools. Some information is free but most information is accessed by paying a fee.

Busy NPs with limited resources or limited time should start their search in PubMed because it is a free database that can be accessed via the Internet from any mobile device (Facchiano & Snyder, 2012b). Natural language or key words can be used for the search by typing in words from your PICOT question (e.g., diabetes). Searches may also be done using controlled vocabulary called medical subject headings (MeSH). In PubMed, when you type in key words or natural language you will automatically get MeSH and you can click on these words and continue the search with these words. You can use built-in filters within PubMed to further refine the search. One example is the clinical queries filter that extracts evidence based on the best study design to answer that PICOT question. Boolean operators include *AND*, *OR*, and *NOT*. They can link key words and further define the search, such as *diabetes care and veterans*. Searches can be further defined using the limit feature. This feature includes many categories such as age, gender, English language, year of publication, and humans or animals. It is important to become familiar with how to do searches efficiently. PubMed offers free tutorials on how to search their database that can be accessed via the homepage.

NPs should investigate gaining access to a health science librarian to aid with searches for evidence. Librarian-provided services have been shown to be effective in saving time for health professionals and providing relevant information for decision making (Perrier et al., 2014). Moreover, studies demonstrated decreased patient length of stay when clinicians requested literature searches related to a patient's case.

What Counts as Evidence?

NPs use a variety of sources of evidence to make clinical decisions regarding diagnoses, treatments, and interventions on a daily basis. Evidence can come from external sources such as published research studies or internal sources such as quality improvement (QI) data or clinical data. What is important to remember is that not all evidence is equally rigorous or applicable to your practice setting or the patient populations you manage. Evidence from a textbook, colleague, or single journal article is not the same as evidence from a systematic review of randomized controlled trials that answers a particular research question. Moreover, the evidence must match the type of clinical question in PICOT format being asked. For example, a synthesis of cohort or case control studies is the highest level of evidence for answering prediction/prognostics questions. Lastly, NPs must be adept at assessing the level, quality, and strength of evidence in order to make a judgment about whether or not to translate that evidence into practice.

Evidence hierarchies exist to help healthcare providers assess the level of evidence based on the type of research design (quantitative or qualitative), summaries of research (e.g., systematic review of quantitative, qualitative, or both), and types of non-research evidence (e.g., clinical practice guideline). In most evidence hierarchies, the strongest evidence is from rigorous scientific research or systematic reviews with or without meta-analysis of single randomized control trials, whereas the weakest evidence is manufacturer recommendations. Evidence hierarchies that contain other evidence types in addition to research studies are most useful to the practicing nurse because many nursing care problems cannot be investigated using research designs such as RCT (Jones, 2010). In this section, select evidence hierarchies from different organizations in nursing and medicine are described.

The American Association of Critical Care Nurses (AACN) created their own evidence-leveling system for all their publications, which is outlined in **Table 2-3** (Armola et al., 2009). The AACN's system is unique in that it includes meta-analysis of multiple controlled trials or meta-synthesis of qualitative studies in the highest level of evidence and manufacturer's recommendations in the lowest level of evidence. All AACN resources include the evidence-leveling system, so practitioners have a reliable guide to assist in determining the strength of evidence.

The Oxford Centre for Evidence-Based Medicine 2011 Levels of Evidence is a hierarchy of evidences described in **Table 2-4**. The OCEBM hierarchy of evidences

Table 2-3 AACN Evidence-Leveling System

Level	Evidence Type
A	Meta-analysis of multiple controlled studies or meta-synthesis of qualitative studies with results that consistently support specific action, intervention, or treatment.
B	Well-designed controlled studies, both randomized and nonrandomized, with results that consistently support a specific action, intervention, or treatment
C	Qualitative studies, descriptive or correlational studies, integrative reviews, systematic reviews, or randomized controlled trials with inconsistent results
D	Peer-reviewed professional organizational standards, with clinical studies to support recommendations
E	Theory-based evidence from expert opinion or multiple case reports
M	Manufacturers' recommendations only

Reproduced from Armola, R. R., Bourgault, A. M., Halm, M. A., Board, R. M., Bucher, L., Harrington, L., ...Medina, J. (2009). AACN levels of evidence: What's new? *Critical Care Nurse 2009, 29*(4), 70–73. © AACN Reprinted by permission.

Table 2-4 OCEBM Levels of Evidence

Type of Question	Level of Evidence
Diagnostic or diagnostic test	1. Systematic review/meta-analysis of RCTs 2. RCTs 3. Nonrandomized controlled trials 4. Cohort study or case-control studies 5. Meta-synthesis of qualitative or descriptive studies 6. Qualitative or descriptive single studies 7. Expert opinion
Prognosis/prediction or etiology	1. Synthesis of cohort study or case-control studies 2. Single cohort study or case-control studies 3. Meta-synthesis of qualitative or descriptive studies 4. Single qualitative or descriptive studies 5. Expert opinion
Meaning	1. Meta-synthesis of qualitative or descriptive studies 2. Single qualitative studies 3. Synthesis of descriptive studies 4. Expert opinion

Reproduced from OCEBM Levels of Evidence Working Group*. (2011). The Oxford Levels of Evidence 2. Oxford Centre for Evidence-Based Medicine. Retrieved from http://www.cebm.net/index.aspx?o = 5653. Reprinted by permission.
* OCEBM Levels of Evidence Working Group = Jeremy Howick, Iain Chalmers (James Lind Library), Paul Glasziou, Trish Greenhalgh, Carl Heneghan, Alessandro Liberati, Ivan Moschetti, Bob Phillips, Hazel Thornton, Olive Goddard, and Mary Hodgkinson

was designed to help busy clinicians, researchers, or patients find the best evidence for a particular type of clinical question (e.g., intervention/diagnosis, prognosis/prediction or etiology, meaning). A clinician who needs to find the best evidence for a treatment clinical query should look for systematic reviews of randomized trials first because they usually provide the most reliable answers. If no evidence is found, the search should continue with individual randomized trials, and so on down the OCEBM Levels of Evidence table.

An important concept raised early in this section, which the OCEBM Levels of Evidence table highlights, is that different types of evidence are appropriate for answering different clinical questions. For example, an NP working in obstetrics may ask the health sciences librarian to do a literature search to answer the question: How do pregnant women (P) with gestational diabetes (I) perceive reporting their blood sugar results (O) to their healthcare providers during both pregnancy and 6 weeks, postpartum (T)? Because this is a meaning PICOT question, the highest level of evidence appropriate for answering this question would be meta-synthesis of qualitative or descriptive studies. Conversely, an NP working in labor and delivery has seen a 3-month spike in postpartum hemorrhage after a practice change from an oxytocin infusion dosage of 80 mg/500 mL to 10 mg/500 mL. The NP should use the PICOT intervention question template to develop a searchable clinical question; and systematic reviews with meta-analysis of RCTs would be the appropriate highest level of evidence to answer the question.

Multiple evidence hierarchies can be overwhelming, so this author created a single general level of evidence hierarchy based on evidence type for the busy NP to refer to when rating the level of evidence (**Table 2-5**). The type of PICOT question each evidence type answers is included.

In practice, there is often a lack of clarity among the terms *level of evidence*, *quality of evidence*, and *strength of evidence* (Jones, 2010). In this section, level of evidence was described and examples of different hierarchies of evidence that can help the NP to rate the level of evidence was provided. Rating the level of evidence is the first in a three-step process for assessing evidence for translation into practice outlined by Jones (2010). The additional steps of assessing quality of evidence and strength of evidence are described in the next section.

Critical Appraisal of Evidence

Critical appraisal of evidence is an important step in the EBP process that comes after the search for best current evidence. Publication of research studies and other types of evidence do not guarantee quality, value, or applicability to

Table 2-5 General Levels of Evidence Hierarchy Based on Evidence Type

Evidence Type	Type of PICOT Question Answered	Level
Systematic review with or without meta-analysis of single randomized control trials	Intervention, Diagnostic	1
Single randomized control trial	Intervention, Diagnostic	2
Systematic review with or without meta-analysis of mixed experimental study designs (RCT or quasi-experimental)	Intervention, Diagnostic	3
Nonrandomized control trial or systematic review of mixed experimental and nonexperimental study designs	Intervention, Diagnostic, Prognosis/prediction, Etiology	4
Observational studies (cohort, case-control)	Intervention, Diagnostic, Prognosis/prediction, Etiology	5
Meta-synthesis or single qualitative or descriptive studies	Prognosis/prediction, Etiology, Meaning	6
Peer-reviewed professional and organizational standards with clinical studies to support recommendations	Intervention, Diagnostic, Prognosis/prediction, Etiology	7
Expert opinion or literature review or peer-reviewed professional and organizational standards without clinical studies to support recommendations	Meaning	8
Manufacturer recommendations	Meaning	9

Critical Appraisal of Evidence

clinical practice. Thus, NPs must have strong research and statistical literacy to critically appraise all types of evidence sources and determine their worth to practice.

There are many types of critical appraisal tools that NPs can use to assess the quality of research and non-research evidence (**Table 2-6**). These tools are designed to help the user systematically examine and critique evidence to determine its validity, clinical significance, and applicability to practice. Critical appraisal tools include

Table 2-6 Critical Appraisal Tools for Different Sources of Evidence

Author	Tools	Research Method	Access
Critical Appraisal Tools by Research Method			
Johns Hopkins Nursing Evidence-Based Practice Research Evidence Appraisal	Research appraisal questions organized by research design	RCTs Meta-analysis of RCTs Quasi-experimental Nonexperimental Qualitative Meta-synthesis of qualitative studies	Dearholt, S., & Dang, D. (2017). *Johns Hopkins Nursing Evidence-based Practice: Models and Guidelines* (3rd ed.). Indianapolis, IN: Sigma Theta Tau.
Melnyk & Fineout-Overholt	Rapid Critical Appraisal (RCA) Checklist; method specific	Case-control Cohort RCTs Systematic reviews Qualitative	Melnyk, B. M., & Fineout-Overholt, E. (2019). *Evidence-based Practice in Nursing and Health Care: A Guide to Best Practice* (4th ed.). Philadelphia, PA: Lippincott Williams & Wilkins.
Centre for Evidence-Based Medicine	Critical Appraisal Sheets	Systematic Prognostic Diagnostic RCT Educational Prescription	https://www.cebm.ox.ac.uk/resources/ebm-tools/critical-appraisal-tools
United Kingdom Critical Appraisal Skills Programme (CASP)	CASP critical appraisal checklists	Systematic reviews RCTs Qualitative research Economic evaluation studies Cohort studies Case-control studies Diagnostic studies Clinical prediction rule	https://casp-uk.net/

(continues)

Table 2-6 Critical Appraisal Tools for Different Sources of Evidence *(continued)*

Author	Tools	Research Method	Access
Critical Appraisal Tools by Research Method			
Critical Appraisal Tools for Clinical Guidelines			
The Agree Collaboration	AGREE II Instrument and My AGREE Plus Software	Clinical practice guideline	https://www.agreetrust.org/
Melnyk & Fineout-Overholt	RCA for Evidence-Based Guidelines	Clinical practice guideline	Melnyk, B. M., & Fineout-Overholt, E. (2019). *Evidence-based Practice in Nursing and Health Care: A Guide to Best Practice* (4th ed.). Philadelphia, PA: Lippincott, Williams & Wilkins.

specific questions based on a particular methodology or research design; therefore, it is important to pick the correct tool based on the type of evidence you are critically appraising.

Johns Hopkins Nursing (Dearholt & Dang, 2017), Melnyk and Fineout-Overholt (2019), Oxford England Centre for Evidence-Based Medicine, and United Kingdom Critical Appraisal Skills Programme (CASP) have created critical appraisal tools for specific research designs and non-research evidence.

The strength of the evidence is determined by synthesizing the information on the level of evidence (hierarchy of evidence) and the quality of evidence (critical appraisal tool) (Jones, 2010). This process begins by organizing the important pieces of information from the completed critical appraisal tools for each evidence source in a meaningful way, which can be done by using a summary of evidence table. Using Word or Excel software, you may create your own table or use **Table 2-7**. If your evidence is solely from experimental studies, you may want to use **Table 2-8**, which is an example of an evidence summary table for RCT/non-RCT created by Facchiano and Snyder (2013). The underlying concept is to choose a table format that will help you organize evidence from multiple studies or sources in the most efficient manner that answers your PICOT question. The summary table should provide a succinct, stand-alone account of the important study/article details that is understandable to anyone viewing the table. The summary of evidence table will form the basis for creating an evidence synthesis table and recommendations described in the next section.

Table 2-7 Summary of Evidence Table

Clinical Question in PICOT Format

Citation	Evidence Type	Sample, Sample Size, Setting	Findings That Help to Answer Clinical Question	Limitations	Evidence Rating	
					Level/Quality	
Author, year, first few words of title	Type of evidence being critically appraised (e.g., systematic review with meta-analysis, RCT, QI study, meta-synthesis clinical practice guideline, expert opinion)	If applicable (e.g., single study) describe the sample, sample size, setting	Describe findings that answer clinical question	Describe limitations that should be considered when assessing the quality of evidence and worth to practice	Identify the level of evidence and, with the first entry, state the evidence hierarchy used	Identify the quality rating of evidence and, with the first entry, state the quality rating system used

Data from JHNEBP Tools

Table 2-8 Evidence Summary Table for Randomized or Nonrandomized Trials

Clinical Question in PICOT Format

Citation	Funding Source	Level of Evidence	Purpose/Research Design	Intervention/Comparison Group	Results	Strengths/Weaknesses	Worth to Practice
Authors and title	Funding agency, note any conflicts	Use level of evidence table from this chapter	Trial's purpose/number of subjects invited to participate, attrition rate, trial length	Describe intervention group and comparison group	Include results that answer clinical question	Critically appraise study using appropriate critical appraisal tool	Clinical significance
Study 1							
Study 2 etc.							

Evidence Synthesis and Recommendations

Evidence synthesis is the next step after organizing the evidence in a meaningful way. This can be done using the evidence synthesis table (**Table 2-9**). This table is organized by number of evidence sources for each level of evidence, overall summary of evidence source results, and overall rating of quality of evidence sources. Strength of evidence is determined from the evidence synthesis table.

Strength of a body of evidence has been defined in terms of quality, quantity, and consistency for intervention studies (Manchikanti, Abdi, & Lucas, 2005). Quality is the extent to which relevant studies for a given topic minimized bias. Quantity includes number of studies that have evaluated the given topic, intervention effect size, and overall sample size across all studies. Consistency reflects the extent to which similar findings are reported from work on a given topic using similar and different study designs.

The JHNEBP Model includes a broadly defined quality of evidence rating scale for research and nonresearch evidence sources (Dearholt & Dang, 2017) that has characteristics of the domains (quality, quantity, and consistency) for rating overall strength of a body of evidence by Manchikanti et al. (2005). For research evidence, a rating of high is defined as The JHNEBP Model includes a broadly defined quality of evidence rating scale for research and non-research evidence sources (Dearholt & Dang, 2017) that has characteristics of the domains (quality, quantity, and consistency) for rating overall strength of a body of evidence by Manchikanti et al. (2005). For research evidence to be considered high quality it needs the following elements: consistency, generalizability, sufficient sample size for study design, adequate control measures, definitive conclusions and consistent recommendations. A rating of good quality research evidence will have some but maybe be missing a few elements of high-quality research evidence. A rating of low or research with a major flaw will have little evidence to support the study with a poorly designed study design, inconsistent results and the inability to draw conclusions. A rating of low or major flaw is considered "little evidence with inconsistent results; insufficient sample size for the study design; conclusions cannot be drawn" (p. 131).

The JHNEBP Model has a *Quality Rating System for Organizational Experience* that can be used to rate the quality of evidence sources from QI, financial evaluation, or program evaluation (Dearholt & Dang, 2017). A high-quality rating has

Table 2-9 Evidence Synthesis

Level of Evidence (LOE)	Total Number of Evidence Sources for LOE	Overall Summary of Evidence Source Results	Overall Rating for Quality of Evidence Sources
Level 1			
Level 2			
Level 3			
Etc.			

The JHNEBP Model has a Quality Rating System for Organizational Experience that can be used to rate the quality of evidence sources from QI, financial evaluation, or program evaluation (Dearholt & Dang, 2017). Similar to the quality of evidence rating scale for research and non- research sources this rating system also looks at the clarity of aims and objectives, formal quality improvement and financial evaluation methods, consistent recommendations and use of supportive evidence. This system also interprets the rating scores as high quality, good quality and poor quality.

Judgments about a body of evidence are used to support recommendations. For example, the strength of evidence (level of evidence + quality of rating of evidence) may be very strong with consistent, high-quality evidence to support a practice change. Conversely, there may be very little strong, consistent, quality evidence, so original research is needed. It is also possible to find good evidence but conflicting results. Thus, a practice change is not recommended until more consistent research evidence becomes available. A pilot of the practice change may be in order if there is good evidence with consistent results from a lower level of evidence sources and quality ratings.

In the next two sections, critical appraisal skills for single intervention studies and clinical practice guidelines are described.

Critical Appraisal of a Single Intervention Study

It is probable as an NP that you will hear about results from a single RCT and ask, "Should I incorporate these findings into my practice?" To answer this question, you should follow the EBP process from the critical appraisal step. Step one is to assess the level of evidence, and based on the evidence hierarchy in Table 2-5, a single RCT is level 2 evidence. Next, read the study abstract to assess if the study is relevant to your practice and the patients in your practice. If the clinical problem is one you encounter frequently, you should read the whole article to determine if the treatment is feasible given the resources in your practice (Vincent et al., 2015). Step two involves an assessment of the quality of evidence. In this, you could use any of the tools for RCTs listed in Table 2-6 under *Critical Appraisal Tools by Research Method*. The next step is to determine the clinical significance. This can be done by looking at number needed to treat (NNT) and absolute relative risk, otherwise known as the effect size. The absolute risk reduction (ARR) compares the event rate in the treatment group to the event rate in the control group. If a study found 80% of patients in the treatment group improved and 20% of patients in the control group improved, the ARR would be 80% – 20% = 60%. The NNT is calculated by dividing 100 by the ARR: 100/60 = 1.6. So, for every two patients exposed to the treatment, one will benefit. After validating the findings from the study, the last step is to determine if patients in your practice mirror the patients described in the study. If this were a real-life example and your patients' values and preferences were open to the treatment, costs were low, and the treatment could be easily adopted into your setting, then you would adopt this new treatment.

Critical Appraisal of a Clinical Practice Guidelines

NPs should be able to rapidly appraise the strength of clinical practice guidelines and the quality of evidence used to create the guidelines. Guidelines should be

> **Box 2-1** AGREE II Instrument
>
> https://www.agreetrust.org/wp-content/uploads/2017/12/AGREE-II-Users-Manual-and-23-item-Instrument-2009-Update-2017.pdf
>
> Data from AGREE Next Steps Consortium (2017). The AGREE II Instrument [Electronic version]. Retrieved , August 8, 2021 from http://www.agreetrust.org.

critically appraised in terms of validity, usefulness, when last updated, and clinical context, including environment and patient values and preferences. Rapid critical appraisal checklists for clinical practice guidelines have been developed by the AGREE Collaboration and Melnyk and Fineout-Overholt (2014). At the bottom of Table 2-6 there is a listing of the tools for appraising clinical guidelines and where they can be accessed.

The AGREE II tool is a free, valid, and reliable 23-item tool that is organized into the domains of scope and purpose, stakeholder involvement, rigor of development, clarity of presentation, applicability, and editorial independence. Each of the 23 items focuses on an area of the clinical practice guideline quality. The AGREE II tool also includes two overall guideline assessment items, where the appraiser rates the overall quality of the practice guideline and makes a determination of whether or not to use the practice guideline (see **Box 2-1**).

My AGREE PLUS allows users to complete individual AGREE II Appraisals, contribute to and coordinate group AGREE II appraisals, save appraisals to a personal library, and share appraisals with colleagues. The AGREE II website http://www.agreetrust.org/agree-ii/ has excellent tutorials on how to use the tool and the software.

Grading recommendation systems have been created to assist the clinician with evaluating the strength of recommendations and the quality of underlying evidence that the clinical guideline is based upon. The strength of a recommendation reflects the extent to which the clinician can be confident that the clinical guideline has the desired effect rather than the undesired effect (Guyatt et al., 2008). A systematic approach in the grading of recommendations is important, to cut down on bias and aid in the interpretation of clinical guidelines developed by experts. Two examples of grading systems are the United States Preventative Services Task Force (USPSTF) and the Grading of Recommendations, Assessment, Development and Evaluations (GRADE) approach that is used by clinical decision-making systems like UpToDate and Cochrane Collaboration.

The USPSTF grading system is displayed in **Table 2-10**. In this system, Grade A is the strongest recommendation, and clinicians should offer this service to their patients. Grade D is the weakest recommendation, and clinicians should not provide this service to patients. There is an additional recommendation of Grade I, which means clinicians should proceed with caution, and patients who want the service need to be aware of the uncertainty of the benefits and harms. Clinicians can visit the website and access free clinical guidelines for many clinical categories (e.g., cancer, heart and vascular diseases, mental health conditions). The guidelines are created by rigorously evaluating clinical research and assessing the merits of preventive measures, including screening tests, counseling, immunizations, and preventive medications. The USPSTF provides a grade for each clinical guideline.

Table 2-10 USPSTF Recommendation Grades and Suggestions

Grade	Grade Definitions	Suggestions for Practice
A	The USPSTF recommends the service. There is high certainty that the net benefit is substantial.	Offer or provide this service.
B	The USPSTF recommends the service. There is high certainty that the net benefit is moderate or there is moderate certainty that the net benefit is moderate to substantial.	Offer or provide this service.
C	The USPSTF recommends selectively offering or providing this service to individual patients based on professional judgment and patient preferences. There is at least moderate certainty that the net benefit is small.	Offer or provide this service only if other considerations support offering or providing the service in an individual patient.
D	The USPSTF recommends against the service. There is moderate or high certainty that the service has no net benefit or that the harms outweigh the benefits	Discourage the use of this service.
I Statement	The USPSTF concludes that the current evidence is insufficient to assess the balance of benefits and harms of the service. Evidence is lacking, of poor quality, or conflicting, and the balance of benefits and harms cannot be determined.	Read the clinical considerations section of USPSTF Recommendation Statement. If the service is offered, patients should understand the uncertainty about the balance of benefits and harms.

USPSTF. (2017). Grade definitions. Retrieved from https://www.uspreventiveservicestaskforce.org/Page/Name/grade-definitions

The GRADE is a method of linking evidence-quality evaluations to clinical recommendations that begin in 2000 (Guyatt et al., 2008). In the GRADE approach, recommendations are classified as strong or weak, according to the balance between desirable effects (health benefits, less burden, cost savings) versus undesirable effects (harms, more burdens, costs). A strong recommendation means that the most informed patients would choose the recommended management, and clinicians can recommend the intervention to patients. Weak recommendations mean the intervention has too many undesirable consequences (Guyatt et al., 2008). The GRADE approach also includes quality of evidence and patient preferences. UpToDate, a clinical decision system, uses the GRADE approach (see **Table 2-11**). In this system, a grade of 1A means a strong recommendation to use this intervention, and the guideline has high-quality evidence backing it. Conversely, a grade of 2C means a weak recommendation with low-quality evidence, and other options should be explored. Both the GRADE Working Group and UpToDate have GRADE resources

Evidence Synthesis and Recommendations **57**

Table 2-11 UpToDate Grading System for Clinical Practice Recommendations

Grade of Recommendation	Clarity of Risk/ Benefit	Quality of Supporting Evidence	Implications
1A Strong recommendation, high-quality evidence	Benefits clearly outweigh risks and burdens, or vice versa.	Consistent evidence from well-performed randomized, controlled trials or overwhelming evidence of some other form. Further research is unlikely to change our confidence in the estimate of benefit and risk.	Strong recommendation, can apply to most patients in most circumstances without reservation. Clinicians should follow a strong recommendation unless a clear and compelling rationale for an alternative approach is present.
1B Strong recommendation, moderate-quality evidence	Benefits clearly outweigh risks and burdens, or vice versa.	Evidence from randomized, controlled trials with important limitations (inconsistent results, methodologic flaws, indirect or imprecise), or very strong evidence of some other research design. Further research (if performed) is likely to have an impact on our confidence in the estimate of benefit and risk and may change the estimate.	Strong recommendation and applies to most patients. Clinicians should follow a strong recommendation unless a clear and compelling rationale for an alternative approach is present.
1C Strong recommendation, low-quality evidence	Benefits appear to outweigh risks and burdens, or vice versa.	Evidence from observational studies, unsystematic clinical experience, or from randomized, controlled trials with serious flaws. Any estimate of effect is uncertain.	Strong recommendation, and applies to most patients. Some of the evidence base supporting the recommendation is, however, of low quality.
2A Weak recommendation, high-quality evidence	Benefits closely balanced with risks and burdens.	Consistent evidence from well-performed randomized, controlled trials or overwhelming evidence of some other form. Further research is unlikely to change our confidence in the estimate of benefit and risk.	Weak recommendation, best action may differ depending on circumstances or patients or societal values.

(continues)

Table 2-11 UpToDate Grading System for Clinical Practice Recommendations *(continued)*

Grade of Recommendation	Clarity of Risk/Benefit	Quality of Supporting Evidence	Implications
2B Weak recommendation, moderate-quality evidence	Benefits closely balanced with risks and burdens, some uncertainty in the estimates of benefits, risks, and burdens.	Evidence from randomized, controlled trials with important limitations (inconsistent results, methodologic flaws, indirect or imprecise), or very strong evidence of some other research design. Further research (if performed) is likely to have an impact on our confidence in the estimate of benefit and risk and may change the estimate.	Weak recommendation, alternative approaches likely to be better for some patients under some circumstances.
2C Weak recommendation, low-quality evidence	Uncertainty in the estimates of benefits, risks, and burdens; benefits may be closely balanced with risks and burdens.	Evidence from observational studies, unsystematic clinical experience, or from randomized, controlled trials with serious flaws. Any estimate of effect is uncertain.	Very weak recommendation; other alternatives may be equally reasonable.

Copyright © (2013) UpToDate, Inc. and GRADE. All rights reserved.

and tutorials that are free and can be accessed at http://www.gradeworkinggroup.org/ and http://www.uptodate.com/home/grading-tutorial, respectively.

Outcomes of the EBP Process

The EBP process should be the core foundation from which all NPs practice. NPs should routinely question practice, describe practice problems using internal evidence (e.g., QI data), formulate clinical questions to answer practice problems in PICOT format, systematically search for external evidence, critically appraise evidence, synthesize evidence, and make recommendations. Outcomes of the EBP process can take the form of research, EBP, QI, and program evaluation. Therefore, a comparison of these outcomes with an example of each is displayed in **Table 2-12**.

Shared Decision Making: An Important Often Missed Part of EBP

Despite the varied definitions of shared decision making (SDM) in the literature (Makoul & Clayman, 2006), Charles, Gafni, and Whelan (1997) first described this collaborative process between patient and provider where information is exchanged, deliberated, and treatment decisions are made. Healthcare reform, including the passage of the Affordable Care Act and subsequent regulations, has spurred healthcare delivery systems to engage patients and families in SDM (Friedberg, Van Busum, Wexler, Bowen, & Schneider, 2013). Existing evidence suggests that SDM benefits patients of all ages and educational levels (Wexler et al., 2015).

Both patient-centered care and evidence-based practices are foundational to the SDM process between providers and patients. Although SDM is the preferred model for engaging patients in the process of decisions about care when more than one reasonable option is available, no option has a clear advantage, or the options have benefits and harms that the patient may value differently (Stacey et al., 2014; Stiggelbout, Pieterse, & De Haes, 2015). Use of this model in practice by clinicians is lacking (Couët et al., 2015; Légaré et al., 2008).

The SHARE Approach is a model for SDM developed by AHRQ (AHRQ, 2016). It is a five-step process that includes exploration and comparison of the benefits, harms, and risks of care options using meaningful provider–patient dialogue. Step 1 is seeking the patient's participation. Step 2 is helping the patient explore and compare treatment options. Step 3 is assessing the patient's values and preferences. Step 4 involves reaching a decision with the patient. Step 5 is to evaluate the patient's decision. In situations where the patient cannot make decisions, the family may participant in each step.

Decision aids (DA) are effective tools to facilitate the SDM discourse between the patient and the provider (Stacey & Légaré, 2015). These tools can be used to prepare the patient to make informed, value-based decisions with their provider. High-quality evidence exists that DA improve patients' knowledge of options and facilitate informed, clear decisions based on preferences (Stacey & Légaré, 2015). Moderate-quality evidence suggests that patients participate more in decision making when using DA. Despite the availability of hundreds of free DA through AHRQ and the Ottawa Hospital Research Institute (OHRI), translation of these tools into

Table 2-12 Comparison of Research, EBP, QI, and Program Evaluation Characteristics

	Research	EBP	QI	Program Evaluation
Definition	Prescribed, methodical, meticulous technique of investigation	A problem-solving process that integrates existing evidence (research, QI), nursing expertise, and patient preferences to guide care decisions	Appraise the efficiency of clinical interventions and provide guidance for achieving quality outcomes, productivity, cost containment	Evaluate a specific program using a well-defined conceptual framework to judge success or failure
Prompted by	Gap in knowledge	New evidence from research	Process breakdown or system failure	Ineffectiveness, inefficiency, new guidelines
Purpose	Generate new knowledge	Integrate best evidence, clinician's expertise, and patient values and preferences to improve health outcomes	Improve system and process of healthcare delivery; real-life experience and data on application of best practices	Provide timely information/data for decision making for particular programs
The Questions	What is the best thing to do?	Are we doing the best thing?	Are we doing the best thing right, all of the time?	Is the thing we are doing successful?
IRB approval	Yes, unless analysis of public data	No, but health systems may require a review to protect their data	No, but health systems may require a review to protect their data	No, but health systems may require a review to protect their data
Sample	Subset of population	Patient population	Unit, service line, institution-wide or health system	Specific programs

	Research	EBP	QI	Program Evaluation
Method	Quantitative or qualitative	Level of evidence matches question asked; assess strength and quality of evidence; make recommendations based on evidence; translate evidence into practice using translation strategies	PDSA Lean Thinking Six Sigma Structure, process, outcome	Quantitative or qualitative
Rigor/Control	Maximum rigor/control	More rigor than QI but not as rigorous as research	Least rigorous	Can be as rigorous as research
Data collection	Follow specific procedures and don't deviate	Research and non-research evidence sources and critically appraise evidence	Pre-data and evaluation, data can come from patient record or surveys	Formative and summative evaluation
Results	Generalizable to population	Recommendation for practice change, clinical research study, or no change	Applicable to the patients studied	Direct, persuasive, or conceptual utilization
Dissemination	Presentation or publish	Presentation or publish	Presentation or publish	Presentation or publication
Example	Emergency department weekend presentation and mortality in patients with acute myocardial infarction (de Cordova, Johansen, Martinez, & Cimiotti, 2017)	Alternate light sources in sexual assault examinations: An evidence-based practice project (Eldredge, Huggins, & Pugh, 2012)	Large-scale implementation of the I-PASS handover system at an academic medical centre (Shahian, McEachern, Rossi, Chisari, & Mort, 2017)	Using the program logic model to evaluate ¡cuídate!: A sexual health program for Latino adolescents in a school-based health center (Serowoky, George, & Yarandi, 2015)

practice is slow. NPs must be the leaders in implementing SDM and DA in the practice setting as part of the EBP process.

Disseminating EBP

Step 6 in the EBP process is disseminating outcomes of the EBP decision or change (Melnyk & Fineout-Overholt, 2019). The goal of disseminating the results of an EBP-driven decision or practice change is to hardwire the change within the organization (Cullen et al., 2018). Internal dissemination can take the form of a brief project summary that is distributed in a newsletter, blog, or the intranet, where NPs and other healthcare staff look for practice updates. Project summaries should include project title, the names and credentials of the project manager/director and team, the purpose, the rationale, a brief synthesis of evidence, practice change, implementation strategies, and evaluation results. External dissemination may include a poster (Forsyth et al., 2010), or podium presentations at local, regional, national, or international conferences, or a publication in a relevant practice journal. Social media can be used to blast the main result on Twitter or Facebook (Flynn et al., 2017).

The Evidence-Based Practice Process Quality (EPQA) guidelines can be used as a reference when writing your EBP project report for external dissemination (Milner, 2016). The guidelines have 34 items ranging from title, abstract, introduction, methods, results, discussion, implementation, and outcomes. Quality improvement methods are often used in EBP practice changes to pilot and evaluate the change. The Doctor of Nursing Practice (DNP) Roadmap is another tool that can be used to plan, implement, evaluate, and disseminate EBP-QI project results (Milner et al., 2019). The Revised Standards for QUality Improvement Reporting Excellence (SQUIRE) 2.0 guidelines have the same major sections as the EPQA and DNP Project Roadmap that authors can follow to ensure high-quality reporting (http://squire-statement.org/).

EBP dissemination may also take the form of disseminating evidence from research studies into practice to increase the use of evidence in practice. A larger-scale example of this is the AHRQ patient-centered outcomes research (PCORI) interventions for dissemination and implementation initiative (Huppert et al., 2019). This AHRQ working group established a framework to prioritize evidence-based practices for dissemination and implementation into clinical practice in the United States. A smaller-scale strategy for increasing the use of evidence in practice is journal clubs. Journal clubs are a recognized, efficient, and effective tool for critically appraising evidence and evaluating its worth to practice (Xiong et al., 2018). Journal clubs can be in-person or virtual, where members critically appraise the evidence and assess its applicability to practice.

Barriers to EBP

If EBP is as much about removing harmful or ineffective practices as it is about implementing robust evidence into practice (Vincent et al., 2015) and it is unethical to practice using evidence-less care (Jones, 2010), why do barriers to EBP continue to exist? Houser and Oman (2010) identified three categories associated with barriers to using evidence in clinical practice that continue to be relevant today (Warren et al., 2016). The first category includes limitations in EBP systems caused by an overwhelming amount of evidence and sometimes contradictory findings in the research. The second category is human factors that create barriers. These factors include lack of knowledge about EBP and skills needed to conduct EBP, nurses' negative attitudes toward research and evidence-based care, nurses' perceptions that research is only for medicine and is a cookbook approach, and patient expectations. The last category identifies the lack of organizational systems or infrastructure to support clinicians using EBP. Causes for barriers in this category include lack of authority for clinicians to make changes in practice, peer emphasis on practicing the way they always have practiced, lack of time during the workday, lack of administrative support or incentives, and conflicting priorities between unit work and research.

The barriers described here may seem overwhelming; however, all healthcare-related disciplines are becoming evidence-based, and professional organizations, accrediting bodies, insurers, and third-party payers are requiring that nurses use evidence to support clinical practices and decision making. Therefore, organizations need to address these barriers and put systems in place to support EBP (Warren et al., 2016). Moreover, NPs with Doctor of Nursing Practice degrees must be EBP leaders who mentor others and promote the EBP process as the foundation upon which practice is built.

Chapter Summary Points

Evidence-based nursing practice is the conscientious, explicit, and judicious use of theory-derived, research-based information in making decisions about care delivery to individuals or groups of patients and considers individual needs and preferences. It is vital to a practice-based profession such as nursing to use the best current evidence from many sources when making clinical decisions. EBP competencies have been described for the NP and should be part of performance evaluation criteria.

There are several steps in the EBP process, beginning with fostering a spirit of inquiry, asking the right clinical question in a PICOT format, finding the best current evidence, critically appraising the evidence, and integrating the synthesis of evidence with patient values and preferences.

Best current research evidence can be found in many web-based electronic databases, such as the Cochrane Database of Systematic Reviews. There are databases for clinical practice guidelines, such as the National Guidelines Clearinghouse. In addition, quantitative, qualitative, and non-research tools specific to study design or evidence type are available to assist clinicians with rapid systematic appraisal of evidence.

The strength of the evidence is determined by synthesizing the information on the level of evidence (hierarchy of evidence) and quality of evidence (critical appraisal tool). An evidence summary table provides a succinct, stand-alone account of the important study/article details and the critical appraisal results. An evidence synthesis table incorporates data from the evidence summary table to make recommendations based on the strength of the evidence.

Existing EBP models can be used to implement and sustain a culture of EBP. These models may aid with translation of evidence into practice. Outcomes of EBP can take the form of NPs collaborating on original research, QI studies, or program evaluation.

Shared decision making and the AHRQ SHARE Approach can be used by NPs to facilitate the incorporation of patient values, preferences, and goals when making care decisions. Existing decision aids for many health conditions or treatments are available for free. NPs should be leaders in adopting this practice.

Disseminating EBP may be done internally or externally. Internal dissemination may take the form of a brief project summary in an organizational newsletter, whereas external dissemination may take the form of a presentation at a local, regional, or national conference or publication. NPs should be leaders in disseminating EBP.

Health systems continue to face the same barriers to implementing and sustaining EBP. NPs need to take an active role in breaking down these barriers, being EBP mentors, and promoting the EBP process as the foundation from which all practice is built.

Seminar Discussion Questions

1. Explain the steps of the EBP process.
2. Write a clinical question in PICOT format for each template type for common practice problems encountered by NPs. Swap answers with a peer and provide feedback.
3. Sign up for clinical practice alerts from the TRIP database in your specialty area.
4. Think about a patient problem you have had in the clinical setting and answer the following:
   a. What formal structures were in place to help you address the problem?
   b. How did you use evidence to investigate the problem?
   c. Did you have time to search for evidence? If not, what were the barriers?
   d. What databases did you access for evidence and why?
   e. Did you use a health sciences librarian to help with your search? Explain why or why not.
5. Go to http://www.guideline.gov and search for chronic pain management clinical practice guidelines. Compare and contrast two guidelines.
6. Find a clinical practice guideline from National Guideline Clearinghouse. Use the AGREE II Plus software to critically appraise the guideline with two or more peers.
7. Find a recent randomized control trial on a topic of interest. Critically appraise the study using a tool from this chapter. Using an evidence hierarchy from this chapter, identify the level of evidence. Enter the relevant data into an evidence summary table. Rate the quality of evidence using the JHNEBP quality rating. Summarize clinical significance using NNT and effective size.
8. Using the databases described in this chapter, find two or more of the following evidence types (research study, QI study, EBP project, or program evaluation). Describe the search process used. After reading the articles, compare and contrast the different methodologies. Did the authors provide support for the selected methodology? Give examples to support your answer.
9. Identify areas where SDM can be used in your practice. Go to https://decision-aid.ohri.ca/ and browse the decision aids by topic. Select a decision aid and write a plan for how it can be incorporated into your practice setting.
10. Compare and contrast strategies for internal and external EBP dissemination.

References

AACN Position Statement on the Practice Doctorate in Nursing. (2004). Retrieved from http://www.aacn.nche.edu/publications/position/DNPpositionstatement.pdf

About Fuld Institute for EBP. (n.d.). Retrieved from https://fuld.nursing.osu.edu/

AHRQ. (2016). *The SHARE approach: A model for shared decision making.* Retrieved from https://www.ahrq.gov/sites/default/files/publications/files/share-approach_factsheet.pdf

Armola, R. R., Bourgault, A. M., Halm, M. A., Board, R. M., Bucher, L., Harrington, L., . . . Medina, J. (2009). AACN levels of evidence: What's new? *Critical Care Nurse, 29*(4), 70–73. Retrieved from https://doi.org/10.4037/ccn2009969

Brouwers, M. C., Kho, M. E., Browman, G. P., Burgers, J. S., Cluzeau, F., Feder, G., . . . Littlejohns, P. (2010). AGREE II: Advancing guideline development, reporting and evaluation in health care. *Canadian Medical Association Journal, 182*(18), E839–E842. doi: 10.1503/cmaj.090449

Charles, C., Gafni, A., & Whelan, T. (1997). Shared decision-making in the medical encounter: What does it mean? (or it takes at least two to tango). *Social Science & Medicine, 44*(5), 681–692. Retrieved from http://www.ncbi.nlm.nih.gov/pubmed/9032835

Couët, N., Desroches, S., Robitaille, H., Vaillancourt, H., Leblanc, A., Turcotte, S., . . . Légaré, F. (2015). Assessments of the extent to which health-care providers involve patients in decision making: A systematic review of studies using the OPTION instrument. *Health Expectations, 18*(4), 542–561. Retrieved from https://doi.org/10.1111/hex.12054

Cullen, L. et al. (2018). *Evidence-based practice in action comprehensive strategies, tools, and tips from the University of Iowa hospitals and clinics.* Indianapolis, IN: Sigma Theta Tau.

de Cordova, P. B., Johansen, M. L., Martinez, M. E., & Cimiotti, J. P. (2017). Emergency department weekend presentation and mortality in patients with acute myocardial infarction. *Nursing Research, 66*(1), 20–27. Retrieved from https://doi.org/10.1097/NNR.0000000000000196

Dearholt, S., & Dang, D. (2017). *Johns Hopkins nursing evidence-based practice: Models and guidelines.* 3rd ed. Indianapolis, IN: Sigma Theta Tau.

DiCenso, A., Cullum, N., & Ciliska, D. (1998). Implementing evidence-based nursing: Some misconceptions. *Evidence Based Nursing, 1*(2), 38–39.

Eldredge, K., Huggins, E., & Pugh, L. C. (2012). Alternate light sources in sexual assault examinations: An evidence-based practice project. *Journal of Forensic Nursing, 8*(1), 39–44. Retrieved from https://doi.org/10.1111/j.1939-3938.2011.01128.x

Evidence-Based Medicine Working Group. (1992). Evidence-based medicine. A new approach to teaching the practice of medicine. *JAMA, 268*(17), 2420–2425.

Facchiano, L., & Snyder, C. H. (2012a). Evidence-based practice for the busy nurse practitioner: Part one: Relevance to clinical practice and clinical inquiry process. *Journal of the American Academy of Nurse Practitioners, 24*(10), 579–586. Retrieved from https://doi.org/10.1111/j.1745-7599.2012.00748.x

Facchiano, L., & Snyder, C. H. (2012b). Evidence-based practice for the busy nurse practitioner: Part two: Searching for the best evidence to clinical inquiries. *Journal of the American Academy of Nurse Practitioners, 24*(11), 640–648. Retrieved from https://doi.org/10.1111/j.1745-7599.2012.00749.x

Facchiano, L., & Snyder, C. H. (2013). Evidence-based practice for the busy nurse practitioner: Part four: Putting it all together. *Journal of the American Academy of Nurse Practitioners, 25*(1), 24–31. Retrieved from https://doi.org/10.1111/j.1745-7599.2012.00751.x

Fain, J. (2014). *Reading, understanding, and applying nursing research.* 4th ed. Philadelphia, PA: F.A. Davis.

Flynn, S. et al. (2017). Leveraging social media to promote evidence-based continuing medical education, *PLOS ONE.* Edited by K. Woolfall, 12(1), p. e0168962. doi: 10.1371/journal.pone.0168962.

Forsyth, D. M. et al. (2010). Disseminating evidence-based practice projects: Poster design and evaluation, *Clinical Scholars Review,* 3(1), pp. 14–21. doi: 10.1891/1939-2095.3.1.14.

Friedberg, M. W., Van Busum, K., Wexler, R., Bowen, M., & Schneider, E. C. (2013). A demonstration of shared decision making in primary care highlights barriers to adoption and potential remedies. *Health Affairs, 32*(2), 268–275. Retrieved from https://doi.org/10.1377/hlthaff.2012.1084

Gawlinski, A., & Rutledge, D. (2008). Selecting a model for evidence-based practice changes: A practical approach. *AACN Advanced Critical Care, 19*(3), 291–300. Retrieved from https://doi.org/10.1097/01.AACN.0000330380.41766.63

Guyatt, G. H., Haynes, R. B., Jaeschke, R. Z., Cook, D. J., Green, L., Naylor, C. D., . . . Richardson, W. S. (2000). Users' guides to the medical literature: XXV. Evidence-based medicine: Principles for applying the users' guides to patient care. Evidence-Based Medicine Working Group. *JAMA, 284*(10), 1290–1296.

Guyatt, G. H., Oxman, A. D., Vist, G. E., Kunz, R., Falck-Ytter, Y., Alonso-Coello, P., . . . GRADE Working Group. (2008). GRADE: An emerging consensus on rating quality of evidence and strength of recommendations. *BMJ* (Clinical Research Ed.), *336*(7650), 924–926. Retrieved from https://doi.org/10.1136/bmj.39489.470347.AD

Hopp, L., & Rittenmeyer, L. (2012). *Introduction to evidence-based practice: A practical guide for nursing*. Philadelphia, PA: F.A. Davis.

Houser, J., & Oman, K. (2010). *Evidence-based practice: An implementation guide for healthcare organizations*. Burlington, MA: Jones & Bartlett.

Huppert, J. S. et al. (2019). Prioritizing evidence-based interventions for dissemination and implementation investments. *Medical Care,* 57, pp. S272–S277. doi: 10.1097/MLR.0000000000001176.

Ingersoll, G. L. (2000). Evidence-based nursing: What it is and what it isn't. *Nursing Outlook, 48*(4), 151–152. Retrieved from https://doi.org/10.1067/mno.2000.107690

Jones, K. R. (2010). Rating the level, quality, and strength of the research evidence. *Journal of Nursing Care Quality, 25*(4), 304–312.

Jordan, Z., Donnelly, P., & Piper, R. (2006). *A short history of a BIG idea: The Joanna Briggs Institute 1996-2006*. Retrieved from https://hekyll.services.adelaide.edu.au/dspace/handle/2440/35988

Jordan, Z., Munn, Z., Aromataris, E., & Lockwood, C. (2015). Now that we're here, where are we? The JBI approach to evidence-based healthcare 20 years on. *International Journal of Evidence-Based Healthcare, 13*(3), 117–120. Retrieved from https://doi.org/10.1097/XEB.0000000000000053

Kitson, A., Harvey, G., & McCormack, B. (1998). Enabling the implementation of evidence based practice: A conceptual framework. *Quality in Health Care, 7*(3), 149–158.

Leeman, J., & Sandelowski, M. (2012). Practice-based evidence and qualitative inquiry. *Journal of Nursing Scholarship: An Official Publication of Sigma Theta Tau International Honor Society of Nursing, 44*(2), 171–179. Retrieved from https://doi.org/10.1111/j.1547-5069.2012.01449.x

Légaré, F., Elwyn, G., Fishbein, M., Frémont, P., Frosch, D., Gagnon, M.-P., . . . van der Weijden, T. (2008). Translating shared decision-making into health care clinical practices: Proof of concepts. *Implementation Science: IS, 3*, 2. Retrieved from https://doi.org/10.1186/1748-5908-3-2

Makoul, G., & Clayman, M. L. (2006). An integrative model of shared decision making in medical encounters. *Patient Education and Counseling, 60*(3), 301–312. Retrieved from https://doi.org/10.1016/j.pec.2005.06.010

Manchikanti, L., Abdi, S., & Lucas, L. F. (2005). Evidence synthesis and development of guidelines in interventional pain management. *Pain Physician, 8*(1), 73–86.

Melnyk, B. M. (2014). Building cultures and environments that facilitate clinician behavior change to evidence-based practice: What works? *Worldviews on Evidence-Based Nursing, 11*(2), 79–80. Retrieved from https://doi.org/10.1111/wvn.12032

Melnyk, B. M. (2016a). An urgent call to action for nurse leaders to establish sustainable evidence-based practice cultures and implement evidence-based interventions to improve healthcare quality. *Worldviews on Evidence-Based Nursing, 13*(1), 3–5. Retrieved from https://doi.org/10.1111/wvn.12150

Melnyk, B. M. (2016b). The doctor of nursing practice degree = evidence-based practice expert. *Worldviews on Evidence-Based Nursing, 13*(3), 183–184. Retrieved from https://doi.org/10.1111/wvn.12164

Melnyk, B. M. and Fineout-Overholt, E. (2019). *Evidence-based practice in nursing and healthcare: A guide to best practice*. 4th ed. Philadelphia, PA: Wolters Kluwer Health.

Melnyk, B. M., Gallagher-Ford, L., Long, L. E., & Fineout-Overholt, E. (2014). The establishment of evidence-based practice competencies for practicing registered nurses and advanced practice nurses in real-world clinical settings: Proficiencies to improve healthcare quality, reliability, patient outcomes, and costs. *Worldviews on Evidence-Based Nursing, 11*(1), 5–15. Retrieved from https://doi.org/10.1111/wvn.12021

Milner, K. A. (2016). Sharing your knowledge: Getting your idea published. *Journal of Infusion Nursing, 39*(5), pp. 297–305. doi: 10.1097/NAN.0000000000000188.

Milner, K., Zonsius, M., Alexander, C., & Zellefrow, C. (2019). Doctor of nursing practice project advisement: A roadmap for faculty and student success. *The Journal of Nursing Education, 58*(12), 728–732. Retrieved from https://doi.org/10.3928/01484834-20191120-09

Newhouse, R. P., Dearholt, S., Poe, S., Pugh, L. C., & White, K. M. (2007). Organizational change strategies for evidence-based practice. *Journal of Nursing Administration, 37*(12), 552–557. Retrieved from https://doi.org/10.1097/01.NNA.0000302384.91366.8f

Newhouse R. P., & Spring B. (2010). Interdisciplinary evidence-based practice. Moving from silos to synergy. *Nursing Outlook, 58*(6), 309–317.

Our mission. (n.d.). Retrieved from https://www.cochrane.org/about-us

Overview | CTEP. (n.d.). Retrieved from https://ctep-ebp.com/about-overview

Perrier, L., Farrell, A., Ayala, A. P., Lightfoot, D., Kenny, T., Aaronson, E., . . . Weiss, A. (2014). Effects of librarian-provided services in healthcare settings: A systematic review. *Journal of the American Medical Informatics Association: JAMIA, 21*(6), 1118–1124. Retrieved from https://doi.org/10.1136/amiajnl-2014-002825

Ragan, P., & Quincy, B. (2012). Evidence-based medicine: Its roots and its fruits. *Journal of Physician Assistant Education: The Official Journal of the Physician Assistant Education Association, 23*(1), 35–38.

Rosswurm, M. A., & Larrabee, J. H. (1999). A model for change to evidence-based practice. *Sigma Theta Tau International, 31*(4), 317–322.

Rycroft-Malone, J., Seers, K., Titchen, A., Harvey, G., Kitson, A., & McCormack, B. (2004). What counts as evidence in evidence-based practice? *Journal of Advanced Nursing, 47*(1), 81–90. Retrieved from https://doi.org/10.1111/j.1365-2648.2004.03068.x

Sackett, D. L., Rosenberg, W. M., Gray, J. A., Haynes, R. B., & Richardson, W. S. (1996). Evidence based medicine: What it is and what it isn't. *BMJ* (Clinical Research Ed.), *312*(7023), 71–72.

Serowoky, M. L., George, N., & Yarandi, H. (2015). Using the program logic model to evaluate ¡cuídate!: A sexual health program for Latino adolescents in a school-based health center. *Worldviews on Evidence-Based Nursing, 12*(5), 297–305. Retrieved from https://doi.org/10.1111/wvn.12110

Shahian, D. M., McEachern, K., Rossi, L., Chisari, R. G., & Mort, E. (2017). Large-scale implementation of the I-PASS handover system at an academic medical centre. *BMJ Quality & Safety*, bmjqs-2016-006195. Retrieved from https://doi.org/10.1136/bmjqs-2016-006195

Stacey, D., & Légaré, F. (2015). Engaging patients using an interprofessional approach to shared decision making. *Canadian Oncology Nursing Journal = Revue Canadienne de Nursing Oncologique, 25*(4), 455–469.

Stacey, D., Légaré, F., Col, N. F., Bennett, C. L., Barry, M. J., Eden, K. B., . . . Wu, J. H. C. (2014). Decision aids for people facing health treatment or screening decisions. *The Cochrane Database of Systematic Reviews, 1*, CD001431. Retrieved from https://doi.org/10.1002/14651858.CD001431.pub4

Stevens, K. R. (2004). *ACE star model of EBP: Knowledge transformation*. San Antonio, TX: Academic Center for Evidence-Based Practice. Retrieved from http://www.acestar.uthscsa.edu

Stiggelbout, A. M., Pieterse, A. H., & De Haes, J. C. J. M. (2015). Shared decision making: Concepts, evidence, and practice. *Patient Education and Counseling, 98*(10), 1172–1179. Retrieved from https://doi.org/10.1016/j.pec.2015.06.022

Titler, M. G., Kleiber, C., Steelman, V. J., Rakel, B. A., Budreau, G., Everett L. Q., . . . Goode, C. J. (2001). The Iowa model of evidence-based practice to promote quality care. *Critical Care Nursing Clinics North America, 13*, 497–509.

Tucker, S. (2014). Determining the return on investment for evidence-based practice: An essential skill for all clinicians. *Worldviews on Evidence-Based Nursing, 11*(5), 271–273. https://doi.org/10.1111/wvn.12055

UptoDate. (2013). Grading Guide. Retrieved from: https://www.uptodate.com/home/grading-guide

Vincent, D., Hastings-Tolsma, M., Gephart, S., & Alfonzo, P. M. (2015). Nurse practitioner clinical decision-making and evidence-based practice. *Nurse Practitioner, 40*(5), 47–54. Retrieved from https://doi.org/10.1097/01.NPR.0000463783.42721.ef

Vratny, A., & Shriver, D. (2007). A conceptual model for growing evidence-based practice. *Nursing Administration Quarterly, 31*(2), 162–170.

Warren, J. I., McLaughlin, M., Bardsley, J., Eich, J., Esche, C. A., Kropkowski, L., & Risch, S. (2016). The strengths and challenges of implementing EBP in healthcare systems. *Worldviews on Evidence-Based Nursing, 13*(1), 15–24. Retrieved from https://doi.org/10.1111/wvn.12149

Wexler, R., Gerstein, B. S., Brackett, C., Fagnan, L. J., Fairfield, K. M., Frosch, D. L., . . . Fowler, F. J. (2015). Decision aids in the United States: The patient response. *International Journal of Person Centered Medicine, 5*(3).

Xiong, L., Giese, A., Pasi, M., Charidimou, A., van Veluw, S., & Viswanathan, A. (2018). How to organize a journal club for fellows and residents. *Stroke, 49*(9). doi: 10.1161/STROKEAHA.118.021728

PART 2

The Nurse Practitioner-Patient Relationship

CHAPTER 3	Family-Focused Clinical Practice: Considerations for the Nurse Practitioner 71
CHAPTER 4	Vulnerable Populations 99
CHAPTER 5	Mental Health and Primary Care: A Critical Intersection 131
CHAPTER 6	Cultural Sensitivity and Global Health..... 155
CHAPTER 7	Chronic Disease Management Models, Pain Management, and Palliative Care.... 187

CHAPTER 3

Family-Focused Clinical Practice: Considerations for the Nurse Practitioner

Susan M. DeNisco

As nurse practitioners, we interface with the patient at the point of care and often neglect to consider the individual in the context of a family unit. It is our moral and ethical obligation to consider the health of families throughout their life cycle. Despite changing demographics, most patients live with family members, and these relationships can strongly influence the health and illness of its members (Bray & Campbell, 2007). It is imperative that we consider family background, structure, and level of function when caring for the individual patient. The information that we glean from the patient will have a significant effect on the health and well-being of the patient, and it has the potential to improve the health of the family unit when the nurse practitioner collaborates with and involves the family in the framework of the treatment plan.

Family Theory

Family health has been studied by a variety of disciplines, including but not limited to psychology, sociology, medicine, anthropology, and economics. Most family theories important to advanced practice nursing have been developed by other disciplines but have been used effectively by nurse practitioners. We do not often think that we are using "theory" when taking a family history or conducting a review of systems in the examination room, but if we study the components of theory, we are better able to understand its practical application in the clinical area. The usefulness of a theory is based on its ability to systematically describe the wide range of relationships between variables in order to generalize the findings (Loveland-Cherry, 2004).

As nurse practitioners, we are continually striving to explain the relationships between symptoms in patients to develop a differential diagnosis. In a simple example, we consider the relationship between chest pain on exertion, back pain, palpitations, and dizziness to help us draw conclusions about coronary heart disease in an individual patient. Similarly, we can use family theory to help expand this differential diagnosis by asking about family risk factors and hereditary causes to assist us in completing the framework of what appears to be coronary heart disease. During the past several decades, nursing literature has emphasized the importance of "family" in nursing practice. Catch phrases such as "family health promotion," "family healthcare nursing," "family interviewing," and "family systems nursing" helped to define family-centered nursing care as an important part of practice (Shajani & Sneel, 2019). According to Denham (2003), a family theory that is meaningful and useful for nurse practitioners must:

- Describe and explain family structure, dynamics, process, and change.
- Describe interpersonal structures and emotional dynamics within the family and the transmission of distress to individuals.
- View the family as the liaison between the individual and culture.
- Describe the process of healthy individuation and differentiation of family members.
- Predict health and pathology within the family.
- Prescribe therapeutic strategies for dealing with family dysfunction, grief, and illness.
- Account for stability and change when viewed within the family's developmental life cycle.

Most of these propositions have been developed out of family social science theories and can be useful for practice.

Application of Macrosystem Family Theory to Clinical Practice

The macrosystem can be described as the larger world in which the family lives and interacts. This can influence the family's overall development and well-being across the family life span. The macrosystem includes social expectations, legal and moral perspectives, and cultural traditions that affect the ways individuals treat and are treated by others. Race, ethnicity, religion, gender, social class, and age may alter the ways individuals and families view themselves and others. The macrosystem serves as a social framework that has unintentional influences on values, attitudes, and behaviors through time. On the other hand, the family's microsystem consists of extended family members, as well as those in the nuclear family, and the roles and expectations that the family holds for its membership.

Structural Approach

All theories, whether at the macrosystem level or microsystem level, have applicability to practice. When the nurse practitioner uses the structural approach to assess the family unit, he or she is considering the position or status of the family in society. Each position has associated social norms or expectations. For example, in most societies a woman in the kinship position of "mother" is expected to act in a nurturing manner toward her child. A social role implies the cluster of expectations or norms for any status position (White & Klein, 2008). An individual may occupy several positions or roles at the same time across the life span. The mother may also be a sister, teacher, wife, volunteer, and daughter simultaneously, which can lead to role strain and conflict.

Interactional Approach

The interactional approach views the family as being constructed by culture and societal norms. Individuals establish their roles and communicate them within the family and to the external environment. It is the way individuals in a family unit frame their behavior. For example, transition to parenthood can be conceptualized when parents form their beliefs about their contributions to parenthood. In a study, new fathers were found to have a greater number of social accounts to justify noninvolvement with childcare activities than the mothers had (White, Klein, & Martin, 2015).

Developmental Approach

The developmental approach considers normal family changes and experiences over the members' lifetime. This framework assesses both individuals and families as a whole unit. The developmental framework has three major theoretical components: (1) individual life span theory, (2) family development theory, and (3) life course theory. All of these components influence each other and must be considered together. Individual life span theory focuses on the genetic development of the individual and factors that affect that development. The family development theory focuses on the systematic and patterned changes experienced by families as experience stages and events of the family life course. Life course theory examines the event history of an individual and how earlier events, such as marriage, influence later outcomes, such as birth or adoption of a child (White, Klein, & Martin, 2015). The developmental approach emphasizes dimensions of time and change in the membership structure of the family, including the change in content of social roles in the family. These events and roles do not necessarily proceed in a given sequence, but rather constitute the sum total of the individual's actual experience.

Application of Microsystem Family Theory to Clinical Practice

Family Systems Approach

Health professionals have applied general systems theory, introduced in 1936 by von Bertalanffy, to the understanding of families for a number of years (Shajani & Sneel, 2019). The general belief of systems theory is that all parts of a system are interconnected. Any change in one family member will affect all family members, and understanding the family is only possible by viewing the whole. The nurse practitioner (NP) that is skilled in collecting and analyzing family data within this framework will consider boundaries within the family and external environment, rules of transformation within the family, positive and negative communication patterns, equilibrium in the family unit, and what the relationships are like within the subsystems of the unit, such as sibling to sibling or parent to child (White, Klein, & Martin, 2015).

Family Stress Theory

Family stress and individual stress must be assessed by focusing on both the individual and family resources and coping skills. The study of stress has emphasized significant events or a pileup of stressors in the individual and family history. Certain normative events such as buying a house, becoming a parent, and changing jobs may occur at the same time as unexpected events such as the death of a parent, infidelity, or divorce. The normative event may be stressful enough; when the compression of unexpected events occurs at the same time, the family unit can become compromised. The NP must consider the general family stressors, specific stressors, and family strengths as identified by the family.

Change Theory

It is well-known that systems of family relationships undergo progressive change. However, a French proverb states, "The more something changes, the more it remains the same." This paradoxical relationship highlights the dilemma frequently faced by families in need of both stability and change (Shajani & Sneel, 2019). Changes in family behavior are dependent on the perception of the problem and may or may not be accompanied by insight. The NP must understand that facilitating change is necessary to help stabilize the family unit in the face of major life events such as death, disability, divorce, natural disasters, and addictions.

Family Resilience and Capacity Models

Resilience is the process of "bouncing back" from life's adversities and difficult experiences. It does not mean that individuals and families do not suffer or experience grief when faced with hardship, but it is a quality that can be learned and developed. In the past decade, Americans have witnessed terrorist attacks, random acts of violence on communities, and losses during the pandemic. Out of these disasters we have seen individual and community efforts to build capacity in order to heal. Health care providers (HCPs), including nurse practitioners, are on the front lines managing the care of patients with COVID-19 in addition to the reality of social distancing and the competing demands of raising family and children. HCPs fear exposure to the virus and transmitting it to family members (Odom-Forren, 2020).

Anxiety and stress common during this pandemic will improve through capacity building. Resilience gives us the ability to combat disturbance of normal family functioning. Strategies to increase family resilience during these times are the integration of self-care practices such as good nutrition, sleep, exercise, practicing mindfulness, and maintaining social connections, all of which will increase coping behavior.

Resilience

Resilience is defined as an individual's or family's abilities to function well and achieve life's goals despite overbearing stressors or challenges that might easily impair the person or family unit (Mullin, 2008). In a concept analysis of older women, attributes of resilience were identified as the ability to achieve, sustain or regain physical or mental health after devastating illness or loss (Felten and Hall, 2001). Wagnild and Young's (1993) theoretical model of resilience describes resilience as an enduring personality characteristic that persists through the human life cycle and moderates the negative effects of stress and promotes adaptation. This model describes five themes that constitute resilience: equanimity, self-reliance, existential aloneness, perseverance, and meaningfulness (Wagnild & Young, 1990). Resilience has also been studied from developmental and environmental perspectives. Environmental factors that influence resilience include social support, which can be described as interactions between the individual, family, and environment (Tusaie & Dyer, 2004). Most researchers agree on the basic nature of resilience but use different terms to define it. The most accepted terms connected to the concept of resilience are *adversity*, *stressors*, *adaptation*, *coping*, *risk factor*, and *protective factor* (Mullin, 2008). Resilience is sometimes conceptualized as the ability to withstand a crisis that is brief in nature, but most often it is associated with the ways an individual or family faces a pervasive social condition such as poverty or a devastating illness or injury.

Resilient individuals preserve hope and construct a meaningful account of their situations (Druss & Douglas, 1988). Resilience is the process of identifying or developing resources and strengths to manage stressors flexibly and gain a positive outcome (Haase, 2004). When they need assistance, resilient individuals reach out to others, including their family, their community, their society, and health professionals (Rabkin, Remien, Katoff, & Williams, 1993). In addition, researchers have identified contributing factors to resilience (Dyer & McGuinness, 1996; Rabkin et al., 1993). Patients with AIDS, for example, have identified social support, excellent medical care, personal resources (e.g., intelligence, education), and access to supplementary services (e.g., visiting nurses, home health aides) as contributing factors to resilience (Rabkin et al., 1993).

In a descriptive correlational study of 71 African-American females with type 2 diabetes, the researcher found that high levels of resilience were significantly correlated with low glycosylated hemoglobin levels, suggesting that resilience may play a role in positive health outcomes (DeNisco, 2011). NPs have an opportunity to consider resilience in the care of minority populations with a chronic illness such as type 2 diabetes. Clinical implications based on the findings of this study include preventing complications of poorly controlled diabetes by recognizing holistic approaches to care that integrate not only the physiological aspects of care but also the psychological aspects of the person, including interventions to help build individual resilience (DeNisco, 2011). **Figure 3-1** depicts a theoretical model of resilience showing the effect of resilience on physiological stressors.

Family Resilience

The system-based resilience model of family stress, adjustment, and adaptation based on the work of McCubbin and McCubbin (1993) is concerned with family development and the family's ability to negotiate change and adapt to stressful life events over time, particularly to stressors such as illness (Kaakinen, Hanson, & Denham, 2010). An approach like this is useful in clinical practice because it analyzes interactions between family members, the family system, and the community or environment to shape the course of family resilience and adaptation.

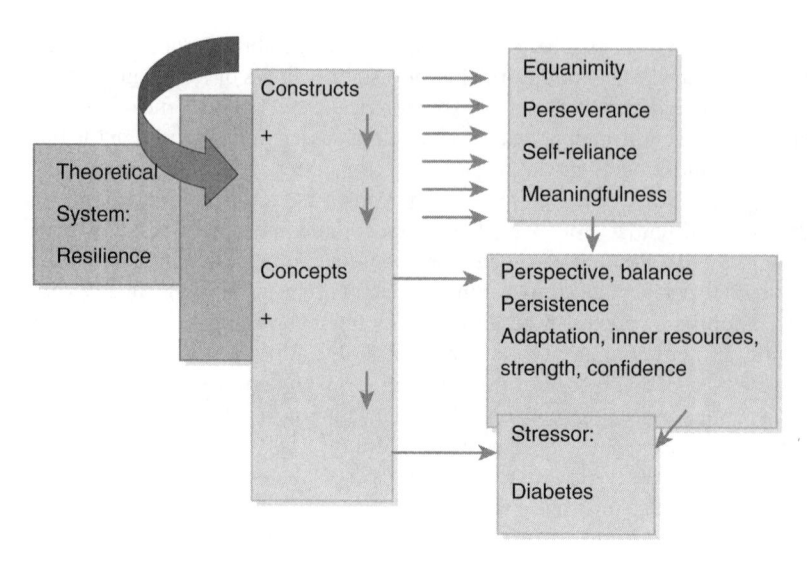

Figure 3-1 Theoretical Model of Resilience

Data from Wagnild, G. M., & Young, H. M. (1993). Development and psychometric evaluation of the resilience scale. *Journal of Nursing Measurement, 1*(2), 165–178. *Journal of Nursing Measurement* by Springer Publishing Company.

Germain and Bloom (1999) wrote that families are more resilient when there is a "fit" between the family and the environment. They note that specific protective factors or positive characteristics of an individual or family help moderate risk factors or negative characteristics that easily become problematic (Germain & Bloom, 1999).

Resilience was identified recently by the Committee on Future Direction for Behavioral and Social Sciences as a research priority for the National Institutes of Health (Singer & Ryff, 2001). The committee addressed the significance of behavioral and psychosocial processes in disease etiology, well-being, and health promotion. Singer and Ryff (2001) point out the need for the increased study of correlates of resilience including protective factors such as optimism, meaning, and purpose, as well as social and emotional support.

Since the 1970s, research on resilience has shifted its focus from the study of personal qualities that predicate positive outcomes to studying the process of resilience, and to foster this in all individuals and develop interventions to promote health (Peterson & Bredow, 2004). The helping professions have been seeking ways to understand the reasons that one individual or family faces insurmountable problems and continues to function well, while others do not. The search to identify the factors of resilience was begun by researchers who focused specifically on children, adolescents, and the elderly (Garmezy, 1993; Gilligan, 2004). Resilient children were seen as having positive temperaments and being easily lovable, autonomous, and intelligent. They were generally seen to have benefited from close relationships with supportive adults or extended family members and others in the community (Garmezy, 1993; Gilligan, 2004).

In a meta-analysis of 24 studies examining the sense of self in children with cancer and in childhood cancer survivors, Woodgate and McClement (1997) found similar themes. Most studies evaluated the psychological functioning of children, including self-esteem and the effect on family functioning and adjustment. It was found that the majority of children with cancer do not have significantly lower self-esteem scores than healthy children (Woodgate & McClement, 1997).

Other studies have focused on resilience in children with asthma (Svavarsdottir & Rayens, 2005; Vinson, 2002). In a descriptive correlational survey study of 235 children with asthma, Vinson (2002) found positive correlations between family environment and child characteristics, as well as between the dependent variables of appraisal, coping, quality of life, and illness indices. The researcher also reported that cohesiveness and adaptability were positively correlated with competence and optimism.

Researchers have also investigated resilience in children with cancer. Hockenberry-Eaton, Kemp, and Dilorio (1994) studied 44 children with cancer receiving outpatient chemotherapy. In this descriptive correlational study, the relationship between the independent variables of childhood cancer stressors (protective factors) and the dependent variables of physiologic and psychological responses to stressors experienced during cancer treatment were examined. Findings revealed that family environment, global self-worth, and social support are protective factors that may influence resilience.

The concept of resilience has also been studied in adolescent populations. In a descriptive correlational study, Rew, Taylor-Seehafer, Thomas, and Yockey (2001) explored relationships among resilience and selected protective factors and which factors were the best predictors of resilience in a convenience sample of 59 homeless adolescents. In another descriptive correlational study, the relationship between adaptive and maladaptive coping correlates to health and illness outcomes in 404 female adolescent athletes who have experienced high levels of stress recently (Yi, Smith, & Vitaliano, 2005).

Resilience has been studied in elderly populations to describe characteristics of resilience. In a qualitative study of elderly women over 85 years of age, nine emerging themes were identified as characteristics of resilience: frailty, determination, hardship, access to care, culture, family support, self-care activities, care of others, and efficiency (Felten & Hall, 2001). The researchers concluded that resilience has implications for healthcare providers to facilitate these traits in order to prevent frailty and disability.

Three other studies were conducted to measure resilience in elderly populations (Adams, Sanders, & Auth, 2004; Becker & Newsome, 2005; Hardy, Concato, & Gill, 2004). In a descriptive qualitative study of 38 African-American participants between the ages of 65 and 91 years, it was found that values such as independence, spirituality, and survival were important factors that shaped responses to chronic illness. Thus, resilience may be a culturally important tool as ethnic minority people age (Becker & Newsome, 2005).

A descriptive cross-sectional study of resilience in 546 community-dwelling older adults found that higher stress levels were negatively correlated ($r = -0.48$, $P < .001$) with lower resilience scores (Hardy et al., 2004). Resilience scores were negatively correlated with depressive symptoms. The authors concluded that more research was needed on the relationship between resilience and future health and functional status as a predication of recovery (Hardy et al., 2004). According to Adams et al. (2004), in a study of 234 elderly participants living in a retirement

Ellen's Story

Ellen Collins is a 63-year-old Jamaican female who has a history of chronic physical problems including type 2 diabetes mellitus, hypertension, asthma, and hyperlipidemia for which she is on numerous medications. Ms. Collins also has a history of depression, but she has maintained well on an antidepressant for a number of years. She visits her primary care provider regularly for the problems mentioned here. Ms. Collins cares for her 87-year-old aunt who has a polymorphic adenoma of the salivary glands. Ms. Collins was also awarded custody of her 13-year-old grandson because her son and daughter-in-law are drug addicts and unable to care for their child. Ms. Collins's youngest son is dually diagnosed with bipolar disorder and alcohol abuse, has had legal problems related to domestic violence, and is currently hospitalized for decompensation of his mental illness.

Despite the myriad adversities, Ms. Collins has a good outlook on life, and she seeks out the support of her healthcare provider and community services. Her chronic health problems are well controlled. She continues to care for her aunt, son, and grandson with a positive attitude and sees hope for the future. She owns her own home, and continues to work with the Department of Children and Families providing foster care for troubled adolescents. She enjoys gardening, raises money for HIV research, and is looking forward to taking her grandson to Niagara Falls this summer.

---

community, loneliness was seen as a risk factor for depression and associated with a smaller social network.

The case study, "Ellen's Story," represents a model case study of resilience.

Family resilience or relational resilience has been defined by Walsh (2016) as having three domains: beliefs systems, family organizational patterns, and communication processes. Walsh redefined resilience as having "reparative" potential on family functioning. The following individual, family, and social factors contribute to family resilience:

- An internal locus of control or the belief that the individual or family is empowered to influence the environment
- Spirituality that fosters personal meaning and a sense of purpose in life
- Downward social comparison
- Positive social supports, including emotional support, informational support, social companionship, and instrumental support

When a nurse practitioner encounters an individual in the healthcare system, the following theoretical assumptions should be kept in mind:

- Some individuals recover or "bounce back" better than expected when faced with an adverse condition (Dyer & McGinness, 1996).
- Positive health outcomes (both physiological and psychological) include the absence of disease or low levels of symptoms or impairments (Heinzer, 1995; Hockenberry-Eaton et al., 1994).
- Resilient individuals have inherent personality characteristics that are protective factors in the face of illness or adversity (Haase, Heiney, Ruccione, & Stutzer, 1999; Jacelon, 1997; Polk, 1997; Woodgate & McClement, 1997).

- Nurse practitioners can be helpful in fostering resilience within individuals, families, and communities (Drummond, Kysela, McDonald, & Query, 2002; Hockenberry-Eaton et al., 1994).

Family Capacity

One of the greatest challenges for many healthcare providers is to address the need for family capacity. If a family has not realized their "capacity" or capabilities, they can face significant obstacles in their day-to-day living. Family capacity-building involves increasing the families' competence in implementing strategies to enhance their development and build their problem-solving skills while increasing their confidence that they are able to do so.

Family capacity can be defined as the extent to which the family needs, goals, strengths, capabilities, and aspirations can meet the family's ability to function to its fullest potential (Dunst & Trivette, 2009). It is the nurse practitioner's responsibility to assess the family's capacity to support the family's health and wellness, as well as prevent illness risks, treat medical conditions, and manage tertiary care needs. Similar to resilience, family capacity can be viewed as the family's ability to adapt and change.

The DeNisco family capacity-building is presented in **Figure 3-2**.

Traditionally, the literature considered children and families as having deficits and weaknesses that needed treatment by healthcare professionals to correct problems, whereas the capacity-building literature believes that families have varied

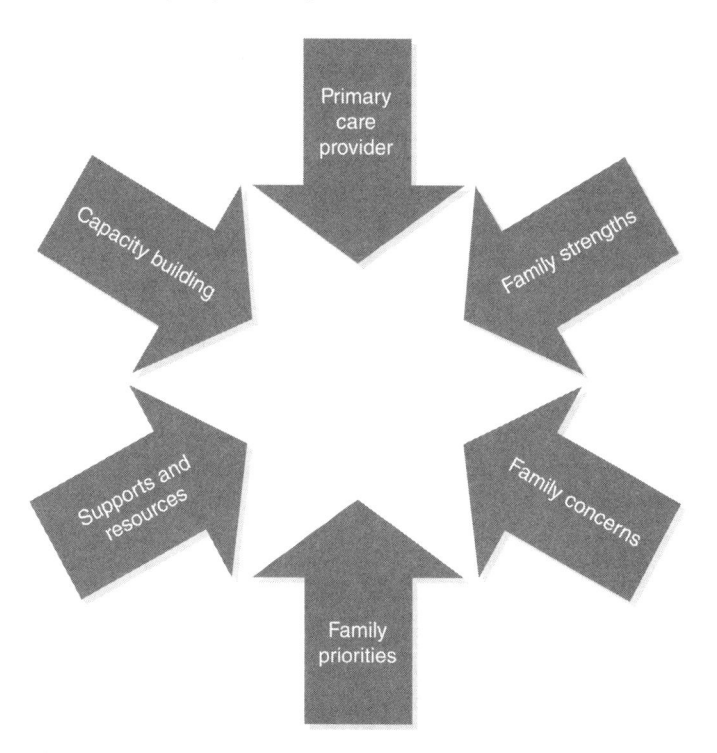

Figure 3-2 The Family Capacity Model

Data from Dunst, C. J., & Trivette, C. M. (2009). Capacity building family systems intervention practices. *Journal of Family Social Work, 12,* 119–143. Reprinted by permission of the publisher, Taylor and Francis Ltd., http://wwwtandf.co.uk/journals and the author.

strengths and assets, and the focus of interventions is on supporting and promoting competence and other positive aspects of family member functioning (Dunst & Trivette, 2009). To understand family capacity, the nurse practitioner needs to understand family structure, function, and roles.

Family Structure, Function, and Roles

There are many clinical family assessment models that the nurse practitioner can use to assess family structure, function, and roles. Some of the popular models are:

- The Calgary Family Assessment (CFAM) (Shajani & Sneel, 2019)
- The Family Assessment and Intervention Model (Kaakinen et al., 2018)
- The Friedman Family Assessment Model (Friedman, 2003)

All three models may have different approaches in their theoretical underpinnings, scope, data collection methods (quantitative or qualitative), and unit of analysis, but they have many similarities. Broadly, these assessment tools are available to expand the clinician's understanding and management of family-wide threats to both physiologic and psychologic health.

There are five key goals of family life:

1. Pass on culture (religion, ethnicity).
2. Socialize young people for the next generation (to be good citizens, to be able to cope in society through going to school).
3. Exist for sexual satisfaction and procreation.
4. Serve as a protective mechanism for family members against outside forces.
5. Provide closer human contact and relations.

Family Structure

The nurse practitioner may use a genogram or "family tree" to gather much of the information regarding family structure. A detailed discussion of the genogram will take place later in this chapter. Family structure can be defined as the organizational framework that determines family membership and the way in which a family is organized according to roles, rules, power, and hierarchies. There is no typical family form in the 21st century. Nurse practitioners need to expand their definitions of the traditional nuclear family (or biological family of procreation) to include alternate forms of family life: the single- or sole-parent family, blended families including stepchildren, grandparents raising grandchildren, communal families, and the lesbian, gay, bisexual, queer, intersexed, transgendered, or twinspirited (LGBT) couple or family (Shajani & Sneel, 2019).

Whether or not you are using a pictorial representation of the family structure such as the genogram or ecomap, the following components should be included in the interview data collection regarding family structure (Bomar, 2004; McGoldrick & Carter, 1999, 2003).

1. Family constellation: Knowledge of who is in the immediate family, who lives in the house, how the individuals are related, and the relationship to extended family and boundaries
2. Family constellation changes: Permanent (birth or death), temporary (illness, hospitalizations, co-parenting in divorced families, homelessness)

3. Individual family members: Age, gender, sexual orientation, ethnicity, race, health problems, occupation, educational level, and cultural/religious beliefs
4. Environmental: Housing or living situation
5. Social support: Stress management, financial support, entitlements such as Medicaid, WIC, food stamps

Family Function

According to Shajani and Snell (2019), family functioning can be defined as the processes by which the family operates as a whole, including communication patterns and manipulation of the environment for problem solving. Each family possesses a distinctive operating system, and it can influence healthcare outcomes. Some specific areas to assess include:

- Activities of daily living: Eating, sleeping, common tasks including family participation in leisure activities and family rituals
- Nutrition: Food insecurity
- Communication patterns: How family members communicate (Is there one spokesperson when articulating healthcare issues?)
- Family perceptions: How illness affects each family member, concerns for other family members, care-seeking behaviors
- Family members' mental health history: Includes substance, tobacco, and alcohol use
- Problem-solving abilities
- Influence and power: Knowledge of who is dominant, subordinate, controlling, abusive, guilt-inducing, the scape-goat, etc.

Family Development

The nurse practitioner must also consider the developmental life cycle for each family that he or she encounters in the clinical setting. Families are shaped by people who share a past and future history together. As contemporary families move through time, there is a normative sequence by which families develop and change. McGoldrick and Carter (2003) have done extensive work on the family life cycle by describing the underlying factors that influence family development as the family expands and contracts by variables such as birth, death, marriage, divorce, adoption, poverty, and catastrophic illness. These events typically cause realignment of the family system to support the entry, exit, and developmental changes of family members through time. Major life-cycle transitions are marked by fundamental changes in the family system itself (second-order changes) rather than rearrangements within the system (first-order changes). McGoldrick and Carter (1999) have designed a classification system of normative stages that typical middle-class American families go through across the life cycle. When reviewing these "normative" stages of the family life cycle, the nurse practitioner must take into consideration societal influences and sweeping changes in the way the family functions. In this day and age, it is hard to conceptualize what is considered a typical family when there are gay and lesbian couples, sole-parent adoptions, dual-career families, grandparents raising grandchildren, cohabiting couples, military families, and foster families.

In the Calgary Family Assessment Model, Shajani and Snell (2019) propose that family developmental assessment includes an overview of the stages, tasks, and attachments that are important to each stage. The nurse practitioner must also keep in mind common health issues that may accompany each stage.

Divorced Families

According to the U.S. Census Bureau (2020), divorce rates in the United States have been declining in recent years, and achieved a record low in 2019. For every 1,000 marriages in the last year, only 14.9 ended in divorce, according to newly released American Community Survey data from the Census Bureau. The drop in the divorce rate is likely to continue in 2021, despite the pandemic. While it is thought the pandemic may have led to some divorces because of quarantine stress, we can speculate that the pandemic may have brought couples closer together. While the divorce rate fluctuates given geographic location, population, income, and educational status, single-parent and divorced families are common in our society and have unique challenges.

The term *divorce* invokes a series of images of bitter custody battles, financial hardship, broken families, vulnerable children, hostility, resentment, and failure to live up to commitments. While these images may be true of some divorces, research shows that most families will experience short-term, moderate effects postdivorce (Bowen, 2012; Demo, 2010). However, it is true that families experiencing divorce are under significant emotional pressure during the transition and must fulfill the same developmental tasks as the two-parent nuclear family, but without all the means. Shortages in time, money, and energy can cause single parents to experience self-doubt and make them feel guilty for not meeting societal expectations of living in a two-parent family (Shajani & Sneel, 2019).

Nontraditional Families

If we consider society a generation ago, the average American family might be defined as a married man and woman with two biological children. Divorce rates were lower, optional single parenthood was rare, and surrogacy and in vitro fertilization by sperm or egg donation were not available. The gay and lesbian community had little hope of raising their own children. Grandparents and extended family members played a supportive role during holidays, special events, and illness, but did not have a major responsibility to the nuclear family. Adoption was closed if available (Lantz, 2012). While societal perceptions of the "traditional family" may still be a certainty for some, this is clearly dependent on age, gender, education, religious beliefs, socioeconomic status, and geographic location. The reality is that less than 25% of U.S. households are considered "traditional."

Single-Parent Families

Single-parent families are recognized as the most common nontraditional family. In 2020, the number of single-parent households decreased slightly from the previous decade trend to 9.8 million, accounting for 25% of families with children in the United States. Father-only families are on the rise, accounting for 2.3 million families, or 5% of all family structures (U.S. Census Bureau, 2020). Single-parent families by divorce or death are under significant pressure for time, space, adequate finances, social control, and tension management. Single parents typically have the ultimate responsibility of paying the bills, disciplining, and caring for the children's physical and emotional needs. This can be especially challenging for the parent who does not have the financial resources, support of the biological parent, or extended family support. Single-parent mothers and fathers also experience societal pressure to live in a "normal family" and feel like failures in meeting the expectations of friends, neighbors, and their extended families (Shajani & Sneel, 2019). In working with single-parent families, it is important for the NP to help the parent explore his or her feelings, develop coping mechanisms, and find community and financial resources to support the parent through issues of custody, visitation, social networks, and effective parenting.

Same-Sex Couple Families

Until recently, gay and lesbian families have been "invisible" in our culture. With changes in the laws recognizing the legal union of same-sex couples, more attention is being focused on these relationships, their structures, challenges, strengths, and issues. In 2019, the American Community Survey (ACS) results showed that 15% of households were headed by same-sex couples with children. By conservative estimates, there are at least 1 million same-sex married or unmarried partner households living with children in the United States. It is estimated that 191,000 children live with same-sex parents. Of these families (U.S. Census Bureau, 2020):

- 72.8% reported having biological children from previous heterosexual relationships or artificial insemination.
- 10.5% reported having stepchildren or adopted children.
- 6% reported having a combination of biological, stepchildren, and adopted children.

While research studies on children raised by gay and lesbian parents are still relatively new, to date, the majority of evidence suggests that children who grow up in families headed by same-sex parents fare as well as children who grow up in families headed by opposite-sex parents. In addition, children who have gay, lesbian, bisexual, or transgender parents do not appear to differ from children who have heterosexual parents in terms of psychological health, social relationships, or cognitive or emotional functioning (Burkholder & Burbank, 2012). State laws and rights of same-sex parents and children vary widely. It is important for the nurse practitioner to understand these differences in order to assist the family to navigate a complicated legal system that may not support the family, or one that may place legal limitations on the family. Child custody issues, adoption rights, and a variety of other rights and benefits offered to married couples, such as insurance coverage and spousal benefits, are not available to same-sex couples. The NP must gain expertise in assessments and interventions that address the unique needs of these families in order to help parents and children to deal with social stress from being perceived as different by other children, or as problematic and threatening by other parents.

Foster Families

Other types of nontraditional families include foster parenting and grandparents raising grandchildren. In 2018, it was estimated that 437,283 U.S. children were in foster care. Forty-six percent of these children were placed in non-relative foster homes, 32% in relative foster homes and smaller percentages lived in group or pre-adoptive homes. Two percent of these children ran away from their placements (Childwelfare Information Gateway, 2020). The nurse practitioner must be cognizant of the intensity of the health and emotional issues that a child residing in foster care may present with; many children have been victims of emotional and physical abuse and have special medical and physiological needs (Lenora, 2009).

In a descriptive study of physical examination findings of 5,181 children taken into protective custody, the researchers found that nearly half (44%) had an identified health problem, including acute infections (otitis media, sexually transmitted diseases), anemia, and lead poisoning. In addition, approximately 5% of the children evaluated for physical abuse were found to have occult fractures not suspected by their caseworkers (Chernoff, Coombs-Orme, Risley-Curtiss, & Heisler, 1994). In another large study of 2,419 children assessed shortly after placement in foster care, almost all (92%) had at least one abnormality on physical examination, including disorders of the upper respiratory tract (66%), skin (61%), genitals (10%), eyes (8%), abdomen (8%), lungs (7%), and extremities (6%). Nearly one-quarter (23%) of younger children failed a developmental screening, and 22% of older children were already receiving special education services before placement. As a result of these evaluations, 53% of the children were referred for further medical services (Flaherty & Weiss, 1990).

Because of the high rate of physical, mental, and developmental problems in foster children, they often require more frequent healthcare visits than most children. Many states require that children newly placed in foster care have a comprehensive health assessment within 30 to 60 days of placement (Simms, 2000). The clinician needs to negotiate a management plan with the foster parents and their children to ensure timely routine health maintenance visits, including close developmental screening and mental health interventions as appropriate. This plan needs to be updated with each patient care encounter and communicated to the caseworker and the foster family. NPs play a significant role in coordinating services for foster children and ensuring they receive care in a timely manner.

Grandparents Raising Grandchildren

Recent U.S. Census reports show that there are more than 13%, or 7 million children being raised in grandparent-headed households (U.S. Census Bureau, 2019). The phenomenon of grandparent caregiving is prevalent among African-American and Latino grandparents: African-Americans and Latino grandparents have a 16.7% and 26.1% chance, respectively, of becoming caregivers for their grandchildren (U.S. Census Bureau, 2019).

The increase in the numbers of grandparents in caregiving roles parallels the increase in the growing number of older adults. According to the federal Administration on Aging (AOA, 2011), it is estimated that the number of adults age 65 and older will make up 20% of the population in the year 2030 as compared to 12% in the year 2000. The grandparenting role is a stressful one; typically, the caregiver attains responsibility for the child secondary to a family crisis where the biological parents cannot effectively care for their child. Factors that may contribute to the shift in parenting include substance abuse, mental health issues, lack of money, incarceration, death, and abuse or neglect of the children. These unexpected life events can cause significant emotional and financial strain on the grandparents as they assume new parenting responsibilities for children.

Grandparents who are primary caregivers usually face a number of challenges, including higher rates of depression, health problems, and fatigue, as compared to noncaregivers or to others their age (Kaakinen et al., 2018). Grandparents often are dealing with their own chronic health issues, may be raising their own adolescent children, and are often providing care for their aging parents. Grandparents report having less time for themselves, experiencing social isolation, and feeling increased financial pressures, especially if they need to reduce their hours at work or draw on their savings in their efforts to provide a home for their grandchildren. Grandchildren are affected, too; research shows that these children have higher rates of asthma, decreased immunity, poor eating and sleep patterns, physical disabilities, and hyperactivity compared to children in parental households (Kaakinen et al., 2018). The nurse practitioner plays a key role in assisting the grandparents to seek out and use existing community resources and social supports to prevent social isolation, ease financial burdens, and promote the health and well-being of the family unit.

Structural Assessment and Family Interviews

Structural assessment tools are helpful to discern the internal and external functioning of the family. Family interviews can be gathered by drawing a genogram, ecomap, or family pedigree. The genogram is essentially a diagram of the family constellation, whereas the ecomap displays the important contacts that are external to the immediate family. The family pedigree is a risk assessment tool for conditions that have familial genetic predisposition.

The relationship between family history and health risks has long been recognized. Indeed, family history is a risk factor for many pediatric and adult onset diseases and disorders. It represents genetic susceptibility, shared environment, common behaviors, and the interactions between and among the family members. The genogram and ecomap are tools that can assist the nurse practitioner in assisting a family as a whole system, as well as assisting the individuals within the family system. The therapeutic relationship between the nurse practitioner and patient can begin in the waiting room, the examination room, or at the hospital beside. When using a genogram or an ecomap, it is impossible to differentiate between its value to the nurse practitioner–patient relationship and its effect on that family or individual. At the most superficial level, either of these tools will give family members a new framework with which to understand themselves as individuals and as an active part of a system (Denham, 2003).

The family pedigree is another interview tool that includes a three-generational assessment of medical conditions in each relative, including specific genetic disorders, birth defects, Down syndrome, and questions about certain behaviors (e.g., alcohol, substance abuse, and tobacco use), as well as questions about consanguinity and ethnicity (Yoon, 2003).

Genograms

A genogram is an assessment tool or clinical method of taking, storing, and processing family information for the benefit of the patient and the family. It is displayed as a graphic representation of family members and their relations over three generations (McGoldrick, 2008). The three-generation family genogram was developed primarily out of the family systems theory and is a popular tool among social workers, psychologists, physicians, and nurses. According to Bowen (2012), people are organized into family systems by age, generation, sex, or other similar features. Where the person fits into the family structure influences the person's functioning, relational patterns, and type of family he or she forms in the next generation. It is also believed that sex and birth order shape sibling relationships and individual characteristics (Rakel & Rakel, 2015). Families repeat themselves over generations in the phenomenon called the transmission of family patterns; what happens in one generation repeats itself in the next, so that the same issues are played out from generation to generation (Bowen, 2012).

The information collected for the genogram may include genetic, medical, social, behavioral, and cultural aspects of the family.

Because the process of creating a genogram involves extensive interviewing, it is a way for the nurse practitioner to establish a therapeutic relationship with the family. Families tend to become engaged in the process of developing the genogram and often gain insight into their potential health issues and missing support systems (Schilsin, 1993). Despite the clear advantages the genogram offers, many primary care clinicians often neglect to use it because it can take up extra time in an already overburdened office schedule (Schilsin, 1993). The genogram does not have to be completed in one sitting but can be started on the initial visit and completed on subsequent visits. While some primary care clinicians may not feel skilled at delving into psychosocial issues and sensitive family matters, nurse practitioners by virtue of their education and experience are poised to assist families to identify strengths as individuals and in a family unit to promote their mutual support and growth. Some key indications for the nurse practitioner to develop a family genogram are represented in **Box 3-1**.

Process of Developing the Genogram

The manner in which a genogram is taken is perhaps more important than what is elicited and the technique of recording. The nurse practitioner needs to be sincere, open-minded, interested, and nonjudgmental, and even occasionally prepared to share anecdotes of his or her own family to put the patient at ease. It is a mutual scientific inquiry with members of a family and they often get enthusiastic about drawing their "family tree" and want it be accurate, complete, and relevant. You may

---

Box 3-1 Key Indicators to Develop a Family Genogram

Depression
Somatic problems (e.g., headache, abdominal pain, chest pain)
Frequent office visits
Poor school or work attendance
Behavioral problems
Problems between family members
Stepfamilies with problems
Obesity, smoking, alcohol, substance abuse
Nonadherence to treatment regimen

use a flip chart, or in a hurried practice setting a pad of paper or progress note. The diagramming of a family genogram must comply with the use of specific symbols to ensure that the family and nurse practitioner have the same understanding and interpretations of the genogram. Authors may vary on symbols used for different nodal events, but all genograms are similar in terms of gathering information on family membership, structure, interaction patterns, and other important information. The genogram does not have to be completed in one session. In general, nurse practitioners working in a primary care setting will see patients and their families over time, and data can be collected and added as a continuous process.

See **Boxes 3-2**, **3-3**, and **3-4** for the three types of family genogram interview data: factual events, expanded events, and relationships.

Understanding and Interpreting the Genogram

Discussion of the completed genogram can offer alternatives to the family for their current behaviors, and it offers a chance to escape from repetitive family patterns if the family views this as helpful. Furthermore, a genogram will help the family make sense of unexplained fears and anxieties about family patterns and illness.

One of the challenges for nurse practitioners is to take the vast amount of information collected during the interview process and consolidate the data into categories that can be analyzed for repetitive relationship patterns between generations. Categorizing the data groups can assist in the identification of the most pertinent

---

Box 3-2 Family Genogram Interview Data: Factual Events

Family composition: Who is the immediate family? Who has the identified health problem?
Who lives with the immediate family, and how are they related?
Dates of births, miscarriages, abortions, and stillbirths
Dates of any adoptions
Dates and causes of deaths
Major illnesses and dates
Dates of marriages, separations, divorces, remarriages, retirements, and relocations

---

Box 3-3 Family Genogram Interview Data: Expanded Events

Religion, ethnic factors, occupations, social class, education, military service
Additional births, abortions, miscarriages, adoptions, and infertility
Congenital abnormalities, mental disabilities, learning problems
Illnesses similar to presenting illness
Cancer, heart disease, hypertension, asthma, hyperlipidemia, diabetes, depression, alcoholism, substance abuse
Common causes of death in that family
Family secrets
Troubles with the law, incest

> **Box 3-4** Family Genogram Interview Data: Relationships
>
> Who is close to whom? Is there too much closeness? Are there "favorites" or "isolates"?
>   Relationships and alliances between:
> - Marriage partners
> - Siblings
> - Children and parents
> - Children and grandparents
>   Boundaries between family members:
> - Permeable
> - Loose
> - Rigid
>   - Power and patterns of avoidance
>   - Patterns of friendships and relationships with work colleagues
>   - Matters that cannot be talked about in the family

> **Box 3-5** Family Genogram Red-Flag Themes
>
> Repetitive patterns between generations, such as alcoholism, drug addiction, divorce, or mental illness
> Chronological coincidences, such as births, marriages, and deaths
> Similarity of names, possible personality resemblances, or identity in upbringing, such as family favorites, family scapegoat
> Cultural, educational, ethnic, and religious backgrounds—differences and similarities
> Family patterns from husband's and wife's relations—similarities and differences
> Family secrets, such as abortions, adoptions, or secret affairs
> Significance of nicknames
> Too much closeness between generations (absence of boundaries)
> Poor or loose contact between the generations, as in cut off
> Inappropriate alliances
> Fighting and domestic abuse

family problem that needs immediate attention. In a family where emotions can be neither recognized nor displayed, distress may present as somatic symptoms resulting in frequent office visits. **Box 3-5** lists themes in a family genogram that should raise a red flag and help you identify problems and patterns that may affect family functioning and individual family members' well-being.

Family Pedigree

Similar to a genogram, a family pedigree is a graphic representation of a person's medical and biological history and is often referred to as the "family tree." Like the genogram, the pedigree is a family history assessment tool developed in an interview with a patient. It includes three generations and involves the use of standardized symbols, which clearly mark individuals affected with a specific diagnosis to allow for easy identification (Yoon, 2003). Advances in genetics and genomics have brought pedigree analysis from the traditional prerogative of genetic specialists into mainstream primary care practice. When appropriately used, a pedigree generated from a family history can be one of the nurse practitioner's most powerful clinical tools for health risk identification, diagnosis, and intervention, yet it provides little insight into family dynamics or the complex context of the patient and family in the community.

Nurse practitioners need a comprehensive, three-generation pedigree that records a patient's medical, social, and environmental history, thereby communicating an expansive scenario for holistic primary care practice. Such a tool can guide the identification of risk factors to inform the patient and family clinical decisions regarding care management strategies, psychosocial support, and education for reproductive decisions, risk reduction, and the prevention, screening, diagnosis, referral, and long-term management of disease. The family pedigree should indicate the age of individuals; if deceased, the age and cause of death; and any relevant health history, illnesses, and age of onset. If any genetic testing has been performed on family members, the results should be indicated on the pedigree. The ethnic background of each grandparent should be listed, as well as any known consanguinity. A general inquiry about more distant relatives should be made in case there is a possible X-linked disorder or autosomal dominant disorder with reduced penetrance (Geonomics Education Programme, 2020).

Whereas the genogram focuses on family relationships and communication patterns, the pedigree is a collection of family health histories and an assessment of disease risk factors. It is used to develop a differential diagnosis for identified familial traits. Family history plays a critical role in assessing the risk of inherited medical conditions and single gene disorders. Certain types of cancer, such as breast cancer and colon cancer, appear more frequently in some families, as do some adverse birth outcomes. Coronary artery disease, type 2 diabetes, depression, and thrombophilias also have familial tendencies (Yoon, 2003).

The U.S. Surgeon General's Family History Initiative was launched in 2004. The goal of this initiative is to educate both healthcare providers and patients about the value of collecting a family history as a screening tool and to increase its use and effectiveness in clinical care by simplifying the collection process and analysis of the family history (Center for Disease, 2020).

Over the past 20 years, the Human Genome Project has afforded us a better understanding of the effect of genetic variation on health and disease. This has furthered research in identifying genotype–phenotype correlations and enhanced the ability to predict those at risk of developing inherited medical conditions (Geonomics Education Programme, 2020). With increased awareness of the importance of using the family history as a screening tool and of the value of preventive measures and increased surveillance, there is hope for improved outcomes.

Although it may be best to take a systematic approach to enquiring about each branch of a family, sometimes this may not be possible in a busy primary care practice. There are some useful general questions, however, that can help the NP to gain a quick overview of the medical conditions in a family. Answers to these questions may trigger a need for drawing out how the people with the condition are related to each other. This would inform a preliminary assessment of whether there is an increased genetic risk that warrants further investigation, a detailed family pedigree,

Chapter 3 Family-Focused Clinical Practice

or specialist referral. **Box 3-6** provides some key questions to ask individuals about their family history.

Figures 3-3 and **3-4** show the process of drawing a family tree and the symbols used.

Box 3-6 Key Questions for a Family History Warranting a Detailed Pedigree

Do you have any concerns about diseases or conditions that seem to run in either your or your partner's side of the family?
Does anyone have a major medical, physical, or mental problem?
Has anyone ever needed treatment in a hospital?
Has anyone ever had any serious illnesses or operations?
How old was this person at diagnosis?
(Avoid just asking "Is everyone well?" because past medical histories may not be offered!)
Have any adults, children, or babies died?
How old were they, and what was the cause of death?
Have there been any miscarriages or babies who were stillborn?

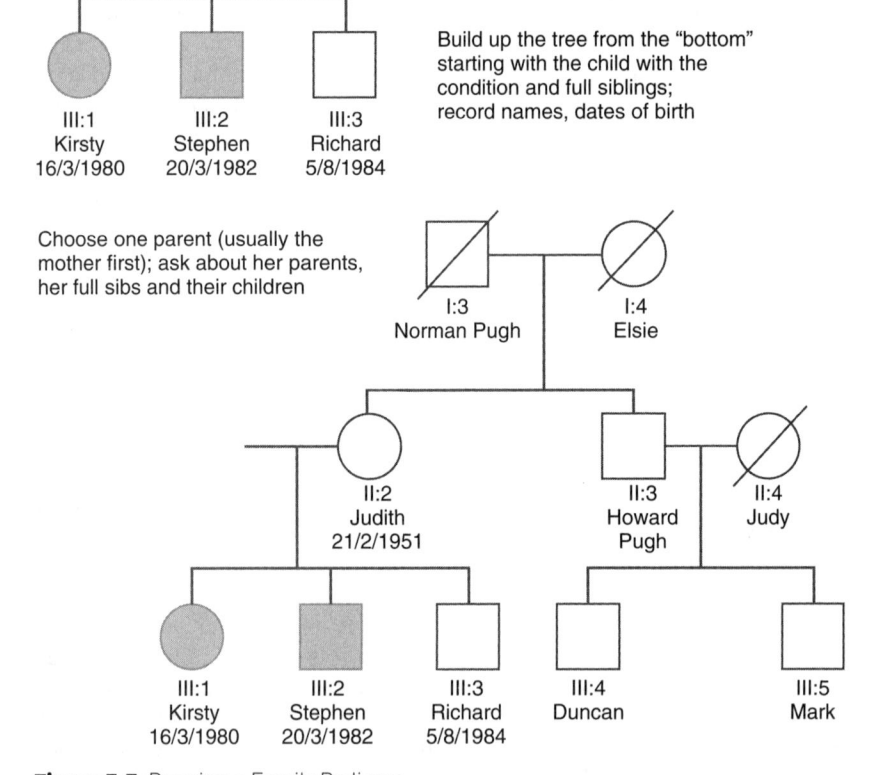

Build up the tree from the "bottom" starting with the child with the condition and full siblings; record names, dates of birth

III:1 Kirsty 16/3/1980
III:2 Stephen 20/3/1982
III:3 Richard 5/8/1984

Choose one parent (usually the mother first); ask about her parents, her full sibs and their children

I:3 Norman Pugh
I:4 Elsie

II:2 Judith 21/2/1951
II:3 Howard Pugh
II:4 Judy

III:1 Kirsty 16/3/1980
III:2 Stephen 20/3/1982
III:3 Richard 5/8/1984
III:4 Duncan
III:5 Mark

Figure 3-3 Drawing a Family Pedigree

Genetic family history pedigree images reproduced with permission from the NHS National Genetics Education and Development Centre.

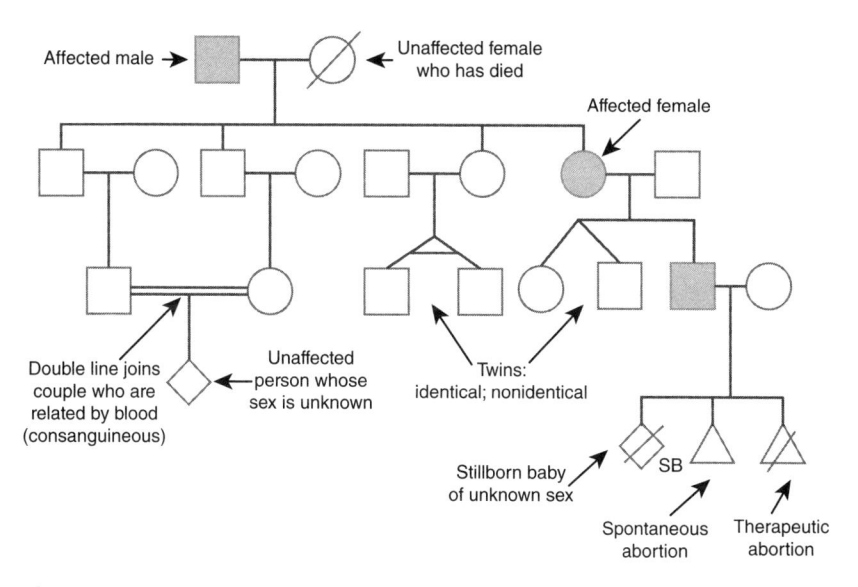

Figure 3-4 Other Pedigree Symbols
Genetic family history pedigree images reproduced with permission from the NHS National Genetics Education and Development Centre.

More samples of pedigree diagrams for healthcare professionals can be found by visiting http://www.geneticseducation.nhs.uk. A PowerPoint presentation showing the process of creating a pedigree as well as exercises to practice making family histories and pedigrees can also be found on this website.

Family Risk Assessment Tools

The screening tool selected should be tailored to the practice setting and patient population, taking into consideration patient education level and cultural background. Whether a pedigree diagram or questionnaire is used, it is important to review and update the family history periodically for new diagnoses within the family as appropriate. A family history screening tool will allow the healthcare provider to stratify levels of risk (Centers for Disease Control and Prevention, 2020). Moreover, the use of a family history screening tool (pedigree or questionnaire) has been shown to increase by 20% the likelihood of detecting a patient at high risk of developing an inherited medical condition compared with medical record review alone (Yoon, 2003). **Box 3-7** lists red flags for genetic conditions that may warrant referral to a genetic specialist (National Coalition for Health Professional Education in Genetics, 2012).

Ecomap

Similar to the genogram, the ecomap is a pictorial representation of a family's contact with larger systems. These systems can include school, work environment, place of worship, healthcare agencies, social support agencies, courts, recreation, housing, and friends. The ecomap is used to clarify reciprocal relationships between family members and the broader community. It provides a way of assessing resources and strengths of family relationships with significant others, organizations, and institutions (Bomar, 2004; Reed, 1994). The ecomap allows the nurse practitioner to view

> **Box 3-7** Red Flags for Genetic Conditions
>
> Family history of a known or suspected genetic condition
> Ethnic predisposition to certain genetic disorders
> Close biological relationship between parents (consanguinity = blood relationship of parents)
> Multiple affected family members with the same or related disorders
> Earlier than expected age of onset of disease
> Diagnosis in less-often-affected sex
> Multifocal or bilateral occurrence of disease (often cancer) in paired organs
> Disease in the absence of risk factors or after application of preventive measures
> One or more major malformations
> Developmental delays or mental retardation
> Abnormalities in growth (growth restriction, asymmetric growth, or excessive growth)
> Recurrent pregnancy losses (> 2)
>
> Reproduced from The National Coalition for Health Professional Education in Genetics (NCHPEG). Available online at http://www.NCHPEG.org.

both the nurturing aspects of a family's world and the family's stress-producing connections. Often the ecomap shows deprivation of resources, which can assist the nurse practitioner in developing an adequate plan of care for the family (Shajani & Sneel, 2019).

Typically a simplified version of the genogram is developed first and can be placed in the center of the ecomap circle. Outer circles represent significant people, agencies, or institutions in the family's context. Lines are drawn between the circles and the family members to depict the nature and quality of the relationships and to show what kinds of resources are moving in and out of the family. Straight lines denote strong or close relationships. Wider or thicker lines show stronger relationships. Straight lines with slashes show stressful or strained relationships. Broken or dotted lines show tenuous, weak, or distant relationships. Arrows are drawn to indicate the flow of energy and resources between people and the environment. The ecomap provides the nurse practitioner with a more integrated perception of the family situation and can be helpful in assisting the family to define goals and increase its use of community resources (Kaakinen et al., 2018).

Family Problem List

Following careful assessment of the individual in the context of the family unit, the nurse practitioner must develop a comprehensive prioritized problem list. The problem oriented medical record (POMR) and the "problem list" date back to the 1960s. They were developed by Dr. Lawrence Weed as a simple way to document and manage important health problems facing a patient (Holmes, 2011). Today, the problem list still exists as an acceptable model of documentation in both paper and electronic medical records. The contents of the problem list may vary from one healthcare organization to the next and may vary depending on the healthcare

provider's preference. In general, nurse practitioners and other primary care providers agree that the problem list should contain the following general information:
- A list of chronic diseases or illnesses
- An ongoing or active problem you are working on with the patient
- A summarization of the most important things about a patient

There is some debate about what diagnosed illnesses are worthy of the problem list. Currently, the decision of which problems are included or excluded remains largely up to the judgment of the practitioner. Some practitioners will exclude certain information because it may "clutter up" the record with extraneous information (e.g., lab results or "sensitive issues" such as sexually transmitted infections or mental health issues). Primary care nurse practitioners provide integrated, accessible healthcare services and are accountable for addressing a large majority of personal healthcare needs, developing a sustained partnership with patients, and practicing in the context of family and community (DeNisco, 2021). In caring for the individual patient in the context of the family unit, it is important for the nurse practitioner to maintain clear documentation of the family's healthcare needs. At a minimum, the problem list should include the following elements: acute self-limiting problems, routine health maintenance issues, allergies, family planning, social problems, and chronic health problems.

Acute self-limiting problems are problems that may be acute or short term. For example, streptococcal pharyngitis is an example of an acute self-limiting problem. Nocturnal leg cramps, upper respiratory infection, and contact dermatitis are other problems that fall into this category. Routine health maintenance refers to health promotion and screening activities that are needed by the patient per age and risk factor analysis. This includes but is not limited to mammograms, annual physical examinations, pap smears, immunizations, and well-child care. Allergies would include allergies to medications, food, dust, and mold. Family planning would address contraceptive needs of the family, including infertility issues. Social problems take into account the toxic history of the patient or family members (e.g., tobacco use, substance abuse, alcohol use). Chronic health problems include long-standing diagnoses the healthcare provider is following (e.g., hypertension, type 2 diabetes, hyperlipidemia, asthma, migraine headaches).

The other category is a net to catch all other problems that may be important to remember as you care for the patient. This may include family problems (death of a family member, mental health issues, school truancy), financial problems (unemployment, entitlements such as food stamps), sexual preferences, and so on.

There are many issues complicating the maintenance of a patient problem list. If the list is messy, unorganized, or partially completed because the healthcare provider did not have time to add problems, the list will not be used effectively. The usefulness of problem lists in the care of the individual patient and family is based on the ability of the nurse practitioner to articulate patient problems (when identified) and follow consistent guidelines that ensure the lists are current and useful.

The family problem list includes these categories:
- Acute self-limiting problems
- Routine health maintenance
- Allergies
- Family planning
- Social
- Chronic problems and other

Family Problem List/Case Study Exercises

Read the following cases and develop a comprehensive problem list for each case. If you do not have enough information to develop a list for each problem category as described in this chapter, propose what questions you would need to ask the patient and family to gather the information you need.

⚲ CASE STUDY ONE

Ms. Belcher is a 48-year-old married white female and has two children and three grandchildren. Ms. Belcher has a long history of schizoaffective disorder and also has chronic medical problems, including type 2 diabetes mellitus, hypertension, and coronary artery disease. She is on a laundry list of medications and visits her primary care provider and psychiatrist regularly. She also attends a day psychiatric program three times a week for socialization and vocational skills. Ms. Belcher has resided at the same low-income housing project for many years. Her husband, who is African-American, also suffers from schizoaffective disorder and has a multitude of chronic health problems and has been hospitalized recently for renal insufficiency. Ms. Belcher's daughters, ages 19 and 15, reside at home and are very important in Ms. Belcher's life. The youngest daughter was hospitalized last year for a new diagnosis of bipolar disorder, and Ms. Belcher was very concerned about this. She was worried that the Department of Children and Families would take her daughter out of the home.

Despite these adversities, Ms. Belcher has an optimistic view regarding her family life and does her best to care for her husband and daughters. She does have moments when she becomes very somatic and visits her healthcare provider frequently for reassurance. Ms. Belcher reaches out to her psychiatric visiting nurse and her primary care provider for support when the going gets tough.

⚲ CASE STUDY TWO

Ms. Dora Roman is a 50-year-old Hispanic female who resides in her car on the streets of Bridgeport. She relocated to Connecticut 1 year ago after she left an abusive relationship with her husband while residing in Florida. Ms. Roman is educated as an LPN and has worked in long-term care settings in the past. She has a history of sarcoidosis and other chronic medical problems. She seeks medical care at the local community health center since relocating to Connecticut and had her medical records sent to Connecticut so she can have continuity of care. Ms. Roman has a sister in Connecticut and uses her house occasionally on the most bitterly cold nights, but mostly sleeps in her car and uses the public beach bath house for hygiene purposes. Since relocating to Connecticut, she has worked seasonally at a Halloween store in the local mall.

Ms. Roman has filled out applications for subsidized housing and Medicaid entitlements for health care, but for unknown reasons she has not been successful in obtaining them. Ms. Roman does not speak to her daughter who lives in Connecticut and feels that she is alone in the world. She has many somatic complaints and seeks narcotics to help her back pain and to "get to sleep in my car."

⚲ CASE STUDY THREE

Ms. Tamika Jenkins is a 30-year-old African-American single mother of three children and resides in an economically disadvantaged housing project in the inner city. She frequently visits the health center with a multitude of complaints typically focused around injury. In the past 6 months, Ms. Jenkins has been seen for a miscarriage, a fractured wrist related to a fall while rollerblading, and a head injury related to an altercation with another woman for unknown reasons. Ms. Jenkins states that her husband is incarcerated and she has no family support. Her mother died of HIV when she was a teenager, and she doesn't speak to her father. When she presents to the health center, she is anxious and despondent and seeks pain medication. She seems to have little insight into her problems. She is currently being investigated by the Department of Children and Families for child neglect.

Seminar Discussion Questions

1. Describe the characteristics that constitute a healthy family.
2. Develop a three-generation family genogram on a partner and build a comprehensive problem list for one family constellation.
3. Draw your family ecomap, and outline the various family relationships to institutions, leisure activities, and agencies. Define which relationships are stress producing and which foster support. Discuss how the individuals in the family are linked to significant people and how they engage in social support.
4. Consider the family capacity model when reading the case of Dora Roman, and outline family strengths, functions, needs, goals, and supports needed to maximize the family potential.

References

Adams, K. B., Sanders, S., & Auth, E. A. (2004). Loneliness and depression in independent living retirement communities: Risk and resilience factors. *Aging and Mental Health*, 8(6), 475–485.

Administration on Aging. (2011). *Aging statistics*. Retrieved from http://www.aoa.gov/AoARoot/Aging_Statistics/index.aspx

Becker, G., & Newsome, E. (2005). Resilience in the face of serious illness among chronically ill African Americans in later life. *Journal of Gerontology*, 60(4), S214–S223.

Bomar, P. (2004). *Promoting health in families: Applying family research and theory to practice*. 3rd ed. Philadelphia, PA: Saunders.

Bowen, M. (2012, October 12). *Bowen theory*. The Bowen Center. Retrieved from http://www.thebowencenter.org/pages/theory.html

Bray, J. H., & Campbell, T. L. (2007). The family's influence on health. In R. Rakel, *Textbook of family medicine* (7th ed.) (pp. 25–34). Philadelphia, PA: Elsevier.

Burkholder, G., & Burbank, P. (2012). Caring for lesbian, gay, bisexual and transsexual parents and their children. *International Journal of Child Birth Education*, 27(4), 12–18.

Centers for Disease Control and Prevention. (2020). *Family health history*. Retrieved from https://www.cdc.gov/genomics/famhistory/knowing_not_enough.htm?CDC_AA_refVal=https%3A%2F%2Fwww.cdc.gov%2Ffeatures%2Ffamilyhealthhistory%2Findex.html

Centers for Disease Control and Prevention. (2020). *Family health history and chronic disease*. Retrieved from https://www.cdc.gov/genomics/famhistory/famhist_chronic_disease.

Chernoff, R., Coombs-Orme, T., Risley-Curtiss, C., & Heisler, A. (1994). Assessing the health status of children entering foster care. *Pediatrics, 93*, 594–601.

Child Welfare Information Gateway. (2020). *Foster care statistics 2018.* Washington, DC: U.S. Department of Health and Human Services, Administration for Children and Families, Children's Bureau. Retrieved from https://www.childwelfare.gov/pubPDFs/foster.pdf

Conway, F. J. (2011). Emotional strain in caregiving among African American grandmothers raising their grandchildren. *Journal of Women and Aging, 23*(2), 113–128.

Demo, D. F. (2010). *Beyond the average divorce.* Thousand Oaks, CA: Sage.

Denham, S. F. (2003). *Family health: A framework for nursing.* Philadelphia, PA: F. A. Davis.

DeNisco, S. (2011). Exploring the relationship between resilience and diabetes outcomes in African Americans. *American Journal of Nurse Practitioners, 23*(11), 602–610. doi: 10.1111/j.1745-7599.2011.00648.x

DeNisco, S. (2021). *Advanced practice nursing: Essential knowledge for the profession. 4th ed.* Burlington, MA: Jones & Bartlett Learning.

Drummond, J., Kysela, G. M., McDonald, L., & Query, B. (2002). The family adaptation model: Examination of dimensions and relations. *Canadian Journal of Nursing Research, 34*(1), 29–46.

Druss, R. G., & Douglas, C. J. (1988). Adaptive responses to illness and disability. *General Hospital Psychiatry, 10*, 163–168.

Dunst, C. J., & Trivette, C. M. (2009). Capacity building family systems intervention practices. *Journal of Family Social Work, 12*, 119–143.

Dyer, J. G., & McGuinness, T. M. (1996). Resilience: Analysis of the concept. *Archives of Psychiatry Nursing, 10*(5), 276–282.

Felten, B. S., & Hall, J. M. (2001). Conceptualizing resilience in women older than 85: Overcoming adversity from illness or loss. *Journal of Gerontological Nursing, 27*(11), 46–53.

Flaherty, E. G., & Weiss, H. (1990). Medical evaluation of abused and neglected children. *American Journal of Diseases of Children, 144*, 330–334.

Friedman, M. Bowden, V. R. & Jones, E. (2003). *Family nursing.* 5th ed. London, UK: Pearson.

Genomics Education Programme. (2019). *Genetics education: Delivering genomics education, training and experience for the healthcare workforce.* Retrieved from https://www.genomicseducation.hee.nhs.uk/

Genomics Education Programme. (2019). *Genomics in primary care.* Retrieved from https://www.genomicseducation.hee.nhs.uk/genomics-in-healthcare/genomics-in-primary-care/#toggle-id-2

Germain, C., & Bloom, M. (1999). *Human behavior in the social environment: An ecological view.* New York, NY: Columbia University Press.

Gilligan, R. (2004). Promoting resilience in child and family social work: Issues for social work and policy. *Social Work Education, 23*, 93–104.

Haase, J. E. (2004). The adolescent resilience model as a guide to interventions. *Journal of Pediatric Oncology Nursing, 21*(5), 289–299.

Haase, J. E., Heiney, S. P., Ruccione, K. S., & Stutzer, C. (1999). Research triangulation to derive meaning based quality of life theory: Adolescent resilience model and instrument development. *International Journal of Cancer Supplement, 12*, 125–131.

Hardy, S. E., Concato, J., & Gill, T. M. (2004). Resilience of community dwelling older persons. *Journal of the American Geriatrics Society, 52*(2), 257–262.

Heinzer, M. M. (1995). Loss of a parent in childhood: Attachment and coping in a model of adolescent resilience. *Holistic Nursing Practice, 9*(3), 27–37.

Hockenberry-Eaton, M., Kemp, V., & Dilorio, C. (1994). Cancer stressors and positive factors: Predictors of stress experienced during treatment for childhood cancer. *Research in Nursing and Health, 17,* 351–361.

Holmes, C. (2011). The problem list beyond meaningful use: The problem with problem list. *Journal of AHIMA* (February), 30–33.

Jacelon, C. S. (1997). The trait and process of resilience. *Journal of Advanced Nursing, 25*, 123–129.

Kaakinen, J. R., Padgett Coehlo, D., Steele, R., & Robinson, M. (2018). *Family health nursing: Theory, practice and research.* 6th ed. Philadelphia, PA: Davis.

References

Lenora, M. (2009). Supporting resilience in foster families: A model for program design that supports recruitment, retention, and satisfaction of foster families who care for infants with prenatal substance exposure. *Child Welfare, 89*(1), 7–29.

Loveland-Cherry, C. (2004). Family health promotion and health protection. In P. Bomar (Ed.), *Promoting health in families* (pp. 61–89). Philadelphia, PA: Saunders.

McCubbin, M. A., & McCubbin, H. I. (1993). Family stress theory and the development of nursing knowledge about family adaptation. In S. Feetham, S. Meister, J. Bell, & C. Gillis (Eds.), *The nursing of families* (pp. 46–58). Newbury Park, CA: Sage.

McGoldrick, M., & Carter, B. (1999). *The expanded family life cycle: Individual, family, and social perspectives.* Boston, MA: Allyn & Bacon.

McGoldrick, M., & Carter, B. (2003). The family life cycle. In F. Walsh (Ed.), *Normal family processes.* New York, NY: Guilford Press.

McGoldrick, M. S. (2008). *Genograms: Assessment and intervention.* New York, NY: W. W. Norton & Company.

Mullin, W. A. (2008). Resilience of families living in poverty. *Journal of Family Social Work, 11*(4).

Odom-Forren J. (2020). Nursing resilience in the world of Covid-19. *Journal of Perianesthesia Nursing, 35*(6), 555–556. doi: 10.1016/j.jopan.2020.10.005

Peterson, S. J., & Bredow, T. S. (2004). *Middle range theories.* Philadelphia, PA: Lippincott Williams Wilkins.

Polk, L. V. (1997). Toward a middle range theory of resilience. *Advanced Nursing Science, 19*(3), 1–13.

Rabkin, J. G., Remien, R., Katoff, L., & Williams, J. B. (1993). Resilience in adversity among long-term survivors of AIDS. *Hospital and Community Psychiatry, 44*(2), 162–167.

Rakel, R. (2007). *Textbook of family medicine.* 7th ed. Philadelphia, PA: Elsevier.

Rakel, R., & Rakel, D. (2015). *Textbook of family medicine.* 9th ed. Philadelphia, PA: Elsevier.

Reed, M. (1994). Digging up family plots: Analysis of axes of variation in genograms. *Teaching Sociology, 22,* 255–259.

Rew, L., Taylor-Seehafer, M., Thomas, N. Y., & Yockey, R. D. (2001). Correlates of resilience in homeless adolescents. *Journal of Nursing Scholarship, 33*(1), 33–40.

Schilsin, E. B. (1993). Use of genograms in family medicine: A family physician/family therapist collaboration. *Family Systems Medicine, 11,* 201–208.

Shajani, Z., & Sneel, D. (2019). Wright and Leahey's *Nurses and families: A guide to family assessment and intervention.* 7th ed. Philadelphia, PA: F. A. Davis.

Simms, M. D. (2000). Health care needs of children in the foster care system. *Pediatrics, 106*(909), 909–918.

Singer, B. H., & Ryff, C. (2001). *New horizons in health: An integrative approach.* Washington, DC: National Academy Press.

Svavarsdottir, E. K., & Rayens, M. K. (2005). Hardiness in families of young children with asthma. *Journal of Advanced Nursing, 50*(4), 381–390.

Tusaie, K., & Dyer, J. (2004). Resilience: A historical review of the construct. *Holistic Nursing Practice, 1,* 3–9.

U.S. Census Bureau. (2019). *Grandparents, American community survey, Table ID S1102.* Retrieved from https://data.census.gov/cedsci/table?q=S1002&tid=ACSST1Y2019.S1002

U.S. Census Bureau. (2019). *U.S. Census Bureau releases CPS estimates of same-sex households.* Retrieved from https://www.census.gov/newsroom/press-releases/2019/same-sex-households.html

U.S. Census Bureau. (2020). *U.S. marriage and divorce rates by state: 2009 & 2019.* Retrieved from https://www.census.gov/library/visualizations/interactive/marriage-divorce-rates-by-state-2009-2019.html

Vinson, J. A. (2002). Children with asthma: Initial development of the child resilience model. *Pediatric Nurse, 28*(2), 149–158.

Wagnild, G., & Young, H. M. (1990). Resilience among older women. *Image: Journal of Nursing Scholarship, 22*(4), 252–255.

Wagnild, G. M., & Young, H. M. (1993). Development and psychometric evaluation of the resilience scale. *Journal of Nursing Measurement, 1*(2), 165–178.

Walsh, F. (2016). *Strengthening family resilience.* 3rd ed. New York, NY: Guilford.

White, J. M., Klein, D. M., & Martin, T. F. (2015). *Family theories.* 4th ed. Los Angeles, CA: Sage.

Woodgate, R., & McClement, S. (1997). Sense of self in children with cancer and in childhood cancer survivors: A critical review. *Journal of Pediatric Oncology Nursing, 14*(3), 137–155.

Wright, L. M., & Leahey, M. (2013). *Nurses and families: A guide to family assessment and intervention.* 6th ed. Philadelphia, PA: F. A. Davis.

Yi, J. P., Smith, R. E., & Vitaliano, P. P. (2005). Stress-resilience, illness, and coping: A person-focused investigation of young women athletes. *Journal of Behavioral Medicine, 28*(3), 257–265.

Yoon, P. S. (2003). Research priorities for evaluating family history in the prevention of common chronic diseases. *American Journal of Preventative Medicine, 24*(2), 128–135.

Additional Resources

Belcher, J. P. (2011). Family capital: Implications for interventions with families. *Journal of Family Social Work, 14,* 68–85.

McKenry, P. (2000). *Families and change: Coping with stressful events and transitions.* 2nd ed. Thousand Oaks, CA: Sage.

Walsh, F. (2002). A family resilience framework: Innovative practice approaches. *Family Relations, 5*(2), 130–137.

CHAPTER 4

Vulnerable Populations

Susan M. DeNisco

Section One: Overview of Vulnerabilities and Disparities

Healthcare disparities generally refers to differences in the quality of health care across individuals or groups in regard to access, treatment options, and preventative services. Vulnerability as a concept originated from a variety of disciplines, including economics, sociology, anthropology, and environmental science. Segments of the global population experience social inequalities and are at risk for poor health outcomes. Nurse practitioners are keenly aware that any individual can become vulnerable at any point in their life. However, it is well documented in the literature that health outcomes and vulnerability fall along a social gradient and that poorer people experience poorer health (Grabovschi, Loignon, & Fortin, 2013; Marmot, 2005). This global phenomenon is seen in low-, middle-, and high-income countries. The World Health Organization (WHO) has been bringing to the forefront a sense of urgency for healthcare leaders to address health inequities across the globe. Health inequities or disparities refers to systematic gaps in health outcomes between different groups of people that are judged to be avoidable and therefore are considered unfair and unjust. It is the inherent human right to primary, secondary, and tertiary medical care, food, housing, and other resources. Primary care nurse practitioners with a strong educational base have a longstanding commitment to cultural competence and social justice. As integral members of the healthcare delivery team, NPs are well positioned for leadership roles in addressing the gaps in health prevention and treatment, and to highlight certain groups as vulnerable populations and attempt to build an understanding of the needs within the various groups.

Social Determinants of Health

The social determinants of health (SDH) are the conditions in which people are born, grow, work, live, and age (Healthy People, 2030). There are four well-established factors that influence individual and aggregate health outcomes, including but not limited to (1) lifestyle and behaviors, (2) genetic factors, (3) social and environmental forces, and (4) medical care. For a brief representation, see **Table 4-1**. Primary care clinicians must be astute at assessing all of these factors, whether seeing a patient at point of care or assessing community needs and developing responsive programs for the particular population in which they serve.

Despite significant medical advances in this country, poor and nonwhite ethnic minorities are ranked lower in health status on numerous measures. According to the Centers for Disease Control and Prevention (CDC), morbidity and mortality rates remain higher for African-Americans who continue to die disproportionally more than whites from chronic disease (CDC, 2017). Reasons for the lower health status ranking may include genetic and gender differences, stereotyping, perceived discrimination, and mistrust of healthcare providers. Language barriers, ineffective use of translators, and lack of cultural humility can influence the nurse practitioner's ability to properly diagnosis and treat patients.

Literacy and Advocacy

Health literacy is a concept grounded in the literature on health promotion and education. Health literacy can be defined as the degree to which individuals have the cognitive and social capacity to access, process, and utilize basic health information and services to maintain good health, make appropriate health decisions, and meet their goals. According to the National Assessment of Adult Literacy, only 12% of adults have proficient health literacy and 14% have below basic health literacy, with 42% reporting health is poor (Kutner, Greenberg, Jin, & Paulsen, 2006). Low literacy has been linked with being underinsured and having poor health outcomes, higher rates of hospitalization, and less frequent use of preventive services. Populations most likely to experience low health literacy are older adults, racial and ethnic minority groups, individuals with low educational levels, those living below the poverty level, and non-native speakers of English (U.S. Department of Health and Human Services [USDHHS], 2020). Individuals with low literacy will find it difficult to navigate the healthcare system, provide accurate health histories, fill out complex forms, and engage in self-care and chronic disease management. According to research studies, persons with limited health literacy skills are less likely to receive preventive measures such as mammograms, Pap smears, colonoscopies, and vaccines

Table 4-1 Social Determinants of Health

Lifestyle	Social/Environmental	Genetic	Medical Care
■ Diet ■ Food ■ Exercise ■ Tobacco use ■ Illicit drug use ■ Unsafe sex ■ Irresponsible motor vehicle use	■ Education ■ Employment ■ Socioeconomic status ■ Food insecurity ■ Social cohesion ■ Quality of housing ■ Crime and violence ■ Discrimination ■ Environmental conditions	■ Predisposed to certain diseases ■ Inherited diseases	■ Access to preventative measures ■ Access to curative measures ■ Health literacy ■ New technology ■ Clinical trials

when compared to those with adequate health literacy skills. Studies have shown that patients with limited health literacy skills enter the healthcare system when they are sicker, which impacts healthcare utilization and cost (USDHHS, 2020).

Advocacy

With advanced education and extensive experience caring for patients and their families, nurse practitioners are equipped to serve as advocates by providing a voice for patients, communities, and the healthcare profession at large. An advocate is defined as an individual or group that pleads, defends, or supports a cause or interest of another. Much of the literature on advocacy comes from nonprofit and special-interest groups that prepare potential advocates to influence public policy. Advocates are often thought of as individuals who lead change through influence and help decision makers work through solutions to problems. At the macrosystem level, advocacy often requires working through formal decision-making bodies to achieve desired goals and outcomes. This process could include working through the "chain of command" within a healthcare organization, state legislature, or other groups at the healthcare system's policy level (Basch, 2014). Ensuring that every individual has access to the health care they need is of paramount importance. Advocacy for social justice and human rights protection for populations who are powerless and dependent on others to address their complex vulnerabilities is a challenge at best. Patients and families often find themselves overwhelmed and lacking the essential information they need to make informed choices. Such vulnerability is cited as a key reason for advocacy at the point of care. At the microsystem level, nurse practitioners must become motivated to act on another's behalf, gain insight into one's self and others, develop cultural skills, and actively engage with diverse groups to promote effectiveness of care (Pacquiao, 2008).

Poverty, Vulnerability, and Resilience

The single, most important determinant of social injustices is poverty and the social and environmental factors that coexist with it. Poverty is a widely recognized global issue and a major determinant of poor health. This association has been extensively studied and verified. It is a growing problem in the United States and in other developed nations, as well as a continuing and devastating problem in the least developed countries (Conway, 2016). The cycle of poverty is more than a socioeconomic issue. It impacts health, well-being, and quality of life for generations to come. Factors that coexist with poverty include poor housing; inadequate nutrition; lack of clean water; increased exposure to violence; fragmented health care; and a higher prevalence of physical illness, mental health issues, and disabilities (Basch, 2014). Despite these well-established linkages, little work has been done to determine what family nurse practitioners can do to address poverty status at point of care and be stewards of sustainable change. For the purposes of this chapter, we will consider poverty in the United States, given the steady influx of immigrants and the projected tipping point at 2040, where minorities will become the numerical majority.

Definition of Poverty

The U.S. Census Bureau uses a set of monetary income thresholds that vary by family size and composition to determine who is in poverty. If a family's total income is less than the family's threshold, then that family and every individual in it is considered as living in poverty. As defined by the federal government, those who make less than the official poverty threshold earn less than $24,000 annually for a family of four. In 2019, 34 million people lived in poverty in the United States at a rate of 10.5% (U.S. Census, 2020). Poverty impacts certain groups disproportionately; single-parent families, women, children, seniors, and the disabled experience greater rates of poverty.

Ethnic Groups and Poverty

Certain ethnic and population groups also face greater challenges than the general population in terms of economic advantage. According to 2019 U.S. census data, the highest poverty prevalence by race is among African-Americans (18.8%), with Hispanics (of any race) having the second-highest poverty rate (15.7%). Whites had a poverty rate of 9%, and Asians 7.3% (U.S. Census Bureau, 2020).

Women and Children Living in Poverty

Poverty does not strike all demographics equally. For example, in 2019, 17.1% of men lived in poverty compared to 21.35% of women (Statsita Research, 2021). Along the same lines, the poverty rate for married couples in 2014 was only 5.4%, but the poverty rate for single-parent families with no wife present was up to 14.9%, and for single-parent families with no husband present 28.2% (Proctor et al., 2015).

According to the National Center for Children in Poverty (NCCP) approximately 15 million children in the United States, or 21% of all children, live in families with incomes below the federal poverty threshold, a measurement that has been shown to underestimate the needs of families (NCCP, 2016). On average, families need an income of about twice that level to cover basic expenses. Using this standard, 43% of children live in low-income families. Children living in poverty are more likely to experience hunger, which has secondary effects of lower reading and math scores, more physical and mental health problems, more emotional and behavioral problems, and a greater chance of obesity (Koball & Yang, 2018).

Elderly and Poverty

While poverty was once far more prevalent among the elderly than among other age groups, today's elderly have a poverty rate similar to that of working-age adults and much lower than that of children. For people aged 65 and older, the 2019 poverty rate declined to 8.9% from 9.7% in 2018, while the number in poverty declined to 4.2 million, down from 4.6 million (U.S. Census Bureau, 2020). Social Security income is often mentioned as a likely contributor to the decline in elderly poverty; however, increases in life expectancy of the elderly over time mean that financial resources have to last longer. At the same time, healthcare and housing costs are on the rise and employer benefit pension plans have decreased. This means seniors face significant insecurity about whether or not their resources are sufficient to cover the duration of their lives after retirement (Borrowman, 2012). In addition, it is well-known that poverty rates among Hispanics and African-Americans age 65 and older are below the threshold when compared to white adults in this age group (Cubanski, Casillas, & Damico, 2015).

Vulnerability and Resilience

Resilience may be an approach to understanding the vulnerability of families and the community in which the nurse practitioner serves. Resilient communities promote or encourage diversity, flexibility, inclusion, and participation among its members. At a systems level, recognition of social values, accepting uncertainty and change, and fostering an educational environment are approaches that facilitate the building of social capacity (deChesney & Anderson, 2020). Understanding the social capacity of a community will help the nurse practitioner identify important differences within communities in terms of access to resources and entitlements for the poor. Individuals with few financial assets may be less resilient, meaning less adaptive to withstanding adversities in terms of poor housing and lack of adequate food, clothing, education, and medical care. Families with low incomes are generally viewed as households with substantial problems putting themselves at risk for homelessness, exposure to violence, school failure, and social deprivation. Helping families assess their strengths in terms of economic resources, problem-solving capabilities, family cohesion, communication, and social support will make them less risk adverse (Orthner, 2004). As individuals and families living in poverty build their resilience and adaptive capacities, positive consequences may be realized in terms of maintaining school attendance, avoidance of violence and crimes, engagement in developmentally appropriate activities, and maintaining stable housing.

Section Two: Overview of Select Special Populations, Direct Care, and Access

Adverse Childhood Events

A large epidemiological research study founded by collaborative researchers from the Centers for Disease Control (CDC) and Kaiser Permanente examined the relationship between adverse childhood experiences (ACEs) and adult health issues in over 17,000 patient members (CDC, 2020). Childhood experiences that have been examined include emotional abuse, physical abuse, sexual abuse, violence against the respondent's mother, living with substance abusing household members, living with mentally ill or suicidal household members, and living with household members who have been imprisoned (CDC, 2020). Results have demonstrated that exposure to one ACE is likely to increase exposure to other ACEs, as well as positively correlate to a large variety of adult illnesses. Adult disease associated with ACEs include cancer, autoimmune conditions, heart disease, chronic obstructive pulmonary disease, alcoholism, depression, and high-risk behaviors (CDC, 2020). Researchers suggest that high-risk behaviors may well be coping strategies used to manage stress associated with surviving ACEs. In the mental health chapter of this book, there is a discussion on the effect of ACEs on the neurocognitive development of children. The ACEs Pyramid, in **Figure 4-1**, can be used as a tool for NPs to use in understanding risk factors that may lead to increased morbidity and mortality later in life.

Nurse practitioners have a unique approach to patients and families and stress both care and cure. Nurse practitioners are in an ideal position to increase the practice of assessing and screening for patients who are survivors of ACEs, and encouraging those who are appropriate for therapy to mental health services. **Box 4-1** provides a sample questionnaire that covers topics from the original ACEs; however,

Chapter 4 Vulnerable Populations

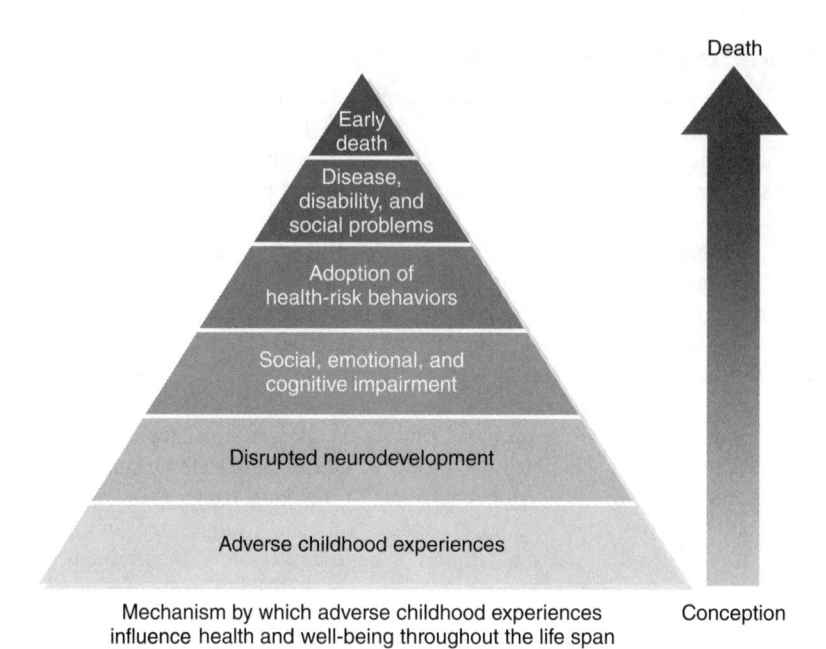

Figure 4-1 ACEs Pyramid

Pyramid levels from bottom to top: Adverse childhood experiences; Disrupted neurodevelopment; Social, emotional, and cognitive impairment; Adoption of health-risk behaviors; Disease, disability, and social problems; Early death.

Mechanism by which adverse childhood experiences influence health and well-being throughout the life span. Conception → Death.

CDC. (2016). About the CDC-Kaiser ACE study. Retrieved from https://www.cdc.gov/violenceprevention/acestudy/about.html.

Box 4-1 BRFSS Adverse Childhood Experience (ACE) Module Prologue (CDC, 2020)

I'd like to ask you some questions about events that happened during your childhood. This information will allow us to better understand problems that may occur early in life, and may help others in the future. This is a sensitive topic and some people may feel uncomfortable with these questions. At the end of this section, I will give you a phone number for an organization that can provide information and referral for these issues. Please keep in mind that you can ask me to skip any question you do not want to answer. All questions refer to the time period before you were 18 years of age. Now, looking back before you were 18 years of age:

1. Did you live with anyone who was depressed, mentally ill, or suicidal?
2. Did you live with anyone who was a problem drinker or alcoholic?
3. Did you live with anyone who used illegal street drugs or who abused prescription medications?
4. Did you live with anyone who served time or was sentenced to serve time in a prison, jail, or other correctional facility?
5. Were your parents separated or divorced?
6. How often did your parents or adults in your home ever slap, hit, kick, punch, or beat each other up?
7. Before age 18, how often did a parent or adult in your home ever hit, beat, kick, or physically hurt you in any way? (Do not include spanking.)
8. How often did a parent or adult in your home ever swear at you, insult you, or put you down?

(continues)

9. How often did anyone at least 5 years older than you, or an adult, ever touch you sexually?
10. How often did anyone at least 5 years older than you, or an adult, try to make you touch them sexually?
11. How often did anyone at least 5 years older than you, or an adult, force you to have sex?

RESPONSE OPTIONS:

Questions 1–4:	1=Yes	2=No	7=DK/NS	9=Refused
Question 5:	1=Yes 9=Refused	2=No	8=Parents not married	7=DK/NS
Questions 6–11:	1=Never 9=Refused	2=Once	3=More than once	7=DK/NS

Free access to review and use survey questionnaires about health and family history are available on the CDC website at https://www.cdc.gov/violenceprevention/acestudy/about.html.

CDC. (n.d.). BRFSS Adverse Childhood Experience (ACE) Module. Retrieved from https://www.cdc.gov/violenceprevention/acestudy/pdf/brfss_adverse_module.pdf

research has uncovered that bullying and witnessing violence in the community are just as, or perhaps more, stressful. Therefore, the NP may prefer to ask the patient about general issues as they relate to the patient's childhood, such as:

- How well do you remember your childhood?
- Are there things that happened to you when you were a child that shouldn't have happened to you or anyone?
- Would you like your children to grow up as you did?
- Sometimes we feel guilty about things that happened to us in the past. Are you feeling any sense of guilt or shame? (Clarke, Schulman, McCollum, & Felitti, 2015)

Transgenerational Trauma

Transgenerational or intergenerational trauma is a wounding from a traumatic event that has effects upon generations after the initial trauma. This type of trauma can occur in individual families, or groups who have experienced genocide, terrorism, natural disasters, etc., as collective trauma. In either case, there can be long-lasting harmful effects on physiological processes in the body, which can cause chronic disease.

An example of this can be found in the Native American population, which suffers from some of the highest health disparities in the United States. The median age of death in South Dakota Native Americans is 58 compared to whites, where 81 years of age is the median (Warne & Lajimodiere, 2015). Native Americans have experienced centuries of inequities adding to the root causes for these poor health disparities. From the 15th to the 19th century, millions of Native Americans died from warfare and infectious diseases, including smallpox which was intentionally spread to the indigenous people by giving them blankets that had been used by smallpox patients (Warne & Lajimodiere, 2015). In the late 1890s up to the 1930s, there were multitudes of off-reservation boarding schools developed to destroy the Native American culture by teaching the children reading, writing, and arithmetic and keeping them away from their parents and tribal culture and customs. Children from ages 4 and up were taken and sent away to boarding schools—their parents often having no choice. These children were exposed to all forms of abuse, homesickness, infectious diseases, lack of love and parenting, and loss of tradition and culture identity, resulting in the deaths of many of these children. Those who survived lack the skills and knowledge to parent, have not been able to heal, and therefore suffer from alcoholism, substance abuse, poverty, depression, and the like. Homicides, suicides, and interpersonal violence injuries beset this population. The trauma has been passed down to the next generation.

Homeless Health Care

According to the National Alliance to End Homelessness, the annual U.S. Department of Housing and Urban Development (HUD) point-in-time count identified 567,715 people experiencing homelessness in 2019. Though the vast majority of the homeless population lived in some form of shelter or in transitional housing at the time of the point-in-time count, approximately one-third lived in a place not meant for human habitation, such as the street or an abandoned building. Subpopulations experiencing homelessness are individuals, which accounts for more than half of the homeless; families are the second-largest subgroup. Other subgroups are those individuals who were chronically homeless, chronically homeless families, veterans, and unaccompanied youth and children. Although most homeless persons live in urban areas, a surprising 16.1% live in rural areas where they sleep in the woods, campgrounds, cars, and abandoned farm buildings.

Defining Homelessness

According to the National Health Care for the Homeless Council (NHCHC, 2020), there is more than one "official" definition of homelessness. Health centers funded by the USDHHS use the following definition:

> A homeless individual is defined in section 330(h)(5)(A) as "an individual who lacks housing (without regard to whether the individual is a member of a family), including an individual whose primary residence during the night is a supervised public or private facility (e.g., shelters) that provides temporary living accommodations, and an individual who is a resident in transitional housing." (NHCHC, 2020)

The Federal Bureau of Primary Health Care expands the definition of homelessness to include the following: an individual may be considered to be homeless if that person is "doubled up," a term that refers to a situation where individuals are unable to maintain their housing situation and are forced to stay with a series of friends and/or extended family members (see **BOX 4-2**). In addition, previously homeless individuals who are to be released from a prison or a hospital may be considered homeless if they do not have a stable housing situation to which they can return. A recognition of the instability of an individual's living arrangements is critical to the definition of homelessness (HRSA, 1999; NHCHC, 2020).

Box 4-2 Assessing for Homelessness at Point of Care

- Patient self-defines as homeless.
- Patient lives place to place.
- Patient lives with family or friends because there is no other option.
- Patient is staying in a place that restricts number of nights (including pays rent by hours, days, or weeks).
- Patient lives in overcrowded situation.
- Patient lives in housing that is based on illegal/unwanted acts (e.g., prostitution).
- Patient is separated from family members because of limited housing choice.

Box 4-3 National Health Care for the Homeless Council Adapted Clinical Guidelines: 10 Areas of Focus

Asthma
Cardiovascular Diseases: Hypertension, Hyperlipidemia, and Heart Failure
Chlamydial or Gonococcal Infections
Chronic Pain
Diabetes Mellitus
General Recommendations for the Care of Homeless Patients
HIV/AIDS
Opioid Use Disorder
Otitis Media
Reproductive Health Care

NHCHC. (2017). Adapted Clinical Guidelines. Retrieved from https://www.nhchc.org/resources/clinical/adapted-clinical-guidelines/

Programs funded by HUD use a different, more limited definition of homelessness that is restricted to individuals living on the streets or in shelters. Advocates of the homeless state that HUD needs to expand its definition to allow communities flexibility in providing cost-effective housing and support services to this currently underserved group.

Clinical Practice Guidelines

With the start of the new millennium, a group of clinicians from the National Health Care for the Homeless Council, in collaboration with the Agency for Health Care Quality and Research (AHCQR), began to adapt clinical practice guidelines for patients who are considered homeless. In 2004, the National Guidelines Clearinghouse placed NHCHC-published guidelines for specific disease processes and general care of the homeless (NHCHC, 2020). There are now nine specific clinical guidelines, as well as a standard clinical practice guideline, to address the special challenges faced by homeless patients that may limit their ability to adhere to a plan of care (see **Box 4-3** and **Table 4-2**). In addition, the NHCHC website provides information on diseases, conditions, and resources for the homeless.

Table 4-2 Health Care for Homeless Patients: Summary of Recommendations

History	Physical Examination
■ Living situation ■ Prior homelessness ■ Acute/chronic illness history ■ Medications ■ Mental illness/cognitive deficit ■ Developmental/behavioral problems ■ Alcohol/nicotine/other drug use ■ Health insurance and other assistance ■ Sexual history—gender identity, sexual orientation, behaviors, partners, pregnancies, hepatitis/HIV/other STIs ■ History and current risk of abuse; emotional, physical, and sexual ■ Legal problems/violence ■ Work history—longest time held a job, veteran status, occupational injuries/toxic exposures ■ Education level ■ Nutrition/hydration—diet, food resources, preparation skills, liquid intake ■ Cultural heritage/affiliations/supports ■ Strengths—coping skills, resourcefulness, abilities, interests	■ Comprehensive exam—at first encounter if possible ■ Serial, focused exams—for patients uncomfortable with full-body, unclothed exam at first visit ■ Special populations—victims of abuse, sexual minorities ■ Dental assessment—age-appropriate teeth, obvious caries, dental/referred pain, diabetes patients
Education, Self-management	**Diagnostic Tests and Screening**
■ Protection from communicable diseases, risk of delayed/interrupted treatment ■ Behavioral change—individual/small group/community interventions, motivational interviewing ■ Education of shelter/clinical staff—regarding special problems/needs of homeless people	■ Baseline labs, including EKG, lipid panel, potassium and creatinine levels, HbA1c, LFTs ■ Asthma—spirometry or peak flow monitoring ■ TB screening for patients living in shelters and others at risk for tuberculosis ■ STI screening—for chlamydia, gonorrhea, syphilis, HIV, HBV, HCV, and trichomonas ■ Mental health—Patient Health Questionnaire (PHQ-9, PHQ-2), MHS-III, MDQ ■ Substance abuse—SSI-AOD ■ Cognitive assessment—Mini-Mental Status Examination (MMSE) ■ Developmental assessment ■ Interpersonal violence—Posttraumatic Diagnostic Scale ■ Forensic evaluation—if strong evidence of child abuse ■ Healthcare maintenance—cancer screening for adults, EPSDT for children

Medications	Follow-up/Outreach and Engagement
■ Simple regimen—low pill count, once-daily dosing where possible ■ Storage/access—in clinic/shelters; if no access to refrigeration, don't prescribe meds that require it. ■ Patient assistance—entitlement assistance, free/low-cost drugs if readily available for continued use ■ Aids to adherence—harm reduction, outreach/case management, directly observed therapy	■ Contact information—phone, email for patient/friend/family/case manager ■ Medical home—to coordinate/promote continuity of health care ■ Frequent follow-up, incentives, nonjudgmental care regardless of adherence ■ Drop-in system—Anticipate/accommodate unscheduled clinic visits ■ Transportation assistance—provide car fare, tokens, help with transportation services ■ Outreach, case management ■ Referrals—linkage with specialists, providers sensitive to underserved populations
Associated Problems and Complications	**Model of Care**
■ No place to heal—efficacy of medical respite/recuperative care, supportive housing ■ Fragmented care—multiple providers ■ Masked symptoms/misdiagnosis ■ Developmental discrepancies ■ Functional impairments—assist with SSI/SSDI applications ■ Dual diagnoses—integrated treatment for concurrent mental illness/substance use disorders ■ Loss of child custody—support for parent of child abused by others, and for abused parent	■ Integrated, interdisciplinary—coordinated medical, dental, and psychosocial services ■ Therapeutic ■ Multiple points of service ■ Flexible service system—walk-ins permitted, help with resolving systems barriers ■ Outreach sites—streets, soup kitchens, shelters, other homeless service sites ■ Clinical standard guidelines ■ Consumer and peer involvement ■ Access to supportive housing

Bonin, E., Brehove, T., Carlson, C., Downing, M., Hoeft, J. Kalinowski, A.,...Post, P. (2010). Adapting your practice: General recommendations for the care of homeless patients. Nashville: Health Care for the Homeless Clinicians' Network, National Health Care for the Homeless Council, Inc. Retrieved from https://nhchc.org/wp-content/uploads/2019/08/GenRecsHomeless2010-1.pdf

Barriers to Health Care for the Homeless

Homeless populations face many barriers to healthcare services. Financial barriers and the ability to get health insurance are obvious. Transportation to medical appointments is problematic, and competing needs for food, shelter, and money take priority. Homeless individuals suffering from mental illness may be paranoid, disorganized, have nontraditional health beliefs, lack social support, and fear authority figures. Conditions living on the street make adherence to medical care problematic in terms of medication storage, inadequate sanitation, and poor nutrition (Montauk, 2006). To help homeless individuals overcome some of these barriers, nurse practitioners must work with a team of healthcare professionals poised to meet this population's unique circumstances. Federal efforts to provide care to homeless populations include bringing services to where homeless populations gather, such as shelters, parks, soup kitchens, transportation centers, and places of worship. Outreach teams, such as the aforementioned, most often are based in healthcare centers where patients can be referred for additional care. Providing bus tokens for transportation, free medication, and a walk-in appointment system are other examples of strategies that can help remove obstacles to care.

Building trust is paramount and can be established by emphasizing patient strengths and capacity. Acknowledging that patients kept their appointment or took the medication prescribed are examples of basic patient assets that should be recognized. The NHCHC guidelines point out that just meeting survival needs while homeless takes resourcefulness, patience, and tenacity.

Substance Use Disorders and Addiction

Substance use is a major public health problem in the United States. According to the Substance Abuse and Mental Health Services Administration (SAMHSA), 60.1% of people age 12 years or older used illicit drugs in the past month, and 20.8% had a substance use disorder (SUD) in the past year (SAMHSA, 2020). Substance use disorders can mimic or coexist with other medical and mental health disorders, and nurse practitioners are in a unique position to provide screening for, urgent care to, and continuity of care for individuals and families who are at risk. Recurrent use of alcohol, tobacco, cannabis, stimulants, hallucinogens, and opioids can have devastating consequences, causing clinically significant impairment, including health problems, disability, and failure to meet major responsibilities at work, school, or home. Reducing SUDs and related problems among adults is critical for mental and physical health, safety, and quality of life. Alcohol use in the United States remains the most widely abused, with marijuana and illicit drug use (including nonmedical use of prescription painkillers) most prevalent (see **Figure 4-2**).

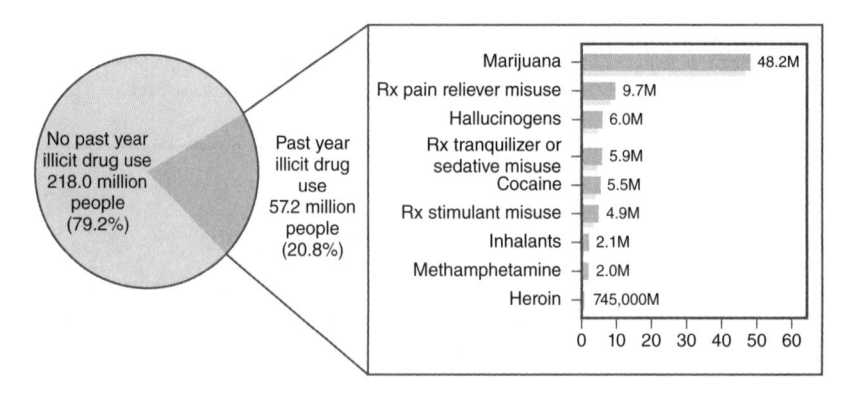

Figure 4-2 Trends in Substance Use Disorders

Substance Abuse and Mental Health Services Administration. (2020). Key substance use and mental health indicators in the United States: Results from the 2019 National Survey on Drug Use and Health (HHS Publication No. PEP20-07-01-001, NSDUH Series H-55). Rockville, MD: Center for Behavioral Health Statistics and Quality, Substance Abuse and Mental Health Services Administration. Retrieved from https://www.samhsa.gov/data/

Impact on Patients

Patients with SUD and addiction have health, emotional, family, social, legal, and spiritual issues that can be troublesome to the patient, the family, and the healthcare provider. Major vulnerabilities include overdose, withdrawal symptoms, unintentional injuries, unintended pregnancy, neonatal complications, long-term health sequela, and disruption to the family unit. SUD is a constellation of cognitive, behavioral, and physiological symptoms that an individual displays, but the person continues to use a harmful substance despite the associated negative consequences. The *Diagnostic and Statistical Manual of Mental Disorders, Fifth Edition* (*DSM-5*), no longer uses the terms *substance abuse* and *substance dependence*; rather, it refers to substance use disorders, which are defined as mild, moderate, or severe to indicate the level of severity, which is determined by the number of diagnostic criteria met by an individual (SAMHSA, 2020).

Addiction

According to the American Society of Addiction Medicine (ASAM, 2019), addiction is a primary, chronic disease of brain reward, motivation, memory, and related circuitry. Dysfunction in these circuits leads to an individual pathologically pursuing reward and/or relief by substance use and other behaviors. Addiction is characterized by the inability to consistently abstain from and control behavior and cravings. It is characterized by diminished recognition of significant problems with one's behaviors and interpersonal relationships, and a dysfunctional emotional response (see **Figure 4-3**). Like other chronic diseases, addiction often involves cycles of relapse and remission. Without treatment or engagement in recovery activities, addiction is progressive and can result in disability or premature death. The term *dependence* implies both psychological craving and physiological symptoms of tolerance and withdrawal.

Vulnerable Populations and SUDs

In addition, the nurse practitioner must be aware of the special populations that are susceptible to substance use disorders. Adolescents are a high-risk population

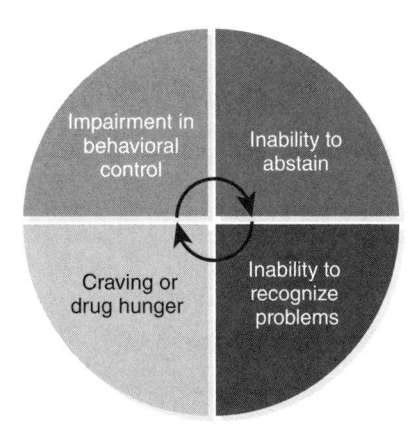

Figure 4-3 Characteristics of Addiction

for marijuana, alcohol, and prescription pain medication obtained from the family medicine cabinet. Drugs used by gay men and men who have sex with men (MSM) at circuit parties can impair judgment and result in risky sexual behavior. Adults that use illicit drugs may have a mental illness they are self-medicating for. As with any population, nurse practitioners working with the LGBT population must practice with competence and sensitivity. It is also important to recognize that chronic pain sufferers who are appropriately prescribed opioids are not substance users or necessarily considered "dependent."

Evaluation

Identifying and treating addiction or SUDs requires proactive assessment, awareness of signs and symptoms associated with abuse, the ability to develop an individual treatment plan, and the willingness to promote community-level policy change as appropriate. Important factors in deciding when and how to treat addiction include the patient's willingness to undergo treatment, the social support network, health insurance coverage, financial resources, programs available in the community, and the provider's skill level in treating addiction. When taking a patient history, the nurse practitioner must be cognizant of the red flags, which can provide clues to areas that will prompt further screening (see **Box 4-4**).

Screening

The U.S. Preventative Services Task Force (USPSTF, 2020) concludes there is sufficient evidence to support screening adolescents, adults, and pregnant women for unhealthy drug, alcohol, and tobacco use. Screening should be instituted when services for accurate diagnosis, effective treatment, and appropriate care can be offered or referred. Nurse practitioners and other healthcare providers have access to many self-report screening tools to assess alcohol misuse, and some are validated for detecting substance abuse. The CAGE questionnaire is thought to be 60–90% sensitive when two or more responses are positive and 40–60% specific for excluding alcohol abuse. The CAGE-AID has been modified for drug use. The CRAFFT test has been validated for screening adolescents for substance-related disorders (Conners & Volk, 2004). It should be noted the screening test is less important than the actual act of the clinician asking the patient about substance use.

Box 4-4 Red Flags for Substance Abuse Disorders

- Family history of alcohol or substance abuse
- Partner who is a substance abuser
- Frequent encounters with the police
- Arrests for driving under the influence (DUIs)
- Behavior changes reported by family members
- Sudden loss of job, financial problems
- Absence from school and work
- Depression or anxiety
- Sleep problems
- Complaints of sexual dysfunction

Management and Treatment of SUDs

Patients who are addicts continue to use substances despite negative consequences. They may be frequently reluctant to stop using even when their plight gets desperate. The nurse practitioner will be most successful in improving their patients' chances for change by understanding their desire to stop or reduce use. The NP can use a wide variety of therapeutic options including but not limited to brief motivational interventions, cognitive behavioral therapy, and targeted pharmacological treatment. Assuring medical and psychological stability is of paramount importance. Decisions regarding outpatient versus inpatient interventions must be considered carefully and long-term monitoring and follow-up care in the community should be part of the treatment plan. Obviously family members and friends are almost always impacted by the addicted patient's tobacco, alcohol, and/or drug use so that the nurse practitioner is in a key position to influence family dynamics and refer patients and families to support programs such as Al-Anon, Nar-Anon, or Alateen.

Refugee and Immigrant Health

The United Nations High Commission for Refugees (UNHCR, 2020) reports an unprecedented 79.5 million people around the world have been forced from home. Among them are nearly 26 million refugees, over half of whom are under the age of 18. Refugees, by definition, are fleeing their countries due to a well-founded fear of being persecuted "for reasons of race, religion, nationality, membership in a particular social group, or political opinion" (CDC, 2013).

By definition, asylum seekers have submitted a claim for refugee status and are waiting for this claim to be accepted or rejected. Refugees and asylees comprise the majority of displaced persons resettled to the United States (CDC, 2013). In the new millennium, nurse practitioners can contribute to improving the quality of life for displaced families, refugees, and immigrants by understanding the needs of new immigrants.

Top Countries of Origin

In 2019, the Syrian Arab Republic was the most common country of origin, with some 6.6 million newly recognized refugees fleeing the conflict there. Crises in Venezuela led to new displacements of almost 3.7 million. The next-largest numbers of new refugees were from Afghanistan, South Sudan, Myanmar, Somalia, Democratic Republic of the Congo, Sudan, Iraq, and the Central African Republic (UNHCR, 2020).

Major Host Countries

According to UNHCR, for the third consecutive year, Turkey hosted the largest number of refugees worldwide, with 3.6 million people (2020). It was followed by Colombia (1.8 million), Pakistan (1.4 million), Uganda (1.4 million), and Germany (1.1 million) (see **Figure 4-4**). In 2019, UNHCR referred 1.1 million refugees to the United States for resettlement. According to the Pew Center for Research (2019), the United States dropped to historic lows for settling refugees during Donald Trump's presidency. The United States had the capacity for 30,000 refugees and

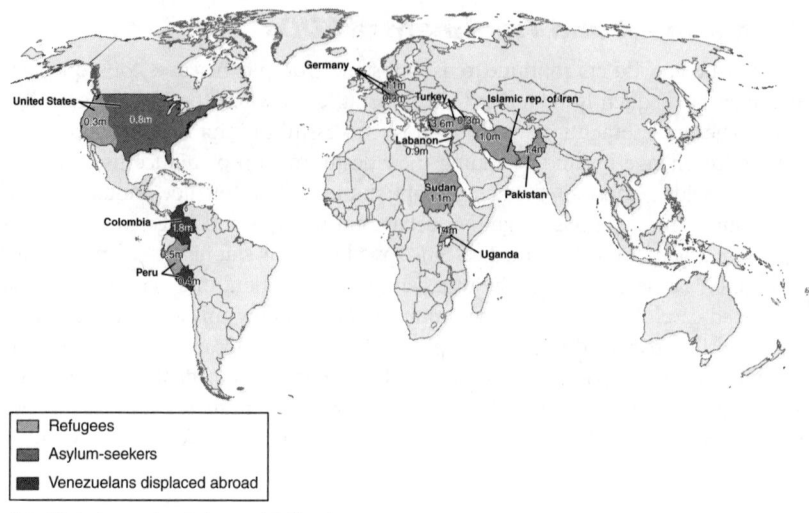

Figure 4-4 Major Host Countries

Data from UNHCR. (2020). Global trends: Forced displacement in 2019. Geneva, Switzerland: Author. Retrieved from https://www.unhcr.org/5ee200e37.pdf

asylum seekers in 2019. Texas, Washington, New York, and California resettled roughly a quarter of all refugees in fiscal 2019. Other states that received at least 1,000 refugees with UNHCR's assistance included Kentucky, Ohio, North Carolina, Arizona, Georgia, and Michigan (Krogstad, 2019).

Resettlement Issues

When refugees arrive in the United States, not only are they leaving what they know, but they are also being introduced to an entirely new culture, language, food, and climate. To support the immediate transition, the U.S. Department of State (USDS, 2021) has cooperative agreements with national resettlement agencies to provide "Reception and Placement" services. Local affiliates of national refugee resettlement agencies arrange food, housing, clothing, employment, counseling, medical care, and other immediate needs for refugees during the first 90 days after arrival. Longer-term transitional support is also available for refugees by the Department of State's Bureau of Population, Refugees, and Migration.

Common Healthcare Issues and Torture

Providing health care for resettled refugees is challenging. It requires knowledge of the health care and social conditions of the country of origin, attention to subtle expressions of acute and chronic illnesses, and a culturally sensitive approach to the individual and family. Historical estimates of the percentage of refugees who endure the trauma of torture have ranged between 5% and 35%. Studies of more recent waves of refugees from Somalia and Ethiopia have indicated torture prevalence rates as high as 69% (Miles & Garcia-Peltoniemi, 2012). Of immigrants from countries where torture is practiced, 6–12% say they have

Table 4-3 Physical and Psychological Morbidities in Refugees

Physical Morbidity	Psychological Morbidity
- Concussive trauma - Suspension, hyperflexion - Ligatures, binding, and compression - Sexual torture and genital mutilation - Burns, electrical shock, and cutting - Injurious environmental factors	- Humiliation and degradation - Extreme fear witnessing torture - Isolation - Sleep deprivation - PTSD sequela from physical torture - Depression

been tortured, but often refugees remain silent about the trauma they experienced (Miles & Garcia-Peltoniemi, 2012). Torture rates are highest in people seeking political asylum and persecution. Of asylum-seeking refugees from Somalia, Ethiopia, Eritrea, Senegal, Sierra Leone, Tibet, and Bhutan, 20–40% report being tortured (Miles & Garcia-Peltoniemi, 2012). The aftermath of witnessing and surviving cruelty and the violence of war leaves many refugees with significant symptoms of psychological distress, including post-traumatic stress disorder (PTSD), depression, and anxiety (Shannon, O' Dougherty, & Mehta, 2012). Chronic pain, post-concussion syndromes, sleep disturbance, and musculoskeletal symptoms can complicate the detection of other infectious and/or chronic conditions. The NP must become astute at identifying victims of torture. Asking direct questions has high sensitivity and specificity. **Table 4-3** represents possible physical and psychological morbidities that individuals may have endured in their home country or refugee camp. Eliciting this information is valuable for legal medical documentation evidence, should the refugee go to court to rule on asylum status, as well as to properly treat and refer the individual so as to reduce disability, pain, and distress.

Other concurrent health problems to consider include oral health problems, tuberculosis, hepatitis B, malaria, lead poisoning, anemia, and malnutrition. Infections such as sexually transmitted diseases (STDs) or intestinal parasites are also common. The NP must evaluate risk factors and potential exposures in the countries of origin. Catch-up vaccinations and cancer screenings, both routine and as indicated by various risk factors, are important parts of complete health care for refugees (CDC, 2019).

Refugee Health Profiles

Health information and refugee health profiles can be an invaluable reference that provides key health and cultural information about specific refugee groups resettling in the United States.

The refugee health profiles information is a collaborative effort between the World Health Organization, the International Organization for Migration (IOM), the United Nations High Commissioner for Refugees, the U.S. Department of State, scientific research, and other sources (CDC, 2017).

The information gleaned from the profiles is provided to assist healthcare providers, public health, and resettlement agencies to facilitate medical screening and

Table 4-4 Refugee Health Profiles

Refugee Topic Information	Refugee Groups Currently Represented
Priority Health Conditions Background Population Movements Health Care and Conditions Pre-arrival Medical Screening of U.S.-bound Refugees Post-arrival Medical Screening Health Information	Bhutanese Refugees Burmese Refugees Central American (Guatemalan, Honduran, Salvadoran) Refugees Congolese Refugees Iraqi Refugees Somali Refugees Syrian Refugees

determine appropriate interventions and services for individuals of a specific refugee group. This comprehensive resource describes the demographic, cultural, and health characteristics of the specific population. It is the responsibility of the NP to gain an understanding of where refugees come from, the circumstances of their displacement, their living conditions during asylum, and the health conditions for which they may be at increased risk (see **Table 4-4**).

Prison Health

The United States is home to 5% of the world's population, but houses 25% of its prisoners. According to statistics from the U.S. Department of Justice (USDJ), approximately 6,899,000 Americans are under correctional supervision, 4,751,400 people were under the supervision of probation and parole, and 2,220,300 individuals were incarcerated in prisons and jails (Kaeble & Cowig, 2018). Currently, 93% of inmates are men and 6.7% are women (Federal Bureau of Prisons, 2021). When factoring in racial disparities, the picture becomes bleak. The statistics on race and incarceration in the United States present an alarming view of a criminal justice system in which people of color are vastly overrepresented and face harsher penalties than their white peers. With an overwhelming number of African-Americans (38.6%) and Latinos (30.1%) in the criminal justice system who already come from impoverished backgrounds, the consequences of their incarceration have a grave impact on their ability to find adequate housing, employment, and health care in the post-incarceration period. Disruption to the family unit is high, with 5 million children under the age of 18 having an incarcerated parent (Annie E. Casey Foundation, 2016).

Healthcare Needs of Prisoners

The healthcare needs of prisoners are diverse and cover the range of conditions found in the general population; however, there tends to be an increased ratio of incarcerated individuals who enter with health problems compounded by alcohol and substance use and a history of general poor health and self-neglect prior to their sentence. Nurse practitioners are in a unique position to intervene at three distinct periods in the incarceration timeline, including identifying risk factors prior to the incarceration, providing direct care during incarceration, and lastly providing

Table 4-5 Incarceration Timeline Risk Factors

Pre-Incarceration Risk Factors	Incarceration Care	Post-Incarceration Stressors
African-American Hispanic Poverty Urban-centered crime Mental illness Substance abuse Homelessness Parent who was incarcerated Failure to complete high school Childhood neglect and abuse	Screening and treatment of infectious disease Health education Preventative health Management of mental health disorders Oral health Managing issues of aging prisoners Encouraging family communication Referring prisoners for internal and external services	Lack of safety net, routine, and boundaries Transition issued to halfway house living Lack of housing Lack of social network Stigma of being a felon Legal barriers Lack of rehabilitation while incarcerated (e.g., acquiring job training, GED) Lack of health care and community services

interventions following the release from prison and transition into society (see **Table 4-5**) (Daniels, 2016).

Clinical Practice Guidelines for Prison Health

The Federal Bureau of Prisons (BOP, 2021) makes clinical practice guidelines available for the public for information purposes and transparency. There are more than 30 healthcare management guidelines including but not limited to the most common health problems prison populations encounter. Infectious disease guidelines include treatment for hepatitis, HIV, MRSA, tuberculosis, and sexually transmitted infections. Mental health guidelines include treatment for depression, bipolar disorder, schizophrenia, and chemical detoxification. Guidelines for management of chronic health problems such as diabetes, asthma, hypertension, and osteoarthritis are also available. The COVID-19 pandemic has prompted new guidelines for monitoring infection rates and vaccine protocols. The BOP also utilizes a medication formulary, which is a list of medications that are considered to be high-quality, cost-effective drug therapy for the population served. The primary goals of formulary management are to optimize therapeutic outcomes, maintain cost-effective care, and ensure drug usage is conducive within the correctional environment.

Interventions for Reintegration Post-Incarceration

Developing a community transition plan is essential for reducing vulnerabilities the prisoner may encounter post-incarceration. As patient advocates, nurse practitioners must assist individuals to achieve their highest level of health and well-being post-incarceration. When working with these populations, understanding the prison discharge process and community resources in your catchment area is essential. Often, ex-offenders find themselves obtaining care through federally

Box 4-5 Transitioning to Life in the Community

Community Transition Checklist for Reentry
- Housing
- Basic Living Needs
- Income Sources
- Medical Care
- Prescriptions
- Mental Health
- Substance Abuse, After Care, and Maintenance
- Disability Benefits and Compensation
- Legal Aid
- Social/Community Supports
- U.S. Veteran Services
- Dental Care
- Vocational Services
- HIV/AIDS Services
- Domestic Violence
- Senior Services
- Offenders: Sex, Female, and Ex-offenders

Data from Federal Bureau of Prisons. (2002). Clinical guidelines for social work professionals: Discharge assistance. Retrieved from https://www.bop.gov/resources/pdfs/discharge.pdf

qualified health centers (FQHCs) in medically underserved communities. Becoming familiar with all the services a FQHC can provide under one umbrella (e.g., internal medicine, dental, mental health, women's health, pharmacy assistance) will make for increased access to services with healthcare providers skilled at working with underserved populations. Working in a team with social and outreach services, the NP can assist the client to identify new social networks and resources to meet basic needs, including but not limited to church groups, legal aid, and vocational services. See **Box 4-5** for an abbreviated community transition checklist for post-incarceration.

Human Trafficking

Millions of persons across the globe are victims of human trafficking (Morris & Vega, 2016). Human trafficking encompasses labor trafficking as well as sex trafficking and includes children, women, and men. The Office of Administration of Children and Families has within it an office that focuses on human trafficking, which likens human trafficking to modern slavery. Action, meaning, and purpose are three facets of criminal activities and exploitation, as depicted in **Figure 4-5**.

All of the vulnerable persons discussed in this chapter are at risk of being targeted for trafficking. Globally, there are approximately 1.2 million children being exploited for sex (Ernewein & Nieves, 2015). Human trafficking for sexual exploitation is one of the most lucrative criminal activities in our time period. Those that are brought here from other countries typically arrive in New York, Miami, or Los Angeles. However, looking within the United States we might think there are more foreign persons being exploited, but that is a false assumption. There are

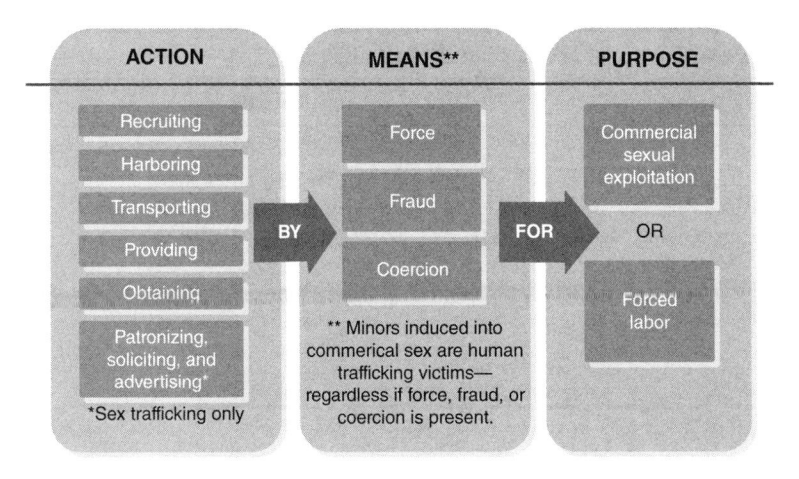

Figure 4-5 Human Trafficking

U.S. Department of Health & Human Services, Office on Trafficking in Persons. (2017). What is human trafficking? Retrieved from https://www.acf.hhs.gov/otip/about/what-is-human-trafficking

more U.S. citizens of all ages being trafficked within our own country (Ernewein & Nieves, 2015).

Gorenstein (2016) reported almost 88% of victims of sex trafficking visit an emergency department at some point. Nurse practitioners are therefore in a prime position to assess patients who may be victims of human trafficking. As mandatory reporters, NPs must recognize and report abuse. Providing confidentiality, safety, and a nonjudgmental manner is crucial to reduce barriers to communication.

Potential indicators of persons being trafficked include having someone with them who appears to be controlling them and the scenario, managing the fear, sadness, bruises and other traumatic injuries, lack of documentation, poor health, discrepancy of behavior and reported age, and generally poor health (Ernewein & Nieves, 2015; Morris & Vega, 2016). Polaris Project (2016) suggests, after assuring the patients of their safety and confidentiality, to ask patients privately where they live and if they are free to come and go as they please, if they have been threatened or harmed, and if they have been forced to have sex or perform sex acts. Useful laboratory testing includes complete blood count, STD testing (including HIV), ova and parasites, hepatitis B and C, as well as tuberculosis. Nurse practitioners need to be astute at identifying the short- and long-term effects of human trafficking on individuals in order to develop a sound treatment (see **Table 4-6**).

Working with social services and law enforcement as a team can assist the NP to help get the victim to safety and into services to assist transitioning to safe housing with long-term treatment for psychological and medical issues. It is imperative that NPs be educated on identifying victims of human trafficking, developing culturally appropriate caring patient/provider relationships, becoming knowledgeable on reporting laws, and assisting colleagues to better identify and refer potential victims. **Box 4-6** has a list of useful telephone numbers for victims and healthcare providers.

Table 4-6 Impact of Sex Trafficking on Victims

Short-Term Effects	Long-Term Effects
<ul><li>Higher risk behaviors (e.g., drug and alcohol abuse)</li><li>Impaired judgment</li><li>Emotional exhaustion</li><li>Depersonalization</li><li>Fear, anxiety, and nervousness</li><li>Muscle tension</li></ul>	<ul><li>Post-traumatic stress disorder</li><li>Trauma bonding</li><li>Severe depression</li><li>Suicidal ideation</li><li>Spiritual questions</li><li>Feelings of being mentally broken</li><li>Sexual dysfunction</li><li>Difficulty establishing/maintaining relationships</li></ul>

Box 4-6 Telephone Numbers for Victims and Healthcare Providers

- The Childhelp National Child Abuse Hotline: (800)-4ACHILD
- National Runaway Safeline: (800)-RUNAWAY
- National Human Trafficking Resource Center: (888)-373-7888

Gender Identity, Expression, and Sexual Preference

Recently, a baby was born in Canada that was not given a genital inspection at birth, which was outside the medical system, and was given a health card by the government with a "U" (unidentified/unknown) for gender/sex (Rahim, 2017). The parent, who identifies as nonbinary, transgender, wants the child to choose a gender identity when ready to. This is likely the first known documentation of an infant to not have a gender/sex assigned upon birth by the choice of the parent(s). Approximately 1.4 million people in the United States identify as transgender (Flores, Herman, Gates, & Brown, 2016). Facebook has over 60 options for choosing gender. Unfortunately, in 2016 there were at least 28 known transgender women reported killed, and the vast majority were of color (Schmider, 2016). Harassment, bullying, assault, homelessness, and health disparities are issues that lesbian, gay, bisexual, transgender, queer, questioning, and intersex (LGBTQ/QI) face daily. Nurse practitioners need to be aware of the issues surrounding children and adults whose gender identity, gender expression, and/or sexual preference(s) are different from the binary, cultural norm that the NP may be comfortable with.

Gender dysphoria is a term that defines a person who has distress with clinical symptomatology because their gender identity is not consistent with the gender assigned at birth. Terminology is critical to be familiar with, to maintain open communication with patients, potential patients, and their significant others. For some, gender may be fluid, as well as sexual partner(s) preference, meaning that one may identify more with female one day and more with male on another day, or may be more attracted to male, female, both, or none at varying times (see **Tables 4-7** and **4-8**).

Health-related disparities are significant in these populations, and sadly many do not seek health care because of fears of being judged or marginalized by

Table 4-7 Commonly Used Gender Identity Terminology (not all-inclusive)

Agender	Does not identify with a gender
Androgynous	Identifies as mixed or neutral gender
Bigender	Identifies as a combination of male and female gender
Cisgender	Identifies with the gender assigned at birth
Gender fluid	Gender is not static, but shifts
Genderqueer	Does not identify with a gender, or falls in between or beyond gender
Pangender	Identifies as all genders

Table 4-8 Commonly Used Sexual Preference or Affectional Orientation Terminology (not all-inclusive)

Asexual	Not attracted to any gender
Bisexual	Attracted to male and female genders, but does not have to be at the same time or with the same intensity
Gay	A male attracted to males
Heterosexual	Attracted to a gender/sex that is not one's own
Homosexual	Attracted to the same gender/sex as one's own
Lesbian	A female attracted to females
Pansexual	Attracted to people regardless of gender, gender identity, or gender expression

healthcare providers and those working in the health system. In addition to the routine health maintenance needs for all children and adults, providers must be aware of health issues that are significantly associated with LGBTQ/QI. These issues include depression, which could be associated with gender dysphoria but may be related to other causes, anxiety, prevention, and/or treatment from being victims of bullying and violence, substance abuse, and suicide attempts. In addition, the provider must be aware of where to refer patients to appropriate mental health specialists, substance abuse counselors, HIV testing and treatment, and specialists for hormone therapy, as well as surgical options for those who are seeking these interventions. As noted earlier, transgender women of color are at high risk of being victims of violence, including homicide, so that providing education regarding safety is a priority if the patient is agreeable to discussing options.

Children and adolescents who are gender nonconforming require support and acceptance of parents/caregivers and healthcare providers (Alegria, 2011). While transient role-play of opposite gender occurs in young children, some may continue to express themselves in nonconforming genders, and a subset may continue to identify as other gender. The NP should be aware of experienced counselors and providers to refer families to so that they can have accurate information and support services if needed. This is very important if there are decisions to be made for an adolescent to transition (Alegria, 2011). It is imperative for NPs to be aware of the distress and dysphoria experienced by many as they move into puberty, because this is a time when severe depression and suicidal attempts may occur (Alegria, 2011). Approximately 50% of gender nonconforming youth do not have the support of their family, and so the risk of abuse, homelessness, substance abuse, and sex work increases (Grossman & D'Augelli, 2007). NPs must be aware of these potential issues and provide compassionate, sincere support in these instances.

Offering an environment in the clinic/office that is safe, inclusive, and nonjudgmental is also paramount. All healthcare providers must be able to put any biases aside. Reflecting on how one views and feels about these issues in advance can help to avoid uncomfortable interactions. If one cannot put biases aside, then it is imperative to know where to refer people to for care. The clinic/office can hang a rainbow flag to show visible support. Another important item is to not assume that anyone (whether adult or child) has a partner or parent(s) who are male, female, or has one or more mothers or fathers. When approaching patients who identify or express themselves as non-cisgender, asking how they would prefer to be addressed is acceptable if done in a considerate manner. Some people may prefer "he" or "she," or perhaps "they" or "ze." Providing care to persons of all backgrounds and beliefs requires NPs to keep up to date with issues facing patients and to continue to reach out to offer assistance with compassion and honesty in a confidential and safe environment.

Lesbian, gay, bisexual, and transgender (LGBT) people experience many specific health-related challenges and disparities. Nurse practitioners are in a unique position to help eliminate these disparities and improve the health of the LGBTQ population. **Box 4-7** provides evidence-based Internet resources to help maximize health outcomes for these individuals and their families.

Box 4-7 Internet Resources for Lesbian, Gay, Bisexual, and Transgender Health

---

- American Association of Family Physicians (LGBTQ) Tool Kit: https://www.aafp.org/family-physician/patient-care/care-resources/lbgtq.html
- Center for Disease Control (LGBT): https://www.cdc.gov/lgbthealth/index.htm
- Johns Hopkins Medicine: Center for Transgender Health & LGBTQ Resources: https://www.hopkinsmedicine.org/diversity/resources/lgbtq-resources.html#students
- National Organization of Nurse Practitioner Faculty (NONPF) Patient Centered Transgender health: A toolkit for nurse practitioner faculty and clinicians: https://cdn.ymaws.com/www.nonpf.org/resource/resmgr/files/transgender_toolkit_final.pdf
- USDHHS Healthy People 2030: LGBT: https://health.gov/healthypeople/objectives-and-data/browse-objectives/lgbt
- World Professional Association for Transgender Health: https://www.wpath.org/resources/general
- USFS Center of Excellence for Transgender Health: https://prevention.ucsf.edu/transhealth

HIV/AIDS

Human immunodeficiency virus (HIV) and acquired immunodeficiency syndrome (AIDS) have been around for almost 100 years that we are aware of (CDC, 2017). The virus is believed to have been spread to humans from chimpanzees during the 1920s in the Republic of Congo. Yet the stigma and discrimination associated with HIV infection remains a huge concern, as well as a reason for many to not get tested and/or not seek health care. Those most at risk for acquiring HIV globally include women, children, men who have sex with men, transgenders, injection drug users, sex workers, and prisoners. These populations are often marginalized and suffer discrimination in many parts of the world. Educating our communities and patients about HIV/AIDS can help to get more people into care early, which can increase their life span, reduce the community viral load, and decrease the stigma associated with HIV/AIDS.

In 1981, there were initial reports of five gay men who were infected with *Pneumocystis carinii* pneumonia (Gottlieb, 2001); and in 1982, there were reports of women being infected, as well as reports of infections from transfusions and vertical transmission (Sepkowitz, 2001). One of the most famous cases of AIDS discrimination occurred in the 1980s. Ryan White, age 13, was infected by a blood transfusion containing HIV. His school prevented him from attending classes, due to unfounded fears of him infecting other students. The case gained much attention, which helped to educate many about HIV. Unfortunately, White died before the Ryan White Comprehensive AIDS Resources Emergency (CARE) Act was passed by Congress (HRSA, 2016), which would have protected him from discrimination.

Globally, in 2018, there were over 37.9 million people living with HIV (Centers for Disease Control and Prevention [CDC], 2021). Twenty-one percent of newly infected people in 2018 were between the ages of 13 and 24 (CDC, 2021). In the 1990s, the addition of protease inhibitors for the treatment of HIV significantly decreased morbidity and mortality of those infected with HIV. Over the past 40 years, with the introduction of prevention options and the advancement of treatments, there are many who view HIV infection as a chronic disease if patients adhere to medication regimens and medical monitoring and visits. However, stigma and discrimination around HIV/AIDS continues across the globe and are the leading barriers to prevention and early treatment (UNAIDS, 2014).

According to the United Nations Programme on HIV/AIDS, "HIV-related stigma refers to the negative beliefs, feelings and attitudes towards people living with HIV, groups associated with people living with HIV (e.g., the families of people living with HIV) and other key populations at higher risk of HIV infection. HIV-related discrimination refers to the unfair and unjust treatment (act or omission) of an individual based on his or her real or perceived HIV status" (UNAIDS, 2014, p. 2). They have been measuring stigma faced by HIV-infected persons internationally for years. The program also guides nations and communities on best practices for reducing the stigma and discrimination facing persons living with or at risk of HIV infection. Emphasis is placed on developing strategies to care for HIV-infected persons and their families, paying close attention to discrimination against women, girls, sex workers, transgenders, and drug users. Programs are targeted to specific groups represented in the community, including families, workplace organizations, and healthcare facilities. Strengthening the legal system to protect the human rights of those infected or at risk of infection with HIV is paramount. Nurse practitioners need to educate their office/clinic staff, colleagues, and communities about the myths and facts of HIV transmission and infection. Maintaining a level of knowledge to most ably serve patients is the best approach, in order to play a part in reducing both the stigma and discrimination fears surrounding HIV/AIDS.

More information on HIV/AIDS is covered in Chapter 8, the Population Health chapter of this book.

Section Three: Developing Population-Based Programs for the Vulnerable

Needs Assessment for a Vulnerable Population

A *needs assessment* is the process of *identifying* and *measuring* areas for improvement in a target population, and determining the methods to achieve improvement. It is different than a list of needs. All of the populations discussed in this chapter, as well as many others not specifically addressed in this book, require initial and periodic assessments of the needs of the population within a certain community. That community may be a local, state, national, or virtual community. For example, it may be within a prison system or a school system. There are different approaches to conducting community needs assessments. All needs assessments begin with target population identification and development of an action plan.

Needs Assessment Framework and Plan

Once you have identified the population of interest, it is necessary to write out the plan, starting with bullet points to develop the framework for the needs assessment. Tasks that need to be considered include the following:

- Formulate a clear description of the population that will be the focus of the needs assessment.
- Create a rationale for why this assessment is being done: What is the purpose and what are the objectives and goals?
- Establish the current problems and the strengths of existing conditions and resources.
- Survey other agencies/organizations in the community to avoid unnecessary overlap in program activities and to identify emerging issues and new resources.
- Interview key informants and community members who have knowledge of or experience with the problem.
- Identify the stakeholders (community members, families, friends, businesses, hospitals, sports organizations, etc.).
- Determine if this needs assessment fits in with a local or state organization's mission and strategic plan. If so, will you be working with someone from that organization in developing and/or implanting the needs assessment?
- Identify who you might collaborate with for best outcomes, if appropriate. For instance, this might require an interprofessional team/committee.

- Discover how the assessment relates to local and global healthcare trends, systems, and policies with the focus on future trends, professional standards, clinical practice guidelines, etc.
- Determine barriers and gaps that exist, to address in the needs assessment.
- Recognize any available resources already in place.

Process Measures

Once you have identified the key issues that the needs assessment will address, it is necessary to decide what process measures will be utilized. For instance, is there a valid survey or questionnaire for data collection, and/or will focus groups be a part of the assessment? Interviews, community forums, public meetings, etc. are all excellent ways to collect information from the community of interest, but you must have the right questions for each key issue that the needs assessment is seeking to assess. Develop a sampling plan for a small pilot group, which will help identify any problem issues that need to be redesigned or addressed prior to the larger sample needs assessment.

Gap Analysis and Results

Using appropriate statistics and analysis for the results of the needs assessment, include the following gap analysis:

- Findings about met and unmet needs from the assessment data
- Information about existing prevention services, resources, funding, and populations served
- Secondary data about availability, accessibility, and appropriateness of existing services for the target population
- Cross reference of needs with existing assets

Consider potential uses of the results; summarize the gap analysis by target population and proposed service needs. Develop an action plan to address the unmet needs of the target population. The action plan should have objectives with corresponding timelines. Short-term, intermediate, and long-term goals should be identified. Recommendations must include budgetary considerations, such as a cost-benefit analysis if appropriate. Be specific, including timelines and people responsible for data collection. Share this information with the key stakeholders and community members to obtain needed support for implementation of the action plan.

Chapter Summary

Given the ever-changing demographic population in the United States and demands for globalization, there is a growing body of knowledge regarding vulnerability and health disparities. Whether your interactions with vulnerable populations is a vocation or an avocation, the rewards are worth the effort put forth to improve the health of those in need. Advocacy is a key role that nurse practitioners can play to benefit patients, families, and communities alike. With advanced education, nurse practitioners have the ability to design, implement, and evaluate individual and population-focused models to ensure that the needs of the vulnerable are met.

Seminar Discussion Questions

1. Which factors make a person or population vulnerable?
2. Is there a specific vulnerable population that you want to learn more about and why?
3. How would you begin developing a needs assessment on a particular vulnerable population?
4. Mary comes in to the urgent care clinic with a broken nose. She appears to be a young teen, perhaps 13 or 14, but says she is 21 years old. She is disheveled and very quiet, answering only with a few words and keeps her eyes downcast. There is a couple (man and woman) who appear to be in their 30s accompanying the girl to be treated. They continue to stare at her and refuse to leave her side. Your attending physician colleague is busy transferring a trauma patient. What are your next steps in specific order?
5. Reach out to an NP working in the prison system or with the homeless. Interview this person about how to approach patients. Does the interviewee deal with legal issues on a daily basis that impede providing health care in the manner preferred?

References

Alegria, C. A. (2011). Transgender identity and health care: Implications for psychosocial and physical evaluation. *Journal of the American Academy of Nurse Practitioners, 23*, 175–182. doi: 10.1111/j.1745-7599.2010.00595.x

American Society of Addiction Medicine. (2019). *Public policy statement: Definition of addiction/short definition of addiction*. Retrieved from https://www.asam.org/docs/default-source/quality-science/asam's-2019-definition-of-addiction-(1).pdf?sfvrsn=b8b64fc2_2

Annie E. Casey Foundation. (2016). *Children of incarcerated parents, a shared sentence: The devastating toll of parental incarceration on kids, families and communities*. Retrieved https://www.aecf.org/resources/a-shared-sentence/

Basch, C. H. (2014). Poverty, health, and social justice: The importance of public health approaches. *International Journal of Health Promotion and Education, 52*(4), 181–187. doi: 10.1080/14635240.2014.894669

Borrowman, M. (2012). Understanding elderly poverty in the U.S.: Alternative measures of elderly deprivation. Schwartz Center for Economic Analysis and Department of Economics, The New School for Social Research, Working Papers Series.

Centers for Disease Control and Prevention. (2013). *Immigrant and refugee health. Refugee health guidelines*. Retrieved from https://www.cdc.gov/immigrantrefugeehealth/guidelines/refugee-guidelines.html

Centers for Disease Control and Prevention. (2017a). *HIV/AIDS*. Retrieved from https://www.cdc.gov/hiv/basics/whatishiv.html

Centers for Disease Control and Prevention. (2017b). QuickStats: Age-adjusted death rates, by race/ethnicity—National Vital Statistics System, United States, 2014–2015. *Morbidity and Mortality Weekly Report, 66*, 375. Retrieved from https://www.cdc.gov/mmwr/volumes/66/wr/mm6613a6.htm

Centers for Disease Control and Prevention. (2017c). *Refugee health profiles*. Retrieved from https://www.cdc.gov/immigrantrefugeehealth/profiles/index.html

Centers for Disease Control and Prevention. (2019). *Vaccination program for US bound refugees*. Retrieved from https://www.cdc.gov/immigrantrefugeehealth/guidelines/overseas/interventions/immunizations-schedules.html

Centers for Disease Control and Prevention. (2020a). *Adverse childhood experiences*. Retrieved from https://www.cdc.gov/violenceprevention/acestudy/about_ace.html

References

Center for Prisoner Health and Human Rights. (2017). *Incarceration in the United States*. Retrieved from http://www.prisonerhealth.org/educational-resources/factsheets-2/incarceration-in-the-united-states/

Clarke, D., Schulman, E., McCollum, D., & Felitti, V. (2015). *Clinical approaches for adult ACE survivors experiencing unexplained physical symptoms and health problems*. Retrieved from http://www.avahealth.org/aces_best_practices/clinical-approaches-for-adults.html

Connors, G. J., & Volk, R. J. (2004). *Self-report screening for alcohol problems among adults*. Retrieved from https://pubs.niaaa.nih.gov/publications/AssessingAlcohol/selfreport.htm

Conway, C. (2016). *UCSF news brief. Poor health: When poverty becomes a disease*. Retrieved from https://www.ucsf.edu/news/2016/01/401251/poor-health

Cubanski, J., Casillas, G., & Damico, A. (2015). Poverty among seniors: An updated analysis of national and state level poverty rates under the official and supplemental poverty measures. *The Henry J. Kaiser Family Foundation*. Retrieved from http://files.kff.org/attachment/issue-brief-poverty-among-seniors-an-updated-analysis-of-national-and-state-level-poverty-rates-under-the-official-and-supplemental-poverty-measures; https://www.healthypeople.gov/2020/data-search/Search-the-Data#topic-area=3499

Daniels, J. (2016). Negotiating the world: Nursing interventions for a vulnerable prison population before and after parole. In M. De Chesnay & B. A. Anderson (Eds.), *Caring for the vulnerable: Perspective in nursing theory, practice, and research* (4th ed.) (chap. 25, pp. 365–380). Sudbury, MA: Jones and Bartlett Publishers.

de Chesnay, M., & Anderson, B. A. (2020). *Caring for the vulnerable: Perspectives in nursing theory, practice, and research*. 5th ed. Sudbury, MA: Jones and Bartlett Publishers.

Ernewein, C., & Nieves, R. (2015). Human sex trafficking: Recognition, treatment, and referral of pediatric victims. *Journal for Nurse Practitioners, 11*(8), 797–803.

Federal Bureau of Prisons. (2021). *Health management resources. Clinical guidelines*. Retrieved from https://www.bop.gov/resources/health_care_mngmt.jsp

Federal Bureau of Prisons. (2021). *Inmate gender*. Retrieved from https://www.bop.gov/about/statistics/statistics_inmate_gender.jsp

Flores, A., Herman, J., Gates, G., & Brown, T. (2016). How many adults identify as transgender in the United States? *The Williams Institute*. Retrieved from https://williamsinstitute.law.ucla.edu/research/how-many-adults-identify-as-transgender-in-the-united-states/

Gorenstein, D. (2016). *Health care takes on the fight against trafficking*. Retrieved from http://www.marketplace.org/2016/03/02/health-care/health-care-takes-fight-against-trafficking

Gottlieb, M. S. (2001). AIDS—Past and future. *New England Journal of Medicine, 344*, 1788–1791.

Grabovschi, C., Loignon, C., & Fortin, M. (2013). Mapping the concept of vulnerability related to health care disparities: A scoping review. *BMC Health Services Research, 13*(1), 1.

Grossman, A. H., & D'Augelli, A. R. (2007). Transgender youth and life-threatening behaviors. *Suicide and Life-Threatening Behavior, 37*, 527–537. doi: 10.1521/suli.2007.37.5.527

Healthy People 2030, U.S. Department of Health and Human Services, Office of Disease Prevention and Health Promotion. Retrieved [cited January, 21, 2021], from https://health.gov/healthypeople/objectives-and-data/social-determinants-health

Homeless Clinician's Network. (2010). *Adapting your practice: General recommendations for the care of homeless patients*, pp. ix–x. Retrieved from http://www.nhchc.org/wp-content/uploads/2011/09/GenRecsHomeless2010.pdf

HRSA. (2016). *About the Ryan White HIV/AIDS program*. Retrieved from https://hab.hrsa.gov/about-ryan-white-hivaids-program/about-ryan-white-hivaids-program

HRSA/Bureau of Primary Health Care. (n.d.). *Health center program terms and definitions*. Retrieved https://www.hrsa.gov/sites/default/files/grants/apply/assistance/Buckets/definitions.pdf

Kaeble, D., & Cowhig, M. (2018). *U.S. Department of Justice: Correctional populations in the United States, 2016*. Retrieved from https://www.bjs.gov/index.cfm?ty=pbdetail&iid=6226

Kaiser Family Foundation. (2017). *The global HIV/AIDS epidemic*. Retrieved from http://www.kff.org/global-health-policy/fact-sheet/the-global-hivaids-epidemic/

Koball, H., Yang, J., et al. (2018). *Basic facts about low-income children. Children under 6 years, 2016*. Retrieved from http://frs.nccp.org/publications/pub_1194.html

Krogstad, J. M. (2019). *Pew Research Center: Key facts about refugees to the U.S*. Retrieved from https://www.pewresearch.org/fact-tank/2019/10/07/key-facts-about-refugees-to-the-u-s/

Kutner, M., Greenberg, E., Jin, Y., & Paulsen, C. (2006). *The health literacy of America's adults: Results from the 2003 National Assessment of Adult Literacy* (NCES 2006–483). U.S. Department of Education. Washington, DC: National Center for Education Statistics.

Marmot, M. (2005). Social determinants of health inequalities. *Lancet, 365,* 1099–1104.

Miles, S. H., & Garcia-Peltoniemi, R. E. (2012). Torture survivors: What to ask, how to document. *Journal of Family Practice, 61*(4), E1–E5.

Montauk, S. L. (2006). The homeless in America: Adapting your practice. *American Family Physician, 74*(7), 1132–1142.

Morris, R., & Vega, C. (2016). Detecting human trafficking: Guidelines for clinicians. *Medscape.* Retrieved from http://www.medscape.org/viewarticle/859358

National Alliance to End Homelessness. (2020). *The of state of homelessness 2020.* Retrieved from https://endhomelessness.org/homelessness-in-america/homelessness-statistics/state-of-homelessness-2020/

National Center for Children in Poverty. (2017). *Child poverty.* Retrieved from http://frs.nccp.org/topics/childpoverty.html

National Health Care for the Homeless Council. (2020a). *What is the official definition of homelessness?* Retrieved from https://nhchc.org/understanding-homelessness/faq/

National Health Care for the Homeless Council. (2020b). *Adapting your practice: Treatment and recommendations for homeless patients.* Retrieved from https://nhchc.org/clinical-practice/adapted-clinical-guidelines/

Orthner, D. (2004). The resilience and strengths of low-income families/Low-income and working-poor families. *Family Relations, 53*(2), S159–S167.

Pacquiao, D. F. (2008). Nursing care of vulnerable populations using a framework of cultural competence, social justice and human rights. *Contemporary Nurse, 28,* 189–197.

Pearson, G. S., Hines-Martin, V. P., Evans, L. K., York, J. A., Kane, C. F., & Yearwood, E. L. (2015). Addressing gaps in mental health needs of diverse, at-risk, underserved, and disenfranchised populations: A call for nursing action. *Archives of Psychiatric Nursing, 29,* 14–18.

Polaris Project. (2016). *2016 Statistics from the National Human Trafficking Hotline and BeFree Textline.* Retrieved from http://www.polarisproject.org/resources/hotline-statistics/human-trafficking-trends-in-the-UnitedStates

Rahim, Z. (2017). Canadian baby given health card without sex designation. *CNN.* Retrieved from http://www.cnn.com/2017/07/04/health/canadian-baby-gender-designation/index.html

Schmider, A. (2016). 2016 was the deadliest year on record for transgender people. *GLADD.* Retrieved from https://www.glaad.org/blog/2016-was-deadliest-year-record-transgender-people

Septowitz, K. (2001). AIDS—The first 20 years. *New England Journal of Medicine, 344,* 1764–1772. doi:10.1056/NEJM200106073442306. Retrieved from http://www.nejm.org/doi/full/10.1056/NEJM200106073442306#t=article

Shannon, P., O' Dougherty, M., & Mehta, E. (2012). Refugees' perspectives on barriers to communication about trauma histories in primary care. *Mental Health in Family Medicine, 9,* 47–55.

Statista Research Department. (2021). *Poverty rate in the US by age and gender in 2019.* Retrieved from https://www.statista.com/statistics/233154/us-poverty-rate-by-gender/#:~:text=In%202019%2C%20the%20poverty%20rate,65%20and%2074%20years%20old

Substance Abuse and Mental Health Services Administration (SAMHSA). (2020). *Key substance use and mental health indicators in the United States: Results from the 2019 national survey on drug use and health.* Retrieved from https://www.samhsa.gov/data/sites/default/files/reports/rpt29393/2019NSDUHFFRPDFWHTML/2019NSDUHFFR1PDFW090120.pdf

UNAIDS. (2014). *Reduction of HIV-related stigma and discrimination.* Retrieved from http://www.unaids.org/sites/default/files/media_asset/2014unaidsguidancenote_stigma_en.pdf

United Nations High Commissioner for Refugees. (2016). *Global trends: Forced displacement in 2016.* Retrieved http://www.unhcr.org/en-us/statistics/unhcrstats/5943e8a34/global-trends-forced-displacement-2016.html

United Nations High Commissioner for Refugees. (2017). *Statistical year book 2015.* Retrieved from http://www.unhcr.org/en-us/statistics/country/59b294387/unhcr-statistical-yearbook-2015-15th-edition.html

U.S. Census Bureau (2020). *Income and Poverty in the United States: 2019.* Retrieved from https://www.census.gov/library/publications/2020/demo/p60-270.html

U.S. Department of Health and Human Services. (2020). *Office of Disease Prevention and Health Promotion health literacy resources quick guide to health literacy*. Retrieved from https://health.gov/our-work/health-literacy/resources

U.S. Department of Health and Human Services, Office on Trafficking in Persons. (2017). *What is human trafficking?* Retrieved from https://www.acf.hhs.gov/otip/about/what-is-human-trafficking

U.S. Department of State. (2021). *The reception and placement program*. Retrieved from https://www.state.gov/refugee-admissions/reception-and-placement/

U.S. Preventative Services Task Force. (2020). *Recommendation topics: A & B recommendations*. Retrieved from https://www.uspreventiveservicestaskforce.org/uspstf/recommendation-topics/uspstf-and-b-recommendations?DESC=1&SORT=D

Warne, D., & Lajimodiere, D. (2015). *American Indians health disparities: Psychosocial influences*. Hoboken, NJ: John Wiley & Sons, Ltd.

World Health Organization. (2017). *Social determinants of health*. Retrieved from http://www.who.int/social_determinants/en/

CHAPTER 5

Mental Health and Primary Care: A Critical Intersection

Anna Goddard and Sara Ann Jakub

Nurse practitioners (NP) are core components to the healthcare team and are more often in primary care provider roles throughout the United States. As primary care providers, NPs can utilize their role as patient advocate, educator, and clinician to comprehensively care for both physical and mental healthcare needs. Mental health and psychosocial morbidities are now surpassing physical health issues, including asthma and diabetes. Several factors contribute to this shift, such as family instability and malfunctioning, stigma associated with mental health, access to care and reimbursement issues, lack of screening, and genetics. The long-standing traumatic impacts from the COVID-19 global crisis, including isolation, loss of financial resources, and overall disruption to life pre-pandemic will be investigated for years to come. Experts have warned that the mental-health effects from COVID-19 will be the "second pandemic" (Owings-Fonner, 2020).

Meanwhile, there is a growing, critical shortage of mental health specialists, especially in child and adolescent psychiatry, with less than < 8,000 providers nationwide, which significantly impedes the ability to meet mental health needs across the nation (Block, 2011; Hornor, 2015; Riddle, 2016). Primary care providers have continued to meet and fill this need as mental health severity has increased over the last decades. Primary care NPs are ideally suited to assist with many of these needs based on their extensive knowledge base and long-term relationships with families. Several national governing and professional bodies such as the American Academy of Pediatrics (AAP), the American Academy of Family Physicians (AFP), the American Association of Nurse Practitioners (AANP), and National Association of Pediatric Nurse Practitioners (NAPNAP) recognize the need to integrate these core essentials of mental health management to ongoing licensing and certification to practice in the field. As value-based care payor systems continue to evolve across the U.S. healthcare system, accountable care organizations have incentivized providing quality mental healthcare screening and management to include evidence-based mental health treatment of patients in primary care.

NP Role in Holistic Care

Behavioral and mental health pathophysiology result in physical, health-related outcomes across a person's lifetime (Anda et al., 2010; Hughes et al., 2017). Historically, in primary care, mental health difficulties were referred out to specialists once identified; these clear delineations between "medical" and "mental health" care have continually diminished over time. NPs must bridge the gap between care with emphasis on integration of the medical and mental health disciplines. This blending of mental health and medical care has required a paradigm shift for many disciplines previously grounded in a division in the mental health field, as well as medical needs in patient care. As the holistic care approach became a critical component of patient-centered care, a continuous shift occurred in training, preparation, and the approach to patients, including a trauma-informed lens with considerations for mental and behavioral health assessment, diagnoses, and management.

Many NPs work as primary care providers as the first-line defense in health maintenance and promotion, disease prevention and diagnosis, and treatment plan management for illness. More than 25% or 1:4 people in the United States have a mental health disorder (National Institute of Mental Health (NIMH, 2021). Early detection of behavioral and mental health concerns becomes critical in preventing future mental health illnesses. The limited amount of mental health resources in the country further contributes to the need for primary care providers to identify, assess, and manage mental health concerns. This said, the NP must have the self-awareness and mindfulness to know when a patient's evaluation or treatment requires knowledge or skills beyond their own training and knowledge base, necessitating referral to another provider for care. However, even when referral to a higher-level of psychiatric services are required, the NP can still play a supportive role in primary care–based psychoeducation, care coordination for comorbidities, and providing community connections and a network for optimal care.

The *Diagnostic and Statistical Manual of Mental Disorders (DSM)*, now in its fifth edition, is a practice handbook that provides healthcare professionals with information on descriptions, systems, and other criteria for diagnosing mental disorders (American Psychiatric Association, 2013). The DSM-V is considered the common language for all healthcare clinicians to make reliable diagnoses and is also used for criteria in ICD-10 coding for billing health claims. Understanding and being able to utilize the DSM-V is an important component of being able to manage mental health concerns in primary care. Risk assessment and learning to evaluate risk are key components for safe, clinical practice. NPs must continue to widen their knowledge base to include competency in managing mental illness symptomatology.

Health Disparities

Little agreement exists in defining and quantifying health disparities or in what qualifies as a disparity in health care, because each entity alters the definition to fit their focus (Carter-Pokras & Baquet, 2002; Smedley & Nelson, 2003). The Centers for Disease Control and Prevention (CDC) provides the most unifying of these agency-specific definitions and considers mental health disparities as "disparities present within the field of public health, health systems, and society" that often fall into one of the following categories: (1) disparities between the attention given mental health and that given to other public health issues of comparable magnitude, (2) disparities between the health of persons with mental illness as compared with that of those without, or (3) disparities between populations with respect to mental health and the quality, accessibility, and outcomes of mental health care (CDC, 2013). Additionally, leading experts often discuss health disparities in relation to social determinants, such as employment, income, housing, and so on, which can influence mental health and access to care (Saffron et al., 2009).

Health disparities are historically tied to inequities in healthcare delivery, often to marginalized communities, and exist in groups of people regarding their level of wellness. Therefore, variants found to trend in one group of people's physical or mental presentation are *health disparities* regardless of the source. Whereas health disparities do not aid in the causal analysis, they are the first essential step in being able to later remedy incongruences in health functioning, specifically in mental health care.

Slight dissimilarities are normative within a group, while individual presentations with health issues and health may vary. Every human is unique; however, NPs can aid their understanding of symptomology by learning what trends are at increased likelihood to occur in various populations. It is important, however, not to utilize such information regarding health disparities typical for one subset as an absolute, resulting in stereotyping and causing notable contradictory evidence in the assessment process.

The general population in America lives 20–30 years longer than adults who have a severe mental health disease, largely due to chronic medical conditions, including pulmonary disease, pneumonia or influenza, lung cancer, diabetes, and cardiovascular disease (NIMH, 2021; Tepper et al., 2017). These comorbidities exist in conjunction with known correlates to mental illness such as substance use, food insecurity, physical consequences to sustained psychotropic medication usage, and adversity. Although chronic health disease tends toward higher use of the healthcare system, individuals with significant mental health disease are 41% more likely to report unmet medical needs (Tepper et al., 2017).

While racial/ethnic minorities in the United States have similar rates of mental health diagnoses, as a group they are more impacted by the negative consequences associated with mental illness. Evidence of the inequitable and higher burden that ethnic minorities face includes higher rates of depression among Blacks (24.6%) and Hispanics (19.6%), with more persistence in duration than white counterparts (NIMH, 2021). Individuals who identify as being of two or more races (24.9%) are most likely to report any mental illness within the past year than any other race/ethnic group, with the second-highest group to exhibit mental health issues being American Indian/Alaska Natives (22.7%), who in turn also report the highest rates of alcohol and post-traumatic stress disorder (PTSD) (APA, 2021). The APA (2021) identified the following barriers for individuals seeking care for mental illness with a greater impact on members of diverse ethnic/racial groups: language barriers, distrust in care systems overall, stigma, no insurance or being underinsured, insufficient safety net support, and absence of diversity and/or culturally competent providers of mental health care.

Continued work toward reducing the barriers to adequate care across all groups, regardless of ethnic/racial identity, is continuously needed for as long as health disparities exist. Health disparities do not exist in a bubble, capable of differentiation between "nature" (genetic) or "nurture" (environmental) causes. Factors exist in our communal, political and environmental structures that influence genetic underpinnings to health in a symbiotic way. Upon identification of an inequitable health-wellness status, a shift toward seeking an immediate remedy is normative. However, solutions vary greatly depending on the specific catalyst(s) for the disparity (Dubiel et al., 2010).

Social Determinants of Health

Social Determinants of Health (SDOH) are conditions in the places we live, learn, work, and play that affect a wide range of health and quality-of-life risks and outcomes (U.S. Department of Health and Human Services [USDHHS], 2020). In the 2008 World Health Organization (WHO) report *"Closing the gap in a generation: Health equity through action on the social determinants of health"* the importance of creating a "more level playing field" in socially driven health outcomes across the world was emphasized and in line with the USDHHS and CDC goals to address determinants of health and mitigating factors through *Health People 2030*.

The USDHHS categorizes SDOH in five main domains that aid in understanding the wide breadth of social factors that impact human health and well-being (**Figure 5-1**).

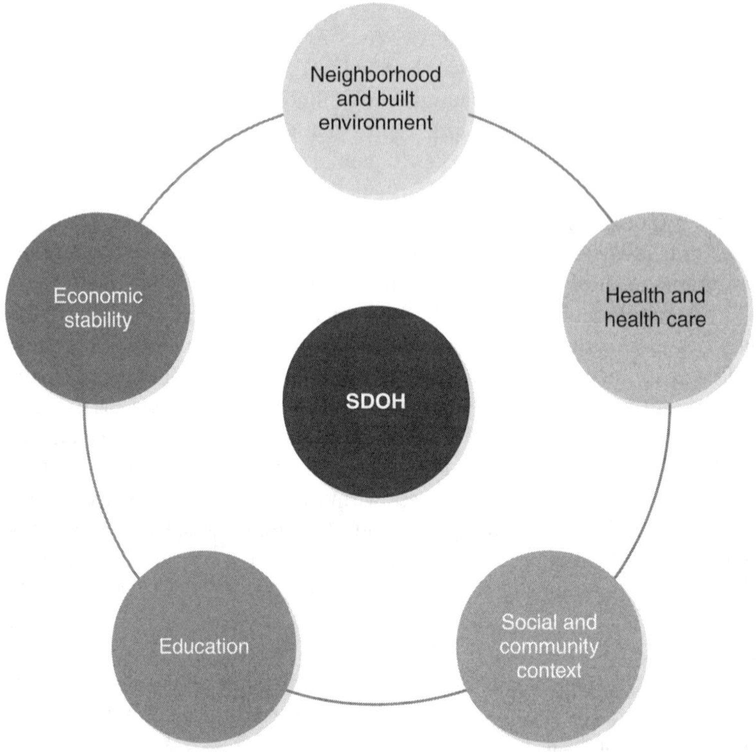

Figure 5-1 The Five Domains of the Social Determinants of Health

U.S. Department of Health and Human Services. (2020). Healthy People objectives: Overview. Retrieved from https://www.healthypeople.gov/2020/topics-objectives/topic/social-determinants-of-health

The five domains of the SDOH are:

1. **Economic Stability:** poverty, housing instability, food insecurity
2. **Education Access and Quality:** high school education, enrollment in higher education, early childhood development and education, language and literacy
3. **HealthCare Access and Quality:** health literacy, access to primary care, access to health services
4. **Neighborhood and Built Environment:** quality of housing, environmental conditions, crime and violence, access to food that helps support healthy eating patterns
5. **Social and Community Context:** social cohesion, incarceration, discrimination, civic participation

Given the vast and differing lives of individuals and environmental interactions, it is essential to evaluate SDOH in parallel. Because people are complex, the evaluation of SDOH factors on each unique individual is essential for improved patient care outcomes. Societal institutions, including family and peers, are typical sources in the creation of social norms for which humans evaluate their social standing and, to an extent, their communal value. This social and community network becomes pivotal, through which the individual gains access or exposure to risk and health behaviors. For example, the likelihood of alcohol use increases if a person resides with an individual who has a pattern of heavy alcohol consumption (Rosenquist et al., 2010). Access to even the general opportunities for healthy development remains influenced by one's social context.

The human body may become more physically sensitive in stressful social situations to those who have experienced systemic or repeated discrimination, thus resulting in increased risk of emotional distress and vulnerability to illness (Guyll et al., 2001). Increased exposure to adversity increases the likelihood of experiencing physical stress, with corresponding mental health–stressed emotional responses, such as depression and anxiety. For example, adolescents who identify as lesbian, gay, bisexual, or trans (LGBT) exhibit increased incidents of depression, self-harm, and suicidality than their heterosexually identified peers, which correlates with the societal stigmatization of sexual identity (Almeida et al., 2009).

Multiple aspects of SDOH connect to mental health functioning and overall wellness. When primary needs such as food, water, shelter, love, and connection are in constant jeopardy, this directly affects the human ability to cope with life's adversities. Exposure to sustained community and interpersonal violence in childhood remains linked to aftereffects in adulthood, with increased risks for substance use, anxiety, depression, and behavioral dysregulation compared to children with only moderate exposure to violence (Margolin et al., 2010). The role of society and the influences inherent within it are not to be discounted as both a possible source of great support and a potential barrier to wellness.

What Is Mental Health?

Mental health has been defined as "a state of well-being in which an individual realizes his or her own abilities, can cope with the normal stresses of life, can work productively and is able to make a contribution to his or her community" (WHO, 2018). One might assume the absence of mental health results in mental illness;

however, the relationship is not that easily causational. Evaluation of mental health is best done through the mindset of a spectrum, with levels of wellness that can be variable over periods. Attempts to measure the level of mental health in the past include scales such as the Global Assessment of Functioning (GAF) where clinicians scored patients 0 (low) to 100 (high), which has been eliminated along with the previous Axis IV from the previous DSM-IV edition. The GAF scale has since been replaced by The World Health Organization Disability Assessment Schedule 2.0 (WHODAS 2.0), which incorporates questions regarding functioning levels in multiple domains to an accumulative score (APA, 2013; Gold, 2014).

What Is Mental Illness?

Mental illness is not the absence of mental health. In the DSM-V, the APA (2013) explains mental illness as "health conditions involving changes in emotion, thinking or behavior (or a combination of these)." Mental illnesses are associated with distress and/or problems functioning in social, work, or family activities. However, the DSM-V cautions users of the manual to refrain from diagnosis simply based on symptom expression, and demand additional assessment for how those diagnostic symptoms actually impact functioning (APA, 2013). Differentiation between mind and body during the assessment process is difficult at best, and considered impossible for most, as the greatest of diagnosticians benefit from a holistic mindset.

Human behavior is complex. It is not easily quantified into perfect categories, given the vast differences found between individuals, including level of insight, motivating factors, and cultural considerations, to name just a few. Endeavors to understand, define, and categorize mental illness has been an active undertaking for many generations. The fifth edition of the DSM, breaking away from the previous axial system, presents a hierarchical structure of diagnosis in order of significance and prioritization listing, to indicate the focus of treatment. Additionally, each mental health diagnosis in the DSM-5 now correlates to the WHO's International Classification of Diseases (ICD-10). In the ICD-10 (2019), section V offers mental and behavioral disorders labeled with F-codes for further differentiation.

> F00-F09 Organic, including symptomatic, mental disorders.
>
> F10-F19 Mental and behavioral disorders due to psychoactive substance use
>
> F20-F29 Schizophrenia, schizotypal and delusional disorders
>
> F30-F39 Mood [affective] disorders
>
> F40-F48 Neurotic, stress-related and somatoform disorders
>
> F50-F59 Behavioral syndromes associated with physiological disturbances and physical factors
>
> F60-F69 Disorders of adult personality and behavior
>
> F70-F79 Mental retardation
>
> F80-F89 Disorders of psychological development
>
> F90-F98 Behavioral and emotional disorders, with onset usually occurring in childhood and adolescence
>
> F99-F99 Unspecified mental disorder

F00* Dementia in Alzheimer disease

F02* Dementia in other diseases classified elsewhere

Cultural differences between diagnosticians and patients can influence the clinical interview, perceptions about appropriate treatment approaches, diagnosis in general, and the impact levels of adherence to treatment interventions (APA, 2013). The DSM-5 intends to maintain a continual progression of updates and future revisions, through the use of a task force with leading experts and research, with the aim of hopefully improving the classification system that practitioners utilize in order to diagnose mental health disorders appropriately. As with most endeavors in research, the assessment and classification practices of mental health disease have improved with time, and the DSM is a living document in constant evolution. Practitioners are encouraged to obtain and review the DSM in its entirety. The main sections of diagnoses in the DSM-5 include:

Neurodevelopmental Disorders

Schizophrenia Spectrum and Other Psychotic Disorders

Bipolar and Related Disorders

Depressive Disorders

Anxiety Disorders

Obsessive-Compulsive and Related Disorders

Trauma- and Stressor-Related Disorders

Dissociative Disorders

Somatic Symptom and Related Disorders

Feeding and Eating Disorders

Sleep-Wake Disorders

Sexual Dysfunctions

Gender Dysphoria

Disruptive, Impulse-Control, and Conduct Disorders

Substance-Related and Addictive Disorders

Neurocognitive Disorders

Personality Disorders

Paraphilic Disorders

Other Mental Disorders

Medication-Induced Movement Disorders and Other Adverse Effects of Medication

Other Conditions That May Be the Focus of Clinical Attention (z-codes)

The most common mental illnesses in a primary care setting include depressive disorders, bipolar disorders, anxiety disorders, and substance abuse, all of which the NP should be familiar with.

Depressive Disorders

Depressive disorders are marked by a presentation of continual depressed mood, with negative tones in the expression of emotion (affect) often, or a decrease in interest/pleasure in the activities of life. Clinical depression is not simply a sad day or period, but rather influences one's perception of their world, negatively alters their thinking and memory patterns, as well as physically, affecting chronic inflammation within the body, to include sleep and diet disturbances (APA, 2013). The depressive disorders impact the individual's ability to find joy in life activities, as well as motivation for connection and social interactions, often leading to social isolation (Steger et al., 2009). Depressive features with an acute grief response is normative in some instances; diagnosticians should also be keen to assess for potential manic, hypo-manic, or mixed-episodes with initial presentation in a depressive state. Cultural considerations include presentation and symptom expression over-prevalence, because some ethnic and racial groups describe emotional pain and depressed mood differently than others. The NP should recognize that many cases of depression go unnoticed in cultures that describe mental health issues in physical terms, because somatic symptoms may be more likely the presenting complaint (APA, 2013).

Types of depressive disorders include disruptive mood dysregulation disorder (DMDD), major depressive disorder, persistent depressive disorder (dysthymia), pre-menstrual dysphoric disorder, substance/medication-induced depressive disorder, depressive disorder due to another medical condition, other specified depressive disorder, unspecified depressive disorder.

Bipolar and Related Disorders

Bipolar disorders are characterized by mood disturbances that are cyclical, with "two poles" that oscillate in episodes from depression to mania. The two most notable types of bipolar disorder, bipolar I and bipolar II, essentially differ in the range between the poles and whether or not a full manic episode has occurred. *Bipolar I disorder* defined by manic episodes that last at least 7 days, or by manic (abnormally elevated mood) symptoms that are severe. Depressive episodes (see major depressive disorder above) occur as well, typically lasting at least 2 weeks, with the possibility of mixed features of the two poles occurring at the same time. Whereas *bipolar II disorder* still has a pattern of episodes of depressive episodes, it is without "full blown" manic episodes, these being replaced by hypomanic episodes (APA, 2013). Manic and hypomanic symptoms include increased impulsivity, decreased need for sleep, racing thoughts and pressed speech in combination with more goal-directed activities that tend toward increasingly irrational decision making than outside of the episode. However, individuals diagnosed with bipolar disorder endorse more significant depressive symptoms than those with unipolar depressive disorders and are more frequently endorse those symptoms as disruptors to quality of life (work, family, etc.) than manic symptoms (Hirschfeld et al., 2003).

Types of bipolar disorders include bipolar I disorder, bipolar II disorder, cyclothymic disorder, substance/medication-indicated bipolar and related disorder, bipolar and related disorder due to another medical condition, other specified bipolar and related disorder, and unspecified bipolar and related disorder.

Anxiety Disorders

Anxiety disorders are rooted in fear in response to a perceived likely threat and apprehension in the form of overwhelming anticipation of future negative events. The autonomic response processes of "fight," "flight," or "freeze" in response to danger, that is perceived to be unavoidable, can result in both avoidance responses of anxiety triggers and their approximations, as well as panic. The DSM-5 highlights how anxiety disorders differ from healthy apprehension to a known stressor, by evaluation of normative developmental responses, as well as in the severity of both levels of anxiety and their duration (APA, 2013). While panic is not an official diagnosis, diagnosticians should also be aware of the availability to add the "panic attack specifier" to a diagnosis within the anxiety disorders category in the DSM.

Criteria for anxiety disorders include intrusive worried thoughts, excessive distress, and complaints of somatic symptoms such as headache, stomachache, nausea and/or vomiting; and with panic, hyperventilation (APA, 2013). Individuals with generalized anxiety disorder (GAD) are less likely to graduate college, and ultimately earn less wages in life (Katzelnick, 2001). Cultural considerations include a higher incidence of GAD in populations that place higher emphasis on cognition rather than physicality. Women are also more likely to experience comorbid anxiety and depression, often comorbid with substance abuse disorders (APA, 2013).

Types of anxiety disorders include separation anxiety disorder, selective mutism, specific phobia, social anxiety disorder (social phobia), panic disorder, agoraphobia, generalized anxiety disorder, substance/medication-induced anxiety disorder, anxiety disorder due to another medical condition, other specified anxiety disorder, and unspecified anxiety disorder.

Substance-Related and Addictive Disorders

The DSM-5 categorizes substance-related and addictive disorders in a separate section from the remaining mental health disorders, but does reference comorbidity with substance abuse for several other illnesses. Substance abuse and mental health are further correlated, in that one can trigger the other, often recognized as a "self-medication" for mental health symptoms (Henwood & Padgett, 2007). Substance-related and addictive disorders include dependence on a drug, periods of intoxication, lack of control in cessation, and in most cases withdrawal symptoms that significantly impact functioning (APA, 2013). Quality treatment includes connection with psychosocial supports, such as family interventions, case management, and collaborative wrap-around support services. Previously referred to as "dual-diagnoses" (individuals with both a mental health and substance abuse diagnosis) require psychoeducational approaches as a baseline standard in treatment (APA, 2013; Henwood & Padgett, 2007).

Types of substance-related and addictive disorders include alcohol-related disorders; caffeine-related disorders; cannabis-related disorders; hallucinogen-related disorders; inhalant-related disorders; opioid-related disorders; sedative-, hypnotic-, or anxiolytic-related disorders; stimulant-related disorders; tobacco-|related disorders; other (or unknown) substance-related disorders; and non-substance-related disorders (gambling disorder).

Suicide

Suicidality, defined as "recurrent thoughts of death (not just the fear of dying), recurrent suicidal ideation without a specific plan, or a suicide attempt or a specific plan for committing suicide" is one of the possible symptom expressions for individuals with a major depressive disorder amongst other diagnoses (APA, 2013). A full assessment of suicidal risk is essential for individuals presenting with outwardly noticeable depressive symptoms. The World Health Organization (WHO) names suicide as the second-leading cause of death in the second and third decade of life, and mental health disorders as the primary catalyst to which depression, substance abuse, psychosis, anxiety, personality disorders, trauma, and eating disorders are most commonly linked (Bachmann, 2018). While the prevalence of suicidality is often daunting to the clinician, with effective screening, assessment, and safety planning it can be addressed. Best practices for primary care providers include routine screening for depression and suicidality, ranging anywhere from annually to as frequently as each visit.

In line with the administration of the Patient History Questionnaire (PHQ-9) and the Columbia Suicide Severity Rating Scale (C-SSRS), a suicidal risk evaluation should include the following questions framed in an age and culturally appropriate language (Kroenke & Spitzer, 2002; Mundt et al., 2013).

1. Do you ever wish you were dead?
2. Do you think about killing yourself?

A "No" response to Question 1 or Question 2 = remaining questions unnecessary
A "Yes" response to Question 1 or Question 2 = engage in ALL the questions

1. Do you have a plan to kill yourself?
2. Do you have means to carry out that plan?
3. Do you intend to carry out the plan to kill yourself?

If Yes to #1 and #2 but all answers are "No" practitioners are to collaborate with the patient, and the caregiver when applicable, on a safety plan (including coping skills, reduction in exposure to triggers, and emergency contact numbers). The inability to execute a safety plan necessitates a mental health professional's assessment for possible hospitalization.

"Yes" responses to any of the subsequent questions (# 3, #4, or # 5) require an immediate assessment by a mental health professional. If a mental health provider is not immediately accessible in an outpatient setting, calling emergency services or having the patient transported to the Emergency Department (ED) would be an appropriate treatment intervention.

Screening

The National Association of Mental Illness (NAMI) has strongly recommended early mental health screening in both the primary care office and in schools. Medical providers are now required to incorporate annual risk assessments for depression, anxiety, and substance use as part of the annual physical exams and are included as defining quality metrics and standards from many professional bodies such as the Agency for Healthcare Research and Quality (AHRQ) and the Centers for Medicaid and Medicare (CMS). In fact, Medicaid now requires screening all Medicaid-eligible children for mental health conditions as a federal mandate under the Early and Periodic Screening, Diagnosis, and Treatment (EPSDT).

Use of screening tools to identify populations at risk for mental health disorders have been implemented in most outpatient and emergency/urgent care facilities as a normative practice. Entities providing psychiatric care must have standard office procedures of their employees around the management of common mental health concerns, as well as a referral guide for mental health services in the community. Identification of informational materials to be used for patients will also be critical, as well as keeping these educational materials updated.

The NIH (2021) calls for routine follow-up surveillance questions with patients to include: (1) "Since the last time I saw you, has anything really scary or upsetting happened to you or your family?" and (2) "Are there times that you worry you won't have enough food to eat or a safe place to stay?" as a start to universal screening for safe environments (Lane et al., 2011). Successful triaging from subsequent screening will be an essential part of any evaluation for mental health concerns. Oftentimes, referral for psychiatric emergencies will be required for emergency evaluations and subsequent treatment. For instance, suicidality, serious threats of violence to others, psychosis, acute substance intoxication, and withdrawal will most likely require emergency referral. Screening will also require consideration for social emergencies that might arise, and clinicians must be willing and able to act on these presentations. Sexual or physical abuse, threat or violence to a child, or family social circumstances that might threaten the well-being or safety of the patient such as domestic violence will require community referrals and mandatory reporting to child and family protective services (Lane et al., 2011).

There are dozens of valid and reliable mental health screening tools available for the NP. While this abundance exists, some screening tools are more reliably used in primary care often due to cost (free to use), ease in utilization, and ongoing evidence-based literature supporting certain screens over others. Ultimately, the NP should be familiar with the screening tools operationalized in the practice in which they work and practice.

Use of the Mental Status Exam

The mental status exam (MSE) is an indispensable tool for the NP and can additionally be used in the assessment of mental illness. The MSE, most often used in the clinical assessment process in neurological and psychiatric disciplines, includes both historical self-report information from the patient as well as observational data from the practitioner. Utilization of the MSE informs on patient functioning level and correlates to various DSM disorders in its ability to distinguish between diagnostic criteria. The MSE aids in continual assessment of functionality, including if symptoms are stable, improving, or worsening. Specific MSE categories can inform to the level of risk for harm to self and others (e.g., thought content including suicidal ideation), while others indicate the capacity of the patient to mitigate possible risk factors or engage in safety planning (e.g., perceptual disturbances including hallucinations) (Snyderman & Rovner, 2009). Included in a mental status exam are items such as homicidal ideation (HI), suicidal ideation (SI), and self-injurious-behavior (SIB). However, once identified, a full risk assessment must be completed.

Complete mental status exams include assessment of a patient on the following 10 criteria: (1) appearance and general behavior, (2) motor activity, (3) speech, (4) mood and affect, (5) thought process, (6) thought content, (7) perceptual disturbances, (8) sensorium and cognition, (9) insight, and (10) judgment.

🔍 CASE STUDY ONE

Cheyenne is a 20-year-old, biracial (African-American and Native American) biologic female, identifies as male, prefers "he/him" pronouns, and resides in a socioeconomically depressed rural community. Cheyenne visits his primary care provider with complaints of poor sleep, intermittent insomnia, and loss of appetite. He completes the Patient History Questionnaire-2 (PHQ-2), indicating he's feeling "down" and in a low mood today and over the last several weeks, triggering completion of the PHQ-9 full questionnaire, in which he also endorsed difficulties concentrating, and thoughts of death. Upon further inquiry, Cheyenne denies active intent to kill himself, citing passive suicidal ideation, "wanting the hurt to stop" in reference to emotional pain from negative responses in response to his gender expression. The assessment indicates that while not currently in imminent risk of suicide, he meets the criteria of a depressive episode. His provider creates a safety plan with him and recommends mental health counseling to manage his depressed mood and prevent escalation of his suicidal risk. If medication management with an antidepressant is deemed appropriate, prescribers would always need to closely monitor for possible manic episodes in case bipolar disorder is emerging with an initial presentation of depression.

Management, Treatment, and Referrals Considerations

Treatment interventions should always include non-medication-based treatments such as guidance, referrals for support and community connections, and evidence-based psychotherapy. While some states allow for full autonomous practice under an APRN license, autonomy does not equal collaboration and consultation in treatment. Patients who have additional mental health concerns are a prime example. The NP should routinely consult on issues beyond the expertise of their own skill-repertoire to include collaboration with psychiatric APRNs who are trained, licensed, and certified in psychiatric care.

Counseling patients, with "talk therapy," remains the primary "prescription" for treatment of mental disorders. Out of the vast modalities of counseling known to exist, those that are evidenced-based, including cognitive behavioral therapy (CBT) and motivational interviewing (MI) demonstrate repeatedly the effectiveness in addressing the most common mental health issues, such as anxiety, depression, substance abuse, and trauma (APA, 2013; Laker, 2007; Riddle, 2016; Snyderman & Rovner, 2009). In a meta-analysis evaluating psychopharmacology effectiveness against CBT for the treatment for anxiety and depression, CBT demonstrated a statistically significant effect overall on anxiety disorders, as well as panic and obsessive-compulsive disorders, with notable advantages in the treatment of depression (Roshanaei-Moghaddam et al., 2011).

Motivational Interviewing (MI) has specifically established credibility in the treatment of substance abuse disorders, including supporting the stages of change models of treatment (Laker, 2007). CBT and MI as a combined approach can further improve outcomes, including reduction in treatment drop-out and overall symptom reduction in the treatment of anxiety disorders, supported by a 2018 meta-analysis of the research literature (Marker & Norton, 2018). Evidence-based interventions such as MI allow for positive engagement with patients currently substance abusing-dependent, many of whom are not currently accessible to a complete abstinence approach (Laker, 2007). Primary care providers are more likely to encounter individuals at various "readiness levels" to addressing addition, and this is considered a normative phase within the substance abuse cycle.

Sometimes, combining psychotropic medication with therapy is needed, especially for ADHD, common anxiety disorders (separation anxiety disorder, social phobia, generalized anxiety disorder), and depression. Evidence from decades of research have consistently found that medication alone does not provide the best treatment when not combined with psychotherapy (Riddle, 2016). Psychotropic medication prescribing in the primary care setting can be safe and effective. However, it must follow key domains, including diagnosis of the disorder, medication, dosing and monitoring parameters, capacity and comfort of the prescriber, and the system of care. The diagnosis in which the patient is seeking care should be sufficiently common for a primary care provider to manage versus a psychiatrist or psychiatric APRN. Furthermore, the diagnosis must be accurate for medication to safely and efficaciously help the patient. Dosing and monitoring of the prescribed medications must be done, including regular, scheduled follow-up appointments, where somatic complaints and vital signs (including height and weight) are monitored.

Trauma

Trauma- and stressor-related disorders in the DSM-5 are the only category of mental health diagnoses that require the prior occurrence of a significant external negative event, and where the occurrence is the source of negative impact on the patient's own symptomology (APA, 2013). Negative life experiences occur all the time as a normative function of life in general. Lay people often utilize the word "trauma" to indicate undesirable situations overall. Trauma as a diagnosis, however, is characterized by a set of responses to highly negative experiences that are perceived to likely result in grave danger, or bring irrevocable harm to self or bystanders. Trauma responses are the human body's best defense system against danger, although when those responses persist, beyond immediate responses for safety, it becomes unsustainable to maintain, and unhelpful for overall functioning (Alexandra et al., 2005; Schick et al., 2013).

Trauma can often be mistaken and misdiagnosed as a variety of disorders, such as ADHD, oppositional behavior, anxiety, depression, bipolar disorder, personality disorders, and somatoform disorders. However, trauma predisposes and contributes to the development of these disorders, so it can be difficult to diagnose and requires close attention to the biopsychosocial history of the individual. For instance, children who are experiencing ongoing trauma and are unable to defend themselves will often present with detachment, numbing, compliance, and fantasy, which often will look like depression, ADHD-inattentive type, and developmental delay (Perry, 2002). Whereas witnesses to violence with ongoing activation of the autonomic nervous system with the "fight, flight, or freeze" response often creates hypervigilance, aggression, anxiety, and other exaggerated responses and are misdiagnosed as ADHD, OCD, conduct disorder, bipolar disorder, and anger management difficulties (Perry, 2002). Evaluation of the family system aids providers in identifying supports, protective factors, as well as the possible risk for mental health disease, including trauma (Schnick et al., 2013). The DSM-5 recognizes several types of trauma- and stressor-related disorders, including reactive attachment disorder disinhibited social engagement disorder, post-traumatic stress disorder, acute stress disorder, adjustment disorders, other specified trauma- and stressor-related disorders, and unspecified trauma- and stressor-related disorders.

Trauma additionally has devastating effects on child development and in acquiring milestones, including tantrums varying from mild to severe, aggression with siblings or other children, and parental detachment (Perry, 2002). School-aged children and adolescents often present with difficulty in skill acquisition, short-term memory loss and difficulty with remembering details, fighting, classroom disruptions, and difficulty with academic schoolwork (Alexandra et al., 2019). SDOH have been found in different populations and are at higher risk of experiencing Adverse Childhood Events (ACEs), which are the precursor events to trauma, due to the social and economic conditions in which they live, learn, work, and play (Block, 2011).

Adverse Childhood Experiences

Adverse childhood experiences (ACEs) is the umbrella term to describe abuse, neglect, and traumatic experiences that occur under the age of 18 years old, now recognized as a public health crisis (Anda et al., 2010). Between 1995–1997, the seminal CDC-Kaiser Permanente Health Appraisal Clinic completed the original ACEs study, where researchers reviewed childhood experiences and current health status and behaviors (Felitti et al., 1998). This study is now recognized as the largest investigation of childhood abuse, neglect, and household dysfunctions, connecting later life health and well-being in adulthood to traumas from childhood. In the original analysis from this study, more than two-thirds of participants reported at least one ACE, with 20% of participants reporting three or more ACEs. The original identified ACES are abuse (physical, emotional, sexual), neglect (physical, emotional), and household dysfunction (mental illness, mother treated violently, divorce, an incarcerated relative, and substance abuse). However, decades of research have now identified additional recognized ACEs, including school and community violence, forced displacements, war, terrorism, political violence, and natural disasters including death and disease, such as COVID-19 (Anda et al., 2006; Burke et al., 2011; Dube et al., 2001; Zarse et al., 2019). More than 10,000 studies have cited the original Kaiser Permanente ACE study, with bodies of research continuing to show the dose–response relationship between higher ACE scores, resulting in higher health outcome risks (Hughes et al., 2017).

Dr. Burke Harris (2014, 2018) brought renewed emphasis to the importance of Felitti et al.'s original study through a now seminal TED Talk and in her book *The Deepest Well,* drawing worldwide discussion on trauma as a major public health crisis. Dr. Harris' work includes helping clinical providers understand the connection between ACEs and the epidemiology of toxic stress on the body, including the neurobiology of negative effects and short- and long-term health consequences if recognition and intervention does not take place. Recently appointed as California's first-ever Surgeon General based on her mission to recognize ACEs as a critical factor in both pediatric and adult health outcomes, Harris announced the ACES Aware Initiative and development of The Bay Area Research Consortium on Toxic Stress and Health (BARC) (ACES Aware, 2020).

Cumulative trauma from ACES is often misdiagnosed as depression, anxiety, or ADHD, and leads to disease, disability, and early death (Felitti, 2009; Felitti & Anda, 2010; Felitti et al., 1998). With both a short- and long-term impact on child and adolescent development, the neurobiological effects of brain abnormalities and stress hormone dysregulation include poor attachment, socialization, and decreased self-efficacy (Perry, 2009; Shonkoff & Garner, 2012). Long-term risk behaviors include smoking, obesity, substance abuse, and promiscuity, and the long-term health-related outcomes identified include death, disease, and disability, major depression, suicide, PTSD, substance use, sexually transmitted disease, cardiovascular disease, cancer, chronic lung, and liver disease (Anda et al., 2010; Garner et al., 2012; Shonkoff & Garner, 2012). Individuals who have experienced cumulative ACEs are more likely to experience social problems such as homelessness, criminal behavior, and unemployment. The "ACE Pyramid" is often used as a conceptual model to understand ACEs in terms of long-term physical and mental health outcomes (**Figure 5-2**).

There are several valid and reliable screens for ACEs. One such screen includes the ACE-Q, which has now been used in a variety of settings and research studies to date (ACES Aware, 2020; Zarse et al., 2019). The ACE-Q is a one-page screener that is free to use and available in several languages with a 17-question child version (0–12 years of age) and a 19-question teen self-report version (13–19 years of age). A score of more or more indicated anticipatory guidance is given, with a score of 1–3 with symptoms, or a score of 4+ indicative of referral for treatment (Anda et al., 2010; Zarse et al., 2019). The Pediatric ACEs Screening and Related Life-events Screener (PEARLS), developed under Dr. Burke's work through BARC, is being implemented statewide in California with translation in 17 languages and

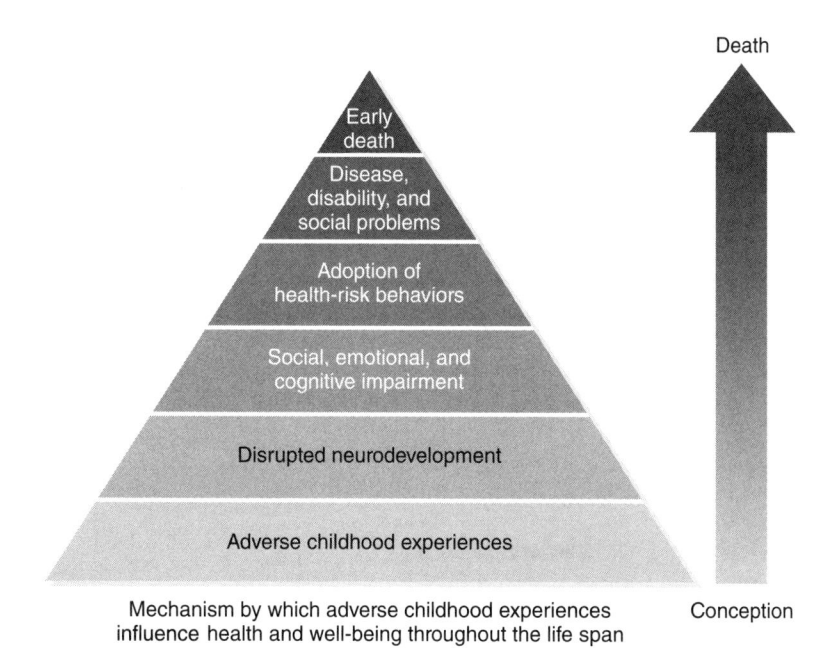

Figure 5-2 ACEs Pyramid

CDC. (2016). About the CDC-Kaiser ACE study. Retrieved from https://www.cdc.gov/violenceprevention/acestudy/about.html

is freely available to providers (ACEs Aware, 2020). Both the ACE-Q and PEARLS can be found at ACES Aware at https://www.acesaware.org/screen/screening-tools/.

Specifics vary on a case-by-case basis; however, the NP requires judgment and knowledge on detecting and treating patients suffering from toxic stress. All patients should be educated about ACEs and toxic stress, especially those at intermediate or high risk. Caregivers should understand the role protective factors can have in buffering the effects of chronic trauma such as nurturing caregiving, maintaining sleep regimens and sleep hygiene, promoting physical activity, and nutrition. Mindfulness and mediation coupled with mental health services are key interventions to combat both ACEs and a chronic, toxic, stress environment.

Trauma-Informed Care

Trauma-informed care requires a "universal precautions" approach, referencing all patients served as presumed to have a history of a traumatic experience (Racine et al., 2020). Being trauma-informed refers to an empathetic, supportive recognition of the background, significance, and needs for individuals who experienced trauma. Trauma-based principles include social connectedness and support systems (including family, religious, and community resources), and an overall recognition that trauma is complex (SAMHSA, 2014, 2018).

NPs must become comfortable with screening and asking questions related to trauma and mental health concerns (such as depression and anxiety) and approach patients in a supportive, nonjudgmental manner. The Substance Abuse and Mental Health Administration (SAMSHA) trauma-informed care approach is based on the framework of "Realize, Recognize, Respond, and Resist Re-traumatization" also referred to as the "4-Rs" (2014, 2018). *Realize* refers to the providers' understanding of the impact of trauma, and that it is not just limited to physical and sexual abuse, carrying neurological, physiological, biological, and psychological effects across the lifetime (SAMHSA, 2018). *Recognize* refers to the signs, symptoms, and presentation of trauma in patients and using open-ended questions in order to assess for potential differentials in physical presentations that may be related to trauma (such as disordered eating, sleep concerns, and developmental delays) (National Child Trauma Stress Network, 2011; SAMHSA, 2014). *Responding* involves knowing both the system and the community to best provide wraparound services for the patient. For example, referral and coordination to the education system, as well as the housing, social support, and community support for an individual, are all required in providing trauma-based management for families. Furthermore, screening, anticipatory guidance, and setting up referral sources should be part of the practices and protocols in the primary care setting. Finally, *resisting re-traumatization* refers to the clinical approach in patient care at both the provider and organizational level.

Pediatric Considerations

Over 8 million U.S. youths (10%) have an impairing psychiatric disorder, with an estimated 1:4 children having a mental health disorder, the most common of which are depression, anxiety, and ADHD (Riddle, 2016). Most of these conditions are initially diagnosed in primary care and are either managed by the pediatric primary care provider or referred for outside services. However, regardless of whether a mental health specialist is sought, most primary care providers initialize or eventually manage psychotropic medications for youths with these conditions.

Children express symptoms in different ways than adults. For example, children may present with irritability or anger versus a depressed mood or affect in a major depressive disorder. Adolescents on the other hand will sometimes present with similar symptoms in younger children or can present with more adult presentation as they reach adulthood. Trauma responses notable in classic post-traumatic stress disorder (PTSD) present very differently in children. For example, reenactment of the traumatic event may occur in acting out similar events in their play, instead of having "flashbacks," as is typical of PTSD. Children's trauma responses differ so greatly from other age groups that the DSM-5 has two separate criteria established: one for children 6 years and older to adulthood, and another for children under the age of 6 years old (APA, 2013).

Pediatric symptomatology often includes disordered eating and sleeping difficulties. Symptom presentation noted in children include rapid eating, lack of satiety, food hoarding, and loss of appetite, as well as difficulty falling asleep, staying asleep, nightmares, insomnias, and parasomnias (sleep terrors, nightmares, rapid eye movement sleep behavioral disorder), especially in pediatric trauma presentations (Burke et al., 2011; Felitti & Anda, 2018; SAMHSA, 2014). Specifically, in patients with known ACEs, providers should also keep in mind that reduced emotional regulation, brain growth, cognitive ability, as well as insulin sensitivity, increased BMI, and hypertension have all been found as adverse associations to childhood trauma (AAP, 2014; Kovachy et al., 2013). Pediatric presentation of mental health concerns can also first present with elimination issues such as constipation, encopresis, or enuresis, as well as accidents in a child who has already been toilet trained (APA, 2013; AAP, 2014). While ruling out organic causes should always be the first consideration in diagnostics, assessing for changes in the home environment or other stressful events in the child's life becomes paramount.

One of the most common valid and reliable assessment and symptom monitoring tools for use in youth aged 4–16 years of age is the Pediatric Symptom Checklist (PSC). Used to identify emotional and behavioral concerns, this 35-item scale for parent/guardians or a self-report version for youth 11 years of age and older is available. An abbreviated 17-item version is also available. The PSC psychosocial screen consists of items scored 0, 1, and 2 between "never," "sometimes," or "often." A cutoff score of 28 or higher indicates psychological impairment. A positive score indicates the need for further evaluation by a health professional (Jellinek et al., 1988).

If physical, emotional, or mental abuse or neglect is suspected with a pediatric or adolescent patient, child protective services must be made as part of state and federal law. All health care providers are required reporters of abuse, and the NP must respond accordingly.

Geriatric Considerations

Later phases of life have great benefits, including insights into life and increased skill sets to manage life's stressors. Sadly, however the "golden years" are at times less bright or positive as one might hope, and can spur exacerbations of preexisting mental illness as well as the development of new concerns. Elder mental health is a subspecialty with unique considerations and challenges. Developmental milestones in this phase of life tend to include levels of declining functioning in multiple domains, as well as increased losses of significant relationships due to death and isolation. Suicide rates for adults 75 years or older are among the highest in the civilized world, with family conflict, serious physical illness, loneliness, and both major and minor depressions associated with suicide in the 75+ group (Waern et al., 2003).

Substance abuse with one's own prescription medication, misuse of drugs, and alcohol remain concerns for the treatment of older generations. Elderly with both mental health conditions and substance abuse are 1.5 to 4.5 times more likely to have an injury due to falling than their same-aged counterparts (Finkelstein et al., 2007). Evidenced-based treatment of mental illness remains effective within the geriatric population, particularly when combined with multidisciplinary, community-based treatment teams (Bartels et al., 2002).

Elder abuse rates in America are sadly quite staggering, with 1 in 10 Americans aged 60 or older reporting some type of abuse or neglect; 60% of the perpetrators are family members of either gender (National Council on Aging, 2021). Mental illness in one or both parties is often correlated with interpersonal-violence, abuse, or neglect, causing significant mental health stress (Sirey et al., 2015).

Importance of Self-Care

The human experience is about connection. It is essential to every phase of development and in each relationship. Gone are the days, in mental health care, of the expectation that providers are "tabla rosa" or "blank slates," with the faulty belief that the provider must remain a detached entity. Being genuinely emotionally present during patient interactions and connecting with true empathy significantly influences the healing process. Scientific advancements in understanding the neurological structures in the process of learning, including "mirror neurons," as well as the hormonal processes of oxytocin, have continued to support the importance of healthy attachments and health. Empathetic practitioners can tap into the body's natural supportive healing processes through the development of positive relationships with their patients. These relationships also benefit the practitioner as well, providing reciprocity in this positive process (Rakel, 2018). However, true honest connection has its inherent vulnerabilities, as empathy requires some level of "feeling" another's experience. When a patient's emotional pain is met with an empathetic response, the practitioner in turn is impacted.

Caring for patients with mental health concerns requires careful balance and self-awareness on behalf of the NP to include mindfulness around compassion fatigue, and possible burn-out and vicarious traumatization, which are common in health care in stressful work environments. *Compassion satisfaction* refers to the positive benefits experienced by the giver in a helping relationship and is the goal of a clinician. Whereas *compassion fatigue* refers to the lower levels of emotional exhaustion and the sense of "care depletion" due to having to provide emotional care routinely, it is easily replenished through supportive measures. *Burn-out* occurs when a helper has extended beyond compassion fatigue levels and has completely depleted their resources to be supportive to others. *Vicarious traumatization* is secondary traumatic stress, when the care provider develops trauma responses (see details in the preceding section) due to exposure, by hearing or processing their patients' actual traumatic experiences during the course of treatment. *Countertransference* is a provider's own emotional reaction to a patient which may impact the quality of care provided if unacknowledged.

⚕ CASE STUDY TWO

Jack is a doctoral-prepared NP who began his first job as a family-based nurse practitioner in a busy urban Federally Qualified Health Center (FQHC) community health center. Jack is required to manage a similar caseload as NPs that are 10 years his senior and more experienced, and often finds himself seeing 4–5 patients an hour, requiring him to work through lunch and after hours to complete his charting. A particular patient Jack sees frequently for asthma maintenance reminds Jack of his best friend in high school who committed suicide. Jack finds his patient similar in sarcastic demeanor, dark humor, and binge-drinking behaviors. Jack continues to assess for suicidality at every visit, but his patient continues to disclose no suicidal risk, and yet Jack finds himself scheduling follow-up appointments sooner than necessary.

Given the innate nature of this process, it is not a sign of weakness to experience emotional impacts from the work, when in a helping profession. The charge then for all providers is to find ways to mitigate the level and severity of negative impacts. Engaging in healthy routines that are helpful includes personal self-care practices (on a systematic level for healthcare administrators) to ensure supportive working conditions, and to collaboratively monitor levels of compassion fatigue, which can serve to actually avoid other concerning effects such as burn-out. Recent studies have found compassion satisfaction to be correlated with good quality sleep, regular exercise, having a life partner, and higher job satisfaction. However, the number of hours worked per day was a significant positive factor for burn-out and increased the occurrence of vicarious traumatization (Wang et al., 2020).

Providers are not alone. There are effective tools to combat the adverse negative effects of caring deeply for others. Open and honest communication with supportive supervisors, colleagues, and mentors reduces isolation. Systems that are structured to encourage such practices also benefit from low levels of burn-out and staff-turnover (Wang et al., 2020). Providers are encouraged to use the following strategies "ABC" anemogram to maintain compassion satisfaction throughout their career. *Awareness:* increase capacity to notice thoughts, feelings, and behaviors that are indicators of advancing work-based stress to compassion fatigue. *Balance:* seek a healthy equilibrium between work and other quality life experiences by creating space activities such as sleep, exercise, meditation, art, and other activities that bring personal joy. *Connection:* seeking positive relationships in all domains of life that bring rejuvenation, including cultivating ones that do not mimic the patient-caregiver dynamic. Caregiving is at best a complicated endeavor. Should practitioners' needs exceed their current self-capacities, self-referral to a mental health provider is encouraged.

Understanding Scope of Practice

Primary care providers routinely provide care for patients with what is considered psychiatric diagnoses. Nurse practitioners both in specialty care and primary care additionally treat these patients across the healthcare system. Currently, there is not an algorithm or "hard-and-fast" rule of when the diagnosis and management of psychiatric symptoms needs to move from primary care to specialty care, including any easy guidance for who should be the primary lead or "caregiver" for these situations. Clinical trainings continue to vary widely across institutions, curricula, degree acquisition, and residencies. All of which contributes to providers' comfort levels and competence in managing certain conditions (Davis et al., 2012). Oftentimes, the national shortage of psychiatric specialists directly limits the availability for consultations and referrals.

Communication between the primary care providers and psychiatric specialists are foundational to optimal patient care. The nurse practitioner is charged with creating and maintaining community provider connections, especially when a patient presentation is outside the NP's scope of practice, training, educational level, or comfort.

♀ CASE STUDY THREE

Pamela is a 9-year-old female student at Lincoln Elementary school. She recently lost her grandmother to COVID-19 and has been in a remote, virtual learning environment for the last 16 months. Pamela used to love school, especially math, and played basketball on the intramural after-school basketball team. Pamela is a registered user for the School-Based Health Center program and has a telehealth appointment for her annual wellness examination. Pamela and her mother log in to her telehealth appointment with her nurse practitioner provider, and Pamela sits next to her mother during the telehealth medical history portion of her wellness examination. Pamela's mother acknowledges difficulty since the loss of their grandmother and reports that Pamela has experienced some grief over the loss, but is otherwise doing "OK." Pamela is visibly withdrawn during the history review with her mother, does not make eye contact with the NP provider, is still in her pajamas at close to lunchtime, and has unwashed, ungroomed hair. The NP asks Pamela if she is going to be playing basketball in the upcoming months or if she has been playing any at home. Her response is a shoulder-shrug. The NP asks Pamela's mother if she would feel comfortable going through the Pediatric Symptom Checklist (PSC) with her during the phone call as part of a routine assessment for mental health in conjunction with the physical exam.

Case Study Discussion Questions

1. What is your next step with this patient?
2. What are you considering as possible diagnoses in this case?
3. How would you manage a risk assessment in this case?

Seminar Discussion Questions

1. What are the most common mental health issues in your own clinical setting?
2. Reflect on any potential personal bias in the assessment and management of mental health or substance abuse difficulties. What are two potential methods to help you address these biases?
3. Create a resource list that includes local 24/7 care, a suicide hotline, domestic violence supports, shelters, alcoholics anonymous, narcotics anonymous, Big Brothers Big Sisters of America, food pantry referrals, any other local resources

that can assist with mental health or act as a social determinant of health presentations to your office.
4. Identify local agencies and community referrals for patients who are:
   a. In psychiatric crisis
   b. In need of social support
   c. Requiring a collaborative to best assist you as the provider

References

ACEs Aware. (2020). *Screening tools*. State of California Department of Health Care Services. https://www.acesaware.org/screen/screening-tools/

Alexandra, C., Joseph, S., Julian, F., Cheryl, L., Margaret, B., Marylene, C., Ruth, D., Rebecca, H., Richard, K., Joan, L., Karen, M., Erna, O., & van der Kook, B. (2005). Complex trauma in children and adolescents. *Psychiatric Annals, 5*, 390. http://doi.org/10.3928

Alexandra, P. (2019). The Importance of Trauma-Informed Schools for Maltreated Children. *BU Journal of Graduate Studies in Education, 11*(1), 22–28. https://files.eric.ed.gov/fulltext/EJ1230310.pdf

Almeida, J., Johnson, R. M., Corliss, H., Molnar, B., & Azarel, D. (2009). Emotional distress among LGBT youth: The influence of perceived discrimination based on sexual orientation. *Journal of Youth and Adolescence, 38*(7), 1001–1014.

American Academy of Pediatrics. (2014). *AAP Trauma Toolkit: Medical home approach to identifying and responding to exposure to trauma*. https://www.aap.org/en-us/Documents/ttb_medicalhome-approach.pdf

American Psychiatric Association. (2013). *Diagnostic and statistical manual of mental disorders* (5th ed.). https://doi.org/10.1176/appi.books.9780890425596

American Psychiatric Association. (2021). *Cultural competency and mental health facts*. https://www.psychiatry.org/psychiatrists/cultural-competency/education/mental-health-facts

Anda, R., Felitti, V., Bremner, J., et al. (2006). The enduring effects of abuse and related adverse experiences in childhood. A convergence of evidence from neurobiology and epidemiology. *Eur Achieves Psychiatry Clinical Neuroscience, 256*(3), 175–186. https://doi.org/10.1007/s0046-005-0624-4

Anda, R. F., Butchart, A., Felitti, V. J., & Brown, D. W. (2010). Building a framework for global surveillance of the public health implications of adverse childhood experiences. *American Journal of Preventative Medicine, 39*, 93–98. http://doi/10.1016/j.amepre.2010.03.015

Bachmann S. (2018). Epidemiology of suicide and the psychiatric perspective. *International Journal of Environment Research and Public Health, 15*(7), 1425. https://doi.org/10.3390/ijerph15071425

Bartels, S., Dums, A., Oxman, T., Schneider, L, Alexopoulos, G., & Jeste, D. (2002). Evidence-based practices in geriatric mental health care. *Psychiatric Services, 53*(11). https://doi.org/10.1176/appi.ps.53.11.1419

Block, R. (2011). *Breaking the silence on child abuse: Protection, prevention, intervention, and deterrence: The U.S. Senate Committee on Health, Education, Labor & Pensions*. Retrieved June 12, 2020 from https://www.help.senate.gov/hearings/breaking-the-silence-on-child-abuse-protection-prevention-intervention-and-deterrence

Burke, N., Hellman, J., Scott, S., Weems, C., & Carrion, V. (2011). The impact of adverse childhood experiences on an urban pediatric population. *Child Abuse Neglect, 35*(6), 408–413. https://doi/10.1016/j.chiabu.2011.02.006

Carter-Pokras, O., & Baquet, C. (2002). What is a "health disparity"? *Public Health Report, 117*, 426–434. https://doi.org/10.1093/phr/117.5.426

Centers for Disease Control and Prevention. (2013). CDC Health Disparities and Inequities Report: United States. *Morbidity and Mortality Weekly Report, 62*(3).

Centers for Disease Control and Prevention. (2021). *Social determinants of health*. https://www.cdc.gov/socialdeterminants/index.htm

Christakis, N., & Fowler, J. (2013). Social contagion theory: Examining dynamic social networks and human behavior. *Stat Med, 32*(4), 556–577.

Davis, D. W., Honaker, S. M., Jones, V. F., Williams, P. G., Stocker, F., & Martin, E. (2012). Identification and management of behavioral/mental health problems in primary care pediatrics: Perceived strengths, challenges, and new delivery models. *Clinical Pediatrics, 51*(10), 978–982.

Dube, S., Anda,., Felitti, V., Chapman, D., Williamson, D., & Giles, W. (2001). Childhood abuse, household dysfunction, and the risk of attempted suicide throughout the life span: findings from the adverse childhood experiences study. *JAMA, 286*(24), 3089–3096. https://doi.org/10.1001/jama.286.24.3089

Dubiel, H., Shupe, A., & Tolliver, R. (2010). The connection between health disparities and social determinants of health in early childhood. *Colorado Department of Public Health and Environment.* https://www.cohealthdata.dphe.state.co.us/chd/Resources/pubs/ECHealthDisparities2.pdf

Felitti, V. (2009). Adverse childhood experiences and adult health. *Academic Pediatrics, 9,* 131–132. https://doi.org/10.1016/j.acap.2009.03.001

Felitti, V., & Anda, R. (2010). The relationship of adverse childhood experience to adult medical disease, psychiatric disorders, and sexual behavior: Implications for healthcare. In R. Linius, E. Vermetten, & C. Pain (Eds.), *The impact of early life trauma on health and disease: The hidden epidemic* (pp. 77–87). Cambridge University Press.

Felitti, V., Anda, R., Nordenberg, D., Williamson, F., Spitz, A., Edwards, V., & Marks, J. (1998). Relationship of childhood abuse and household dysfunction to many of the leading causes of death in adults: The adverse childhood experiences study. *American Journal of Preventative Medicine, 14,* 245–248. https://doi.org/10.1016/s0749-3797(98)00017-8

Finkelstein, E., Prabhu, M., & Chen, H. (2007). Increased prevalence of falls among elderly individuals with mental health and substance abuse conditions. *The American Journal of Geriatric Psychiatry, 15*(7), 611–619. https://doi.org/10.1097/JGP.0b013e318033ed97

Garner, A., Shonkoff, J., Siegel. B., Dobbins, M., Earls, M., Garner, A., Wood, D., et al. (2012). Early childhood adversity, toxic stress, and the role of the pediatrician: Translating developmental science into lifelong health. *Pediatrics, 129* (1), e224–e231. https://doi.org/10.1542/peds.2011-2662

Gold, L. (2014). DSM-5 and the assessment of functioning: The World Health Organization Disability Assessment Schedule 2.0 (WHODAS 2.0). *Journal of the American Academy of Psychiatry and the Law Online, 42*(2), 173–181.

Guyll, M., Matthews, K., & Bromberger, J. (2001). Discrimination and unfair treatment: Relationship to cardiovascular reactivity among African American and European American women. *Health Psychology, 20*(5), 315–325.

Harris, N. (2014). *How childhood trauma affects health across the lifetime* [Video file]. TED. https://www.ted.com/talks/nadine_burke_harris_how_childhood_trauma_affects_health_across_a_lifetime?utm_campaign=tedspread&utm_medium=referral&utm_source=tedcomshare

Harris, N. (2018). *The deepest well: Healing the long-term effects of childhood adversity.* New York: Houghton, Mifflin, Harcourt.

Henwood, B., & Padgett, D. (2007). Reevaluating the self-medication hypothesis among the dually diagnosed. *American Journal of Addiction, 16*(3), 160–165. doi: 10.1080/10550490701375368

Hirschfeld, R. M., Calabrese, J., Weissman, M., Reed, M., Davies, M., Frye, M., Keck, P., McElroy, S., McNulty, J., & Wagner, K. (2003). Screening for bipolar disorder in the community. *Journal of Clinical Psychiatry, 64*(1), 53–59. doi: 10.4088/jcp.v64n0111

Hornor, G. (2015). Childhood trauma exposure and toxic stress: What the PNP needs to know. *Journal of Pediatric Health Care, 29,* 191–198. https://dx.doi.org/10.1016/j.pedhc.2014.09.006

Hughes, K., Bellis, M. A., Hardcastle, K. A., Sethi, D., Butchart, A., Mikton, C., Dunne, M., et al. (2017). The effect of multiple adverse childhood experience on health: A systematic review and meta-analysis. *Lancet Public Health, 2*(8), e356–366. https://doi.org/10.1016/s2468-2667(17)30118-4

Jellinek, M., Murphy, J., Robinson, J., et al. (1988). Pediatric Symptom Checklist: Screening school-age children for psychosocial dysfunction. *Journal of Pediatrics, 11*(2), 201–209. http://psc.partners.org

Katzelnick, D. J., & Greist, J. H. (2001). Social anxiety disorder: An unrecognized problem in primary care. *Journal of Clinical Psychiatry, 62,* Suppl 1:11-5; 15–16.

Kovachy, B., O'Hara, R., Hawkins, N., Gershon, A., Primeau, M. M., Madej, J., & Carrion, V. (2013). Sleep disturbance in pediatric PTSD: Current findings and future directions. *Journal of Clinical Sleep Medicine, 9*(5), 501–510. doi:10.5664/jcsm.2678

Kroenke, K., & Spitzer, R. L. (2002). The PHQ-9: A new depression and diagnostic severity measure. *Psychiatric Annals, 32,* 509–521.

References   **153**

Laker, C. (2007). How reliable is the current evidence looking at the efficacy of harm reduction and motivational interviewing interventions in the treatment of patients with a dual diagnosis? *Journal of Psychiatric Mental Health Nursing, 14*(8), 720–726. doi: 10.111/j.1365-285.2007.01159.x

Lane, W., Bair-Merritt, M., & Dubowitz, H. (2011). Child abuse and neglect. *Scandinavian Journal of Surgery, 100*(4), 264–272. doi: 10.1177/14574969111000406

Margolin, G., Vickerman, K. A., Oliver, P. H., & Gordis, E. B. (2010). Violence exposure in multiple interpersonal domains: Cumulative and differential effects. *Journal of Adolescent Health, 47*(2), 198–205.

Marker, I., & Norton, P. J. (2018). The efficacy of incorporating motivational interviewing to cognitive behavior therapy for anxiety disorders: A review and meta-analysis. *Clinical Psychology Review, 62*, 1–10. doi: 10.1016/j.cpr.2018.04.004

Mundt, J. C., Greist, J. H., Jefferson, J. W., Federico, M., Mann, J. J., & Posner, K. (2013). Prediction of suicidal behavior in clinical research by lifetime suicidal ideation and behavior ascertained by the electronic Columbia-Suicide Severity Rating Scale. *The Journal of Clinical Psychiatry, 74*(9), 887–893. doi: 10.4088/JCP.13m08398

National Child Trauma Stress Network. (2011). *Complex trauma in children and adolescents.* http://www.nctsn.org/trauma-types/complex-trauma

National Council on Aging. (2021). *Elder abuse.* https://www.ncoa.org/public-policy-action/elder-justice/elder-abuse-facts/

National Institute of Mental Health. (2021). Mental illness. https://www.nimh.nih.gov/health/statistics/mental-illness.shtml

Owings-Fonner, N. (2020). Telepsychology expands to meet demand. *Monitor on Psychology, 51*(4). https://doi.org/10.1037/e514482018-001

Perry, B. (2002). Childhood experiences and the expression of genetic potential: What childhood neglect tells us about nature and nurture. *Brain and Mind, 3*, 79–100.

Perry, B. D. (2009). Examining child maltreatment through a neurodevelopmental lens: Clinical applications of the neurosequential model of therapeutics. *Journal of Loss and Trauma, 14*, 240–255. https://doi.org/10.1080/15325020903004350

Racine, N., Killam, R., & Madigan, S. (2020). Trauma-informed care as a universal precaution: Beyond the adverse childhood experiences questionnaire. *JAMA Pediatrics, 174*(1), 5–6. doi: 10.1001/jamapediatrics.2019.3866

Rakel, D. (2018). *Compassionate connection: The healing power of empathy and mindful listening.* New York, NY: Norton & Company, Incorporated, W.W.

Riddle, M. (2016). *Pediatric psychopharmacology for primary care* (2nd ed.). American Academy of Pediatrics. Illinois: AAP.

Rosenquist, J., Murabito, J., Fowler, J., & Christakis, N. (2010). The spread of alcohol consumption behavior in a large social network. *Ann Intern Med, 157*(7), 426–433. https://doi.org/10.7326/0003-4819-152-7-101004060-00007

Roshanaei-Moghaddam, B., Pauly, M. C., Atkins, D. C., Baldwin, S. A., Stein, M. B., & Roy-Byrne, P. (2011). Relative effects of CBT and pharmacotherapy in depression versus anxiety: Is medication somewhat better for depression, and CBT somewhat better for anxiety? *Depression & Anxiety, 28*, 560–567. https://doi.org/10.1002/da.20829

Schick, M., Morina, N., Klaghofer, R., Schnyder, U., & Muller, J. (2013). Trauma, mental health, and intergenerational associations of Kosovar families 11 years after the war. *European Journal of Psychotraumatology, 4* (1). doi:10.3402/ejpt.v4i0.21060

Shonkoff, J., & Garner, A. (2012). The lifelong effects of early childhood adversity and toxic stress. *Pediatrics, 129*(1), e232–e246. https://doi/10.1542/peds.2011-2663

Sirey, J. A., Berman, J., Salamone, A., DePasquale, A., Halkett, A., Raeifar, E., Banerjee, S., Bruce, M., & Raue, P. (2015). Feasibility of integrating mental health screening and services into routine elder abuse practice to improve client outcomes. *Journal of Elder Abuse & Neglect, 27*(3), 254–269. https://doi.org/10.1080/08946566.2015.1008086

Snyderman, D., & Rovner, B. (2009). Mental status exam in primary care: A review. *American Family Physician, 80*(8), 809–814.

Steger, M., Oishi, S., & Kashdan, T. B. (2009). Meaning in life across the life span: Levels and correlates of meaning in life from emerging adulthood to older adulthood. *The Journal of Positive Psychology, 4*(1),43–52. http://dx.doi.org/10.1080/17439760802303127

Substance Abuse and Mental Health Services Administration. (2014). *SAMHSA's concept of trauma and guidance for a trauma-informed approach.* HHS Publication No. (SMA). Rockville, MD: Substance Abuse and Mental Health Services Administration. Available at http://www.trauma informedcareproject.org/resources/SAMHSA%20TIC.pdf

Substance Abuse and Mental Health Services Administration. (2018). *Trauma-informed approach and trauma-specific interventions.* https://www.samhsa.gov/nctic/trauma-interventions

Tepper, M., Cohen, A., Progovac, A., Ault-Brutus, A., Leff, H., Mullin, B., Cunningham, C., & Le Cook, B. (2017). Minding the gap: Developing an integrated behavioral health home to address health disparities in serious mental health. *Psychiatric Services, 68*(12), 1217–1224. https://doi.org/10.1176/appi.ps.201700063

U.S. Department of Health and Human Services. (2020). Healthy people objectives: Social determinants of health. https://health.gov/healthypeople/objectives-and-data/social-determinants-healt/literature-summaries

Waern, M., Rubenowitz, E., & Wilhelmson, K. (2003). Predictors of suicide in the old elderly. *Gerontology, 49*, 328–334. https://doi.org/10.1159/000071715

Wang, J., Okoli, C., He, J., Feng, F., Li, J., Zhuang, L., & Lin, M. (2020). Factors associated with compassion satisfaction, burnout, and secondary traumatic stress among Chinese nurses in tertiary hospitals: A cross-sectional study. *International Journal of Nursing Studies, 102.* https://doi.org/10.1016/j.ijnurstu.2019.103472

World Health Organization. (2018). *Closing the gap in a generation: Health equity through action on the social determinants of health.* Commission on Social Determinants of Health. https://www.who.int/social_determinants/en

Zarse, E., Neff, M., Yoder, R., Chambers, J., Chambers, R., & Schumacher, U. (2019). The adverse childhood experiences questionnaire: Two decades of research on childhood trauma as a primary cause of adult mental illness, addiction, and medical diseases. *Cogent Medicine, 6*(1), 1–9. https://doi/10.1080/2331205X.2019.1581447

CHAPTER 6

Cultural Sensitivity and Global Health

Michelle A. Cole and Christina B. Gunther

Introduction

One of the most noted fundamental teachings in many of the world's religions is commonly referred to as the Golden Rule. The Golden Rule, "Do unto others as you would have them do unto you," is likely the most familiar moral value in Western culture (Stanglin, 2005). The rule has a strong connection to many religions, including Christianity, Buddhism, Judaism, and Islam. Despite the origin, the tenet of the Golden Rule guides us to treat others as we would like to be treated. Its foundation is the reciprocity of kindness and human giving; however, it may have some unintended shortcomings when applied to the provision of patient care.

There is an assumption that people who resemble us or speak our language are the same and should be treated as we would like to be treated. As the providers of direct care to individuals and populations, nurse practitioners (NPs) must consider how those they provide care for want to be treated. This consideration differs from the Golden Rule, in which we treat others in a manner that is acceptable to our standards and beliefs without consideration of the individual's preferences. Stepping away from viewing circumstances from our own perspective to the patient's perspective is a critical step in the care of others in a diverse world. Putting aside an imperialistic attitude of thinking, one knows what is best for others, and taking the time to know what is significant to individuals and communities, is an important step in developing a successful patient–NP relationship (Ott & Olson, 2011).

Care should not be based on the paternalistic of what "I think is best" or "what I would want for myself" but instead shifted to the perspective of the person receiving care. In an effort to be a NP who also strives to serve as a global citizen, one should adapt the perspective offered by the Platinum Rule. According to the urban dictionary, the Platinum Rule "Do unto others as they would have you do unto them, not as you would have them do unto you" (*Urban Dictionary: Platinum Rule*, n.d.) steps above the Golden Rule. Using the Platinum Rule, the practitioner takes on an active role, asking the patient how they want to be treated and listening to their preferences. This approach meets the patient where they are and considers their unique viewpoint, needs, and values. While practitioners may feel challenged by this approach, providing what the other wants and needs, this is an opportunity to connect with the patient to determine how the two, patient and provider, can work to develop mutual goals, a plan, and outcomes that reflect what is important in meeting the patient's needs (Vetto, 2015). The general principles that often drive the day-to-day decisions and actions of nurse practitioners need reconsideration for the diverse and unique populations they serve.

As the United States is becoming more diverse, healthcare providers are caring for individuals and groups who have varied perspectives; many are distinct from the mainstream healthcare system. Many healthcare providers, including NPs, do not identify themselves with any one particular culture; however, they often do view their patients and families as having cultural traits (Matteliano & Street, 2012). The notion that our own cultural and societal norms can be applied to the general population can create obstacles and barriers in caring for patients. These beliefs are a result of personal, professional, and educational socialization. Ethnocentrism impedes the delivery of culturally competent nursing care (Dayer-Berenson, 2014). Not understanding others, or having limited information about another group, can lead primary care providers to make false assumptions that could potentially be harmful, hurtful, and destructive. Believing that the culture one is most familiar with is the cultural standard does not afford providers the opportunity to comprehend and appreciate the needs of others. Critical to understanding the perspective of others is the willingness of NPs to acknowledge their own beliefs and recognize that other individuals' values are cogent despite being different from their own (Dayer-Berenson, 2014). Considering the viewpoint of others is the first step to comprehending the ideals from the eyes of others and the avoidance of unfounded assumptions and biases.

Implicit bias has become increasingly more acknowledged in the field of nursing. Hall et al. (2015) determined that most healthcare providers appear to have implicit bias, with many holding negative attitudes toward people of color. We all have biases influenced by the environment that surrounds us. As FitzGerald and Hurst (2017) show, a positive relationship exists between healthcare provider bias and lower quality care of patients, resulting in disparities in health outcomes. Recognizing implicit biases requires a willingness to measure them through tools such as the Implicit Associations Test (IAT) and a willingness to disrupt any biases discovered. Engaging in ongoing exercises that directly target self-awareness abilities (McIntosh, 2015), such as noticing inner thought patterns or reframing any stereotyped ideas of diverse others, help to disrupt implicit biases. In doing this, the NP will be better prepared to relate to patients with multicultural backgrounds and avoid any unintentional discriminatory practices.

It is important to note that implicit biases must be recognized and disrupted before adaptive behaviors can take place (Hagiwara et al., 2019). To uncover any held implicit biases, take an IAT through Project Implicit at https://implicit.harvard.edu/implicit.

Global Diversity

The world is becoming increasingly more diverse. Globalization brings diversity and affects societies as cultures, values, and traditions transcend into new territory. The U.S. population is becoming increasingly more ethnically and socioculturally varied. With more that 40% identifying as non-Hispanic white in 2019, with an expected increase to 50% by 2044, the United States is projected to become more diverse in the coming decades (Budiman, 2020). The data highlight the changes in population and increasing diversity of the United States. Considering the United States as a "melting pot" or the blending together of various cultures to form one, is not considering the unique qualities of the various cultures of the population. Instead, looking at the U.S. society as a "tossed salad," where the diversity of the culture is valued for what it contributes to the whole, embraces a more culturally aware viewpoint. As advanced practice nurses, NPs are challenged to respond to this "tossed salad" culture by providing care for the health and wellness needs of the population. Disparities in health care limit quality health care and contribute to unnecessary costs. Disparities amount to approximately $93 billion in excess medical care costs and $42 billion in lost productivity per year (Turner, 2018). Reducing disparities can contribute to social and economic gains. "To remain competitive in a global economy, we need the full creative and economic potential of all our people. Greater racial equity will not only improve individual lives, it will increase the size of the economic pie for everyone" (Turner, 2018).

Leininger's theory on diversity and universality implies that for a caregiver's work to be meaningful and relevant, transcultural knowledge and competencies are imperative to guiding decisions and actions for effective and successful outcomes (Tomey & Alligood, 2002). Leininger's theory is suitable for application to the care of diverse populations. Her theory states that the provision of care needs to be harmonious with an individual's or group's cultural beliefs, practices, and ideals (Sitzman & Eichelberger, 2004). With the impact of globalization, primary care providers must possess sensitivity, compassion, and competence to care for individuals and communities from diverse cultural backgrounds. To effect positive health promotion activities and influence positive healthcare outcomes of individuals and communities, healthcare providers must understand and appreciate the importance of culturally competent care (Sitzman & Eichelberger, 2004). NPs are charged with integrating cultural care into practice through a comprehensive clinical approach, role modeling, policy development, performance, evaluation, and use of the advanced nursing process (McFarlane & Eipperle, 2008). The advanced practice NP has an obligation to develop the skills necessary to be a culturally competent practitioner.

Cultural Competency and Clinical Education

Cultural competency is an essential component to be infused into professional practice. Professional nursing organizations recognize the need for nurses, at all levels, to respond to the diversity in the population. The American Association of Colleges of Nursing (AACN), in the *Essentials of Baccalaureate Education for Professional Nursing Practice*, states, "The professional nurse practices in a multicultural environment and must possess the skills to provide culturally appropriate care" (2008, p. 6). The *Essentials of Master's Education of Advanced Practice Nurses* includes cultural competence as an essential component of the advanced practice nurse's educational preparedness (AACN, 1994). Cultural sensitivity and awareness are concepts guiding the practice of the Doctorate of Nursing Practice prepared nurse (AACN, 2006).

Cultural competency is a crucial component of the educational preparedness of nurses, and the inclusion of cultural sensitivity and awareness into the curriculum will promote cultural competency within the profession of nursing. Many definitions of cultural competence exist that are routinely debated in the literature. The definition for the purposes of this chapter comes from Garneau and Pepin's (2015) constructive definition that outlines the concept as a "continuum of knowledge not as a shift in knowledge" (p. 9). Their definition supports the notion that gaining cultural competence skills is a lifelong journey that must be a continual learning process.

Medical and nursing academics are infusing cultural competence preparation into their educational curricula. Nursing organizations include culture in practice standards and curricular requirements. The American Nurses Association (ANA), in the third edition of *Nursing: Scope and Standards of Practice* (NSSP), introduced the Standard of Culturally Congruent Practice. The standard, outlines nursing practice that is congruent with cultural diversity and inclusion principles (Marion et al., 2016).

> The standard, outlines nursing practice that is congruent with cultural diversity and inclusion principles (Marion et al., 2016). In order to provide culturally competent care, the nurse must possess evidenced base knowledge that is congruent with the chosen cultural ideals, views and practices of the patient, families and other stakeholders. Nurses are poised to design and lead culturally congruent care, and services for diverse populations to improve access to care with the intention of promoting positive health care outcomes and reducing health care disparities

The ANA Culturally Congruent Standard infers that the Platinum Rule is the foundation for their position, stating that the preferred preferences of the healthcare consumer are applied. The ability of the nurse to move away from their viewpoint to the viewpoint of others was a perspective of inclusive care to individuals with diverse backgrounds. Setting the bar for the delivery of culturally congruent care, the standard was developed after considering many social constructs in our current society.

The standard has 20 principles, with 12 for the registered nurse. Additional principles are included for the graduate nurse and the advanced practice nurse (**Box 6-1**).

The AACN essentials outline the required curriculum requirements and student learning outcomes, which include cultural competency. Nursing and medical faculty are charged to develop teaching strategies to achieve the set standards over the curriculum recognizing that cultural competence is a developmental process. In an effort to design the graduate nursing curriculum to meet these expectations, faculty have collaborated with community leaders to develop recommendations for the development of competencies for graduate nursing curricula (Axtell et al., 2010). Recommendations for graduate students are to practice self-awareness, increase knowledge of different cultures, promote cross-cultural communication and advocate for all regardless of race or ethnicity. The inclusion of the community to assist in the development of the graduate nurse was viewed as a positive strategy in the development and projected outcomes of the identified objectives (Axtell et al., 2010). Caring for individuals necessitates understanding the influence of culture

Box 6-1 ANA Standard 8: Culturally Congruent Practice and Associated Competencies

The registered nurse practices in a manner that is congruent with cultural diversity and inclusion principles.

Competencies for the registered nurse:

1. Demonstrates respect, equity, and empathy in actions and interactions with all healthcare consumers.
2. Participates in lifelong learning to understand cultural preferences, worldview, choices, and decision-making processes of diverse consumers.
3. Creates an inventory of one's own values, beliefs, and cultural heritage.
4. Applies knowledge of variations in health beliefs, practices, and communication patterns in all nursing practice activities.
5. Identifies the stage of the consumer's acculturation and accompanying patterns of needs and engagement.
6. Considers the effects and impact of discrimination and oppression on practice within and among vulnerable cultural groups.
7. Uses skills and tools that are appropriately vetted for the culture, literacy, and language of the population served.
8. Communicates with appropriate language and behaviors, including the use of medical interpreters and translators in accordance with consumer preferences.
9. Identifies the cultural-specific meaning of interactions, terms, and content.
10. Respects consumer decisions based on age, tradition, belief and family influence, and stage of acculturation.
11. Advocates for policies that promote health and prevent harm among culturally diverse, under-served, or under-represented consumers.
12. Promotes equal access to services, tests, interventions, health promotion programs, enrollment in research, education, and other opportunities.
13. Educates nurse colleagues and other professionals about cultural similarities and differences of healthcare consumers, families, groups, communities, and populations.

Additional competencies for the graduate-level prepared registered nurse:

1. Evaluates tools, instruments, and services provided to culturally diverse populations.
2. Advances organizational policies, programs, services, and practices that reflect respect, equity, and values for diversity and inclusion.
3. Engages consumers, key stakeholders, and others in designing and establishing internal and external cross-cultural partnerships.
4. Conducts research to improve health care and healthcare outcomes for culturally diverse consumers.
5. Develops recruitment and retention strategies to achieve a multicultural workforce.

Additional competencies for the advanced practice registered nurse:

1. Promotes shared decision-making solutions in planning, prescribing, and evaluating processes when the healthcare consumer's cultural preferences and norms may create incompatibility with evidence-based practice.
2. Leads interprofessional teams to identify the cultural and language needs of the consumer.

Reproduced from American Nurses Association (ANA). (2015). *Nursing: Scope and standards of practice* (3rd ed.). Silver Spring, MD: Nursebooks.org.

on their healthcare situation. Approach the individual without preconceived assumptions to avoid treating persons with common backgrounds the same. Each individual should have input into their healthcare choices, incorporating their cultural preferences.

> "We have been traveling over seas and providing care in our back yards to divers populations for years. Every patient encounter we experience must be looked at as a cultural encounter. Exercise self awareness as you work with patients. Ask questions, don't make assumptions and negotiate the best plan of care for each individual and family." (Cole, M. & Gunther, C., 2021)

The NP must be aware of the secondary elements of diversity in these situations that are not typically considered to be a cultural encounter. Loden and Rosener (1991) first developed the "dimensions of diversity" model to incorporate elements of diversity such as religion, sexual orientation, education, gender, age, and socioeconomic class, among others. Asking questions that incorporate the broader elements of diversity will make the patient encounter and healthcare outcomes more successful.

Cultural Awareness

"We don't see the world the way it is. We see the world the way we are."

—Anais Nin

Cultural awareness is being knowledgeable about one's own thoughts, feelings, and sensations, as well as the ability to reflect on how these can affect one's interactions with others (Giger et al., 2007). One's perceptions of "what is" are connected to our interpretation of the world, our experiences, values, and beliefs. To deliver care that is culturally sensitive, the NP needs to have an appreciation of the culturally relevant facts about a client and the provision of care. Giger and Davidhizar's "transcultural assessment model" includes six cultural phenomena that influence healthcare delivery (Giger, 2017).

Communication

Language or communication patterns are a significant part of how information is transferred in the healthcare setting. Communication, however, extends beyond linguistics and includes the process of communication. "Nurses need to have not only a working knowledge of communication with clients of the same culture, but also a thorough awareness of racial, cultural, and social factors that may affect communication with persons from other cultures" (Giger, 2017, p. 20).

> While conducting a health needs assessment in a remote area of the Dominican Republic near the Haitian border, the NP stopped in a corner market looking for candles. The power in this region was unstable so the electricity was often out. The NP, having learned Spanish in Guatemala, used the

Guatemalan word for candles when asking for the item. The shopkeeper smiled and told her she had requested "bombs'" when the electricity was out.

Regionalism can affect the transmission of information from patient to NP. The NP must ask the translator to investigate any colloquialisms, unfamiliar terms, or words with several meanings. Further questioning may be necessary to avoid cultural miscommunication. Describing the intent of the question to the translator will also assist in circumventing miscommunication.

Space

Personal space is the area that surrounds an individual and his or her level of comfort, which may vary from one individual to another. Space should consider sensory aspects including olfactory, sensory, auditory, and visual, all of which can have cultural implications.

> After discussing the pathology report, the NP reached out and embraced the young female patient. The NP, feeling her embrace was not welcomed, later reflected on the gesture. The gesture, intended to be a measure of comfort, was not positively received by the client. The client, from a culture where touch is limited, felt that the NP was intrusive, especially when distressing news was recently discussed.

Social Organization

Social organizations are structured groups that have a pattern of behaviors and set norms, beliefs, and values that influence the persons within the group. Examples include family, religious groups, communities, and organizations. Race and ethnicity may also be considered a social organization.

Time

The concept of time can have different implications based on a person's cultural view. Culture can impact one's relationship to time—past, future, or present orientation. Future orientation considers the future in present-day terms, past orientation has a connection to the past. New changes are based on what was considered in the past. Present orientation is focused on the current time. Understanding a client's orientation to time can be helpful in determining possible reasons for motivation, compliance, and participation.

> The toddler came into the office with several layers of clothing. The day was warm and comfortable. The mother stated, "My baby has a cold." Believing that the source of the cold was from the cool evening air that the infant was exposed to was a literal belief that the mother held from her past; the "chill was caught."

Environmental Control

The relationship between a person, the environment, and health and wellness determines the person's environmental control. Considerations of environmental control include the locus of control. *The client verbalized that the illness was in God's hands and* they did not have any control. Alternative therapies are more frequently considered in Western medicine. In 2012, approximately 30% of adults and approximately 12% of children were using some form of complementary and alternative medicine (CAM) (National Center for Complementary and Integrative Health [NCCIH] and the National Center for Health Statistics, 2012). Mind and body practices, such as yoga and mindfulness, have increased according to a 2017 National Health Interview Survey (NHIS) (*More Adults and Children Are Using Yoga and Meditation*, 2018)

> The scent of lavender was present in the hospital room. The patient applied the essential oil to her temples to relieve the tension headache she was experiencing.

Biological Variations

Biological variations exist and should be considered when caring for individuals and groups. A person's body structure, hair, and skin color are variable and have genetic and ethnic connections. In addition, this framework considers nutritional preferences. Genetics (the study of heredity) and genomics (the study of genes and their functions) are part of the NP's practice. Some genetic conditions are more likely to occur in a particular group; however, one cannot assume that a biological variation exists based on an individual's culture or ethnicity. For example, in the United States, sickle cell anemia is most prevalent in the African-American population due to ancestral origins.

> A young African-American mother brought her toddler in for a physical exam. She reported her daughter was pale and she expressed concern that her daughter might have sickle cell disease, like her brother. She was told as a young child their family had "bad cells" and her fear of her daughter having the disease was frightening. Upon further examination of the child, it was determined she had iron deficiency anemia, a condition common in toddlers who consume excessive amounts of cow's milk, and not sickle cell disease caused by a genetic mutation.

In contrast, some conditions such as hypertension are more prevalent in non-Hispanic black adults (*Facts About Hypertension, CDC,* 2020), but may be unrelated to race. In a review of the racial differences in hypertension (Lackland, 2014), racial disparities of hypertension in African-Americans remain unclear. Many of the standardized norms used in healthcare have been determined based on white data and may not be appropriately applied to all groups (Giger, 2017). Considering the many non-genetic factors that impact hypertension, including access to health care, early identification and treatment, and follow-up care, as well as geographic differences in the United States (*Facts About Hypertension, CDC,* 2020), it cannot be determined that one's race is the sole cause of this condition. There are complex interactions between genetics, social, and environmental determinants.

> An infant from China was adopted by American parents. The infant is brought in for a well child visit and the height, weight and head circumference is obtained and plotted on the CDC (Centers for Disease Control and Prevention) growth charts. All of the baby's anthropometric measures are under the 5th percentile. When considering the expected growth of

the infant, using the CDC growth charts, the NP should identify that the percentiles are used to assess the size and growth patterns of children in the United States and not in China. While ethnic and race defined growth charts are no longer recommended for use (Jones & Schulte, 2019), the child's growth should be monitored over time with consideration to the child's ethnicity and geographical origin, which will provide information to the child's growth assessment.

It is important to note that biological racial differences do not exist, despite resistance to the concept by some in the healthcare field. The Human Genome Project, an international effort to map the human genome, concluded in April 2003 (NHGRI, 2020). Among the outcomes of the project is the understanding that only 0.1% genetic difference exists between any two individuals—any two individuals have 99.9% identical DNA (Mersha & Abibi, 2015). The issue arises when race and ethnicity are used interchangeably, as they often are in the United States. While race does not include a biological component, ethnicity can. Race describes the phenological traits of individuals, most notably skin color, whereas ethnicity encompasses "biological factors, geographical origins, historical influences, as well as shared customs, beliefs, and traditions among populations that may or may not have a common genetic origin" (Mersha & Abibi, 2015, p. 2). It is, therefore, more crucial for the NP to ask questions of ancestry in order to discover any possible genetic conditions.

A helpful visual highlighting the 99.9% similarities in DNA across races can be found here: https://sitn.hms.harvard.edu/flash/2017/science-genetics-reshaping-race-debate-21st-century.

Hofstede's Cultural Dimensions Theory

Geert Hofstede developed a framework for cross-cultural communication that describes the effects of a society's culture on the values of its members. Understanding the culture's values can provide a clearer understanding of how to relate to the culture. Although Hofstede's work focused on the influence of culture on the values in the workplace, the information obtained can be applied to other settings. Applying Hofstede's model on national culture to the healthcare industry equips the provider with insight about culture and fosters opportunities to recognize the uniqueness of another culture through a comparison perspective. (Hofstede's model on national culture can be found at https://geerthofstede.com/culture-geert-hofstede-gert-jan-hofstede/6-dimensions-organizational-culture.)

Cultural Humility

Culture has many different components that shape who we are and how we interact with the world. It is dynamic and multifaceted. Each of us has our own personal culture evolving from not only our own ethnic background but also our gender, age, socioeconomic status, life experiences, and so on (California Health Advocates, 2007; Office of Minority Health [OMH], 2011b; Tervalon & Murray-Garcia, 1998). Reading and learning about other cultures is a worthwhile endeavor; however, it is unlikely that one can become competent in every culture. Being aware of this limitation, the concept of "cultural humility" is perhaps a better term to assist the NP in improving meaningful relationships with patients, coworkers, and others.

In the *Handbook of Humility: Theory, Research, and Applications* (2016), Mosher and colleagues describe cultural humility as placing a priority on "developing mutual respect and partnership with others" (p. 91). This requires self-awareness and reflection as a lifelong process to develop a respectful relationship with patients. It also requires the provider to be flexible and humble in order to be open to the cultural dimensions of each patient encounter. Values associated with cultural humility include openness, appreciation, and acceptance, in addition to flexibility (Luluquisen, Schaff, & Galvez, n.d.).

Further, it is important for the NP to focus on both interpersonal and intrapersonal components of cultural humility—realizing one's own limitations in understanding cultural backgrounds and being open to the "other" (Mosher et al., 2016). One needs to be acutely aware of the potential power imbalances that can occur in the healthcare expert–patient interaction. By continually working to be open, flexible, appreciative, and accepting of their patients, in addition to striving to avoid any imbalance of power, NPs can create meaningful partnerships with patients and communities to develop treatment plans, and individual and community goals to improve health. Practicing lifelong self-awareness and reflection will assist the NP to be a culturally sensitive healthcare provider.

In an effort to educate healthcare providers (NPs, physicians, PAs) about delivering culturally sensitive care, *A Physician's Guide to Culturally Competent Care* was developed by the U.S. Department of Health and Human Services, Office of Minority Health (OMH, n.d.). It contains nine Cultural Competency Curriculum Modules (CCCMs), including Standards for Culturally and Linguistically Appropriate Services in Health Care (CLAS standards), which are available for free at https://cccm.thinkculturalhealth.hhs.gov/. CME credits can be earned.

The objectives for this educational program are for NPs, PAs, and physicians to:

- Define issues related to cultural competency in medical practice.
- Identify strategies to promote self-awareness about attitudes, beliefs, biases, and behaviors that may influence the clinical care.
- Devise strategies to enhance skills toward the provision of care in a culturally competent clinical practice.
- Demonstrate the advantages of the adoption of the CLAS standards in clinical practice.

In many of the modules are patient cases and scenarios that require the healthcare provider to reflect upon what is being presented by the case, as well as how the reader feels about the situation. The fictional practice setting includes a profile of the community and the patients that are seen at the setting. The vast majority of the populations are white, non-Hispanic, who have at least a high school education; however, there are many migrant farm workers who use the practice, as well as Native Americans. The providers and support staff come from a variety of ethnic backgrounds and take different approaches to their practice. The practice setting is in need of much improvement, to work more efficiently and to provide culturally competent care to their patients. Through the learning modules, the healthcare provider is encouraged to consider what the patient's perspective is, to be more sensitive to one's own attitudes, including biases and the behaviors they may have displayed that affect patient care. **Box 6-2** represents eight essential elements to consider in developing a culturally competent healthcare provider.

Box 6-2 Eight Elements of Cultural Competence for Primary Healthcare Providers

1. Examine your values, behaviors, beliefs, and assumptions.
2. Recognize racism and the institutions or behaviors that breed racism.
3. Engage in activities that help you to reframe your thinking, allowing you to hear and understand other worldviews and perspectives.
4. Familiarize yourself with core cultural elements of the communities you serve.
5. Engage clients and patients to share how their reality is similar to, or different from, what you have learned about their core cultural elements.
6. Learn, and engage your clients to share, how they define, name, and understand disease and treatment.
7. Develop a relationship of trust with clients and coworkers by interacting with openness, understanding, and a willingness to hear different perceptions.
8. Create a welcoming environment that reflects the diverse communities you serve.

Nova Scotia Department of Health. (2005). A cultural competence guide for primary health care professionals in Nova Scotia. Halifax, Nova Scotia: Author.

Cultural Competence and the Clinician

Nurse practitioners are poised to lead initiatives to implement the strategies to meet the challenge of fulfilling national standards of cultural competence in health care. Since there are hundreds of ethnic groups in our society with diverse needs, there is no one specific intervention for each health issue. Developing the NP to provide cultural care by enhancing/developing one's competency is a process which can be developed using the steps in **Box 6-3**.

Schools of nursing and organizations recognize the need to promote cultural awareness and sensitivity and provide opportunities for enhancing the practice of nursing (AACN, 2008). The American Association of Colleges of Nursing (2008) calls for the need for cultural competence education in graduate nursing to address the diverse needs of patients and minimize disparities in health. Once healthcare providers identify their own need for cultural growth, they can engage themselves in a variety of actions to increase their cultural competence on an individual level. This engagement calls for self-reflection and acknowledgment that their own beliefs, values, and attitudes may affect the care they provide to others. The NP can take a "cultural approach," being cognizant of "cultural variations" that will be advantageous to the patient as a management plan is developed for the individual. Each encounter should be approached as unique. Clustering values, beliefs, and behaviors from a cultural group and applying them to all persons of that culture does not consider the multiple variables that may influence an individual's cultural uniqueness. The following example demonstrates misinterpretation of communication style.

> Elsu, a 76-year-old Native American male, arrived at the clinic for reevaluation of hypertension. The nurse assessing the patient felt that Elsu was "not truthful." The nurse expressed the concerns to the practitioner in charge of his care. Upon entering the room, the practitioner noticed

> **Box 6-3** Process for Competency Enhancement/Development
>
> The following steps apply to the nursing process for the purpose of enhancing or developing one's own nursing competencies. The steps include:
> - Assessment of one's own competencies
> - Diagnosis of competency gaps, i.e., competencies in need of further refining or development
> - Establish competency goal or goals, e.g., time frame within which competency will be more fully enhanced or developed
> - Create plan to achieve competency goal
> - Implement competency goal enhancement/development plan
> - Establish an ongoing program to evaluate self-progress, attainment of competency benchmark, and increasing mastery of the competency
>
> Note: Tools used to achieve new competencies include continuing education, professional reading, attendance at lectures, TED talks, seeking input and guidance from respected consumers, peers, colleagues, current or past mentors, as well as methods using newer technologies, e.g., videotaping and analysis of performance in practice.

Republished with permission of OJIN: The Online Journal of Issues in Nursing, from [Implementing the new ANA standard 8: Culturally congruent practice, Marion, L., Douglas, M., Lavin, M., Barr, N., Gazaway, S., Thomas, L., & Bickford, C., 22(1), 2016]; permission conveyed through Copyright Clearance Center, Inc

that Elsu avoided eye contact and participated minimally in conversation. The nurse who initially encountered the patient viewed his behaviors as untrusting. Elsu, being a Native American, is quiet and reserved when meeting new people. Eye contact, for the Native American, is considered a sign of disrespect and hence is avoided. The nurse assumed that Elsu's communication style had a different and undesirable meaning.

While one viewpoint of illness may be disease oriented, another perspective may focus on non-biomedical causes of disease. In an ethnographic study examining mental illness, distinct differences were noted between ethno-racial groups. The Euro-American group viewed mental illness with a disease-oriented perspective, whereas the Latino and African American population were critical of mental health services and interpreted mental illness from a non-biomedical perspective (Carpenter-Song et al., 2010). While this is an example of the variations that may exist between cultures, it highlights various perspectives that exist within the population.

Patterns of culturally incompetent care from providers affects patient care outcomes and may widen the healthcare disparities gap (Birkhäuer et al., 2017; Wasserman et al., 2019). Health disparities are linked to social, economic, and environmental disadvantages causing a difference in one's well-being (Office of Disease Prevention and Health Promotion, 2020). *Healthy People 2030* identifies populations who experience barriers to health care at higher rates than the general population. These groups include Hispanics, African-Americans, those with low levels of education, and the poor. The COVID-19 pandemic of 2020 further revealed these health disparities. For example, data collected in the United States during March 2020 of the pandemic showed that 33% of hospitalized patients were Black and African-American, although Blacks and African-Americans only make up 13% of the total population in the United States (Aubrey, 2020; Garg, Kim, Whitaker, et al., 2020).

These disparities among populations have long been known to healthcare institutions. The American College of Physicians (2010) in a position paper, *Racial and Ethnic Disparities in Health Care,* discuss the disparities and poor health care that exist among racial and ethnic groups. The American College of Physicians (2010) made several recommendations to reduce the disparities that affect health and wellness. Progress was made yet inequities continue to exist, and in 2021, the American College of Physicians released "A Comprehensive Policy Framework to Understand and Address Disparities and Discrimination in Health and Health Care." The recommendations strongly emphasize the role of policymakers in addressing the disparities in health and health care. In addition to the framework, three additional policy papers address disparities and discrimination (Serchen et al., 2021a, 2021b, 2021c, 2021d).

Culturally competent care providers can influence the health of the population by reducing the barriers that negatively impact health. Cultural sensitivity and awareness are important steps to understanding the complex issue of racial and ethnic health disparities.

Culture Awareness and Cultural Sensitivity

The acknowledgment and appreciation of the existence of differences in attitudes, beliefs, thoughts, and priorities in the health-seeking behaviors of different patient populations is critical. Cultural awareness is having the knowledge or information about what is unique or the same among various cultures. In contrast, cultural sensitivity is the individual's attitude about themselves or others and their desire to learn about the cultural aspects of others (Schim, Doorenbos, Benkert, & Miller, 2007). In an effort to meet the needs of communities and populations, we need to be open to learning about the unique characteristics they possess. Being aware and sensitive will allow us the ability to see beyond what the accepted norm within our society. Cultural sensitivity is when we are able to appreciate the situation from another's perspective and value the viewpoint of others, despite it being different from our own.

"The ANA supports the notion of self-reflection for understanding own cultural beliefs to avoid both conscious and unconscious biases toward others." (Marion et al., 2016).

Implicit bias occurs when actions based on stereotypes and prejudice are taken without intention. Individuals are unaware that their actions may have an unintended negative impact on others. To improve the awareness of one's bias the Implicit Association Test (IAT) https://implicit.harvard.edu/implicit/ is a resource that can facilitate awareness and encourage self-reflection. Reflection is a resource that supports a progressive journey in developing improved self-awareness and addressing any implicit bases that one may have. The opportunity to consider how the NP's individual experience, culture, and values can impact their response and actions to others through self-awareness is an important part of culturally sensitive care.

What Determines Cultural Competence?

Many theoretical and methodological models exist that attempt to determine cultural competence. Schim, Doorenbos, Miller, and Benkert (2003) describe a theoretical model of cultural competence with three components: the circumstance in which the clinician incorporates the cultural diversity experience; the clinician's awareness of his or her reactions to people who are different; and lastly, examining attitudes and cultural bias toward other sociocultural groups. Based on this description and the cultural competence model developed by Schim and Miller (as cited in Schim et al., 2003), the Cultural Competence Assessment (CCA) was developed. The CCA tool is a method of measuring cultural competence behaviors (CCB) and cultural awareness and sensitivity (CAS).

In contrast, the *Purnell Model for Cultural Competence* (Purnell, 2002) uses a methodological approach to determine cultural competence. The basic assumptions of the model derive from multidisciplinary theories including organizational, administrative, communication, and family development, as well as anthropology, sociology, psychology, and several others. The model has evolved to include 12 domains in a framework that assist the NP in developing cultural competence abilities.

International education scholar Darla Deardorff developed the Pyramid Model of Intercultural Competence (2006, 2009), which includes requisite attitudes necessary to develop cultural competence. These attitudes include respect, openness, and curiosity and discovery. Respect includes valuing other cultures and cultural diversity; openness is a measure of withholding judgment of other cultures and diversity; curiosity and discovery allow for tolerating ambiguity and uncertainty. See **Figure 6-1**.

Measuring our cultural competency aids in our understanding and responsiveness to the components of care crucial for meeting the needs of the diverse populations that NPs serve. Using a tool such as the CCA will give educators, mentors, and primary care providers the opportunity to evaluate their progress in, or journey into, cultural competency.

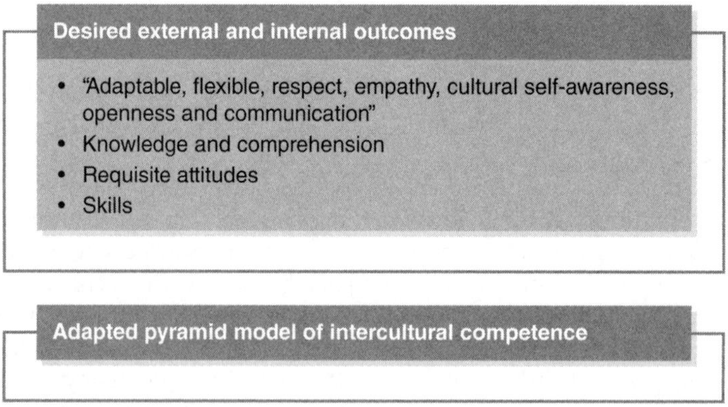

Desired external and internal outcomes

- "Adaptable, flexible, respect, empathy, cultural self-awareness, openness and communication"
- Knowledge and comprehension
- Requisite attitudes
- Skills

Adapted pyramid model of intercultural competence

Figure 6-1 Pyramid Model of Intercultural Competence

Data from Deardorff, D. (2006). Identification and Assessment of Intercultural Competence as a Student Outcome of Internationalization. *Journal of Studies in International Education, 10*(3), 241-266.

A personal self-assessment tool for the primary healthcare provider can offer insight into the cultural competence of the care provider (see **Box 6-4**). This quantitative tool requires the clinician to reflect on various areas of the cultural provision of care. Although there are no right or wrong answers, responding that "I rarely or never do" may suggest limitations in the ability to "demonstrate beliefs, attitudes, values, and practices that promote cultural competence within healthcare delivery programs" (Nova Scotia Department of Health, 2005, p. 19).

Box 6-4 Promoting Cultural Competence in Primary Health Care

I. Physical Environment, Materials, and Resources
  A. I ensure the printed and posted information in my work environment reflects the diversity and literacy of individuals or families to whom I provide service.
II. Communication Styles
  A. When interacting with individuals and families who do not have spoken English proficiency, I always keep in mind that:
    1. Spoken English proficiency does not reflect literate English proficiency or language of origin proficiency or literacy.
    2. Limited ability to speak the language of the dominant culture has no bearing on ability to communicate effectively in one's mother tongue.
    3. Limitations in English proficiency do not reflect mental ability.
  B. I use bilingual and/or bicultural staff trained in medical interpretation when required or requested.
  C. For individuals and families who speak languages other than English, I attempt to learn and use key words in their language so I am better able to communicate with them during assessment, treatment, or other interventions.
  D. I understand the cultural context for naming disease and try to be respectful of this in my interactions. (In some cultures, there is stigma associated with terminal disease, sexually transmitted disease, and/or communicable diseases. In some cultures, this stigma is avoided by naming the disease by its attributes, rather than its medical name (e.g., AIDS is sometimes named "the sleeping sickness").
  E. I can provide alternatives to written communication if required or preferred.
III. Social Interaction
  A. I understand and accept that family is defined in a variety of different ways by different cultures (e.g., extended family members, kin, godparents).
  B. Even though my professional or moral point of view may differ, I accept individuals and families as the ultimate decision makers for services and supports affecting their lives.
  C. I understand that age, sex, and life-cycle factors need to be considered in interactions with individuals and families. For instance, a high value may be placed on the decisions of elders, the role of eldest male or female in families, or roles and expectations of children within the family.

(continues)

D. I accept and respect that male–female gender roles may vary among different cultures and ethnic groups (e.g., which family member makes major decisions for the family).

IV. Health, Illness, and End-of-Life Issues
   A. I understand that the perceptions of health, wellness, and preventive health services have different meanings to different cultural or ethnic groups.
   B. I intervene in an appropriate manner when I observe other staff or clients within my program or agency engaging in behaviors that are not culturally competent.
   C. I screen resources for cultural, ethnic, or racial stereotypes and/or inclusion before sharing them with individuals and families served by my program or agency.
   D. I am aware of the socioeconomic and environmental risk factors that contribute to the major health problems of culturally, ethnically, and racially diverse populations served by my program or agency.
   E. I avail myself to professional development and training to enhance my knowledge and skills in the provision of services and supports to culturally, ethnically, racially, and linguistically diverse groups.
   F. I advocate for the review of my program or agency's mission statement, goals, policies, and procedures to ensure that they incorporate principles and practices that promote cultural and linguistic competence.

Nova Scotia Department of Health. (2005). *A cultural competence guide for primary health care professionals in Nova Scotia.* Halifax, Nova Scotia: Author.

Cultural Immersion Experiences

Cultural competency, infused into the skill set of all NPs, is a starting point for the reduction of disparities that exist within our healthcare system. Increasing cultural competence among providers will facilitate the goal of decreasing the healthcare disparities gap (Doorenbos et al., 2005). Cultural immersion experiences have been cited as a method to increasing cultural awareness and sensitivity (Green et al., 2011; Johns & Thompson, 2010; Jones et al., 2010; Larson et al., 2010). When individuals interact with various culturally diverse groups, their own beliefs regarding a cultural group will be affected and thus prevent stereotyping (Campinha-Bacote, 2003). A substantial portion of the literature on cultural immersion experiences affecting cultural awareness and sensitivity relates to students within the educational setting. Inclusion of service learning activities that increase the cultural sensitivity and awareness of students is a means to addressing the needs of our society. Students are likely to gain global attitudes and perspectives when schools of nursing include global experiences in their curriculum (Riner, 2011). This preparation will develop a sensitivity to and appreciation of cultures in an effort to provide high-quality care across various settings. The following is a reflection of a graduate student who participated in a clinical immersion experience in Central America:

> One of the things that really affected me while we were in Guatemala was seeing the number of children that were unable to go to school because

they had to work to help support their families. Growing up in the United States, our culture prides itself on education for all children. However, going to Guatemala and speaking with children who actually cannot go to school because they have to work really struck a chord with me. It is so easy for Americans to live in their little bubble because many have no idea what it is like to not have that option. In other words, we can complain about school because there is little risk that school won't be there for us. We see it as our inherent "right." Then there are the kids in Guatemala that are longing to go to school who are denied because their family needs them to help put food on the table. Kids who are 6, 7, and 8 years old, who, in America, would be doing homework, are instead out on the street selling bracelets at 10 pm at night in order to help their families. Talk about perspective! It really helps me to appreciate all the educational opportunities I have been and still am being given. (Regina, graduate student)

Cultural awareness and sensitivity improvements can be directed toward practicing providers within the healthcare setting. Communication and cultural awareness education can infuse a healthcare provider's communication skills with empathy, a nonjudgmental approach to patients, enhanced awareness of self, and awareness of his or her own nonverbal communication (Thomas & Cohn, 2006). To care for the population in a culturally competent manner, NPs should see themselves on a journey growing and cultivating distinctive experiences, which will lead toward achieving cultural competence (Campinha-Bacote, 2003). This journey provides the opportunity to learn and appreciate the uniqueness of culture. In the following excerpt, a nurse educator speaks about her journey to develop cultural competency:

As an educator I prided myself in having knowledge to share with others. Reflecting on years of direct patient care, caring for individuals and groups of various cultural and ethnic backgrounds, I was humbled by what I still did not know. It is when I examined my cultural competence that I began to realize that I will not "achieve" cultural competence but will be on a journey forever to reach competency. Each interaction I have with others will increase my understanding, my sensitivity, and my awareness. I will approach others with openness and nonjudgment as I persist in my efforts along the journey. (Carolina, nurse faculty)

Demystifying the Cultural Competence Puzzle

Cultural awareness training may be helpful in increasing cultural awareness, yet it is not an easy fix to improving outcomes for disparate populations. Sequist and colleagues (2010) in a randomized control study noted that primary care clinicians had increased awareness of racial disparities after an intensive 12-month program consisting of cultural competency training and race-stratified performance feedback. This training did not improve important aspects of disease control for black diabetic patients in the program, suggesting a need for further interventions (Sequist et al.,

2010). Awareness of cultural aspects of a particular group can be insightful, aiding in increased understanding, but it is not until the provider recognizes the influence of culture on a person's existence that it is significant. A partnership between a NP and client could assist in developing a greater understanding and appreciation of the culturally specific needs of the client in the context of his or her population. As expressed by the graduate student below, having one piece of the cultural competence puzzle is not enough:

> We talked about various cultures in the cultural nursing course, but it had little meaning to me. I am a NP student who has not encountered much diversity in my life. As a future NP, I know I need cultural skills to be effective in my role. But is having the knowledge I learned in class enough?

In a 2010 qualitative study, Erwin et al. (2010) examined the barriers and opportunities of Latino women to obtain health screenings and interventions. The study found that country of origin and their current geographical location affected their experiences with healthcare systems and access to services. Several cultural themes emerged, including the influence of "machismo" and putting the family before themselves. The effects of these culturally based influences can present as barriers to women obtaining healthcare services (Erwin et al., 2010). Cultural influences, such as the (American/U.S.) approach where women are encouraged to care for themselves and seek health promotion services, may be regarded as a method of empowerment in one culture, yet perceived as a barrier in other cultures.

For the Latino woman who depends on the input of her husband to receive care, it is in the best interest of the woman to involve her husband in the decision-making process regarding care decisions. By considering the Latino family's views as the preferred approach to health care, the healthcare team may have greater success in meeting the family's healthcare needs.

The following case study is representative, in that it involves a Guatemalan male in the implementation of care for his infant child:

> Ana, a mother who walked 90 minutes to the clinic in a developing country, brought her 3-month-old baby, Alessandra, to the clinic our team sponsored. The mother reported she was told to bring her baby home to die; the doctors in her country could not help her. When Alessandra arrived at the clinic, she was just over 3 pounds, nearly 2 pounds less than her birth weight. The team, after assessing the baby, determined that she was drinking cow's milk and had severe gastrointestinal and cutaneous symptoms. The team developed a feeding plan utilizing soy-based formula. When the team discussed the plan with the mother, it was apparent that the father of the baby needed to consent to the outlined plan. Ana was not able to make the decision for her baby. A community leader, who served as the liaison between team and family, facilitated the communication of the plan to the father, who consented. It was through the use of the community leader and a nonjudgmental approach, incorporating cultural considerations into the plan, that a successful plan was created for Alessandra. (Ellen, public health nurse)

In an article describing the fasting practices of women during pregnancy and breastfeeding, the differences between some practicing Muslim women and U.S. standards were discussed (Kridli, 2011). In a culture where pregnant women are encouraged to "eat for two," caregivers may find that the practice of fasting during pregnancy or breastfeeding is strange or wrong. It is important for the NP to take the time to understand the significance of fasting in the spiritual life of the Muslim woman. It is when healthcare providers can accept and appreciate the cultural uniqueness of an individual that they can then adapt the provision of care to meet the needs of the patient. The following case scenario is an example of how the nurse practitioner helped the patient with strong religious beliefs navigate his care in a complex health system:

> As a nurse practitioner I often need to reassess my own ability to reframe the ability to accept my patients' beliefs regarding healthcare treatments as well as their spirituality. It is sometimes difficult when we feel strongly that current practices are the only viable option for patients to choose, particularly when their choice is almost always one that will significantly alter the ability to survive. Religious beliefs can stir up much passionate argument for insisting patients do things "our" way. I will touch upon this in my short story.
>
> George was a middle-aged gentleman who came in yearly for his physical examination. He was doing very well in keeping his cholesterol in check with diet and a low dose statin and was up to date with immunizations. Until one recent visit, there were no other significant healthcare-related issues. At that visit George described feeling so fatigued he could hardly get through his workday as a manager for a large home goods store. He said he was bruising easily, and was very concerned, as was I. I knew that George was a Jehovah's Witness, and we had in his file his official document regarding no blood transfusions. I have some members of my family who are also Jehovah's Witnesses, so I was well aware of all the details and scriptural support for this belief. Unfortunately, his blood work returned showing a severe pancytopenia. I convinced him to go for the consultation with the hematologist we worked closely with, assuring him I would be his advocate for him to be the main director of his own healthcare treatment plan once he was fully assessed and treatment options were discussed. Being an advocate, I also had to speak with the hematologist before George went there so he could understand what issues could cause tension within their patient–physician relationship during this time of turmoil. Unfortunately, it did appear that George had aplastic anemia.
>
> We are working to find the cause, and he has opted to use complementary and alternative therapies instead of blood transfusions. The hematologist made George sign a document that released him from liability regarding George's decisions; however, he is still working with us for the time being. George is well aware of the possibility of dying without getting transfused, and he strongly holds to his belief system. As his primary care provider, I try to be supportive, as well as honest, when discussing his current status and his options. I have found that I am often being an advocate for George among the staff and other providers, using opportunities to correct inaccurate understanding regarding Jehovah's Witnesses.

Incorporating a cultural assessment or the collection of relevant cultural data relating to a patient's diagnosis or health concern is vital in the care of diverse populations (Campinha-Bacote, 2003). It is important to consider the biological, physical, and physiological cultural variations that may influence the physician's ability to conduct an appropriate and correct physical evaluation (Purnell, 1998, as cited in Campinha-Bacote, 2003). Significant cultural data should be gathered, adapted prior to and during the evaluation, and used in the planning and implementation of care. Goldbach, Thompson, and Hollaren Steiker (2011) discuss the importance of cultural consideration in the care of Latinos with substance abuse. The Latino culture values family orientation, *familismo,* and respect, *respeto,* in their lives. The inclusion of culturally specific aspects of care, along with acculturation, were identified as considerations when treating adolescents with substance abuse (Goldbach et al., 2011). Current strategies or approaches that do not include culturally specific strategies may be ineffective in meeting the unique needs of a specified population. To care for the adolescents, the practitioner must care for the family, use respect, and understand the psychosocial adjustment to the society in which the adolescent lives.

To understand health, it must be examined from the viewpoint of the individual or family. Health must not be gauged by others; the information must come directly from the person or community and be related to their specific circumstances (Kagan, 2008). To be effective practitioners caring for individuals, communities, and populations of need, it is important to use awareness and sensitivity, authentic listening, trust, partnerships, and commitment. It is when we strive for cultural competence that we are able to improve the lives of others.

Language and Communication

The Institute of Medicine (IOM, 2003) report, *Unequal Treatment: Confronting Racial and Ethnic Disparities in Health Care,* illustrates the importance of cross-cultural communication. Effective culturally sensitive communication will lead to patient satisfaction, adherence, and thus favorable patient outcomes, as seen in **Figure 6-2**. Faulty communication and a lack of consideration of the sociocultural factors will lead to poor patient outcomes and racial and ethnic disparities in care (IOM, 2003). To be an effective communicator, the NP must possess curiosity, empathy, respect, and humility (IOM, 2003) during interactions with individuals and communities. It is when providers ask questions and listen to the response that assumptions can be avoided.

The Office of Minority Health (OMH) was established in 1986 in response to the increased awareness regarding poor health outcomes in racial and ethnic

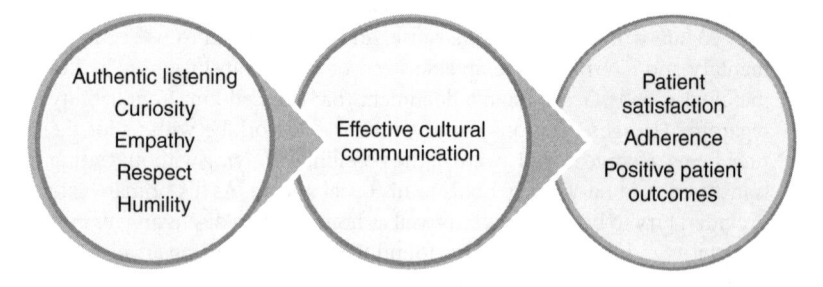

Figure 6-2 Communication Model

minority populations in the United States (OMH, 2011a). CLAS standards were developed by the OMH for healthcare systems to use in order to provide the best care possible for the diverse patient populations seeking care in the United States. These standards were recently enhanced, and the goals are to (1) advance health equity, (2) improve quality, and (3) help eliminate healthcare disparities. Providing services that are adapted to an individual's cultural and language preference can aid in positive patient outcomes. The 15 CLAS standards guide the NP and other healthcare providers to the recommended language and communication processes in healthcare settings that will enhance patient care outcomes (OMH, n.d.). For example, the NP should know the qualifications of the interpreter, interpreters must be trained in their role, and the clinician should speak directly to the patient and not the interpreter. The Think Cultural Health initiative contains educational resources to aid in the development of healthcare providers and organizations and have e-learning modules (https://www.thinkculturalhealth.hhs.gov/index.asp).

Listening

An important element of communication must not be overlooked: listening. Listening is an important yet underused skill. Patients express a desire to be listened to by their healthcare providers more than anything else (Berman & Chutka, 2016). Listening is an essential part of the appreciation and awareness of the viewpoints and feelings of others and is inherently connected to quality of life (Kagan, 2008). It is especially beneficial to employ therapeutic listening when working with individuals or groups from other cultures.

One study illustrated the benefit of listening and gaining insight into the lives of immigrant women (Belknap & VandeVusse, 2010). Using active listening, the researchers were able to identify emerging themes related to the lived experience of the women. Interventions and support related to the themes can be developed based on the knowledge obtained from listening sessions. The NP must become familiar with culturally competent organizations in the community to assist families. Partnering with the community and listening to their needs can assist the NP with the assessment, development, and implementation of interventions for the specified community. The listener, by providing a safe environment, allows the individual or group to feel secure to voice their expression. It is essential for the listener to be nonjudgmental, accepting, and negate all preconceived ideas, prejudices, and negative attitudes (Shipley, 2010). It is through active listening that the provider is receptive to discovering the needs and desires of others. NPs are often seen as the care providers that hear the patient. Most times, they have the ability to truly listen to the patient's voice, and this has significant implications in the cultural considerations of care.

The ETHNIC mnemonic represented in **Box 6-5** has been identified as a tool to assist the primary care provider in obtaining a history that encourages the inclusion of the patient's cultural perspective.

Trust

There is mistrust of the healthcare system by minority patients. Their mistrust is connected to treatment refusal for a variety of reasons including discontentment with the patient–provider relationship (Birkhäuer et al., 2017). As part of the most honest and ethical profession (ANA President Proud of Nurses for Maintaining #1 Spot in Gallup's 2019 Most Honest and Ethical Professions Poll, ANA, 2020), NPs

> **Box 6-5** The ETHNIC Mnemonic
>
> **E: *Explanation***
> What do you think may be the reason you have these symptoms? What do friends, family, or others say about these symptoms? Do you know anyone else who has had or who has this kind of problem? Have you heard about/read/seen it on TV/radio, or in a newspaper? (If the patient is unable to offer an explanation, ask the patient what is most concerning about the problem.)
>
> **T: *Treatment***
> What kinds of medicines, home remedies, or other treatments have you tried for this illness? Is there anything you eat, drink, or do (or avoid) on a regular basis to stay healthy? Tell me about it. What kind of treatment are you seeking from me?
>
> **H: *Healers***
> Have you sought any advice from alternative/traditional or folk healers, friends, or other people (nondoctors) for help with your problems? Tell me about it.
>
> **N: *Negotiate***
> Negotiate options that will be mutually acceptable to you and your patient and that do not contradict, but rather incorporate, your patient's beliefs.
>
> **I: *Intervention***
> Determine an intervention with your patient. This may include incorporation of alternative treatments, spirituality, and healers, as well as other cultural practices (e.g., foods eaten or avoided both in general and when sick).
>
> **C: *Collaboration***
> Collaborate with the patient, family members, other healthcare team members, healers, and community resources.

Reproduced with permission from Patient Care: The Practical Journal for Primary Care Physicians. Special Issue: Caring for Diverse Populations: Breaking Down Barriers, 34(9), 189. Patient Care is a copyrighted publication of Advanstar Communications Inc. All rights reserved.

are in a position to establish trusting and meaningful relationships with individuals, groups, and communities. Many of the skills necessary to build cultural awareness and sensitivity are instrumental in establishing trust: empathy, respect, listening, and a nonjudgmental approach. Taking time to build a rapport will aid in the development of trust and build relationships between the provider and the patient community. The following displays examples of a trusting relationship between a NP and a high-risk patient:

> Jana is an African-American mother of a 2-year-old, recently paralyzed child. The child suffered the injuries during a motor vehicle accident in which her maternal grandmother was under the influence of an illegal substance. Jana herself is a recovering from a substance use disorder and former sex worker who is starting to make great strides in her life. She is working and independently living in a small apartment with her daughter. As the NP overseeing her care in the hospital setting, I have the tremendous responsibility of working with the mother, with the mutual goal of discharging the daughter home.
>
> The initial discharge was complex. There were many considerations: ventilator, G-tube feedings, wheelchair, and nursing, to highlight several. As I discussed the

plan with the discharge coordinator, we were encountering obstacle after obstacle to meeting our goal. Was the home accessible? Was it safe? Did the mother have adequate support? We updated the mother frequently with the progress (or lack of progress). One morning the mother was angry and started to voice her concerns in a loud and disruptive manner; she said she "had it" with "all of you." After calming her and listening to her concerns it was apparent that she did not trust that we were truly trying to discharge her daughter to home. She felt the obstacles were hiding what she felt we considered the "true" issue: that she was unfit, due to her past history, to provide care to her daughter. Despite displaying the skills and behaviors that could support her daughter's needs, Jana felt that the staff saw her as an unfit parent. I was shocked. I thought we had a professional relationship that fostered trust, but what I did not understand was how Jana's life events affected her ability to trust us and voice her concerns. I learned, after caring for Jana and her daughter, that experiences can affect a person's perception and reaction. As an NP, I need to ensure that patients and their families are able to trust me as their care provider. I need to find ways to better understand them and their experiences.

Trust and privacy were major themes that emerged in a 2012 study examining the provision of health-related services to bisexual men (Dodge et al., 2012). Perception of others, confidentiality, and trusting relationships influenced their likelihood of seeking healthcare services. Fearing that their privacy and trust will be violated, many marginal groups may distance themselves from the healthcare services they require. This separation leads to continued disparities in the provision of care and negatively affects their health and well-being.

Global and race-based medical mistrust were high among black women who have sex with black women in a recent study (Brenick, Romano, Kegler, & Eaton, 2017). Individuals with mistrust have less engagement in health care, which is of concern for the health and well-being of this identified population. Stigma from race or sexual orientation, although low in the study, should be considered to reduce disparities and promote engagement in health care.

Trust can influence health. Another study examining the relationship of trust between patients with type 2 diabetes and their physicians demonstrated that trust was related to patient outcomes. The authors concluded that "trust in physicians could contribute to improvements in patient outcomes over time" (Lee & Lin, 2011, p. 411). When caring for populations, trust is essential to building a caring relationship, and having trust in a relationship is an important aspect of care that can improve health outcomes. If a provider is culturally competent, it will positively impact the treatment adherence of the patient and the quality of care (Davey, Waite, Nuñez, Niño, & Kissil, 2014).

Nurse practitioners are viewed as being skillful in developing trusting relationships with patients. The trust is developed by learning about the patient's family, culture, and socioeconomic needs; developing and using cultural tools; and incorporating nursing tenets from professional training.

Community Partnerships

When providing care to marginalized or culturally based populations, establishing a relationship with the community is essential. Partnership, defined as two or more individuals or groups working together for a shared goal, is a key element to community engagement. Meade, Meanard, Therival, and Riveria (2009) discuss the importance of community partnerships in the development and adaptation of sustainable breast health education and outreach programs for Haitian women. The partnership worked on the unique needs of the community and included cultural, educational, and literacy considerations. The development of a partnership affords the ability to determine factors that affect health and to develop approaches to maximize health and wellness. Partnerships with community leaders and community gatekeepers are essential features to the success of outreach initiatives (Meade et al., 2009).

An example of a lack of partnerships within the healthcare setting was presented in a 2009 study examining the use of CAM in the treatment of autism spectrum disorder (ASD) in the United States and China. An interesting finding from this study revealed that only 22.4% of respondents informed their doctors about CAM use to treat ASD. The study suggests that the participants did not inform their physician of the CAM use because they felt that the Western physician would not allow CAM nor believe its effectiveness (Wong, 2009). Lack of trusting partnerships can lead to continued healthcare disparities.

In a study exploring the influence of NPs on the delivery of culturally competent care, NPs stated that collaborating with other members of the healthcare team, as well as patients, was effective in the delivery of culturally competent care. Working with patients to meet their identified needs was a priority for the NP, as well as for the patient. Addressing other impending concerns was completed by negotiation and partnering.

In a 2011 study of Native American men and HIV, barriers to HIV/AIDS care were presented. Many of the barriers were related to and contributed to the disparity in the provision of care to Native American men. The participants in this study identified that using indigenous outreach workers would be an effective approach to the prevention and intervention efforts (Burks, Robbins, & Durtschi, 2011). They also expressed the importance of inclusion of traditional healing practices into the provision of HIV/AIDS services. Establishing partnerships with community leaders and outreach workers could improve the health of the community by addressing their needs with a culturally focused approach.

In addition, Saha and colleagues (2013) found that minority HIV patients who had a provider who scored toward the middle or high ranges of cultural competence were more likely to be on antiretrovirals than patients who had a provider who scored low in cultural competence. Again, this study shows that the cultural competence of the healthcare provider is connected to healthcare quality and outcomes of patients.

Pulling It All Together

Caring for patients and addressing and adapting care to meet the cultural needs of patients takes a holistic approach. When care is provided in a culturally sensitive manner, it extends beyond the medical concerns presented. The inclusion of social, spiritual, lifestyle, societal, and familial aspects of the individual is imperative to determining and responding to the patient's needs. Having a holistic approach means to look at the patient's complete life, not just focus on an illness.

The LIAASE, a general cultural competence tool, is a helpful structure to guide the provider in providing care that is sensitive to the individual's culture and preferences (see **Box 6-6**).

Language and Communication **179**

Box 6-6 The LIAASE: A General Cultural Competence Tool

Learn Read literature from other cultures. Identify your own biases and stereotypes.	**Avoid Polarization** Solicit other options or points of view. Ask what perspective a person from a different background would have.
Inquire Ask questions to clarify and understand information. Dig deeper to find reasons for behaviors or attitudes. Frame inquiries as searches for answers, showing a willingness to learn. Do not judge or interpret actions or speech; verify that what you understand is correct. Speak clearly; avoid slang, colloquial expressions, and large, complex words.	Curb the impulse to defend your point of view or opinion. Agree to disagree on differences in values. **Show Empathy** Listen not just to the words, but to the feelings behind the words. Acknowledge and validate powerful emotions when expressed.

State Your Needs and Expectations
It is important to set a respectful tone for the interaction. Let people know what you want and what you consider unacceptable behavior. In this way, assumptions, conflict, and/or resentment can be avoided.

Reproduced from Nova Scotia Department of Health and Wellness. (2005). *A cultural competence guide for primary health care professionals in Nova Scotia.* Retrieved from http://www.healthteamnovascotia.ca/cultural_competence/Cultural_Competence_guide_for_Primary_Health_Care_Professionals.pdf. Used by permission of Nova Scotia Department of Health and Wellness.

In the following case scenario, the NP uses components of the LIAASE tool as she develops a culturally competent plan of care for the patient.

Using the LIAASE Tool to Provide Culturally Sensitive Care

While working in a busy OB/GYN clinic as a new FNP, I was quickly moving my novice skill level to advanced due in part to the resident physicians' avoidance of the clinic. It was also a wonderful place to provide culturally sensitive care. We had a large number of patients from Haiti and Guatemala, in addition to almost every other country. One day I went into an examination room and found a pleasant young couple waiting for a new OB examination. The woman was covered in a very colorful sari and was smiling, but quiet and deferential to her equally pleasant husband.

He very nicely told me that since I was the only female provider in the clinic that day that they had requested I do her initial intake and examination. I loved doing the new OB visits, so that was not the challenge—the challenge was in trying to do a pelvic exam and get a PAP smear and ultrasound with all that clothing. Saris can be worn in different colors to represent different meanings. For instance, yellow can typically be worn for the first 7 days postpartum, and paisley can be worn as a symbol of fertility. The couple was pleased that I managed to get all the necessary portions of the examination done while maintaining the woman's privacy. We developed a mutually understanding and respectful partnership during a time of joy for this newly pregnant couple in what could have been disastrous if the provider who attended to them was not culturally sensitive.

Evaluation

When working with individuals or groups, there is a need to evaluate the outcomes of the interventions, including the evaluation of those we partner with. Outcome evaluations should be culturally sensitive; they should use wording and terms that the community or individual would understand within the context of their culture. It is important to receive feedback from the community or individual on whom the intervention focused. Do they perceive the intervention as useful or beneficial? After using focus groups to determine the best interventions to use in a community-based intervention program for Mexican American women, Ingram et al. (2012) used a participatory evaluation process to adapt to the needs of the women in the community. The authors, using the women's responses, were able to understand the behavioral and knowledge changes as a result of the program's interventions. Their responses revealed why they adapted their behaviors and showed the barriers they encountered when following the intervention recommendations (Ingram et al., 2012). Their input was valuable to gaining their perspective on the significance of the interventions as well as their perceived barriers, thus contributing an important aspect of program evaluation. When examining the outcomes of a program or intervention, cultural influences must be considered when applying meaning to the results (Issel, 2009).

Evaluation is the ability to reflect on our care as NPs in an effort to gain greater clarity on the provision of culturally competent care. It serves as a time to ask if the care was what the patient needed or desired. In our role, this feedback ensures that we are evaluating not only the care provided but also ourselves as care providers. In summary, nurse practitioners must respond to the unique and distinct needs of the diverse and ever-changing society. Attention to cultural variations, as well as societal factors influencing health, must be considered to care for an increasingly diverse population. Cultural awareness and sensitivity are critical to the achievement of culturally competent care.

Seminar Discussion Questions

1. Identify your own cultural beliefs and values.
2. Discuss the variety of cultures in your professional practice.
3. Reflect on your cultural journey. What do you consider as obstacles to achieving cultural competence? What strategies can be employed to overcome the barriers?
4. Describe a situation or circumstance when cultural factors influenced the care of an individual or family. Were culturally sensitive interventions/approaches

implemented? If yes, please describe. If interventions/approaches were not based on the individual's or family's cultural preferences, how could the encounter have been adapted to meet the unique cultural needs?
5. What method or strategy could be implemented to evaluate the integration of cultural strategies during a patient encounter?

References

American Association of Colleges of Nursing. (1994). *The essentials of master's education for advanced practice nursing.* http://www.aacn.nche.edu/education-resources/MasEssentials96.pdf

American Association of Colleges of Nursing. (2006). *The essentials of doctoral education for advanced nursing practice.* http://www.aacn.nche.edu/publications/position/DNPEssentials.pdf

American Association Colleges of Nursing (2008). *Cultural Competency in Baccalaureate Nursing Education.* Retrieved from: https://www.aacnnursing.org/Portals/42/AcademicNursing/CurriculumGuidelines/Cultural-Competency-Bacc-Edu.pdf

American Association of Colleges of Nursing. (2008). *The essentials of baccalaureate education for professional nursing practice.* http://www.aacn.nche.edu/education-resources/BaccEssentials08.pdf

American College of Physicians. (2010). *Racial and ethnic disparities in health care* (Policy paper). Author.

American Nurses Association [ANA]. (2012). *Diversity awareness mission statement.* Retrieved from http://nursingworld.org/MainMenuCategories/ThePracticeofProfessionalNursing/Improving-Your-Practice/Diversity-Awareness/Mission-Statement.html

American Nurses Association [ANA]. (2015). *Nursing: Scope and standards of practice* (3rd ed.). Silver Spring, MD: Nursebooks.org.

American Nurses Association [ANA]. (2016). *Nurses rank #1 most trusted profession for 15th year in a row.* http://www.nursingworld.org/FunctionalMenuCategories/MediaResources/PressReleases/Nurses-Rank-1-Most-Trusted-Profession-2.pdf

American Nurses Association [ANA]. (2020). ANA president proud of nurses for maintaining #1 spot in Gallup's 2019 most honest and ethical professions poll. https://www.nursingworld.org/news/news-releases/2020/american-nurses-association-president-proud-of-nurses-for-maintaining-1-spot--in-gallups-2019-most-honest-and-ethical-professions-poll/

Aubrey, A. (2020). CDC hospital data point to racial disparity in COVID-19 cases. *National Public Radio.* https://www.npr.org/sections/coronavirus-live-updates/2020/04/08/830030932/cdc-hospital-data-point-to-racial-disparity-in-covid-19-Cases

Axtell, S. A., Avery, M., & Westra, B. (2010). Incorporating cultural competence content into graduate nursing curricula through community-university collaboration. *Journal of Transcultural Nursing, 21,* 183–191. doi:10.1177/1043659609357633

Belknap, R. A., & VandeVusse, L. (2010). Listening sessions with Latinas: Documenting life contexts and creating connections. *Public Health Nursing, 27,* 337–346. doi:10.1111/j.1525-1446.2010.00864.x

Birkhäuer, J., Gaab, J., Kossowsky, J., Hasler, S., Krummenacher, P., Werner, C., & Gerger, H. (2017). Trust in the health care professional and health outcome: A meta-analysis. *PloS one, 12*(2), e0170988.

Berman, A. C., & Chutka, D. S. (2016). Assessing effective physician-patient communication skills: "Are you listening to me, doc?". *Korean Journal of Medical Education, 28*(2), 243–249. https://doi.org/10.3946/kjme.2016.21

Betancourt, J. R., Green, A. R., Carrillo, J. E., & Anaaeh-Firempong II, O. (2003, July–August). Defining cultural competence: A practical framework for addressing racial/ethnic disparities in health and health care. *Public Health Reports, 118,* 293–302.

Boutin-Foster, C., Foster, J., & Konopasek, L. (2008). Viewpoint: Physician, know thyself: The professional culture of medicine as a framework for teaching cultural competence. *Academic Medicine, 83,* 106–111. doi:10.1097/ACM.0b013e31815c6753

Brenick, A., Romano, K., Kegler, C., & Eaton, L. A. (2017). Understanding the influence of stigma and medical mistrust on engagement in routine healthcare among black women who have sex with women. *LGTB, 4*(1). doi:10.1089/lgbt.2016.0083

Budiman, A. (2020). Americans are more positive about the long-term rise in U.S. racial and ethnic diversity than in 2016. *Pew Research Center.* https://www.pewresearch.org/fact-tank/2020/10/01/americans-are-more-positive-about-the-long-term-rise-in-u-s-racial-and-ethnic-diversity-than-in-2016/

Burks, D. J., Robbins, R., & Durtschi, J. P. (2011). American Indian gay, bisexual, and two-spirit men: A rapid assessment of HIV/AIDS risk factors, barriers to prevention, and culturally sensitive intervention. *Culture, Health & Sexuality, 13*(3), 283–298.

California Health Advocates. (2007). *Are you practicing cultural humility? The key to success in cultural competence.* http://www.cahealthadvocates.org/news/disparities/2007/are-you.html

Campinha-Bacote, J. (2003). Many faces: Addressing diversity in health care. *Online Journal of Issues in Nursing, 8.* http://www.nursingworld.org/MainMenuCategories/ANAMarketplace/ANAPeriodicals/OJIN/TableofContents/Volume82003/No1Jan2003/AddressingDiversityinHealthCare.aspx

Carpenter-Song, E., Chu, E., Drake, R. E., Ritsema, M., Smith, B., & Alverson, H. (2010). Ethno-cultural variations in the experience and meaning of mental illness and treatment: Implications for access and utilization. *Transcultural Psychiatry, 47*(2), 224–251. https://doi.org/10.1177/1363461510368906

Centers for Disease Control and Prevention. (2020). *Facts about hypertension.* https://www.cdc.gov/bloodpressure/facts.htm

Corazzini, K. N., Lekan-Rutledge, D., Utley-Smith, Q., Piven, M. L., Colon-Emeric, C. S., Bailey, D., Anderson, R. A., et al. (2006). The golden rule: Only a starting point for quality care. http://www.ncbi.nlm.nih.gov/pmc/articles/PMC1636677

Davey, M. P., Waite, R., Nuñez, A., Niño, A., & Kissil, K. (2014). A snapshot of patients' perceptions of oncology providers' cultural competence. *Journal of Cancer Education, 29*(4), 657–664.

Dayer-Berenson, L. (2014). *Cultural competencies for nurses: Impact on health and illness* (2nd ed.). Jones & Bartlett Learning.

Dodge, B., Schnarvs, P. W., Gonclaves, G., Majebranche, D., Martinez, O., Reece, M., & Fortenberry, J. D. (2012). The significance of privacy and trust in providing health-related services to behaviorally bisexual men in the United States. *AIDS Education and Prevention, 24,* 242–256.

Erwin, D. O., Trevino, M., Saag-Harfouche, S. G., Rodriguez, E. M., Gage, E., & Jandorf, L. (2010). Contextualizing diversity and culture within cancer control interventions for Latinas: Changing interventions, not cultures. *Social Science & Medicine, 71,* 693–701. http://ac.els-cdn.com.silk.library.umass.edu

FitzGerald, C., & Hurst, S. (2017). Implicit bias in healthcare professionals: a systematic review. *BMC Medical Ethics, 18*(1), 1–18.

Garg, S., Kim, L., Whitaker, M., et al. (2020). Hospitalization rates and characteristics of patients hospitalized with laboratory-confirmed coronavirus disease 2019—COVID-NET, 14 States, *MMWR Morb Mortal Wkly Rep 2020; 69*:458–464. http://dx.doi.org/10.15585/mmwr.mm6915e3 external icon

Garneau, A. B., & Pepin, J. (2015). Cultural competence: A constructivist definition. *Journal of Transcultural Nursing, 26*(1), 9–15.

Giger, J. N. (2017). *Transcultural nursing: Assessment and intervention* (7th ed.). https://pageburstls.elsevier.com/#/books/9780323399920/

Giger, J., Davidhizar, R., Purnell, L., Harden, J., Phillips, J., & Strickland, O. (2007). American Academy of Nursing Expert Panel Report: Developing cultural competence to eliminate health disparities in ethnic minorities and other vulnerable populations. *Journal of Transcultural Nursing, 18*(2), 95–102.

Goldbach, J. T., Thompson, S. J., & Hollaren Steiker, L. K. (2011). Special considerations for substance abuse intervention with Latino youth. *Prevention Researcher, 18*(2), 8–11.

Green, S. S., Comer, L., Elliott, L., & Neubrander, J. (2011). Exploring the value of an international service-learning experience in Honduras. *Nursing Education Perspectives, 12,* 302–307.

Hagiwara, N., Elston Lafata, J., Mezuk, B., Vrana, S. R., & Fetters, M. D. (2019). Detecting implicit racial bias in provider communication behaviors to reduce disparities in healthcare: Challenges, solutions, and future directions for provider communication training. *Patient Education and Counseling,* S0738399119301429. https://doi.org/10.1016/j.pec.2019.04.023

References 183

Hall, W. J., Chapman, M. V., Lee, K. M., Merino, Y. M., Thomas, T. W., Payne, B. K., Coyne-Beasley, T., et al. (2015). Implicit racial/ethnic bias among health care professionals and its influence on health care outcomes: A systematic review. *American Journal of Public Health, 105*(12), e60–e76. https://doi.org/10.2105/AJPH.2015.302903

Hyattsville, MD: National Center for Health Statistics. Howell, W. L. (2012).

Ingram, M., Piper, R., Kunz, S., Navarro, C., Sander, A., & Gastelum, S. (2012). Salud sí: A case study for the use of participatory evaluation in creating effective and sustainable community-based health promotion. *Family & Community Health, 35,* 130–138. doi:10.1097/FCH.0b013 e31824650ed

Institute of Medicine. (2003). *Unequal treatment: Confronting racial and ethnic disparities in health care.* Washington, DC: National Academy Press. http://www.nap.edu/openbookphp?record_id=12875&page=200

Issel, L. M. (2009). *Health program planning and evaluation* (2nd ed.). Jones & Bartlett Learning.

Johns, A., & Thompson, C. W. (2010). Developing cultural sensitivity through study abroad. *Home Health Care Management Practice, 22,* 344–348. doi:10.1177/1084822 309353153

Jones, E. D., Ivanov, L. L., Wallace, D., & VonCannon, L. (2010). Global service learning project influences culturally sensitive care. *Home Health Care Management Practice, 22,* 464–469. doi: 10.1177/1084822310368657

Jones, V., & Schulte, E. E. (2019). Comprehensive health evaluation of the newly adopted child. *Pediatrics, 143*(5), e20190657. https://doi.org/10.1542/peds.2019-0657

Kagan, P. N. (2008). Feeling listened to: A lived experience of human becoming. *Nursing Science Quarterly, 21*(1), 59–67. doi:10.1177/0894318407310779

Kridli, S. (2011). Health beliefs and practices of Muslim women during Ramadan. *MCN, the American Journal of Maternal Child Nursing, 36,* 216–221. doi:10.1097/NMC.0b013e3182 177177

Lackland, D. T. (2014). Racial differences in hypertension: Implications for high blood pressure management. *The American Journal of the Medical Sciences, 348*(2), 135–138. https://doi.org/10.1097 /maj.0000000000000308

Larson, K. L., Ott, M., & Miles, J. M. (2010). International cultural immersion en vivo reflections in cultural competence. *Journal of Cultural Diversity, 2,* 44–50.

LaVeist, T., Gaskin, D., & Richard, P. (2009). *The economic burden of health inequalities in the United States.* Washington, DC: Joint Center for Political and Economic Studies. http://www.jointcenter.org/hpi/sites/all/files/Burden_Of_Health_FINAL_0.pdf

Lee, Y., & Lin, J. L. (2011). How much does trust really matter? A study of the longitudinal effects of trust and decision-making preferences on diabetic patient outcomes. *Patient Education and Counseling, 85,* 406–412. doi:10.1016/j.pec.2010.12.005

Levin, S. J., Like, R. C., & Gottlieb, J. E. (2000). Appendix: Useful clinical interviewing mnemonics. *Patient Care: The Practical Journal for Primary Care Physicians.* Special Issue: *Caring for Diverse Populations: Breaking Down Barriers, 34*(9), 189.

Loden, M., & Rosener, J.B. (1991). *Workforce America.* Homewood, IL: Business One Irwin.

Luluquisen, M., Schaff, K., & Galvez, S. (n.d.). Alameda County Public Health Department Community Assessment Planning & Education Unit. *Cultural competence and cultural humility* [PowerPoint presentation]. http://www.acphd.org/media/133120/modii_slides_cultural_competency.pdf

Marion, L., Douglas, M., Lavin, M., Barr, N., Gazaway, S., Thomas, L., & Bickford, C. (2016). Implementing the new ANA standard 8: Culturally congruent practice. *OJIN: The Online Journal of Issues in Nursing, 22*(1). doi:10.3912/OJIN.Vol22No01PPT20. https://ojin.nursingworld.org/MainMenuCategories/ANAMarketplace/ANAPeriodicals/OJIN/TableofContents/Vol-22-2017/No1-Jan-2017/Articles-Previous-Topics/Implementing-the-New-ANA-Standard-8.html

Matteliano, M. A., & Street, D. (2012). Nurse practitioners' contributions to cultural competence in primary care settings. *Journal of American Academy of Nurse Practitioners, 24,* 425–435.

McFarlane, M. M., & Eipperle, M. K. (2008). Culture care theory: A proposed practice theory guide for nurse practitioners in primary care settings. *Contemporary Nurse, 28*(1/2), 46–63.

McIntosh, P. (2015). Extending the knapsack: Using the white privilege analysis to examine conferred advantage and disadvantage. *Women & Therapy, 38*(3–4), 232–245.

Meade, C. D., Meanard, J., Therival, C., & Riveria, M. (2009). Addressing cancer disparities through community engagement: Improving breast health among Haitian women. *Oncology Nursing Forum, 36,* 716–723. doi:10.1188/09.ONF.716-722

Mersha, T. B., & Abebe, T. (2015). Self-reported race/ethnicity in the age of genomic research: its potential impact on understanding health disparities. *Human genomics, 9*(1), 1–15.

Mosher, D.K. et al. (2016) Handbook of Cultural Humility, Edited By Everett L. Worthington Jr., Don E. Davis, Joshua N. Hook Chapter Six: Humility Routledge. Retrieved https://doi.org/10.4324/9781315660462

National Center for Complementary and Integrative Health [NCCIH]. (2018). *More adults and children are using yoga and meditation.* https://www.nccih.nih.gov/news/press-releases/more-adults-and-children-are-using-yoga-and-meditation

National Human Genome Research Institute [NHGRI]. (2020). The human genome project. https://www.genome.gov/human-genome-project

Nova Scotia Department of Health. (2005). *A cultural competence guide for primary health care professionals in Nova Scotia.* Halifax, Nova Scotia: Author.

Office of Disease Prevention and Health Promotion. (2020). *Healthy People 2030.* http://healthypeople.gov/2020/about/DisparitiesAbout.aspx

Office of Minority Health. (n.d.). *A physician's practical guide to culturally competent care.* https://cccm.thinkculturalhealth.hhs.gov

Office of Minority Health. (n.d.). *National CLAS standards.* https://www.thinkcultural health.hhs.gov/Content/clas.asp#clas_standards

Office of Minority Health. (2011a). *About OMH.* http://minorityhealth.hhs.gov/templates/browse.aspx?lvl=1&lvlID=7

Office of Minority Health. (2011b). *What is cultural competency?* http://minority health.hhs.gov/templates/browse.aspx?lvl=2&lvlID=11

Ott, B. B., & Olson, R. M. (2011). Ethical issues of medical missions: The clinicians' view. *HEC Forum, 23*(2), 105–113. doi:10.1007/s10730-011-9154-9

Purnell L. The Purnell Model for Cultural Competence. J Transcult Nurs. 2002 Jul;13(3):193-6; discussion 200-1. doi: 10.1177/10459602013003006. PMID: 12113149.

Riner, M. E. (2011). Globally engaged nursing education: An academic program framework. *Nursing Outlook, 59,* 308–317. doi:10.1016/j.outlook.2011.04.005

Saha, S., Korthuis, P. T., Cohn, J. A., Sharp, V. L., Moore, R. D., & Beach, M. C. (2013). Primary care provider cultural competence and racial disparities in HIV care and outcomes. *JGIM: Journal of General Internal Medicine, 28*(5), 622–629.

Schim, S. M., Doorenbos, A., Benkert, R., & Miller, J. (2007). Culturally congruent care: Putting the puzzle together. *Journal of Transcultural Nursing, 18,* 103–110. doi:10.1177/1043659606298613

Schim, S. M., Doorenbos, A. Z., Miller, J., & Benkert, R. (2003). Development of a cultural competence assessment instrument. *Journal of Nursing Measurement, 11*(3), 29–40.

Sequist, T. D., Fitzmaurice, G. M., Marshall, R., Shaykevich, S., Marston, A., Safran, D. G., & Ayanlan, J. Z. (2010). Cultural competency training and performance reports to improve diabetes care for black patients. *Annals of Internal Medicine, 152*(4), 40–46. http://web.ebscohost.com.silk.library.umass.edu/ehost/pdf

Serchen, J., Doherty, R., Atiq, O., & Hilden, D. (2021a). A comprehensive policy framework to understand and address disparities and discrimination in health and health care: A policy paper from the American College of Physicians. *Annals of Internal Medicine.* https://doi.org/10.7326/m20-7219

Serchen, J., Doherty, R., Atiq, O., & Hilden, D. (2021b). Understanding and addressing disparities and discrimination affecting the health and health care of persons and populations at highest risk: A position paper of the American College of Physicians. https://www.acponline.org/acp_policy/policies/understanding_discrimination_affecting_health_and_health_care_persons_populations_highest_risk_2021.pdf

Serchen, J., Doherty, R., Atiq, O., & Hilden, D. (2021c). Understanding and addressing disparities and discrimination in education and in the physician workforce: A position paper of the American College of Physicians. https://www.acponline.org/acp_policy/policies/understanding_discrimination_in_education_physician_workforce_2021.pdf

Serchen, J., Doherty, R., Atiq, O., & Hilden, D. (2021d). Understanding and addressing disparities and discrimination in law enforcement and criminal justice affecting the health of at-risk persons and populations: A position paper of the American College of Physicians. https://www.acponline.org/acp_policy/policies/understanding_discrimination_law_enforcement_criminal_justice_affecting_health_at-risk_persons_populations_2021.pdf

Shipley, S. D. (2010). Listening: A concept analysis. *Nursing Forum, 45*(2), 125–134.

Sitzman, K., & Eichelberger, L. W. (Eds.). (2004). *Understanding the work of nurse theorists.* Jones and Bartlett.

Stanglin, K. D. (2005). The historical connection between the Golden Rule and the second greatest love command. *Journal of Religious Ethics, 33*(2), 357–371.

Tervalon, M., & Murray-Garcia, J. (1998). Cultural humility versus cultural competence: A critical distinction in defining physician training outcomes in multicultural education. *Journal of Health Care for the Poor and Underserved, 9*(2), 117–125.

Thomas, V. J., & Cohn, T. (2006). Communication skills and cultural awareness courses for healthcare professionals who care for patients with sickle cell disease. *Issues and Innovations in Nursing Education, 53,* 480–488.

Tomey, A. M., & Alligood, M. R. (2002). *Nursing theorists and their work* (5th ed.). Mosby./Elsevier.

Turner, A. (2018). *The business case for racial equity: A strategy for growth.* Altarum. https://altarum.org/RacialEquity2018

Urban dictionary: Platinum rule. (n.d.). Urban Dictionary. https://www.urbandictionary.com/define.php?term=Platinum Rule

Vetto, J. T. (2015). Reflections: Cancer education and "the platinum rule." *Journal of Cancer Education, 32*(1), 206–207. https://doi.org/10.1007/s13187-015-0907-z

Wasserman, J., Palmer, R. C., Gomez, M. M., Berzon, R., Ibrahim, S. A., & Ayanian, J. Z. (2019). Advancing health services research to eliminate health care disparities. *American Journal of Public Health, 109*(S1), S64–S69.

Wong, V. C. (2009). Use of complementary and alternative medicine (CAM) in autism spectrum disorder (ASD): Comparison of Chinese and Western culture. *Journal of Autism & Developmental Disorders, 39*(3), 454–463. doi:10.1007/s10803-008-0644-9

CHAPTER 7

Chronic Disease Management Models, Pain Management, and Palliative Care

Mary Lou Siefert, Sylvie Rosenbloom, Elizabeth Ercolano, and Jean Boucher

Introduction

This chapter provides a brief overview of palliative care and chronic disease management. The advanced practice nurse (APN) role and relationship between chronic disease and palliative care symptom management are discussed in the context of quality of life for patients with serious illness and its effect on their families. Additionally, information pertinent to the goals of care and transitions of care are discussed. Some key national organizations instrumental in providing palliative care resources and guidelines are described and presented. Symptom management in palliative care is reviewed, and resources are provided for further information and up-to-date symptom management guidelines. Finally, a case study is presented to pull the elements of chronic disease and palliative care together in the context of advance practice nursing.

Palliative Care Definition and Background

Palliative care is both a philosophy and a structure for the delivery of care. There are many definitions of palliative care. Common themes through most definitions are (1) the addressing of symptoms to relieve and prevent suffering and improve the quality of life of patients and families in the face of serious illness, (2) the inclusion of the patient and family caregivers, (3) facilitation of autonomy, and (4) access to information and the choice with an interprofessional team approach to the delivery of care. These themes do *not* preclude treatment of the underlying condition or illness (World Health Organization, 2015). The overall goal of palliative care is to provide symptom management, prevent and treat suffering, and maintain or improve quality of life for the patient and the family members at any time and is not based on the patient's prognosis (Center to Advance Palliative Care [CAPC], 2021; Centers for Medicare & Medicaid Services [CMS], 2008; National Consensus Project [NCP] for Quality Palliative Care, 2018).

Although palliative care grew out of the hospice movement, it is not the same as hospice care. Hospice care has a defined focus on end-of-life care. It is provided to patients with serious illnesses with a limited prognosis who are *not* receiving treatment with a curative or life-prolonging intent. Palliative care is often misunderstood and defined as hospice care by both healthcare professionals and the general public (*Oxford Textbook of Palliative Nursing*, 2010). Many healthcare professionals and the general public hold the same misconception that all palliative care is hospice care and that one is the same as the other. Misconceptions and misunderstandings about palliative care can be detrimental to the successful implementation and delivery of palliative care, and thus detrimental to patients and their families such that quality of life is compromised. Healthcare professionals, and patients and families, are often hesitant to discuss palliative care because of the misconception that it must be end-of-life care and that other disease-focused treatments with curative intent cannot be administered concurrently with palliative care. While hospice care falls under the larger umbrella of palliative care, hospice care is not representative of the whole of palliative care; rather hospice care can be understood as including elements of palliative care or as a type of palliative care provided to patients and families as patients near death, and therefore hospice care has a distinct focus on end-of-life care (see **Figure 7-1**). Provision of both palliative care and hospice care result in improved patient outcomes in terms of symptom management, satisfaction, and death at the patient's place of preference; cost savings can be achieved with reduced hospital admission costs; and some evidence suggests life may be prolonged (Meier, 2011). Palliative care can be provided at any time during one's life or disease trajectory, does not preclude treatment of an underlying illness or disease with a curative or life-prolonging intent, and does not and should not only be provided as end-of-life care.

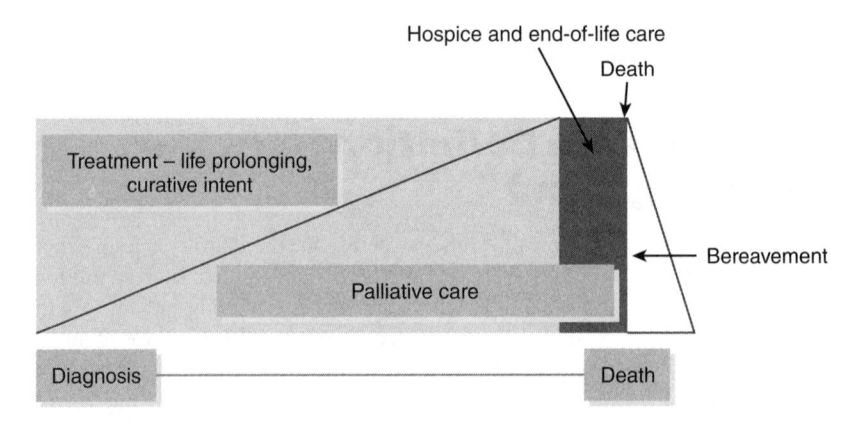

Figure 7-1 Palliative and Hospice Care

Data from Parikh, R. B., Kirch, R. A., Smith, T. J., & Temel, J. S. (2013). Early specialty palliative care--translating data in oncology into practice. *The New England Journal Of Medicine, 369*(24), 2347-2351.

Goals of Care

One principal component of palliative care is having goal-setting discussions with patients and their caregivers. A goal-oriented process encourages communication and decision-making, reduces patient uncertainty, and promotes the identification of the health outcomes a patient desires to achieve (Waldrop & Meeker, 2012). Discussion about goals also encourages patients and families to identify facilitators that will help patients reach their goals and barriers that may prevent goal attainment. Identification of specific and measurable health-related goals that are congruent with and address the patient's and family's quality of life (QOL) needs is associated with greater success in goal achievement. However, frequently patients and their healthcare providers are reluctant to have conversations about goals of care particularly in the context of advanced disease with a poor prognosis or when physical and emotional symptoms overwhelm patients (Wright et al., 2008). Therefore, it is most helpful for APNs to engage patients and their caregivers in discussions about their care preferences and goals of care *early* in the delivery of palliative care services.

Care Transitions

Care transitions represent changes in treatment approaches and philosophy due to progression or remission of a disease. Care transitions also represent changes in the level of complexity of healthcare services. For most patients, care transitions are associated with uncertainty, worry, and related physical, functional, and social adjustments (Bakitas, 2017). Advanced practice nurses play a central role in supporting patients and their caregivers through care transitions to reduce uncertainty, increase knowledge, and promote self-management. The APN providing palliative care must be vigilant and constantly monitor the patient for changes in condition. This requires ongoing assessment and evaluation of the patient and the response to interventions. Goals of care will change as a disease progresses or the responses to treatments change. Transition times can occur rather quickly, taking only minutes to hours, or may occur more slowly, and take days to weeks or longer. The transition times are opportunities for APNs to reassess the goals of care and promote key palliative care objectives of symptom management, advocate for patients and families, and facilitate consults with the palliative care interdisciplinary team (Dahlin et al. 2016; McCorkle et al., 2015).

Quality of Life

For the purposes of this chapter, quality of life (QOL) will be defined using the conceptual model of QOL developed and extensively used and tested by Ferrell and colleagues (Ferrell, 1996; Ferrell, Dow, & Grant, 1995; Ferrell, Grant, Padilla, Vemuri, & Rhiner, 1991). Ferrell and colleagues (1991, 1995) defined QOL as including four domains—the physical, psychological, social, and spiritual areas of one's life. Each of the four domains contains different concepts, concerns, types of distress, and symptoms that fall within each domain (**Figure 7-2**). The areas within each domain may vary slightly depending on a specific illness or symptom. For example, for the patient with breast cancer, the model has been revised slightly to

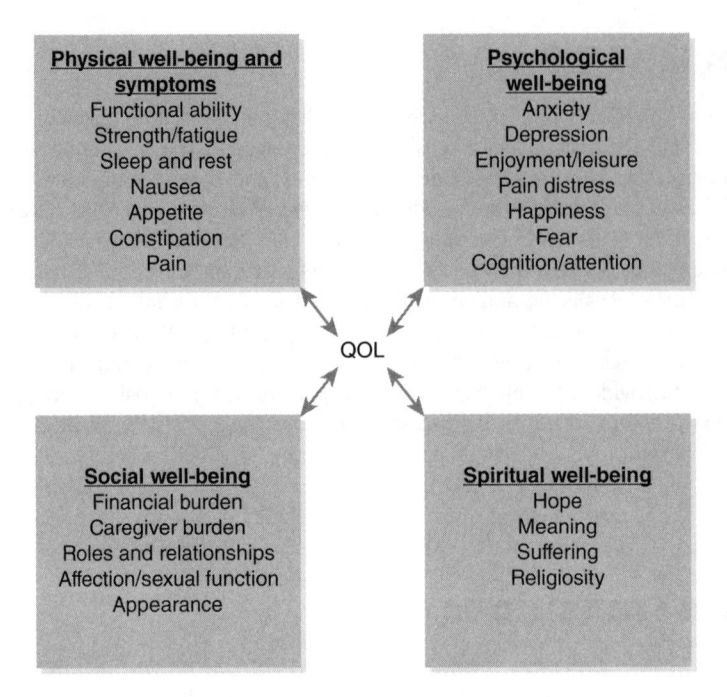

Figure 7-2 Quality of Life (QOL) Model

Physical well-being and symptoms
- Functional ability
- Strength/fatigue
- Sleep and rest
- Nausea
- Appetite
- Constipation
- Pain

Psychological well-being
- Anxiety
- Depression
- Enjoyment/leisure
- Pain distress
- Happiness
- Fear
- Cognition/attention

Social well-being
- Financial burden
- Caregiver burden
- Roles and relationships
- Affection/sexual function
- Appearance

Spiritual well-being
- Hope
- Meaning
- Suffering
- Religiosity

Reproduced from Ferrell, B.R., & Grant, M. (2000). Quality-of-life model. Duarte, CA: City of Hope National Medical Center. Reprinted with permission. Available online at http://prc.coh.org

include menstrual change/fertility within the physical domain in the QOL model (Ferrell et al., 1996). Another example of a difference in the model is the inclusion of strength and fatigue in the physical domain in the QOL model for pain (Ferrell et al., 1991). A large systematic review of qualitative literature (3,589 articles) was conducted to ascertain the aspects of QOL that are important from patients' perspectives. Eight were identified: physical, personal autonomy, emotional, social, spiritual, cognitive, health care, and preparatory (McCaffrey et al., 2016). The findings in this more recent review are congruent with the domains and concepts contained in the model developed by Ferrell and colleagues.

Quality of life is a multidimensional concept, and when one dimension of QOL is affected, other dimensions are also affected. For example, when the physical domain or dimension of QOL is affected by pain, the psychological and social domains may also be affected. One may not only be distressed by the physical presence of pain but may also experience psychological distress by feeling anxious or depressed about the meaning of the pain. One may also feel unable to engage with friends or family socially due to the unpleasant and uncomfortable nature of the pain. Persons with pain can therefore feel socially isolated because they are unable to enjoy time with friends and family due to the distress associated with both the physical and psychological symptoms associated with the pain. The lack of social engagement can thus also negatively impact their psychological distress; therefore, it is understandable why one area of distress in the QOL model can have a profound impact in other areas of QOL. When

APNs provide interventions to address symptoms in more than one area of QOL, patients showed stronger outcomes than if only one area of QOL was targeted by nurses (McCorkle et al., 2009).

National Organizations

There are a number of national palliative care–focused organizations and each has a slightly different focus, mission, and goals. However, they all foster and support the implementation and delivery of high-quality palliative care through the provision of various resources and activities. A few of these organizations that the APN will find helpful are highlighted here. The reader is encouraged to seek further information from and about any of the organizations and the affiliates listed here, as well as others they may find helpful. The websites are included in the text, and information is regularly updated for each of the organizations described here.

The National Coalition for Hospice and Palliative Care (The Coalition) (http://www.nationalcoalitionhpc.org/) was founded in 2001 and originally consisted of four member organizations. Today, The Coalition is comprised of 13 national professional organizations and has subsequently grown to include tens of thousands of interdisciplinary healthcare professional members, including nurses, physicians, chaplains, pharmacists, physician assistants, social workers, and other professionals from the 13 member organizations. The Coalition was originally founded to communicate, coordinate, and collaborate around issues related to hospice and palliative care and has five strategic priority areas identified in 2021 as quality, advocacy, payment, research, and workforce. The current goals (2021) of The Coalition are to:

> *Coordinate* and *communicate* a shared national vision about the importance of high quality palliative care in multiple settings including hospice, hospitals, and in the community. *Educate* the public and policy makers about the need for high quality palliative care for people living with serious illness and the need for high quality hospice care for those facing the end of life. *Collaborate* on public policies to improve the care of people living with serious illnesses and their loved ones. To *facilitate* the National Consensus Project for Quality Palliative Care (NCP) to establish and implement high quality clinical practice guidelines in all settings. (National Coalition for Hospice and Palliative Care, 2021a)

The National Consensus Project (NCP) is a task force of The Coalition that began in 2002 and whose purpose is to develop guidelines through an evidence-based review process, and to promote and implement these guidelines in order to assist in the delivery of consistent high-quality palliative care. The NCP has developed and disseminated four editions of the Clinical Practice Guidelines for Quality Palliative Care in 2004, 2009, 2013, and 2018. The National Quality Forum (NQF) has used these guidelines as a framework for the NQF Preferred Practices and they have been used to guide policy by healthcare providers and consumers in defining and understanding quality palliative care (National Coalition for Hospice and Palliative Care, 2021b). In January 2017, The Coalition announced that the Hospice and Palliative Nurses Foundation (HPNF) (one of the member organizations of The Coalition) was awarded a grant from the Gordon and Betty Moore Foundation to support The Coalition's efforts to develop community-based guidelines for quality palliative care modeled on the NCP Clinical Practice Guidelines for Quality Palliative Care (2013). The websites for The Coalition, its member organizations, and task forces provide a vast amount of additional information and resources that are updated regularly for those who desire more detailed information about the efforts, recommendations, and guidelines introduced here.

The Center to Advance Palliative Care (CAPC) was established in 1999 as a National Program Office of the Robert Wood Johnson Foundation. Since 2006, it has been supported by a consortium of foundations and individuals, and in 2015 it became a membership organization. It is affiliated with the Icahn School of Medicine at Mount Sinai in New York City. CAPC is a major resource supporting the development and quality of care for people with serious illness through education, collaboration, technical support, and essential tools. The website (https://www.capc.org) provides a wealth of information and education for providers, institutions, payors, and policy makers. Members have access to additional resources.

The End of Life Nursing Education Consortium (ELNEC) is a national and international education project originally founded with a large grant from the Robert Wood Johnson Foundation in 2000 to improve palliative care. It is currently funded by a large number of institutions and organizations, including the National Cancer Institute (NCI). ELNEC provides education about palliative care to nurses and other healthcare professionals. It has provided education in palliative care with a distinct focus on end-of-life care nationally in all 50 states, and internationally in 100 countries. Recently, ELNEC has made undergraduate and graduate curricula available to Schools of Nursing, with over 52,000 students completing the online course. The ELNEC course content is comprehensive, uses a train-the-trainer model, and has grown to include not only the original core course but specialty-focused courses such as those for students, APNs, pediatric, critical care, and geriatric nurses, among other courses. To date (2021), over 1,256,506 nurses and other healthcare professionals have been educated in ELNEC. The reader is encouraged to thoroughly review the ELNEC website (https://www.aacnnursing.org/ELNEC) with the regularly updated resources and course information available there.

Nurses and Palliative Care

Nurses make up the largest group of healthcare professionals. The latest estimates of the U.S. Department of Labor Bureau of Labor Statistics indicate there are 2,982,280 nurses (excluding nurse practitioners, midwives, and anesthetists) and 200,600 nurse practitioners employed in the country (https://www.bls.gov/oes/tables.htm#3). In the hospital setting, nurses are the primary frontline professional caregivers. Although much nursing time is spent with documentation and indirect care away from the patient, nurses spend a significant amount of time with patients and families (Hendrich, Chow, Skierczynski, & Lu, 2008; Westbrook, Duffield, Li, & Creswick, 2011). Nurses spend more time and advocate for patients especially when palliative care services at end of life are needed (Paice, 2015; Thacker, 2008). Additionally, they are well-positioned as healthcare professionals to assess, intervene, and refer patients to other healthcare professionals as needed and as appropriate for palliative care services. Advance practice nurses will encounter patients with palliative care needs across all healthcare settings and along the continuum of patient care. Advance practice nurses are by definition and in their advanced practice role able to *not only* assess and intervene on a basic nursing level but are also allowed to diagnose, treat, and prescribe within the scope of the state statutes governing nursing practice. According to the American Nurses Association (2021):

> Nursing is both an art and a science; a blending of the heart and mind. At the core is the fundamental respect for human dignity and sensitivity for a patient's needs. Nursing requires specialized knowledge and a broad range of skills to meet the diverse and complex needs of their patients. There is a unifying tenet that each nurse possesses in their ability to care for each patient; while the use subjective and objective data to assess and develop a treatment plan is the foundation of practice nurses also consider the patients biopsychosocial needs to provide holistic patient centered care.

Nurses, and specifically APNs, are the ideal healthcare providers to deliver and coordinate palliative care services to patients and their families. Nurses have played a pivotal role in the original development of palliative care as it grew from the hospice movement. The hospice movement was started in Great Britain in the 1960s by Dame Cicely Saunders, who was first a nurse and a social worker before becoming a physician. In the early 1970s, Florence Wald, MSN, FAAN, former Dean at the Yale School of Nursing, was instrumental in opening The Connecticut Hospice, the first hospice in the United States, in New Haven, Connecticut in 1971. Nurses are educated to be clinicians, leaders, educators, administrators, and researchers and are therefore in an excellent position to contribute to palliative care at all levels (Paice, 2015).

The APN must have adequate knowledge and a good understanding of the evidence to support palliative care delivery. Knowledge and skills are needed related to: obtaining a thorough patient history, conducting an excellent and comprehensive physical assessment, appropriate interventions and the concepts related to intervening early to relieve and prevent distress related to symptoms, and addressing QOL needs for patients and their families. It is not an expectation that nurses would or should be able to provide all palliative care without pulling in the expertise of their colleagues in other disciplines. Just as QOL is multidimensional, palliative care, because it addresses all domains of QOL, is intended to include an interdisciplinary healthcare team with expertise in areas in addition to nursing, including those disciplines and professionals who attend to the spiritual needs of patients and their families. Palliative care teams typically include nurses, physicians, social workers, and spiritual or religious professionals. Teams often also include pharmacists, psychologists, dieticians, and volunteers.

Chronic Diseases

Chronic diseases (CD) are the leading causes of disability and death in the world (WHO, 2020). The Centers for Disease Control and Prevention (CDC) defines CD as any health condition impacting one's quality of life and lasting more than one year (CDC, 2021b). Approximately 90% of the United States' healthcare expenditure is attributed to CD, approximating $3.5 trillion annually (CDC, 2021a).

194   **Chapter 7** Chronic Disease Management Models

Chronic diseases are responsible for roughly 60% of all deaths (CDC, 2021a). The top seven leading chronic diseases in the United States include (CDC, 2021):

1. Heart disease
2. Cancer
3. Chronic lung disease
4. Stroke
5. Alzheimer disease
6. Diabetes
7. Chronic kidney disease

Individual lifestyle choices are the top contributing causes of CD. Sedentary lifestyle, tobacco use disorder, poor nutrition, and excessive alcohol intake will lead to the development of certain CD (CDC, 2020; Raghupathi & Raghupathi, 2018). People with CD can develop other issues and conditions such as social isolation, depression, and anxiety, leading to poorer QOL. Patients with heart failure, chronic obstructive pulmonary disease, and hospitalized patients with CD have higher rates of depression and anxiety (Fattouh et al., 2019; Mathew et al., 2019; Zhang et al., 2019).

Another compounding issue affecting CD is that of healthcare disparities. Lack of access to health care, including health promotion and education on disease prevention, can affect the management of, and contribute to the development and/or worsening of, CD. Many APNs choose to practice in rural and underserved areas with lack of accessibility, bridging the gap in health care for this population (Xue et al., 2019). The APN is in a unique position to enhance population health by improving the overall health of people with CD. Patient education is an area of expertise of APNs. Advanced practice nurses spend much of the patient encounter providing education on diseases, health promotion, and lifestyle changes needed to achieve optimal health.

Chronic Diseases and the Role of the NP
Self-Management Programs

Self-management programs (SMP) are recommended for people with CD (CDC, 2020; Healthy People 2020, 2020). Teaching patients with CD how to self-manage their condition can enhance patients' QOL and lead to improved health outcomes (Healthy People 2020, 2020). The CDC (2018a) offers various SMPs and tool kits for healthcare providers. These resources can be utilized by NPs, allowing them to develop various SMPs, enhancing the care of patients with CD. Self-management programs can be offered in various formats, such as small groups, individualized, or online. An example of a successful small group SMP is the National Diabetes Prevention Program (NDPP) (CDC, 2021a). This CDC program, developed in 2010, was instituted to address the increased incidence of obesity and pre-diabetes and prevent or delay the development of diabetes in these patients (CDC, 2021b). A 10-year follow-up study of the NDPP showed that participants of the program were 33% less likely to develop diabetes compared to those who did not participate (CDC, 2021b). People are more likely to discuss health issues and successful strategies that are helpful in managing their CD with other individuals who have similar issues. Sharing ideas with one another can incite people to try new tactics that may help self-manage their CD and improve their health.

The SMP developed by Dr. Kate Lorig, RN, for people with CD at Stanford University is a highly endorsed program by the National Council on Aging (BeWell Stanford, 2021; National Council on Aging, n.d.). Stanford University, funded by grants from the Robert Wood Johnson and Archston Foundations, has been offering numerous SMPs for people with CD to help patients cope with fatigue, pain, and isolation (Stanford Medicine, 2021). The SMPs are offered in small groups, as well as in online formats (Stanford Medicine, 2021). Stanford's SMPs are weekly workshop classes, offered over six weeks, focusing on chronic pain management, healthy eating, exercises, medication, and also providing emotional support (Self-management Resource Center, 2021). Additionally, these programs are conveniently offered in churches, community centers, libraries, and hospitals (Self-management Resource Center, 2021). Advanced practice nurses with leadership skills can develop and implement such programs in the community where they practice.

Community Health Workers

Community health workers (CHWs) are laypersons with an interest in improving community health. CHWs can be "go-to" people between the healthcare agency and the community and are successfully used with patients with various CDs, to improve patient health and empower patients to become active participants in their health (Kyounghae Kim et al., 2016). Additionally, the study conducted by Kyounghae Kim and colleagues (2016) revealed that participants increased their confidence in the CHW, allowing for the development of a trusting relationship. When CHWs with CD lead a SMP, group participants are more likely to discuss their health issues and divulge their failures and successes (Brownstein & Allen, 2015). CHWs can be used to provide health education, help patients navigate the healthcare system, provide social support and counseling, and are cost-effective (Kyounghae Kim et al., 2016).

NPs can lead SMPs or educate CHWs in specific areas, allowing them to be able to lead small groups of individuals with common health issues. Having CHWs run a SMP for people with CD can bridge healthcare gaps and improve population health. The CDC offers various tool kits to aide NPs in developing such programs (Brownstein & Allen, 2015).

As the population ages, the healthcare burden of CD will only increase. NPs have the necessary skills to impact population health. Nurse practitioners who provide SMP in the community can improve patients' self-efficacy and empower them to actively partake in their care. Additionally, NPs can train CHWs to offer SMPs or other educational programs in the community, thus increasing the patients' understanding of CDs and leading them toward a path to optimal health. When managing chronic non-cancer pain, NPs need to remain current on evidence-based pharmacologic treatment options, as well as non-pharmaceutical modalities.

The next section will provide an overview of palliative care and symptom management that needs to be considered with all patients who have CD. Having goals-of-care discussions about palliative care options including end-of-life care early on in the disease process will allow patients and families to have improved QOL and permit their advanced directives to be carried out, ensuring their wishes are upheld.

Symptom Management

The symptom experience can negatively impact QOL. This experience includes not only the number, type, and severity of symptoms, but also the distress associated with the symptoms. In people with cancer, where the majority of the symptom management research has been conducted and reported, it is well-established that multiple co-occurring symptoms are associated with increased distress, decreased function, and decreased survival (Cleeland, 2007; Degner & Sloan, 1995; Kurtz, et al., 2000). In the context of serious illness, patients usually experience more than one symptom from the illness and the treatments, thus increasing the symptom burden and negative impact on one's QOL. Patients with illnesses other than cancer, such as cardiac disease, dementia, and HIV/AIDS, also experience a high symptom burden. The *essence* of palliative care aims to relieve suffering, and involves excellent symptom management. Comorbidities, particularly in the elderly and aging population, contributes to the existence of multiple co-occurring symptoms. In addition to pharmacologic management for symptoms, psychosocial and spiritual care are also needed, and thus interdisciplinary care is required to optimally address symptom distress.

Common symptoms especially in palliative care during end-of-life care include pain, anorexia, other gastrointestinal-related symptoms, dyspnea, fatigue, anxiety and depression, and loss of function. Many other symptoms can exist especially at end of life and the authors refer the readers to the symptom management literature for end-of-life care for a more complete discussion of end-of-life symptoms. The management of all symptoms is beyond the scope of this chapter, and we will highlight some of the more common symptoms for patients who need palliative care services. For the purposes of this chapter, we will review some of the evidence-based practices for the assessment and treatment of pain, anorexia, dyspnea, fatigue, anxiety, and depression. We also refer the reader to other sources for up-to-date clinical practice guidelines and evidence-based practices for symptom management (see **Box 7-1**).

Pain

Pain is a common symptom, affecting up to two-thirds of those with an advanced cancer diagnosis (van den Beuken-van Everdingen, et al., 2016) and many patients with chronic disease (CD). It is described as an unpleasant sensory and emotional experience, associated with actual or potential tissue damage (Merskey, 1986) and interferes with QOL. It is important to remember that pain is *whatever the patient says it is* (Pasero & McCaffery, 2012).

In the 1990s, the United States experienced an increase in prescription opioid overdose deaths, with a second and third wave occurring in 2010 and 2013, respectively (CDC, 2021c). Since then, the CDC has been dedicated to combating the opioid crisis by assessing usage trends and providing states with resources to improve data collection. Additionally, the CDC is assisting healthcare systems and providers by supplying them with various data tools to ameliorate evidence-based decision-making and improve opioid prescribing and patient safety (CDC, 2021c).

All nurses have an ethical responsibility to assess pain and relieve the suffering caused by it. In order to appropriately relieve pain and suffering, NPs must conduct a full pain assessment and provide individualized evidence-based interventions. The

Box 7-1 Symptom Management and Palliative Care Resources

BeWell Stanford: Self-managing chronic disease
https://bewell.stanford.edu/self-managing-chronic-disease
Symptom Interventions and Guidelines (Oncology Nursing Society)
https://www.ons.org/practice-resources/pep
and
https://www.ons.org/explore-resources?source=1506&display=source&sort_by=created&items_per_page=50
Centers for Disease Control & Prevention – Self-management education program for chronic disease management
https://www.cdc.gov/learnmorefeelbetter/programs/index.htm
Clinical Practice Guidelines for Dyspnea (American Thoracic Society)
https://www.thoracic.org/professionals
National Comprehensive Cancer Network (NCCN) Clinical Practice Guidelines -Supportive Care
https://www.nccn.org/professionals/physician_gls/default.aspx#supportive
City of Hope Pain and Palliative Care Resource Center
http://prc.coh.org
National Coalition for Hospice and Palliative Care
http://www.nationalcoalitionhpc.org
World Health Organization—Palliative Care
http://www.who.int/mediacentre/factsheets/fs402/en
Hospice and Palliative Nurses Association (most resources are limited to members only)
https://advancingexpertcare.org
End-of-Life Nursing Education Consortium (ELNEC)
https://www.aacnnursing.org/ELNEC
Center to Advance Palliative Care
https://www.capc.org
Self-Management Resource Center
https://www.selfmanagementresource.com/programs/small-group/chronic-disease-self-management/
Dementia/Agitation/Confusion The Confusion Assessment Method for ICU (CAM-ICU)
https://www.cochranelibrary.com/cdsr/doi/10.1002/14651858.CD013126/full
Montreal Cognitive Assessment (MOCA)
https://geriatrictoolkit.missouri.edu/cog/MoCA-8.3-English-Test-2018-04.pdf
Constipation
https://www.cancer.gov/about-cancer/treatment/side-effects/constipation/gi-complications-hp-pdq#_39_toc
Pain management guidelines resource
https://prc.coh.org/NRE%20Pain%20Card%20revised%2010.17.17.pdf
Edmonton Symptom Assessment Scale
http://cancercaresoutheast.ca/sites/default/files/files/resource/edmonton_symptom_assessment_system.pdf
Memorial Symptom Assessment Scale
https://www.midss.org/content/memorial-symptom-assesment-scale-%E2%80%93-short-form-msas-sf

(continues)

> **Box 7-1** Symptom Management and Palliative Care Resources *(continued)*
>
> **Performance Assessment Tools:**
> ECOG Performance Tool for Cancer
> http://www.npcrc.org/files/news/ECOG_performance_status.pdf
> Functional Assessment Staging Tool (FAST) for Dementia
> https://www.compassus.com/sparkle-assets/documents/functional-assessment-staging-fast.pdf
> Palliative Performance Staging (PPS)
> https://www.mypcnow.org/fast-fact/the-palliative-performance-scale-pps

NP, as a prescriber, needs to be familiar with the various types of pain (nociceptive, visceral, somatic, and neuropathic) and the respective evidence-based treatment guidelines. Not only does the NP need to be familiar with the evidence for pharmacologic agents, they need to be cognizant of the evidence for non-pharmaceutical modalities. If the NP is considering an opioid for moderate to severe pain, the benefits, risks, and side effects, including the risk for addiction, need to be discussed with the patient. Patient education regarding the proper way to take the medication, including dosage and side-effect management, must be provided. Additionally, best practices regarding opioid prescribing need to be followed. These best practices include accessing the prescription drug monitoring program prior to writing a prescription and developing a pain contract with the patient, which includes periodic assessments to ensure that the patient is not misusing. These assessments usually include random pill counts and urine toxicology screens (Dowel et al., 2016).

Pain may be described as acute or chronic. Acute pain is most often the result of an injury or trauma and is expected to resolve over a relatively short period of time. Chronic pain is usually associated with CD, including cancer, will generally last over an extended period of time (more than 6 months), and have a negative impact on QOL, functionality, and other symptoms. Optimal management of chronic pain requires palliative care and multidisciplinary and multimodal approaches, including pharmacologic and non-pharmacologic modalities, and interventional procedures when appropriate (Paice, Portenoy, Lacchetti, et al., 2016).

Treatment and attention to pain is imperative and may require more expertise or knowledge than an NP in an area other than palliative care may possess, unless the NP has acquired additional education and skills in palliative or end-of-life care, or pain management. Therefore, adequate pain management often requires the expertise of those who are specialists in the field of pain management and end-of-life care. Pain management with opioids requires ongoing monitoring and careful follow-up. APNs who provide pain management should maintain their professional education in the areas of safe opioid prescribing and their knowledge of local prescribing and reporting requirements. A brief overview of basic principles for pain management follows. The NP is encouraged to consult with colleagues who specialize in pain management, for management of pain in patients with unrelieved and complex pain.

A pain assessment is best obtained by a self-report when possible and should include cultural considerations. A thorough pain assessment should include the following: location, intensity, pattern, quality, length of time, aggravating or alleviating factors/treatments, meaning of the pain—history of past experiences, and psychosocial and functional assessments. Because pain has a negative effect on QOL and function, it is important to thoroughly assess all domains of QOL. Only once a thorough assessment is conducted can the NP continue to properly evaluate the pain and provide interventions to relieve or manage the pain. Further evaluation includes a careful physical exam, paying attention to the area of pain and underlying medical diagnoses if known. Diagnosis of the pain may involve evaluation with laboratory or imaging studies. When considering diagnostic testing, the NP must carefully contemplate and weigh the risk versus benefit in terms of physical and emotional distress, the additional discomfort and financial burden to the patient and family, and ultimately try to determine if the results of the test(s) will change the course of treatment and improve the symptom—in this case, pain. The diagnostic test(s) under consideration may be beneficial in determining an adequate treatment. However, in some cases the physical, emotional, and financial distress may outweigh the diagnostic benefit.

Adequate pain management may require very advanced techniques and can include pharmacologic and non-pharmacologic methods. Pharmacologic treatments may include opioid and non-opioid medications. The NP prescribing medications for pain relief must be knowledgeable about the methods of actions, including the metabolism of the drug, side effects and interactions with other medications. Acetaminophen and non-steroidal anti-inflammatory drugs (NSAIDs) are two common examples of non-opioid medications used in the management of pain. Acetaminophen is metabolized in the liver and can cause liver dysfunction in doses greater than 3 grams per day. Caution must be used with NSAIDs in patients with bleeding risks and renal dysfunction. Additionally, NSAIDs have a direct local effect on the gastric mucosa that can result in gastrointestinal irritation and bleeding. Common opioids and opioid-like drugs include codeine, fentanyl, hydrocodone, hydromorphone, methadone, morphine, oxycodone, oxymorphone, and tramadol. All opioids cause constipation, sedation, and respiratory depression. Many patients also experience nausea, diaphoresis, pruritus, and urinary retention with opioid use. Opioid rotation can be used when the side effects are not well tolerated or the pain is unrelieved after the dose of an opioid is appropriately titrated upward. Opioid rotation can involve the use of many different opioids until an effective opioid and dose are found (Pasternak, 2014).

Adjuvant medications include steroids, antidepressants, and anticonvulsion medications. Anti-depressants and anti-convulsive medications can be used to treat neuropathic pain (Lussier & Portenoy, 2015). Steroids can also be helpful in treating neuropathic pain, bone pain, and other types of pain, particularly pain resulting from inflammatory processes.

The National Cancer Institute (NCI) (2020) provides an evidence-based comprehensive overview of the use of cannabis as a treatment for people with cancer-related symptoms, including pain. The overview provided by the NCI is updated regularly and is a good resource for the APN. The evidence is weak for cannabis for pain management, although many patients may ask about the use of it to treat pain. It is helpful for the NP to be aware of the current evidence, recommendations, and regulations regarding the use of cannabis.

Non-pharmacologic interventions such as radiation therapy, neurological procedures, surgery and other interventional procedures require the NP to consult and refer patients to colleagues who are specialists in the related interventional areas. Other non-pharmacologic interventions for pain management include those that target the physical, psychosocial, and existential distress associated with pain. The

NP should collaborate with colleagues such as physical therapists, social workers, chaplains, psychotherapists, and others who can assist the patient and family with techniques and interventions to address functional limitations and distress related to pain. Techniques to address pain, functional limitations, and psychosocial and spiritual distress can help address areas of QOL that are affected by pain (Cheville & Basford, 2014; Dusenbury & Tatu, 2017; Meyer & Ring, 2019; Syrjala et al., 2014; Taylor, S. F., & Melroy, M. K., 2017).

Anorexia/Cachexia

Anorexia and cachexia are common in many advanced illnesses, especially cancer. Both are experienced together by up to 80% of all patients with cancer and are associated with a negative impact on QOL and survival. Anorexia is a loss of appetite and desire to eat associated with a reduced intake (Tarricone et al., 2016; Schack & Wholihan, 2019). Cachexia is due to a lack of nutrition and involves muscle wasting, weight loss, is associated with fatigue and is common in advanced cancer and other illnesses (Schack & Wholihan, 2019). Anorexia and cachexia are usually difficult to treat. Causes can vary from the illness to different treatments. A careful and thorough assessment includes a patient history of involuntary weight loss, other comorbid conditions or deficiencies, a physical exam to assess for wasting and weakness, skin conditions, and gastrointestinal problems. Laboratory tests may be helpful to identify deficiencies. Interventions are not always successful. When possible, remove or treat the underlying causes. Referrals to dieticians may be considered. Individualized interventions are most appropriate. There is some evidence for appetite stimulants; however, these are not always helpful especially in advanced illness (Dev, Del Fabbro, & Bruera, 2007). When considering the impact of anorexia and cachexia for patients, the NP must consider the social and cultural importance that is often placed on food and mealtimes. Eating is frequently a social event, even when dining at home, and includes more than simply eating for nourishment. Meal planning, preparation, and sharing in the meal are not enjoyed by those affected by anorexia and cachexia.

Dyspnea

Dyspnea is a very common, distressing symptom experienced by patients with respiratory illnesses such as lung cancer and chronic obstructive pulmonary disease (COPD), cardiac disease, and other serious and advanced illnesses. It severely impacts functionality and QOL (Mularski et al., 2013; Sung et al., 2017; Weingaertner et al., 2014; Yancy et al., 2006). Dyspnea is a subjective and multidimensional symptom experience and is defined by the American Thoracic Society (Mularski et al., 2013) as the "sustained and severe resting breathing discomfort that occurs in patients with advanced, often life-limiting illness and overwhelms the patient and caregivers' ability to achieve symptom relief" (p. S100). The experience causes anxiety for patients and their caregivers and is a common cause of emergency department visits. A dyspnea crisis occurs with a changing severity of the underlying dyspnea, a chaotic environment with caregiver stress, and the patient's own physical, psychosocial, and spiritual distress. It is characterized by fear, anxiety, and increased shortness of breath (Mularski et al., 2013). The assessment of dyspnea is best accomplished with a self-report by the patient as with all symptoms, because the self-report is the most valid and reliable form of assessment. Patients can respond to a yes or no query ("Are you short of breath?") to determine the presence of dyspnea. However, it is recommended to perform an assessment that encompasses more than a yes or no to obtain an accurate assessment of this multidimensional symptom and to use at least a numeric rating scale such as a 1–10 analog scale to assess the severity of dyspnea so that the patient's response to treatment can also be assessed (Dorman, Byrne, & Edwards, 2007; Pang et al., 2014; Crombeen & Lilly, 2020). In addition to assessing the actual dyspnea, the NP must assess the patient's functional status and anxiety.

Respiratory rate, oxygenation, and extent of disease may not correlate with the patient's experience or report of dyspnea (Blouin, Fowler, & Dahlin, 2008; Donesky, D., 2019; Myers & Dudgeon, 2011). The causes of dyspnea can range from various physiological reasons including neurological disturbances and severe anemias, to infiltration, obstruction, or compression of the respiratory tract, cardiac insufficiency, and other symptoms such as pain and anxiety (Crombeen & Lilly, 2020). Be sure to think about the patient's goals of care, and risk versus benefit, when ordering tests. When weighing the risk and benefit of diagnostic tests used to determine the causes of dyspnea, the NP must always consider the importance of respecting the patient's wishes for care and if the results of the tests will change the course of treatment and provide benefit to the patient.

Management of dyspnea and respecting patients' goals of care can be challenging. When possible, reverse the underlying cause and always provide symptom management (Blouin et al., 2008). Pharmacologic interventions that can be beneficial in reducing the sensation of dyspnea and its related distress include the use of opioids, bronchodilators, steroids, and anxiolytic agents; oxygen use may be beneficial in the setting of hypoxia. Nonpharmacologic interventions include providing a calm environment, breathing exercises such as pursed lip breathing, attending to caregiver and patient anxiety, and using a fan or open window to provide a sense of air flow (National Comprehensive Cancer Network [NCCN], 2021). The readers are directed to clinical practice guidelines that are regularly updated at the American Thoracic Society website (https://www.thoracic.org/statements/health-care.php) and the National Comprehensive Cancer Network Guidelines for Palliative Care (NCCN, 2021).

Caregivers who observe their loved ones' experience of dyspnea can also experience distress and anxiety. It is important to consider the caregivers' distress and related needs. To help alleviate caregiver distress, provide support including resources for coping, information and education about the patient's dyspnea, and ways to treat the dyspnea.

Fatigue

Fatigue is the most commonly reported symptom by those with cancer, reported by 60%–100% of patients (even in fairly healthy patients), and is prevalent and distressful in other diseases as well, such as cardiac disease and respiratory illnesses (Brissot, Gonzalez-Bermejo, Lassalle, Desrues, & Doutrellot, 2006; O'Neil-Page, E. Anderson, P., & Dean, G., 2015; Mitchell et al., 2014; Siefert, 2010; Stridsman, Müllerova, Skär, & Lindberg, 2013). Fatigue is worse in those with advanced COPD, with respiratory symptoms or heart disease and COPD, and in heart disease without COPD (Stridsman et al., 2013).

Fatigue is a subjective sense of tiredness and may have a sudden or gradual onset and has a high inverse correlation with functional status. Fatigue may occur as a single symptom; however, it is frequently associated with other symptoms such as insomnia, depression, and pain. Fatigue may be caused by the underlying disease and/or its treatments, but often the etiology of fatigue is not known or well understood. Medications, as well as other symptoms, can contribute to fatigue. A complete history and assessment should include a careful assessment of contributing factors and other symptoms, and lab tests if appropriate, to rule out anemias or other physiologic causes of fatigue. The assessment of fatigue is most accurate by obtaining a subjective patient self-report using an analog (1–10) scale similar to a pain scale. However, since fatigue often occurs with other symptoms and is associated with poor QOL and functional status, a full symptom assessment including QOL should be considered. Treatment of underlying causes when possible should be taken into account, and if other symptoms are contributing to the fatigue, such as depression and insomnia, they should also be treated. If it is considered safe and appropriate, instruct the patient and caregiver about activities such as short periods of walking. Rest alone does not relieve fatigue. Instruction should also include good sleep hygiene techniques combined with daytime activity conservation and management techniques such as priority setting and readjustment of priority tasks and activities, and monitoring of activities and fatigue (Mitchell et al., 2014; O'Neil-Page et al., 2015).

Fatigue in the cancer population has been well studied and reported over the past two decades in patients with various cancer diagnoses, receiving chemotherapy and or radiation therapy, and in the post-treatment period. It is well established that short periods of activity such as a home-based or supervised exercise or activity program, even 10 to 20 minutes a day of activity such as walking, can help mitigate fatigue in patients who are physically able to participate in an exercise program (Mitchell et al., 2014). The optimal dose and intensity of an exercise or activity program has not been determined. However, it is recommended that, if tolerated, patients maintain or start some type of physical activity as tolerated and safe.

Anxiety

Anxiety is subjective feelings of uneasiness and apprehension (Salman et al., 2019). Although anxiety is a normal response to life events and is common in acute and chronic illness, anxiety usually co-occurs with pain and dyspnea and may peak as patients experience illness-related transitions they feel unprepared to handle. Anxiety has been associated with decreased learning, impaired decisions, and patients' inability to perform or complete illness-related tasks (Salman et al., 2019). Advanced practice nurses in the palliative care setting need to routinely assess for anxiety in order to intervene early to reduce and control its effects on patients' QOL. They can take the lead in identifying and acting upon evidence-based psychosocial approaches that can best target anxiety. The interdisciplinary team approach to anxiety management supports a range of evidence-based modalities with proven efficacy to treat anxiety, including cognitive-based therapies, mindfulness-based interventions, psychoeducation interventions, and psychopharmacology (Ercolano, 2017).

Depression

It is expected that in the course of the illness trajectory, most individuals experience intermittent short-lived sadness or feelings of helplessness or hopelessness. Not all instances of advanced disease or CD will result in clinical depression (Katon, Lin, & Kroenke, 2007). Prolonged sadness greater than 2 weeks, however, may indicate a clinical depression, which is also accompanied by sleep disturbance, body aches, appetite changes, concentration problems, social isolation, and thoughts of hurting oneself or others (Salman et al., 2019). Anxiety and depression often coexist with overlapping physical, emotional, and mental symptoms (Ercolano, 2017). In the course of progressive disease, the decline of physical function, loss of social roles, and increasing pain may exacerbate symptoms of depression. In the palliative care, non-psychiatric setting, brief screening measures are now routinely used to assess for depressive symptoms or clinical depression. These brief screening measures, including the Hospital Anxiety and Depression Scale (HADS), Beck Depression Inventory (BDI), or the Physicians Health Questionnaire 9 (PHQ-9), will alert NPs to underrecognized or untreated depression and provide a foundation for referrals to other disciplines with specific expertise in psychosocial management (Zigmond & Smith, 1983; Kroenke, Spitzer, & Williams, 2001). For example, behaviorally oriented interventions that encourage expression of feelings, reduce social isolation, and help with negative cognitive distortions have demonstrated efficacy. Psychopharmacology has shown efficacy in both the treatment of depression and pain in advanced disease and may be used as an adjunct to psychotherapies or other behavioral therapies (Ercolano, 2017).

Conclusion

Palliative care is a growing field in health care that has evolved from the earlier hospice movement. Palliative care is, at its essence, excellent symptom management utilized at *any time* with CD or a serious illness to relieve suffering and maintain or improve QOL for patients and their families. Similar to hospice care, excellent palliative care requires a multidisciplinary approach. Advance practice nurses and nurse practitioners play a key role in the implementation and delivery of palliative care to patients and their families.

♀ CASE STUDY

Mr. Mendez is a 76-year-old Latino gentleman admitted to the hospital for his third acute episode of COPD exacerbation in the past few months. The patient has symptoms of severe dyspnea requiring continuous oxygen at home. The patient uses a walker to ambulate, but notes he becomes quite fatigued after ambulating from the bedroom to his bathroom. Mr. Mendez's wife states that he has lost his appetite with a noticeable weight loss of 12 pounds that has occurred in the last 3 months. His wife notes the patient demonstrates anxiety at times at night with insomnia. Mr. Mendez requires home care support with the visiting nurse, including assistance with medication management and a home health aide for his activities of daily living.

Mr. Mendez is homebound, has visits occasionally with his church minister at home, and has two children who live within an hour's driving distance from his home.

Mr. Mendez has been told by his clinicians in the hospital that his COPD condition has progressed to a severe state based on his symptoms and diagnostic testing (chest X-ray and pulmonary function testing). The patient has no advanced care directives or plan in place. Mr. Mendez is worried about his wife managing his illness at home, which causes her anxiety and is concerned about what will happen to her when he is no longer around. The interdisciplinary care team including the nurse, physician, social worker, and case manager determine that Mr. Mendez has a life-limiting illness that requires consideration of a palliative care consult to discuss the patient's goals of care for advanced care planning, including transition of care.

Seminar Discussion Questions

1. Referencing the previous case study, what would be the next steps to take with regard to introducing palliative care to the patient and family?

   According to the palliative care best practices based on the National Consensus Project Domains (2018) and National Quality Forum Preferred Practices (2006), the steps include processes and structure of care that involve a comprehensive care plan with goals of care conversations about advanced care planning, decision making, and consideration of the patient's goals, preferences, and values.

   A comprehensive plan of care includes an assessment of the patient and family. An interdisciplinary team can include medicine, nursing, social work, chaplain, pharmacist, physical therapy, occupational therapy, nutrition, and other allied care services (National Consensus Project Domains, 2018; National Quality Forum Preferred Practices, 2006). Quality assessment includes timely and thorough communication of the patient's goals of care, including preferences, values, and clinical information for assuring continuity of care during transition of care (You, Fowler, & Heyland, 2014). Performance assessment of function and cognition should be documented continuously using tools such as ECOG for cancer, Palliative Performance Scale (any patient), and Functional Assessment Staging Scale for dementia.

   Goals of care conversations include setting up a meeting to discuss with Mr. Mendez and his family his goals or wishes, preferences, and values regarding his current medical condition. Important aspects include providing a systematic approach in asking the patient what he understands about his illness, and asking permission to discuss the nature of his condition including in what detail he would like to know about his prognosis and illness using simple language in small chunks (avoiding medical jargon), building rapport, listening, and providing empathy. The patient should be asked about his wishes, preferences, and values that are important to him. The patient and family also need to be asked about their fears and concerns. Important goals, wishes, values, and preferences should be taken into consideration in developing the plan of care. The plan of care should be discussed regarding advanced care planning (ACP), including advanced care directives and surrogate designations. The ACP discussion involves asking and documenting the patient and family wishes about care setting for palliative and end-of-life care including advanced care directives. Education on the process of the disease, prognosis, and benefits and burdens of potential interventions need to be discussed with the patient and family to make informed decisions about Mr. Mendez's care. Patients and families, such as Mr. Mendez's, should be asked about introducing palliative care and hospice care programs as options (National Consensus Project Domains, 2012; National Quality Forum Preferred Practices, 2006).

2. What are the important aspects of care that need to be addressed based on palliative care best practices?

Based on National Consensus Project Domains (2018) and National Quality Forum (NQF) Preferred Practices (2006), aspects of care include assessment of physiological, psychological, social, and spiritual components by the interdisciplinary team. Physiological aspects of care involve the patient's activities of daily living, symptom management, and maintaining physical comfort. Management of Mr. Mendez's dyspnea, fatigue, anxiety, insomnia, and loss of appetite with anorexia includes a timely assessment using standardized scales in a safe and effective manner to a level acceptable to patient and family, with documentation.

Psychological aspects of care involve Mr. Mendez's fears, worries, and concerns. Psychological reactions involve the patient and family, including stress, anticipatory grief, and coping. Symptom management of the patient's anxiety or other related symptoms should be addressed with safe, effective interventions. The family will also need a plan of care that involves grief and bereavement for at least 13 months after Mr. Mendez's death. Untoward behavioral disturbances or maladaptive coping may require psychological consultation for evaluation and counseling (National Consensus Project Domains, 2012; National Quality Forum Preferred Practices, 2006).

Social aspects of care involve ongoing communication by the interdisciplinary team with the patient and family to identify social needs and respond to assessments of religious, spiritual, and existential concerns. Information on spiritual care services and counseling should be provided while encouraging Mr. Mendez to talk to his own clergy minister for support.

Cultural aspects of care should be assessed with patient and family. Mr. Mendez may have certain preferences based on an assessment of his preferences in decision making, disclosing information, dietary preferences, language, family communication, and supportive measures such as complementary and alternative medicines. The interdisciplinary team needs to ask Mr. Mendez and his family about what they need to know about their cultural preferences and values as important patient factors in his care (National Consensus Project Domains, 2012; National Quality Forum Preferred Practices, 2006).

Ethical/legal considerations (Prince-Paul & Daly, 2019) include aspects of care that involve respecting the patient's goals, preferences, and choices within the limits of applicable state and federal laws and current acceptable standards of medical care. An advanced care directive that documents the surrogate/decision maker in accordance with state law should be in place. Documentation of patient/surrogate preferences for goals of care should be transferrable across hospital, community, and emergency service settings. Such documentation ensures that the patient/surrogate wishes are maintained when transitions of care occur across acute, short-term, long-term, and home care settings. Documentation within health records needs to also adhere to the Health Insurance and Portability and Accountability Act (HIPAA) regulations to ensure patient privacy (National Consensus Project Domains, 2012; National Quality Forum Preferred Practices, 2006).

3. What is the role of the nurse in caring for Mr. Mendez and his family?

The role of the APN involves providing physiological, psychological, sociocultural, and ethical/legal aspects of care to Mr. Mendez as previously outlined in this case study. The APN works within an interdisciplinary team that provides care focused on communication with patient and family about providing care that meets their goals while reducing symptom burden, alleviating stress, and enhancing comfort and well-being.

Goals of care (GOC) discussions offer important ways in which persons can communicate with healthcare providers, including nurses, and family members about their wishes in advanced care planning about the type of care desired while honoring personal choices, values, and beliefs (Kaldijian et al., 2008). Despite a perceived societal culture of persons not wanting to have GOC conversations with clinicians, including advanced care planning and end-of-life care, studies have shown that patients want to have these conversations sooner, including hearing about options and using a systematic, interprofessional team approach (Bach et al., 2009; Gesme & Wiseman, 2011; Legare et al., 2011). Studies have shown that earlier conversations reduce stress, anxiety, and depression in the relatives of the elderly (Detering et al., 2010) including use of early palliative and less aggressive care that resulted in patients with non-small-cell lung cancer living almost 3 months longer (Temel et al., 2010). Evidence supports the provision of early communication regarding serious illness and GOC conversations including EOL preferences for improved care outcomes involving better quality of life, less life-sustaining treatments near death, consistency of care with patient preferences, and improved bereavement outcomes for families (Bernacki & Block, 2014).

APNs require training on effective communication skills within an interdisciplinary team approach. Evidence reveals barriers to communication of GOC conversations include inadequate healthcare provider training, documentation and exchange of patient values and goals, and misperceptions of increasing anxiety and depressions in patients (Bernacki & Block, 2014). Barriers identified by hospital-based clinicians involve patient-related and family-member factors in difficulty accepting a poor prognosis, difficulty understanding the limitations and complications of life-sustaining treatments, disagreements among family member on GOC, and patient incapacity to make decisions. Such barriers require a tailored approach to address individualized approaches to GOC conversations that involve a team approach by healthcare providers. An interprofessional team approach of healthcare providers can be effective (Reeves et al., 2008), including physicians and nurses, by improving communication training to initiate and participate in GOC conversations within their professional role and scope of practice (Schroder, Heyland, Jiang, Rocker, & Dodek, 2009). Such preparation includes effective communication skills on best practice approaches involving assisting patients with understanding their illness, building rapport, providing empathy, listening, and discussing prognosis (Bernacki & Block, 2014).

Systematic approaches to GOC conversations that can be used with patients such as Mr. Mendez and family include use of cognitive maps or mnemonic tools that are useful to implement within a healthcare provider team approach with patients and families. An important cognitive map communication mnemonic for use as a process for sharing in a GOC conversation meeting is the use of S.P.I.K.E.S: Setting, Perception, Invitation, Knowledge, Emotions, Summary (Bailey et al., 2000). The setting includes a private quiet area where the healthcare interdisciplinary team, patient, family, and/or surrogate decision maker can meet. The setting should allow for the ability to communicate with seating, proper eye contact, and verbal interaction. Patient perception can be addressed by asking patients what has been told to them about the medical situation, including thoughts and understanding of their illness. This invitation also includes asking the patient permission about discussing the medical condition as more global or in greater detail based on what the patient wants to know about the condition. Knowledge includes giving information in small chunks while ascertaining understanding periodically, using simple language in layperson terms (avoiding medical jargon) while acknowledging the uncertainty of the prognosis. Addressing emotions includes asking about patient fears and worries while providing empathy and pauses for emotions as important. A summary of the goals of care and plan for future conversation or next steps should occur at the conclusion of the meeting (You et al., 2014).

The R.E.M.A.P. framework can be a useful tool for nurses in transitions in GOC conversations (Childers, Back, Tulsky, & Arnold, 2017). Reframe can be used in asking about feelings regarding how the patient and family think things are going. Expect emotion and empathize; ask permission to talk about what the patient and family are worried about, while recognizing their concerns and what this means to them. Map out patient goals or values, including what is most important to persons like Mr. Mendez and his family, such as future goals and future concerns. Aligning with goals or values includes listening and verbalizing back to patients about what is most important, including a plan proposing to help with those important goals (Vitaltalk.org, 2017).

The NURSE statements are another useful cognitive map for nurses to respond to emotion in articulating empathy. Naming the emotion can include stating, "It sounds like you are frustrated." The understanding statement acknowledges, "Help me understand what you are thinking" and respecting the person in stating, "You really have been trying to follow the instructions," or through praise in "I think you have done a great job with this." Supporting includes a powerful statement such as "I will do my best to make sure you have what you need" while exploring in asking, "Could you say more about what you mean when you say that. . .?" (Vitaltalk.org, 2017).

Lastly, the nurse can provide continuity of care through assessment, education, and support that impacts quality of palliative care (Ferrell & Coyle, 2010). The End-of-Life Nursing Education Curriculum (ELNEC, 2021) addresses the role of the nurse in palliative care involving aspects of care, as summarized previously, guided within the context of a QOL framework developed by Ferrell and Coyle (2010). Nurses also have a therapeutic presence (Krammer, Hanks-Bell, & Cappleman, 2011) to address existential concerns about personal meaning, maintaining hope (Cotter & Foxwell, 2019; Ferrell & Coyle, 2010), spiritual needs, and realistic expectations for patients such as Mr. Mendez and his family (Ferrell & Coyle, 2010).

References

American Nurses Association (ANA). (2021). *What is nursing?* Retrieved on February 5, 2021 from https://www.nursingworld.org/practice-policy/workforce/what-is-nursing/

Bach, V., Ploeg, J., & Black, M. (2009) "Nursing roles in end-of-life decision making in critical care settings," Western Journal of Nursing Research, vol. 31, no. 4, pp. 496–512.

Bailey, W. F., Buckman, R., Lenzi, R., et al. (2000). SPIKES—A six-step protocol for delivering bad news: Application to the patient with cancer. *Oncologist, 5,* 302–311.

Bakitas, M. A. (2017). On the road less traveled: Journey of an oncology palliative care researcher. *Oncology Nursing Forum, 44*(1), 87–95.

BeWell Stanford. (2021). Self-managing chronic disease. *Stanford University Human Resources, BeWell.* Retrieved on January 3, 2021 from https://bewell.stanford.edu/self-managing-chronic-disease/

Bernacki, R. E., & Block, S. D. (2014). American College of Physicians high value care task force. Communication about serious illness care goals: A review and synthesis of best practices. *JAMA Internal Medicine, 174*(12), 1994–2003.

Blouin, G., Fowler, B. C., & Dahlin, C. (2008). The national agenda for quality palliative care: Promoting the National Consensus Project's domain of physical care and the National Quality Forum's preferred practices for physical aspects of care. *Journal of Pain & Palliative Care Pharmacotherapy, 22*(3), 206–212.

Brissot, R., Gonzalez-Bermejo, J., Lassalle, A., Desrues, B., & Doutrellot, P. L. (2006). Fatigue and respiratory disorders. *Annales De Readaptation Et De Medecine Physique: Revue Scientifique De La Societe Francaise De Reeducation Fonctionnelle De Readaptation Et De Medecine Physique, 49*(6), 320.

Brownstein, J. N., & Allen, C. (2015). Addressing chronic disease through community health workers. *Centers for Disease Control and Prevention.* Retrieved on December 31, 2020 from https://www.cdc.gov/dhdsp/docs/chw_brief.pdf

Center to Advance Palliative Care. (2021). *About palliative care* (n.d.). Retrieved January 21, 2021 from https://www.capc.org/about/palliative-care/

Centers for Disease Control and Prevention. (2018). *National diabetes prevention program.* U.S. Department of Health and Human Services. Retrieved on December 21, 2020 from https://www.cdc.gov/diabetes/prevention/about.htm

Centers for Disease Control and Prevention. (2018a). *Self-management education: Learn more. Feel better.* U.S. Department of Health and Human Services. Retrieved on December 19, 2020 from https://www.cdc.gov/learnmorefeelbetter/sme/index.htm

Center for Disease Control (2021) National Center for Chronic Disease and Health Promotion: About Chronic Disease. Retrieved from: https://www.cdc.gov/chronicdisease/about/index.htm

Centers for Disease Control and Prevention. (2021a). *National diabetes prevention program.* U.S. Department of Health and Human Services. Retrieved on December 21, 2020 from https://www.cdc.gov/diabetes/prevention/about.htm

Centers for Disease Control and Prevention. (2021b). *Research Behind the National Diabetes Prevention Program.* Retrieved from https://www.cdc.gov/diabetes/prevention/research-behind-ndpp.htm

Centers for Disease Control and Prevention. (2021c). Opioids: *Understanding the epidemic.* U.S. Department of Health and Human Services. Retrieved on February 1, 2021 from https://www.cdc.gov/opioids/basics/epidemic.html

Centers for Medicare & Medicaid Services (CMS). (2008). Medicare and Medicaid programs: Hospice conditions of participation; final rule. *Federal Register. Vol 73.* Washington, DC: Accessed March 2, 2021 from: https://www.govinfo.gov/app/details/FR-2008-06-05/08-1305

Cheville, A. L., & Basford, J. R. (2014). Role of rehabilitation medicine and physical agents in the treatment of cancer-associated pain. *Journal of Clinical Oncology, 32*(16), 1691–1702.

Childers, J., Back, A., Tulsky, J., & Arnold, R. (2017). REMAP. *Journal of Oncology Practice.* doi:10.1200/JOP.2016.018796. [Epub ahead of print]

Cleeland, C. S. (2007). Symptom burden: Multiple symptoms and their impact as patient-reported outcomes. *Journal of the National Cancer Institute (Monographs), 37,* 16–21.

Cotter, V. T., & Foxwell, A. M. (2019). The meaning of hope in the dying. In B. R. Ferrell & (Eds.), *Oxford textbook of palliative nursing.* 5th ed. (chap. 30, pp. 379–389). New York, NY: Oxford University Press.

Crombeen, A. M., & Lilly, E. J. (2020). Management of dyspnea in palliative care. *Current Oncology, 27*(3), 142–145.

Dahlin, C., Coyne, P. J., &. Ferrell, B. R. (Eds.). (2016). *Advanced practice palliative nursing.* New York, NY: Oxford University Press.

Degner, L. F., & Sloan, J. A. (1995). Symptom distress in newly diagnosed ambulatory cancer patients and as a predictor of survival in lung cancer. *Journal of Pain & Symptom Management, 10*(6), 423–431.

den Beuken-van Everdingen, M. H., Hochstenbach, L. M., Joosten, E. A., Tjan-Heijnen, V. C., & Janssen, D. J. (2016). Update on prevalence of pain in patients with cancer: Systematic review and meta-analysis. *J Pain Symptom Mgmt,* 51:1070–1090.e9.

References

Detering, K. M., Hancock, A. D., Reade, M. C., et al. (2010). The impact of advance care planning on end of life care in elderly patients: Randomised controlled trial. *BMJ, 340,* c1345.

Dev, R., Del Fabbro, E., & Bruera, E. (2007). Association between megestrol acetate treatment and symptomatic adrenal insufficiency with hypogonadism in male patients with cancer. *Cancer, 110*(6), 1173–1177.

Donesky, D. (2019). Dyspnea, cough and terminal secretions. In B. R. Ferrell, & J. Paice (Eds.), *Oxford textbook of palliative nursing* (5th ed.) (chap. 16, pp. 217–229). New York, NY: Oxford University Press.

Dorman, S., Byrne, A., & Edwards, A. (2007). Which measurement scales should we use to measure breathlessness in palliative care? A systematic review. *Palliative Medicine, 21*(3), 177–191.

Dowel, D., Haegerich, T., & Chou, R. (2016). CDC guideline for prescribing opioids for chronic pain – United States, 2016. *Centers for Disease Control and Prevention.* http://dx.doi.org/10.15585/mmwr.rr6501e1

Dusenbury, A. H., & Tatu, W. J. (2017). Physical therapy. In P. J. Coyne, B. Bobb, & K. Plakovic (Eds.), *Conversations in palliative care* (4th ed.) (chap. 28, pp. 287–294). Pittsburgh, PA: Hospice and Palliative Nurses Association. End-of-Life Nursing Education Consortium (ELNEC) FACT SHEET (October 2020). Last accessed February 5, 2021 from https://www.aacnnursing.org/Portals/42/ELNEC/PDF/ELNEC-Fact-Sheet.pdf

End-of-Life Nursing Education Fact Sheet. Retrived from: https://www.aacnnursing.org/Portals/42/ELNEC/PDF/ELNEC-Fact-Sheet.pdf

Ercolano, E. (2017). Psychosocial concerns in the postoperative oncology patient. *Seminars in Oncology Nursing, 33*(1), 74–79. doi:10.1016/j.soncn.2016.11.007

Fattouh, N., Hallit, S., Salameh, P., Choueiry, G., Kazour, F., & Hallit, R. (2019). Prevalence and factors affecting the level of depression, anxiety, and stress in hospitalized patients with a chronic disease. *Perspectives in Psychiatric Care, 55*(4), 592–599. https://doi-org.sacredheart.idm.oclc.org/10.1111/ppc.12369

Ferrell, B., Grant, M., Padilla, G., Vemuri, S., & Rhiner, M. (1991). The experience of pain and perceptions of quality of life: Validation of a conceptual model. *Hospice Journal, 7*(3), 9–24.

Ferrell, B. R. (1996). The quality of lives: 1,525 voices of cancer. *Oncology Nursing Forum, 23*(6), 909–916.

Ferrell, B. R., Dow, K. H., & Grant, M. (1995). Measurement of the quality of life in cancer survivors. *Quality of Life Research, 4*(6), 523–531.

Ferrell, B. R., Grant, M., Funk, B., Garcia, N., Otis-Green, S., & Schaffner, M. L. (1996). Quality of life in breast cancer. *Cancer Practice, 4*(6), 331–340.

Ferrell, B. R., & Coyle, N. (Eds.). (2010). *Oxford textbook of palliative nursing* (3rd ed.). New York, NY: Oxford University Press.

Gesme, D. M., & Wiseman, M. (2011). Advance care planning with your patients. *Journal of Oncology Practice, 7*(6), e42–e44.

Healthy People 2020. (2020). Evidence-based resource summary. *Office of Disease Prevention and Health Promotion.* Retrieved on January 3, 2021 from https://www.healthypeople.gov/2020/tools-resources/evidence-based-resource/self-management-education-chronic-disease-self

Hendrich, A., Chow, M. P., Skierczynski, B. A., & Lu, Z. (2008). A 36-hospital time and motion study: How do medical-surgical nurses spend their time? *Permanente Journal, 12*(3), 25–34.

Kaldjian, Lauris & Jones, Elizabeth & Wu, Barry & Forman-Hoffman, Valerie & Levi, Benjamin & Rosenthal, Gary. (2008). Reporting Medical Errors to Improve Patient Safety: A Survey of Physicians in Teaching Hospitals. Archives of internal medicine. 168. 40-6. 10.1001/archinternmed.2007.12.

Kaldjian, L. C., Curtis, A. E., Shinkunas, L. A., & Cannon, K. T. (2011). Goals of care toward the end of life: A structured literature review. *American Journal of Hospital Palliative Care.* doi:2550111

Katon, W., Lin, E., & Kroenke, K. (2007). The association of depression and anxiety with medical symptom burden in patients with chronic medical illness: *General Hospital Psychiatry, 29*(2), 147–155.

Krammer, L. M., Hanks-Bell, M. J., & Cappleman, J. (2011). Therapeutic presence. In J. Panke & P. Coyne (Eds.), *Conversations in palliative care* (3rd ed.) (chap. 17). Philadelphia, PA: Hospice and Palliative Nurses Association.

Kroenke K., Spitzer R. L., & Williams J. B. W. (2001). The PHQ-9. Validity of a brief depression severity measure. *Journal of General Internal Medicine, 16,* 606–613.

Kurtz, M. E., Kurtz, J. C., Stommel, M., Given, C. W., & Given, B. A. (2000). Symptomatology and loss of physical functioning among geriatric patients with lung cancer. *Journal of Pain and Symptom Management, 19*(4), 249–256.

Kyounghae Kim, Choi, J. S., Eunsuk Choi, Nieman, C. L., Jin Hui Joo, Lin, F. R., Gitlin, L. N., & Hae-Ra Han. (2016). Effects of Community-Based Health Worker Interventions to Improve Chronic Disease Management and Care Among Vulnerable Populations: A Systematic Review. *American Journal of Public Health, 106*(4), e3–e28. https://doi.org/10.2105/AJPH.2015.302987

Légaré, F., Stacey, D., Gagnon, S., et al. (2011). Validating a conceptual model for an inter-professional approach to shared decision making: A mixed methods study. *Journal of Evaluation in Clinical Practice, 17*(4), 554–564.

Lussier, D., & Portenoy, R. K. (2015). Adjuvant analgesics. In N. Cherny, M. Fallon, S. Kaasa, R. K. Portenoy, & D. C. Currow (Eds.), *Oxford textbook of palliative medicine* (5th ed.) (chap. 9.7, pp. 577–589). Oxford, UK: Oxford University Press.

Mathew, A., Yount, S., Kalhan, R., & Hitsman, B. (2019). A Preliminary Study of Relations with Smoking Status and Disease Impact. *Nicotine & Tobacco Research,* 21(5), 686–690. doi:10.1093/ntr/nty102

McCaffrey, N., Bradley, S., Ratcliffe, J., & Currow, D.C. (2016). What aspects of quality of life are important from palliative care patients' perspectives? A systematic review of qualitative research. *Journal of Pain and Symptom Management, 52*(2), 318–328. doi:10.1016/j.jpainsymman.2016.02.012

McCorkle, R., Dowd, M., Ercolano, E., Schulman-Green, D., Williams, A.-l., Siefert, M. L., Schwartz, P., et al. (2009). Effects of a nursing intervention on quality of life outcomes in post-surgical women with gynecological cancers. *Psycho-Oncology, 18*(1), 62–70. doi:10.1002/pon.1365

McCorkle, R., Jeon, S., Ercolano, E., Lazenby, M., Reid, A., Davies, M., Gettinger, S., et al. (2015). An advanced practice nurse coordinated multidisciplinary intervention for patients with late-stage cancer: A cluster randomized trial. *Journal of Palliative Medicine, 18*(11), 962–969. doi:10.1089/jpm.2015.0113

Meier, D. E. (2011). Increased access to palliative care and hospice services: Opportunities to improve value in health care. *Milbank Quarterly, 89*(3), 343–380. doi:10.1111/j.1468-0009.2011.00632.x

Mersky, H. (1986). Classification of chronic pain: Descriptions of chronic pain syndromes and definitions of pain terms. *Pain, 3*(Supplement Pt.2) S1–S226.

Merskey, H. (1986) Classification of chronic pain. Descriptions of chronic pain syndromes and definitions of pain terms. Prepared by the International Association for the Study of Pain, Subcommittee on Taxonomy. (1986). Pain. Supplement, 3, S1 -S226.

Meyer, M-A. & Ring, M. (2019). Complementary and integrative therapies in palliative care. In B. R. Ferrell, & J. Paice (Eds.), *Oxford textbook of palliative nursing* (5th ed.) (chap. 28, pp. 361–370). New York, NY: Oxford University Press.

Mitchell, S. A., Hoffman, A. J., Clark, J. C., DeGennaro, R. M., Poirier, P., Robinson, C. B., & Weisbrod, B. L. (2014). Putting evidence into practice: An update of evidence-based interventions for cancer-related fatigue during and following treatment. *Clinical Journal of Oncology Nursing, 18*(6), 38–58. doi:10.1188/14.CJON.S3.38-58

Mularski, R. A., Reinke, L. F., Carrieri-Kohlman, V., Fischer, M. D., Campbell, M. L., Rocker, G., White, D. B., et al. (2013). An official American Thoracic Society workshop report: Assessment and palliative management of dyspnea crisis. *Annals of the American Thoracic Society, 10*(5), S98–S106. doi:10.1513/AnnalsATS.201306-169ST

Myers, J., & Dudgeon, D. (2011). Dyspnea. In S. Y. a. E. Bruera (Ed.), *Oxford American Handbook of Hospice and Palliative Medicine* (pp. 169–180). New York, NY: Oxford University Press.

National Cancer Institute. (2020). Cannabis and cannabinoids (PDQ®)–Health Professional Version. Last accessed February 20, 2021 from https://www.cancer.gov/about-cancer/treatment/cam/hp/cannabis-pdq

National Coalition for Hospice and Palliative Care. (2021a). *Cooperation. Communication. Collaboration.* Retrieved February 5, 2021 from https://www.nationalcoalitionhpc.org/

National Coalition for Hospice and Palliative Care. (2021b). *Strategic priorities.* Retrieved February 5, 2021 from https://www.nationalcoalitionhpc.org/strategic-priorities/

National Comprehensive Cancer Network. (2021). *Clinical practice guidelines in oncology (NCCN Guidelines®): Palliative care.* Retrieved March 3, 2021 from https://www.nccn.org/professionals/physician_gls/pdf/palliative.pdf

References

National Consensus Project (NCP) for Quality Palliative Care. (2018). *Clinical practice guidelines for quality palliative care* (4th ed.). Retrieved March 3, 2021 from https://www.nationalcoalitionhpc.org/wp-content/uploads/2018/10/NCHPC-NCPGuidelines_4thED_web_FINAL.pdf

National Council on Aging. (n.d.). *Chronic disease self-management programs.* National Council on Aging. Retrieved on January 3, 2021 from https://www.ncoa.org/healthy-aging/chronic-disease/chronic-disease-self-management-programs/

National Quality Forum. (2006). *A national framework and preferred practices for palliative and hospice care quality.* Washington, DC: Author. Retrieved from http://www.qualityforum.org/publications/2006/12/A_National_Framework_and_Preferred_Practices_for_Palliative_and_ Hospice_Care_Quality.aspx

O'Neil Page, E., Anderson, P., & Dean, G. (2015). Fatigue. In B.R. Ferrell, N. Coyle, & J. Paice (Eds.), *Oxford textbook of palliative nursing* (4th ed.) (pp. 154–166). New York, NY: Oxford University Press.

Oxford Textbook of Palliative Nursing. (2010). (B. R. Ferrell & N. Coyle Eds. 3rd ed.). New York, NY: Oxford University Press.

Paice, J. (2015). Introduction to palliative nursing care. In B. Ferrell, N. Coyle, & J. Paice (Eds.), *Oxford textbook of palliative nursing* (4th ed.) (pp. 3–10). New York, NY: Oxford University Press.

Paice, J. A., Portenoy, R., Lacchetti, C., Campbell, T., Cheville, A., Citron, M., et al. (2016). Management of chronic pain in survivors of adult cancers: American Society of Clinical Oncology clinical practice guideline. *J Clin Oncol,* 34(27), 3325–45.

Pang, P. S., Collins, S. P., Sauser, K., Andrei, A.-C., Storrow, A. B., Hollander, J. E., Mebazaa, A., et al. (2014). Assessment of dyspnea early in acute heart failure: Patient characteristics and response differences between Likert and visual analog scales. *Academic Emergency Medicine: Official Journal of the Society for Academic Emergency Medicine,* 21(6), 659–666. doi:10.1111/acem.12390

Pasero, C. & McCaffery, M. (2012) Pain Care. American Society of PeriAnesthesia Nurses 1089-9472/doi:10.1016/j.jopan.2011.11.002

Pasternak, G. W. (2014). Opiate pharmacology and relief of pain. *Journal of Clinical Oncology,* 32(16), 1655–1661. doi:10.1200/JCO.2013.53.1079

Prince-Paul, M. J., & Daly, B. (2019). Ethical considerations in palliative care. In B. R. Ferrell & J. Paice (Eds.), *Oxford textbook of palliative nursing* (5th ed.) (chap. 70, pp. 824–836). New York, NY: Oxford University Press.

Raghupathi, W., & Raghupathi, V. (2018). An empirical study of chronic diseases in the United States: A visual analytics approach. *International journal of environmental research and public health,* 15(3), 431. https://doi.org/10.3390/ijerph15030431

Reeves, S., Zwarenstein, M., Goldman, J., et al. (2008). Interprofessional education: Effects on professional practice and health care outcomes. *Cochrane Database System Reviews, 1,* CD002213.

Salman, J, Wolfe, E., & Patel, S. K. (2019). Anxiety and depression. In B. Ferrell & J. Paice (Eds.), *Oxford textbook of palliative nursing* (5th ed.) (pp. 309–318). New York, NY: Oxford University Press.

Schack, E., & Wholihan, D. (2019). Anorexia and cachexia. In B. R. Ferrell, N. Coyle, & J. Paice (Eds.), *Oxford textbook of palliative nursing* (5th ed.) (chap. 11, pp. 140–148). New York, NY: Oxford University Press.

Schroder, C., Heyland, D., Jiang, X., Rocker, G., & Dodek, P. (2009). Canadian researchers at the end of life network. Educating medical residents in end-of-life care: Insights from a multicenter survey. *Journal of Palliative Medicine,* 374, 1196–1208.

Self-management Resource Center. (2021). *Chronic disease self-management.* Self-management Resource Center. Retrieved on January 3, 2021 from https://www.selfmanagementresource.com/programs/small-group/chronic-disease-self-management/

Siefert, M. L. (2010). Fatigue, pain, and functional status during outpatient chemotherapy. *Oncology Nursing Forum,* 37(2), e114–e123. doi:10.1188/10.ONF.114-123

Stanford Medicine. (2021). *Stanford studies online self-management for people with chronic disease.* Stanford University. Retrieved on January 3, 2021 from https://www.selfmanagementresource.com/programs/small-group/chronic-disease-self-management/

Stridsman, C., Müllerova, H., Skär, L., & Lindberg, A. (2013). Fatigue in COPD and the impact of respiratory symptoms and heart disease—a population-based study. *COPD,* 10(2), 125–132. doi:10.3109/15412555.2012.728642

Sung, M. R., Patel, M. V., Djalalov, S., Le, L. W., Shepherd, F. A., Burkes, R. L., Leighl, N. B., et al. (2017). Evolution of symptom burden of advanced lung cancer over a decade. *Clinical Lung Cancer, 18*(3), 274–280, e276. doi:10.1016/j.cllc.2016.12.010

Syrjala, K. L., Jensen, M. P., Mendoza, M. E., Yi, J. C., Fisher, H. M., & Keefe, F. J. (2014). Psychological and behavioral approaches to cancer pain management. *Journal of Clinical Oncology, 32*(16), 1703–1711.

Tarricone, R., Ricca, G., Nyanzi-Wakholi, B., & Medina-Lara, A. (2016). Impact of cancer anorexia-cachexia syndrome on health-related quality of life and resource utilisation: A systematic review. *Critical Reviews in Oncology/Hematology, 99*, 49–62. doi:10.1016/j.critrevonc.2015.12.008

Taylor, S. F., & Melroy, M. K. (2017). Occupational therapy. In P. Coyne, B. Bobb, & K. Plakovic (Eds.), *Conversations in palliative care* (4th ed.) (chap. 27, pp. 279–286). Pittsburgh, PA: Hospice and Palliative Nurses Association.

Temel, J. S., Greer, J. A., Muzikansky, A., et al. (2010). Early palliative care for patients with metastatic non-small-cell lung cancer. *New England Journal of Medicine, 363*, 733–742.

Thacker, K. S. (2008). Nurses' advocacy behaviors in end-of-life nursing care. *Nursing Ethics, 15*(2), 174–185. doi:10.1177/0969733007086015

van den Beuken-van Everdingen, et al. (2016). Update on Prevalence of Pain in Patients With Cancer: Systematic Review and Meta-Analysis. Journal of Pain Symptom Management Jun;51(6):1070-1090.e9. doi: 10.1016/j.jpainsymman.2015.12.340. Epub 2016 Apr 23. PMID: 27112310.

Vitaltalk.com. (2017). *Nurse statements for articulating empathy*. Retrieved from http://vitaltalk.org/guides/responding-to-emotion-respecting/

Waldrop, D. P., & Meeker, M. A. (2012). Communication and advanced care planning in palliative and end-of-life care. *Nursing Outlook, 60*(6), 365–369. doi:10.1016/j.outlook.2012.08.012

Weingaertner, V., Scheve, C., Gerdes, V., Schwarz-Eywill, M., Prenzel, R., Bausewein, C., Simon, S. T., et al. (2014). Breathlessness, functional status, distress, and palliative care needs over time in patients with advanced chronic obstructive pulmonary disease or lung cancer: A cohort study. *Journal of Pain and Symptom Management, 48*(4), 569–581, e561. doi:10.1016/j.jpainsymman.2013.11.011

Westbrook, J. I., Duffield, C., Li, L., & Creswick, N. J. (2011). How much time do nurses have for patients? A longitudinal study quantifying hospital nurses' patterns of task time distribution and interactions with health professionals. *BMC Health Services Research, 11*(1), 319. doi: 10.1186/1472-6963-11-319

World Health Organization. (2015). *Palliative care*. Retrieved from http://www.who.int/mediacentre/factsheets/fs402/en/

World Health Organization. (2020). *Chronic disease and health promotion*. World Health Organization. Retrieved on January 3, 2021 from https://www.who.int/chp/about/integrated_cd/en/

Wright, A. A., Zhang, B., Ray, A., Mack, J. W., Trice, E., Balboni, T., Prigerson, H. G., et al. (2008). Associations between end-of-life discussions, patient mental health, medical care near death, and caregiver bereavement adjustment. *JAMA, 300*(14), 1665–1673. doi:10.1001/jama.300.14.1665

Xue, Y., Smith, J., & Spetz, J. (2019). Primary care nurse practitioners and physicians in low-income and rural areas, 2010–2016. *Journal of the American Medical Association, 321*(1), 102–105.

Yancy, C. W., Lopatin, M., Stevenson, L. W., De Marco, T., & Fonarow, G. C. (2006). Clinical presentation, management, and in-hospital outcomes of patients admitted with acute decompensated heart failure with preserved systolic function: A Report from the Acute Decompensated Heart Failure National Registry (ADHERE) Database. *Journal of the American College of Cardiology, 47*, 76–84. http://dx.doi.org/10.1016/j.jacc.2005.09.022

You, J. J., Fowler, R. A., & Heyland, D. K. (2014). On behalf of the Canadian Researchers at the End of Life Network (CARENET). Just ask: Discussing goals of care with patients in hospital with serious illness. *Canadian Medial Association Journal, 186*(6), 425–432. doi:10.1503/cmaj.121274

Zhang, R., Huang, J., Shu, Q., Wu, L., Zhang, Q., & Meng, Y. (2019). Improvement in quality of life of Chinese chronic heart failure patients with neuropsychiatric complications over 12-months post-treatment with Metoprolol. *Medicine, 98*(4). http://dx.doi.org/10.1097/MD.0000000000014252

Zigmond, A. S., & Smith, R. P. (1983). The hospital anxiety and depression scale. *Acta Psychiatrica Scandinavica, 67*(6), 361–370.

PART 3

Clinical Education for the Nurse Practitioner

CHAPTER 8	Quality, Safety, and Prescriptive Authority	215
CHAPTER 9	Clinical Education: The Role of the Student, Faculty, and Preceptor	237
CHAPTER 10	Case Presentation, Consultation, and Collaboration in Primary Care	255
CHAPTER 11	Clinical Prevention/Community and Population Health	277
CHAPTER 12	Electronic Health Record and Impact on Healthcare Outcomes	305
CHAPTER 13	Telehealth: Increasing Access to Health Care	327

CHAPTER 8

Quality, Safety, and Prescriptive Authority

Sylvie Rosenbloom, Linda S. Morrow, and Tammy A. Testut

An Introduction to Quality

Healthcare quality and safety has taken great leaps in the past decade. Major stakeholders have set quality in health care as a priority in the fight for safe and quality patient care provision. Whether you practice in primary care, acute care, or in the community, quality measures are those benchmark criteria that set the standards for not only patient care but also for accreditation and payment. Gone are the days when quality was measured in days of stay or episodes of care. Quality care is a direct reflection of the patient-centered model of care, and patient outcomes are at the top of the list when it comes to validating or verifying the provision of care and overall prevention of illness.

Florence Nightingale was probably the first quality improvement expert in the healthcare field (Riddle, 2010). She tracked hospital death rates, which included a depiction of unnecessary military deaths caused by unsanitary conditions. Nightingale was an innovator in the collection, tabulation, interpretation, and graphical display of descriptive statistics (Riddle, 2010; Sheingold & Hahn, 2014). She was at the forefront of a specialty that previously hadn't been considered a major initiative in the overall provision of care.

Quality has been known by a multitude of terms since the 19th century. Many refer to quality initiatives as Quality Improvement (QI), Continuous Quality Improvement (CQI), and Quality Assurance (QA), but there are notable differences among these various initiatives (Varkey et al., 2007; Green, 1991):

> Quality Improvement (QI) activities are designed to improve performance by using an intentional approach to the continuous study and improvement of the processes used to provide services to meet the needs of the individual and others. Continuous Quality Improvement (CQI) is the agency's ongoing effort to manage performance, motivate improvement, and capture lessons learned in areas that may or may not be measured as part of accreditation. It is a continuous effort to improve the efficiency, success, value, or performance of services, processes, capacities, outcomes

and consequences. Quality Assurance (QA) refers to the gamut of evaluation activities intended to ensuring compliance with minimum quality standards. The primary aim of quality assurance is to demonstrate that a service or product fulfills or meets a set of requirements or standards.

Today, quality and safety are the driving forces for improvement in all healthcare arenas. There is a current consensus that quality initiatives in any healthcare setting are crucial to the success and failure of its overall systems. The role of quality improvement in any healthcare setting has moved from a luxury to a necessity.

This chapter will briefly review quality and safety issues and initiatives and conclude with an overview of safe prescribing.

Quality in Doctoral Education

Healthcare and educational standards both have an extreme focus on outcome measures to allow for a conscious awareness and act of qualifying and quantifying the provision of service. Within a doctoral education for Advanced Nursing Practice, essential elements and foundational outcome competencies are followed.

The Essentials of Doctoral Education for Advanced Nursing Practice delineate curricular elements and foundational outcome competencies. There are eight foundational competencies deemed essential for all DNP graduates regardless of whether they are preparing for a clinical, administrative, or academic role. The eight DNP Essentials are from the American Association of Colleges of Nursing [AACN], 2006:

1. Scientific Underpinnings for Practice
2. Organizational and Systems Leadership for Quality Improvement and Systems Thinking
3. Clinical Scholarship and Analytical Methods for Evidence-Based Practice
4. Information Systems/Technology and Patient Care Technology for the Improvement and Transformation of Health Care
5. Health Care Policy for Advocacy in Health Care
6. Interprofessional Collaboration for Improving Patient and Population Health Outcomes
7. Clinical Preventive and Population Health for Improving the Nation's Health
8. Advance Nursing Practice

Essential II focuses on organizational and systems leadership for quality improvement and systems thinking. This essential highlights the need for DNP graduates to "be proficient in quality improvement strategies and in creating and sustaining changes at the organizational and policy levels," to "ensure accountability for quality of health care and patient safety for populations with whom they work," and to be prepared to "lead quality improvement and patient safety initiatives in health-care systems" (AACN, 2006, p. 9).

U.S. Healthcare System

The U.S. healthcare system places a high priority on prevention of illness, early diagnosis, treatment of disease, and the use of advanced interventions to improve the physical and mental health of its population (Agency for Healthcare Research and Quality [AHRQ], 2019). The Patient Protection and Affordable Care Act mandated the establishment of a National Strategy for Quality Improvement in Health Care (the National Quality Strategy, or NQS), as part of the goal of increasing access to high-quality, affordable health care for all Americans. Opportunities to improve healthcare services involve addressing the six dimensions of quality.

> The National Quality Strategy's six priorities address the range of quality concerns that affect most Americans: making care safer by reducing harm caused in the delivery of care; ensuring that each person and family are engaged as partners in their care; promoting effective communication and coordination of care; promoting the most effective prevention and treatment practices for the leading causes of mortality, starting with cardiovascular disease; working with communities to promote wide use of best practices to enable healthy living; and making quality care more affordable for individuals, families, employers, and governments by developing and spreading new health care delivery models. (AHRQ, 2019, p. 13)

Unfortunately, there have been inequalities in the access to care, resulting from poor communication, lack of patient–provider relationships, and/or low health literacy among U.S. residents. Social determinants of health (SDOH) have been brought to the forefront of nursing and other healthcare professions. Doctorally prepared nurses are part of the commitment to promote health equity in the 21st century, by assessing SDOH and the overall care of a diverse population (Thornton & Persaud, 2018).

The Agency for Healthcare Research and Quality (AHRQ) has devised three basic questions to guide Americans to improved health care:

1. What is the status of healthcare quality and disparities in the United States?
2. How have healthcare quality and disparities changed over time?
3. Where is the need to improve healthcare quality and reduce disparities greatest?

In the AHRQ 2019 National Healthcare Quality and Disparities Report, the number of Americans with access to health care has shown a dramatic improvement. Quality of health care shows a consistent level of improvement but varies across the National Quality Strategy (NQS) priorities. Areas such as effective treatment, patient safety, person-centered care, and healthy living indicate improvement overall with a continued focus on specific disparity reduction.

Coordination, which is the process of promoting communication and coordination of care across the care continuum, "measures have lagged behind other priorities in overall performance" (AHRQ, p. 2).

> Transformation and the changes required will not be easy—at the individual or systems level. Individually, it requires an examination of one's own knowledge, skills, and attitudes and whether that places you as ready to contribute or resist the coming change. At an organizational level, it requires an analysis of mission, goals, partnerships, processes, leadership, and other essential elements of the organization and then overhauling them, thus disrupting things as we know it. The reality is that everyone's role is changing—the patients', physicians', nurses', and other healthcare professionals'—across the entire continuum of care. Healthcare professionals will

be successful when they collaborate and come to understand and leverage their unique contributions to patient care and the healthcare system at large. Nurse practitioners are poised to lead new initiatives and coordinate patient centered care. (Salmond & Echevarria, 2017)

Institute of Medicine Quality Reports

The three major reports related to healthcare quality include the Institute of Medicine's (IOM's) National Roundtable on Health Care Quality report, *The Urgent Need to Improve Health Care Quality* (Chassin & Galvin, 1998); *To Err Is Human* (IOM, 2000); and the IOM's *Crossing the Quality Chasm* (2001). In the IOM National Roundtable report, the contributors concluded that the U.S. healthcare system had serious and widespread issues affecting the delivery of quality care. It was noted that there was underuse, overuse, and misuse of healthcare practices which was stored under the umbrella of fraud and abuse. These three categories of use included various healthcare testing and interventions that were viewed, compared, and contrasted to the quality and safety of patient care.

When *To Err Is Human* was published, it garnered the attention of healthcare providers and policy makers, as well as consumers (Ransom et al., 2019; Taylor-Sullivan, 2013). Highlighted in the report were specific individual cases of preventable errors and startling statistics related to harm inflicted upon patients from the healthcare system's unacceptable, and often preventable, mistakes.

Shortly after *To Err Is Human* was published, *Crossing the Quality Chasm* was released by the IOM and contained a framework for improving the healthcare system. The six dimensions of quality health care are (IOM, 2000):

1. Safe—avoidance of injuries
2. Effective—provision of services based on scientific findings and abstinence of services to patients not likely to benefit
3. Efficient—avoidance of waste
4. Timely—reduction of delays for patients receiving care
5. Patient centered—provision of care based on patient needs, preferences, and value systems
6. Equitable—delivery of quality care irrespective of personal characteristics

Outcome measurements can indicate how well an organization or individual is doing in relation to these six dimensions. Examples of outcome measurements include percentages of adverse events, use of evidence-based practice guidelines, cost of care, wait times, patient satisfaction scores, and disparities in health care by gender or race (Ransom et al., 2019).

Attributes of quality care include (Ransom et al., 2019):

- Technical performance—The skill of medical providers in performing procedures and interventions
- Management of interpersonal relationships—Maintenance of a good patient–client relationship
- Amenities—Latest technology and equipment, wide range of services, best nurses and physicians, and most personalized care
- Access—Availability of necessary resources (e.g., prompt access to providers)

- Responsiveness to patient preferences—Respectful of complementary and alternative therapies and being culturally sensitive
- Equity—Provision of the same healthcare options to all individuals
- Efficiency—Wise use of resources
- Cost-effectiveness—Good value for the money; in other words, dollars spent to enhance health outcomes

Professional Accountability and Teamwork

For quality initiatives to be successful, it is imperative to have leadership and all stakeholders promoting a culture of quality. Doctorally prepared Nurse Practitioners (NPs) are poised to be in leadership roles either formally or informally; therefore, understanding the basic components of leadership and quality is essential. Scholtes, Joiner, and Streibel (2018) identified eight principles of quality leadership:

1. Having the customer as the focus of quality efforts
2. Exhibiting great passion for quality in the organization
3. Acknowledging and appreciating structure at work
4. Creating efficient work processes by reducing variation and instituting quality control measures
5. Fostering unity of purpose so all who work in an organization are clear about the vision
6. Examining systems for defects, and not placing blame on the individuals working within the confines of the system
7. Working collaboratively across disciplines
8. Offering initial training and continuing education to maintain the culture of quality in the organization

Leaders can also develop a culture of safety, or *just culture* in the work environment (AHRQ, n.d.). In a *just culture,* there is an understanding of the differences between human error, at-risk behaviors, and zero tolerance for reckless behaviors. This approach is viewed as being more balanced in that staff can be held accountable for errors in particular situations in the healthcare environment. Achieving a culture of safety needs to be a systemwide commitment, and the ability of the doctorally prepared NP to foster collegial and collaborative teamwork is an asset to the culture of quality and safety.

In addition to putting the leadership quality principles into practice in the work environment, the doctorally prepared NP should also evaluate his or her own practice outcomes. Outcome measurements as indicators of quality health care have largely been associated with medical interventions and treatments; however, nurse-sensitive patient outcomes have also been developed as indicators of quality associated with nursing care (Zaccagnini & Pechacek, 2021). The doctorally prepared NP bases interventions on physiological, psychosocial, functional, behavioral, and knowledge-focused parameters (Zaccagnini & Pechacek, 2021). Numerous quality indicators can be used for outcome measurements, including such indicators as total number of patients meeting standardized goals (e.g., HgA1C < 7.0, SBP mm Hg < 120, and DBP mm Hg < 80), patient satisfaction, patient adherence to treatment regimens, and immunization rates.

Quality and Safety Education for Nurses

The Quality and Safety Education for Nurses (QSEN) initiative, funded by the Robert Wood Johnson Foundation, has resources for the practicing NP, as well as for NP nursing students (The Quality and Safety Education for Nurses [QSEN], 2021). The goal of QSEN is to develop curricula and competencies in patient-centered care, teamwork and collaboration, evidence-based practice, quality improvement, safety, and informatics in an effort to continuously improve the quality and safety of healthcare systems (QSEN, 2021).

The QSEN initiative aids in the NP's ability to analyze, synthesize, and use findings from credible evidence-based research to enhance one's own practice. The program meets the IOM challenge of preparing future nurses and fostering lifelong learning and advancement with the knowledge, skills, and attitudes to meet the ever-changing needs of health care (QSEN, 2021). The QSEN initiative has developed knowledge, skills, and attitudes for safety that are meant to minimize the risk of harm to patients and providers through both system effectiveness and individual performance (see **Tables 8-1** and **8-2**).

Table 8-1 QSEN Knowledge, Skills, and Attitudes for Safety

Knowledge	Skills	Attitudes
Describe human factors and other basic safety design principles, as well as commonly used unsafe practices (such as work-arounds and dangerous abbreviations) Describe the benefits and limitations of selected safety-enhancing technologies (such as barcodes, computer provider order entry, and electronic prescribing) Evaluate effective strategies to reduce reliance on memory	Participate as a team member to design, promote and model effective use of technology and standardized practices that support safety and quality Participate as a team member to design, promote, and model the effective use of strategies to reduce risk of harm to self and others Promote a practice culture conducive to highly reliable processes built on human factors research Use appropriate strategies to reduce reliance on memory (such as forcing functions, checklists)	Value the contributions of standardization and reliability to safety Appreciate the importance of being a safety mentor and role model Appreciate the cognitive and physical limits of human performance

(continues)

Knowledge	Skills	Attitudes
Delineate general categories of errors and hazards in care Identify best practices for organizational responses to error Describe factors that create a just culture and culture of safety Describe best practices that promote patient and provider safety in the practice specialty	Communicate observations or concerns related to hazards and errors to patients, families, and the health care team Identify and correct system failures and hazards in care Design and implement micro-system changes in response to identified hazards and errors Engage in a systems focus rather than blaming individuals when errors or near misses occur Report errors and support members of the healthcare team to be forthcoming about errors and near misses	Value own role in reporting and preventing errors Value systems approaches to improving patient safety in lieu of blaming individuals Value the use of organizational error reporting systems
Describe processes used to analyze causes of error and allocation of responsibility and accountability (such as root cause analysis and failure mode effects analysis)	Participate appropriately in analyzing errors and designing, implementing, and evaluating system improvements	Value vigilance and monitoring of care, including one's own performance, by patients, families, and other members of the healthcare team
Describe methods of identifying and preventing verbal, physical, and psychological harm to patients and staff	Prevent escalation of conflict Respond appropriately to aggressive behavior	Value prevention of assaults and loss of dignity for patients, staff, and aggressors
Analyze the potential and actual impact of national patient safety resources, initiatives, and regulations	Use national patient safety resources: - For own professional development - To focus attention on safety in care setting - To design and implement improvements in practice	Value relationship between national safety campaigns and implementation in local practices and practice settings

Reprinted from Publication title, Vol /edition number, Cronenwett, L., Sherwood, G., Barnsteiner J., Disch, J., Johnson, J., Mitchell, P., Sullivan, D., Warren, J. , Quality and safety education for nurses. *Nursing Outlook,* 55(3)122–131., Copyright (2007), with permission from Elsevier.

Table 8-2 QSEN Knowledge, Skills, and Attitudes for Quality Improvement

Knowledge, skills, and attitudes for quality improvement, which are used in monitoring the outcomes of care processes and use improvement methods to design and test changes to continuously improve the quality and safety of healthcare systems.

Describe strategies for improving outcomes of care in the setting in which one is engaged in clinical practice Analyze the impact of context (such as access, cost, or team functioning) on improvement efforts	Use a variety of sources of information to review outcomes of care and identify potential areas for improvement Propose appropriate aims for quality improvement efforts Assert leadership in shaping the dialogue about and providing leadership for the introduction of best practices	Appreciate that continuous quality improvement is an essential part of the daily work of all health professionals
Analyze ethical issues associated with quality improvement Describe features of quality improvement projects that overlap sufficiently with research, thereby requiring IRB oversight	Assure ethical oversight of quality improvement projects Maintain confidentiality of any patient information used to determine outcomes of quality improvement efforts	Value the need for ethical conduct of quality improvement
Describe the benefits and limitations of quality improvement data sources, and measurement and data analysis strategies	Design and use databases as sources of information for improving patient care Select and use relevant benchmarks	Appreciate the importance of data that allows one to estimate the quality of local care
Explain common causes of variation in outcomes of care in the practice specialty	Select and use tools (such as control charts and run charts) that are helpful for understanding variation Identify gaps between local and best practice	Appreciate how unwanted variation affects outcomes of care processes
Describe common quality measures in the practice specialty	Use findings from root cause analyses to design and implement system improvements Select and use quality measures to understand performance	Value measurement and its role in good patient care

Analyze the differences between micro-system and macro-system change	Use principles of change management to implement and evaluate care processes at the micro-system level	Appreciate the value of what individuals and teams can to do to improve care
Understand principles of change management	Design, implement, and evaluate tests of change in daily work (using an experiential learning method such as Plan-Do-Study-Act)	Value local systems improvement (in individual practice, team practice on a unit, or in the macro-system) and its role in professional job satisfaction
Analyze the strengths and limitations of common quality improvement methods	Align the aims, measures, and changes involved in improving care	
	Use measures to evaluate the effect of change	Appreciate that all improvement is change but not all change is improvement

Reprinted from Publication title, Vol /edition number, Cronenwett, L., Sherwood, G., Barnsteiner J., Disch, J., Johnson, J., Mitchell, P., Sullivan, D., Warren, J. , Quality and safety education for nurses. *Nursing Outlook, 55*(3)122–131., Copyright (2007), with permission from Elsevier.

Patient-Centered Care

Patient-centered care focuses on the need for the provider to view patients as partners who have input into healthcare decisions. Knowledge and skills specific in this area include analyzing one's own and the healthcare team's limitations in providing culturally sensitive care and collaborating and communicating as a team member to have successful patient outcomes. Value and respect are key components of the attitude aspect of patient-centered care. One of the key values can be related to the ability of the NP to use interprofessional consultations and referrals to obtain solutions for patients' issues, whether they are disease related or associated with psychosocial problems.

One of the well-known models in the acute care setting is the Planetree Model (Planetree Organization, 2020). This comprehensive approach to patient-centered care was founded in 1978 by Angelica Thieriot after she experienced the depersonalized effects of being a patient as well as a care provider for her spouse and son. The model encompasses mind, body, and spirit for healing the patient. The focus of the health care in this model centers around the patient. Family members, caregivers, professionals—anyone in contact with the patient—must be sensitive to the patient's need for respect and control, and provide warm and supportive care. Patient-centered care takes place in the office, clinic, and even during volunteer activities, as described by Tracy, NP:

Tracy's Story

I used to volunteer in a community center in a low-income area in Queens, New York. The neighborhood population consisted of a significant number of elderly people who lived at or near the poverty level. While at the community center, I was asked by a concerned woman to "check in" on her neighbor. This neighbor was described as "all alone" and possibly incapable of properly caring for herself. Later that week, I knocked on the neighbor's door with the intention of inviting her to

(continues)

join our community center. I introduced myself and the reason for my visit. While I was speaking to her about our center, I noticed her apartment was dark, cluttered, and dirty. She told me she lived alone with no family to speak of, had difficulty walking due to being overweight, and had tripped and fallen in her home a number of times. Additionally, she had difficulty seeing and hearing and was agoraphobic. Thus, she relied on neighbors to "pick up" groceries for her. She was scared every day of being without food or falling and not being able to get up again.

This elderly woman was identified as being socially isolated, at risk for falls, and unable to adequately care for herself as a result of limited resources (financial or otherwise). I spoke to her about going to the hospital, both for medical evaluation as well as for referral for needed services. She agreed. While hospitalized, it was determined she had hypothyroidism, contributing to her significant weight gain and loss of hearing. She was started on thyroid replacement. Her hearing eventually improved, and she lost weight, improving her mobility. She was also diagnosed with cataracts and has since undergone bilateral cataract surgeries, improving her vision. While hospitalized, she was deemed eligible for Medicaid and can now afford her medication and healthcare services. As a Medicaid recipient, she is eligible for home care services. An aide visits her 5 days a week and assists with her cooking and ambulation outside the home. She has also started coming to our meetings at the community center. It was through identification of an individual in need and referral to appropriate services that we were able to create an improved quality (and safety) of life for this woman.

Communication and Care Coordination

Care coordination is a key concept that lays the foundation for successful care across the care continuum. As part of the healthcare team, NPs have a concerted responsibility to promote effective communication, to foster greater outcomes of care. According to the Institute for Healthcare Improvement (IHI), "Care coordination delivers health benefits to those with multiple needs, while improving their experience of the care system and driving down overall health care (and societal) costs" (Craig, Ebey, & Whittington, 2011, p. 2). Part of care coordination is the ability to communicate with multiple members of the team, including the patient and family members.

Communication between the patient, healthcare providers, and members of the healthcare team is essential for obtaining excellent outcomes by allowing an interprofessional approach to caring for the patient. The Enhanced Calgary Cambridge Guide is one of the tools used in healthcare universities and colleges to enhance communication skills between providers and patients (Kurtz, Silverman, Benson, & Draper, 2003). Although this model was originally developed for medical students, it has been adapted for a variety of health-related professionals, including veterinarians and pharmacists, and it is well-suited to depict the communication used to develop the nurse practitioner–patient relationship. This type of communication encourages open discussion (led by the healthcare provider) that allows the patient to tell his or her story. Clarification occurs when the listener verifies any ambiguous areas of the story. Respect is paramount, and the listener is taught to use empathy and explore the patient's perspective and expectations. It will take time before the student or novice NP becomes proficient at integrating the physical examination and patient interview components into the full assessment.

An example of the integration of patient-centered care as part of NP practice is apparent in the following case, as explained by an experienced NP.

Jane's Story

I met Mr. L. in my heart failure clinic for the first time in January this year, soon after he moved from Florida to live with his granddaughter (an RN at a nearby emergency department). He was 83 years old and had NYHA Class III heart failure symptoms. He had turned down any home care services because his granddaughter was able to take care of all his needs. I set him up for telehealth services. On the third visit, I invited our palliative care APRN to a joint appointment to introduce him to the palliative care team. At that time, he made it very clear that he wanted to die at home when the time came. Our palliative care APRN provided whatever he needed to live independently at home—hospital bed, oxygen for prn use, and a "fat spoon" (because he had difficulty using utensils to feed himself from his rotator cuff injury that he suffered from a fall a year earlier). We also allowed the granddaughter to decide how much of his heart failure medicines to give him due to great fluctuation in his blood pressure.

During his last outpatient visit in early March, he told me that he had fallen three times and no longer had enough energy to make his bed (according to his granddaughter, he was a very proper man and making the bed was a very important daily function that he insisted on doing). He also started choking when he ate. At this time, I had a very honest talk with him acknowledging that I knew he wanted to die at home, but I told him that it was no longer safe for him to stay at home during the day by himself (due to falling and choking). He clearly was in class IV HF. I told him that we could help make him comfortable and safe if he agreed to be admitted to the inpatient hospice service. To my surprise, it was almost a relief for him to hear that, and he instantly agreed. His granddaughter supported his decision. Since he had met with our palliative care team, they accepted him into our inpatient hospice unit directly from the outpatient clinic.

Mr. L. was a deeply religious person and he was happy to have a daily chaplain visit, and repeatedly said to the chaplain that he had a good life and that he was at peace and ready to "go home" to see his wife and a deceased son. His sister visited from New Jersey, and his son came from Maine to be with him. I tried to go visit him daily. He was always smiling and always had a relative by his bedside. Two weeks later, he died peacefully with his family by his side. We respected his wishes, supported him, and transitioned him to an appropriate level of care when his health deteriorated. He trusted me and the palliative care APRN. With his cooperation, I think he received the most ideal end-of-life care. I still get choked up when I think of him. He was such a gentleman, and I was happy to be involved in his care.

Quality Improvement Planning

Although it may seem as though QI was introduced and perfected within the acute care hospital setting, it is as important in tertiary care sites as it is in outpatient clinics and private practices. The NP needs to acquire the specific skills to identify gaps in care and areas for improvement, recognize appropriate tools to use to measure variations, and collaborate to institute change based on the best practices found in the literature. Once change is implemented, it is vital to evaluate its effectiveness and make alterations as necessary. The change process is seen along a continuum where checks and revisions are necessary for the improvement to stay viable.

The purpose of any QI initiative is to improve the performance of existing processes, as well as to plan new ones. There are many ways to approach change within any organization, whether the change is small or large in scale.

One common QI methodology is the Plan-Do-Study-Act (PDSA) framework. The PDSA framework is an effective method for sustaining continuous change in an organization (Deming, 1986). Dr. W. Edwards Deming is known as the father of quality. Deming showed that by reducing waste, repetitive work, and staff turnover, organizations can improve quality and customer satisfaction. The PDSA process can be used to initiate a change in practice for ensuring quality. The key to this conceptual framework is to develop rapid cycles of change to sustain momentum in changing behaviors, procedures, and policies as quickly as possible. The four stages to a PDSA cycle are:

Plan: Plan the change to be tested or implemented.

Do: Carry out the test or implement change.

Study: Study data before and after the change and reflect on what was learned.

Act: Plan the next change cycle or plan implementation.

A PDSA cycle involves testing the improvement ideas on a small scale before introducing the change on a large scale. By building on the learning from the test cycles in a structured and incremental way, a new idea can be implemented with a greater chance of success. Barriers to change are often reduced when different people are involved in trying something out on a small scale before implementation on a larger scale. The model is not meant to replace change models that organizations may already be using, but rather to accelerate improvement. This model can improve many different healthcare processes and outcomes, such as those related to health behavior and quality. Within the PDSA framework, nurse managers and NPs must ensure a collaborative approach with other disciplines to meet the current challenges throughout the healthcare system (Younger, 2020).

An example follows in the next case study.

Quality Initiatives

At our institution, we use the Plan-Do-Study-Act (PDSA) method for quality improvement efforts. Our HIV clinic manager had identified opportunities for improvement in a few key areas of routine patient health maintenance. The healthcare providers and staff did not believe that the sample of charts reviewed were accurate. Once the top three quality indicators were identified that did not meet benchmark standards, a team meeting was held to discuss the current flow for patients in the clinic. Input was obtained as to where inconsistencies in care might be occurring, along with suggestions for improvement.

Three separate quality efforts were developed to improve (1) the number of patients getting annual tuberculosis testing, (2) the number of females having gynecological examinations and PAP testing, and (3) the number of patients getting vaccinated for hepatitis B, if nonimmune. Each of these three indicators had a number of interventions that were agreed upon by the multidisciplinary team in an attempt to achieve 100% adherence.

Interestingly, there were multiple things that contributed to the top three problems. For instance, at the time of the chart reviews, there was no area to document if the patient had had a positive tuberculosis screen, thereby nullifying the need for further skin testing. This issue was easily remedied by amending the electronic medical record (EMR) and adding a field for this documentation. Regarding the gynecological exams and PAP testing, we found that many of our patients did not visit our gynecology clinic and instead had their own provider outside of our institution, so we made note and started to get release forms to be able to share information with the outside provider. In addition, as the NP, I had experience in basic gynecology and offered to do the PAPs and STD testing for anyone who needed it during their routine HIV care visit. As for the hepatitis B vaccinations, we instituted an alert in the patient's EMR that required the healthcare provider and follow-up RN to note that the patient needed a vaccination as well as an area to document if the patient had declined the vaccination for whatever reason.

This team approach worked well, not only for quality improvement but the unique contributions that make efforts really work well when there is interprofessional collaboration.

Safety

A basic concept such as safety initially may not appear to require much elaboration; however, when you consider the lack of standardization and monitoring in many practice settings, the need to continually work on safety issues is quite apparent. In 2002, The Joint Commission established its National Patient Safety Goals (NPSGs) program. The NPSGs were developed to assist accredited organizations to focus on specific areas of concern regarding patient safety. The Joint Commission is also responsible, with the help of the safety advisory board made up of multiple healthcare specialties, for determining the highest priority patient safety issues (The Joint Commission, 2021). According to Ransom et. al, 2019, the Joint Commission also endorses patient safety as a goal to avoid any harm or suffering as a result of any healthcare intervention. Fortunately, errors do not always reach the patient, or they may not cause harm if they reach the patient. It is important to identify issues of concern, strive for transparency in reporting errors, and design and implement safety systems to prevent further errors.

An example of this is given by Nancy, FNP:

Nancy's Story

I remember sitting in the advanced health assessment course and listening to the professor discuss the significance of taking a good history from a patient. I distinctly remember her saying that a good history will give you most of the information you need. I have followed this advice in my practice, and it has proven to be invaluable, particularly in a situation where I treated a gentleman for diabetes.

The patient is a 68-year-old African-American male with an extensive history including type 2 diabetes mellitus (T2DM), hypertension, coronary artery disease, hyperlipidemia, and stage 2 chronic kidney disease. His T2DM is well controlled with a hemoglobin A1c of 6.7 on a regimen of sitgliptin (Januvia), Metformin, and

(continues)

bedtime detemir (Levemir). Generally, he checks his blood glucose 1–2 times a day, and results range between 90 mg/dL and 150 mg/dL. He is on many other medications for his other co-morbidities and is under the care of a cardiologist.

During a visit in March, the patient stated to me that he felt fine. In fact, that morning he had a visit with his cardiologist who also told the patient that he was doing well. The patient had not had any recent bloodwork drawn, but he did have a log book of blood sugars that seemed to be fairly well controlled, albeit slightly higher than his previous averages. His blood pressure in the office was noted to be significantly lower than his norm. It was only after a period of time during our office visit (something that thankfully as a nurse practitioner I am allowed to have with my patients) that the patient mentioned that twice earlier in the week his legs had "given out" while he was walking. He insisted that he did not fall but rather "went down to his knees" and afterward was able to pull himself up. He also denied any change in level of consciousness, speech, paresthesias, pain, or injury of any kind. His physical exam was unremarkable other than a lower than usual BP.

Still, it was not something that I was willing to let go of that easily. Despite the patient's insistence that he was fine and was not concerned, it bothered me. I told him that having his legs "give out" was not okay and that we had to get to the bottom of it. He had not checked his blood sugars at the time the events occurred, but he denied having any symptoms of hypoglycemia. We began to review all of his medications (an extensive list, definitely a case of polypharmacy), and he mentioned that he didn't feel that his blood sugars were as good since he had started taking the "white Januvia" which his wife (a certified nursing assistant) had reassured him was probably the generic form that had been substituted. As the prescriber, I was aware that there is no generic form of Januvia and that all Januvia would be described as pink, red, or brown. Thus, I asked the patient to return home and bring back the bottle of pills (he had a 3-month supply of these and had been taking them for the past 45 days). The patient returned with his bottle, and there was a pharmacy label clearly printed and marked as Januvia 100 mg that had been applied over each bottle of Losartan 100 mg. (He actually had three bottles all labeled the same way.) The patient was receiving an additional antihypertensive medication and he was already on a beta blocker, a thiazide diuretic, a calcium channel blocker, and an ACE inhibitor. I sent him for labs that afternoon and told him to stop his Metformin and hold on any (real) Januvia until I called him the next day. The next day the laboratory results confirmed an acute deterioration in his kidney function (with a GFR of 28 ml/min and creatinine of 2.7 mg/dL, most likely caused by hypoperfusion related to his hypotension).

I explained to the patient that this was most likely the reason for his leg weakness. He was instructed to keep himself well hydrated with water over the next few days and to refrain from taking the Metformin, Januvia, and any over-the-counter non-steroidal anti-inflammatory such as ibuprofen until his kidney function tests returned to baseline. One week later, I rechecked his kidney function and it had returned to baseline. His medications were resumed; his blood sugars and blood pressure returned to baseline levels.

Later, when I discussed the case with the endocrinologist that I work for, she insisted that she would never have discovered the underlying reason for this man's leg weakness. I insisted that she would have, but she was emphatic about it. "No," she said, "I would never have been that thorough with his history."

I feel that it was because I had the time to spend with this patient that he had a successful outcome. I also felt that my professor's words of wisdom regarding a thorough history served as my "inner voice" that warranted delving further into this man's issue. I saw the patient a few weeks ago and he is doing great.

Informatics

An area of focus for quality and safety education for nurses is informatics. Electronic medical records or electronic health records (EHRs) are the standard in many hospitals and practice sites; however, not all sites can afford to implement EMR/EHRs due to the costs associated with the initial purchase, implementation, and ongoing support and maintenance. Measures to quantify costs versus benefits can indicate a significant cost savings and error prevention related to implementation of EMRs. In fact, the Centers for Medicare and Medicaid Services (CMS) has an active program incentivizing providers to use EMR and electronic prescribing.

Another important area that relates to informatics is the vast amount of communication and education available to patients and healthcare providers who use technology. There are many evidence-based clinical decision support resources to aid healthcare practitioners in making the best decisions at the point of care. Certainly all of these avenues bring potential benefits to health care. It is important to always remember that strict measures need to be undertaken to safeguard patient privacy at all times.

Today, many health centers are connected to outpatient clinics and private provider practices. The benefit of access to EMRs is to be able to provide the best coordinated care to patients, without having to wait to obtain medical records and results from another department or site. The challenge is to ensure all safety measures are in place to prevent any lapse in patient privacy.

TeamSTEPPS

There are many tools for organizations to use to measure outcomes and develop methods to improve safety and quality. A comprehensive program has been developed and updated by the AHRQ (About TeamSTEPPS, 2019). This system for healthcare professionals is focused on developing a culture of safety. TeamSTEPPS is an evidence-based teamwork system to improve communication and teamwork skills among healthcare professionals. It is a source for ready-to-use materials and a training curriculum to successfully integrate teamwork principles into all areas of your healthcare system. Scientifically rooted in more than 20 years of research and lessons from the application of teamwork principles, TeamSTEPPS was developed by the Department of Defenses' Patient Safety Program in collaboration with the AHRQ.

This approach uses assessment and training tools to develop teams that work to improve patient outcomes. Clear roles and responsibilities are emphasized, as well as methods to improve communication, thereby reducing conflicts. Barriers to achieving and maintaining a culture of safety and quality are addressed. There are six regional training centers that provide intensive training to master trainers who can offer training to healthcare centers on TeamSTEPPS. Information can be found on the AHRQ TeamSTEPPS website.

Prescriptive Authority

Registered nurses (RNs), as patient advocates, are in a unique position to consider which medication may be best for the patient and confer with the prescribing provider. Advanced Practice Registered Nurses (APRNs), however, have a greater role in pharmacotherapeutics than the RN. Advanced practice registered nurses receive additional training in the area of pharmacotherapeutic in their educational curriculum and require additional knowledge regarding prescriptive authority. Furthermore, extensive knowledge is essential regarding pathophysiology of diseases and medical diagnosis to allow for rational drug selection. Knowing if a medication can be legally prescribed in the state of practice, if the APRN can prescribe it and how to write prescriptions are central to all prescribing APRNs.

Prescriptive authority for APRNs varies depending upon the state of practice. It is imperative that APRNs be aware of their scope of practice in the state which they practice. Additionally, APRNs need to recognize that health organizations may have their own regulations regarding prescriptive authority. There are numerous states that have independent practice, including full prescriptive authority and states that require some form of collaboration with or supervision by a physician (National Council of State Boards of Nursing [NCSBN], 2020). This list is updated yearly in the January issue of the *Nurse Practitioner* journal and the *Journal for Nurse Practitioners'* legislative update.

The graduate APRN needs to apply for registration with the Drug Enforcement Agency (DEA) in order to prescribe any controlled substances. Additionally, certain states require the APRN to obtain a controlled substances registration. Because there is no national legislation regarding prescriptive authority, safety issues can arise. Prescription Drug Monitoring Programs (PDMPs) which are electronic monitoring systems for tracking prescriptions of controlled substances have been around for a while with its first inception in New York State in 1918 (Centers for Disease Control and Prevention [CDC], 2020; Bulloch, 2018). Currently, 49 states, the District of Columbia, and Guam have implemented PDMPs, with Missouri being the only state without such a program (Bulloch, 2018). Utilizing the PDMPs, now mandatory in most states, allows the prescriber and pharmacist to review all prescriptions for controlled substances that have been filled for each patient, the date the prescription was filled, the prescriber who ordered the medication, the medication strength, the number of prescribed pills and the location filled. In reviewing the PDMP, APRNs can assess for potential narcotic misuse red flags, such as controlled substances issued by various providers, prescriptions filled from different pharmacies, as well as the frequency of obtaining such medications. For the new APRN or for the APRN who travels from state to state, keeping abreast of prescriptive practice guidelines and legislative issues is of paramount importance. It has been shown that since the implementation of the PDMP verification mandate prior to prescribing opiates, there has been a significant reduction in the prescribing of opiates (Danovich et al., 2019).

The APRN needs to be aware of state Medicaid formularies and tiered medications and be cognizant that patients may attempt to fill prescriptions out of state because issues may arise if the state does not acknowledge prescriptions written by APRNs. Another consideration is the dispensing of samples left by pharmaceutical representatives, which may not be allowed in a specific institution nor by the state licensing board. Again, APRNs must know the rules and regulations in their state and institution.

All prescribers need to be aware of the guidelines issued by the U.S. Food and Drug Administration (FDA) that describe acceptable relationships between pharmaceutical companies' representatives with prescribers, including the types of gifts that can be given to prescribers that are not patient care–related items, and what types of interaction can occur when healthcare prescribers have continuing education events. There are codes and guidelines developed by the Pharmaceutical Research and Manufacturers of America (PhRMA) that address pharmaceutical companies' interactions with patient groups, healthcare centers, professionals, and direct-to-consumer advertising (PhRMA, n.d.). However, not all companies must comply with these guidelines because participation is voluntary. Additionally, healthcare institutions will also have their own rules, which the APRN needs to abide by.

The prescribing APRN has responsibilities when writing prescriptions. These include:

- Generic versus brand-name drugs: Know generic names of all the medications prescribed.
- Treatment guidelines and new medications: Attend continuing education programs on medication updates and subscribe to professional newsletters that provide updates on medications (The Prescriber's Letter, etc.).
- Formularies: Maintain a list of the most common formularies, as well as a list of low-cost pharmacies' generic medications.
- Failed therapies: Closely monitor all patient medications, including past medications, and when and why any have been discontinued.
- Disease control: How stable is the patient on the currently prescribed regimen? Is the patient being adherent? Are medication side effects being monitored? Are the patient's health outcomes achieved? For example, regarding blood pressure, hemoglobinA1c, etc.
- Food and Drug Administration position: It is the prescribing APRN's responsibility to stay abreast of the FDA's warnings, recalls, and pertinent information on medications you may prescribe.

Other issues that the prescribing APRN needs to consider include the following:

- State Medicaid formularies
- Formulary tiered/preferred medications
- Out-of-state prescriptions
- Emergency controlled substance (Schedule II) dispensing
- Sample dispensing
- Drug substitutions

Electronic Prescribing (E-prescribing)—Prescription Writing

Electronic prescribing (E-prescribing) is a component of the electronic health record (EHR). E-prescribing has been shown to decrease medication errors, such as inaccurate dosing, wrong medication being dispensed because of illegible writing, and incomplete prescriptions (Franklin & Puaar, 2020; Hodgkinson et al., 2017). E-prescribing programs can alert the prescriber of drug–drug interactions, avoiding potential adverse events. Additionally, patient allergies can be cross-checked with the newly prescribed medication, and the prescriber can be alerted as needed.

As stated earlier, writing a prescription is a process that not only requires considerable knowledge of pharmacology but also includes the need to have extensive knowledge about the pathophysiology of disease and comorbid conditions. Not only does the prescriber need to write an appropriate prescription, but laboratory and diagnostic testing pertaining to illness and pharmacology need to be accurately monitored and interpreted. Additionally, knowledge about the patient's age, gender, lifestyle, allergies, medical history, and current medications, including adherence and management of side effects need to be considered.

Patient Safety and Medication Errors

Common errors can involve patient-related mistakes; pharmacy-related errors; look-alike drugs; and errors in dosage, strength, concentration, and misleading abbreviations, to name a few. Although there has been a decrease in dosage, strength, concentration, and abbreviation errors with the advent of E-prescribing, patient-related mistakes and pharmacy-related error can still occur. Pharmacy-related errors can occur when the wrong medication is dispensed. Patient-related mistakes can occur as a result of misunderstanding dosing directions as well as adherence. Medication adherence is another essential component of prescription writing that the prescribing APRN needs to monitor. The definition of patient adherence to a medication treatment plan is the extent to which the patient continues the agreed-upon treatment plan under limited supervision when faced with conflicting demands, as distinguished from compliance or maintenance. Medication adherence can be intentional and non-intentional. Inadequate adherence to medication regimens can result in the inaccurate assessment of the drug's utility, toxicity when given or taken incorrectly, disease exacerbations and progression, and increased acute care admissions. It is critical for the prescribing APRN to review the patient's medication list at every encounter. By taking a patient-centered approach, which consists of involving the patient in the development of the treatment plan, medication adherence can be increased. The APRN is the expert in patient education, as well as goal-setting and using a patient-centered approach to ensure adherence with pharmaceutical regimens. Methods to assess for adherence to the prescribed plan can include:

1. Medication refill dates
2. Patient self-report
3. Patient diaries
4. Pill counts
5. Patient contracts
6. Measurement of drug titers found in body fluids
7. Electronic medication monitors

The Agency for Healthcare and Quality (AHRQ) encourages patients to ask their healthcare provider(s) questions if there are any concerns or doubts about the treatment plan, inquire about side effects, keep a medication list, bring a list of all medications currently being taken to all healthcare provider visits, and notify providers about medication allergies (AHRQ, n.d.).

In addition, prescribers should be aware of the official "Do Not Use" list developed by The Joint Commission regarding abbreviations that should not be used, to avoid medication errors (The Joint Commission, 2017). See **Table 8-3**.

Writing a Prescription: What to Include?

The following items need to be included on a prescription (see **Figure 8-1**). Not all states will require all components (some may not require a DEA number on non-scheduled medication prescriptions):

- Patient's full name, address, date of birth
- Prescriber's full name and address
- Drug Enforcement Agency number (DEA)
- National Provider Identification number (NPI)

Table 8-3 Official "Do Not Use" List[1]

Do Not Use	Potential Problem	Use Instead
U, u (unit)	Mistaken for "0" (zero), the number "4" (four), or "cc"	Write "unit"
IU (International Unit)	Mistaken for "IV" (intravenous) or the number "10" (ten)	Write "International Unit"
Q.D., QD, q.d., qd (daily) Q.O.D., QOD, q.o.d., qod (every other day)	Mistaken for each other Period after the "Q" mistaken for "I" and the "O" mistaken for "I"	Write "daily" Write "every other day"
Trailing zero (X.0 mg)* Lack of leading zero (.X mg)	Decimal point is missed	Write "X mg" Write "0.X mg"
MS MSO$_4$ and MgSO$_4$	Can mean morphine sulfate or magnesium sulfate Confused for one another	Write "morphine sulfate" Write "magnesium sulfate"

[1]Applies to all orders and all medication-related documentation that is handwritten (including free-text computer entry) or on preprinted forms.
*Exception: A "trailing zero" may be used only where required to demonstrate the level of precision of the value being reported, such as for laboratory results, imaging studies that report the size of lesions, or catheter/tube sizes. It may not be used in medication orders or other medication-related documentation.
© The Joint Commission, 2017. Reprinted with permission.

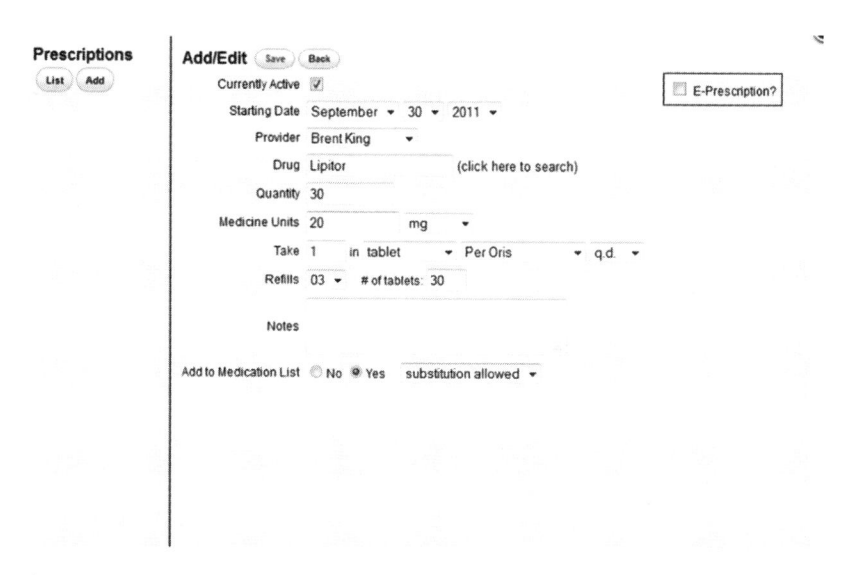

Figure 8-1 An e-prescription sample.

- Nurse practitioner license number
- Drug name
- Drug strength and dosage form
- Directions for use
- Quantity to be dispensed (written out long-hand if for narcotic)
- Refill instructions
- Substitution rights
- Signed and dated

Chapter Summary

In summary, the APRN needs to be equipped with the knowledge and skills necessary to lead the way in supporting a culture of safety and quality regardless of the practice setting. Understanding the tools and processes needed for quality and safety improvement to adequately utilize them to improve patient care and optimize outcomes is a vital component for the practice-based APRN.

Seminar Discussion Questions

1. The mission of AHRQ is to improve the quality, safety, efficiency, and effectiveness of health care for Americans. Review the AHRQ website and examine current initiatives, research findings and reports, and funding for grants.
2. Various quality improvement methodologies are used in clinical practice. Compare and contrast these methodologies.
3. Care coordination occurs throughout the span of the care continuum. Explore the concept of care coordination in your setting and beyond. Consider how you may enhance your NP role in care coordination.
4. Conduct a quality improvement project utilizing the PDSA methodology.
5. There are many patient safety organizations in existence. Explore these organizations and discuss their relevance for improving patient safety.
6. Consider how you can be a champion for patient safety in your organization.
7. Review the laws and regulations regarding nurse practitioners writing schedule II and III medications in your state.

References

About TeamSTEPPS. (2019). Agency for Healthcare Research and Quality, Rockville, MD. Retrieved from https://www.ahrq.gov/teamstepps/about-teamstepps/index.html

Agency for Healthcare Research and Quality. (n.d.). *Patient safety network*. Retrieved from http://psnet.ahrq.gov

Agency for Healthcare Research and Quality. (2019). *National healthcare quality and disparities reports and 5th anniversary update on the national quality strategy*. Retrieved from https://www.ahrq.gov/research/findings/nhqrdr/nhqdr19/index.html

American Association of Colleges of Nursing. (2006). *The essentials of doctoral education for advanced nursing practice*. Retrieved from https://www.aacnnursing.org/DNP/DNP-Essentials

References

Bulloch, M. (2018). The evolution of the PDMP. *Pharmacy Times*. Retrieved on January 14, 2021 from https://www.pharmacytimes.com/contributor/marilyn-bulloch-pharmd-bcps/2018/07/the-evolution-of-the-pdmp

Centers for Disease Control and Prevention. (2020). *Prescription drug monitoring systems*. Retrieved from https://www.cdc.gov/drugoverdose/pdmp/index.html

Chassin, M. R., & Galvin, R. W. (1998). The urgent need to improve health care quality. *Journal of the American Medical Association, 280*(11), 1000–1005.

Craig, C., Eby, D., & Whittington, J. (2011). *Care coordination model: Better care at lower cost for people with multiple health and social needs*. IHI Innovation Series white paper. Institute for Healthcare Improvement.

Danovich, D., Greenstein, J., Chacko, J., Hahn, B., Ardolic, B., Ilyaguyev, B., & Berwald, N. (2019). Effect of New York State electronic prescribing mandate on opioid prescribing patterns. *Journal of Emergency Medicine, 57*(2), 156–161. https://doi.org/10.1016/j.jemermed.2019.03.052

Deming, W. E. (1986). *Out of the crisis*. Cambridge, MA: MIT.

Franklin, B. D., & Puaar, S. (2020). What is the impact of introducing inpatient electronic prescribing on prescribing errors? A naturalistic stepped wedge study in an English teaching hospital. *Health Informatics Journal, 26*(4), 3152–3162. https://doi.org/10.1177/1460458219833112

Green D. K. (1991). Quality improvement versus quality assurance?. *Topics in Health Record Management, 11*(3), 58–70.

Hodgkinson, M. R., Larmour, I., Lin, S., Stormont, A. J., & Paul, E. (2017). The impact of an integrated electronic medication prescribing and dispensing system on prescribing and dispensing errors: A before and after study. *Journal of Pharmacy Practice & Research, 47*(2), 110–120. https://doi.org/10.1002/jppr.1243

Institute of Medicine. (2000). *To err is human: Building a safer health system*. National Academy Press.

Institute of Medicine. (2001). *Crossing the quality chasm: A new health system for the 21st century*. National Academy Press.

Joint Commission. (2020). *Facts about the official "do not use" list of abbreviations*. Retrieved from https://www.jointcommission.org/facts_about_do_not_use_list/

Joint Commission. (2021). *Facts about the national patient safety goals*. Retrieved from https://www.jointcommission.org/facts_about_the_national_patient_safety_goals/

Kurtz, S. M., Silverman, J. D., Benson, J., & Draper, J. (2003). Marrying content and process in clinical method teaching: Enhancing the Calgary-Cambridge Guides. *Academic Medicine, 78*(8), 802–809.

National Council of State Boards of Nursing. (2020). *APRN consensus model: Can CNPs prescribe independently*. Retrieved from https://www.ncsbn.org/5411.htm

Phillips, S. J. (2020). 32nd Annual APRN Legislative Update. *The Nurse Practitioner, 45*(1), 28–55. doi:10.1097/01.NPR.0000615560.11798.5f

PhRMA. (n.d.). Principles and guidelines. *Pharmaceutical Research and Manufacturers of America*. Retrieved from https://www.phrma.org/Codes-and-guidelines

Planetree Organization. (2020). *Planetree pioneers*. Retrieved from www.planetree.org

Quality and Safety Education for Nurses. (2021). *Graduate QSEN Competencies*. Retrieved from https://qsen.org/competencies/graduate-ksas/

Ransom, E., Joshi, M., Nash, D., & Ransom, S. (2019). *The healthcare quality book: Vision, strategy, and tools* (2nd ed.). Foundation of the American College of Healthcare Executives.

Riddle, L. (2010). *Florence Nightingale by Cynthia Audain, 1998*. Retrieved from http://www.agnesscott.edu/lriddle/women/nitegale.htm

Salmond, S., & Echevarria, M. (2017). Healthcare transformation and changing roles for nurses. *Orthopedic Nursing, 36*(1), 12–25.

Scholtes, P., Joiner, B., & Streibel, B. (2018). *The TEAM handbook* (3rd ed.). Oriel.

Sheingold, B., & Hahn, H. (2014). The history of healthcare quality: The first 100 years 1860–1960. *International Journal of Africa Nursing Sciences*. doi:10.1016/j.ijans.2014.05.002

Taylor-Sullivan, D. (2013). In S. DeNisco & A. Barker (Eds.), *Advanced practice nursing: Evolving roles for the transformation of the profession* (2nd ed.). Jones & Bartlett Learning.

Thornton, M., & Persaud, S. (2018). Preparing today's nurses: Social determinants of health and nursing education. *OJIN: The Online Journal of Issues in Nursing, 23*(3), Manuscript 5. doi:10.3912/OJIN.Vol23No03Man05

U.S. Department of Justice and Drug Enforcement Administration: Diversion Control Division. (2021). *State prescription drug monitoring systems*. Retrieved from https://www.deadiversion.usdoj.gov/

Varkey, P., Reller, M. K., & Resar, R. K. (2007). Basics of quality improvement in health care. *Mayo Clinic Proceedings, 82*(6), 735–739. Retrieved from https://sacredheart.idm.oclc.org/login?url=https://www.proquest.com/scholarly-journals/basics-quality-improvement-health-care/docview/216873932/se-2?accountid=28645

Younger, S. (2020). Leading advanced practice nursing in complex health care systems. *Nursing Administration Q, 44*(2), 127–135.

Zaccagnini, M., & Pechacek, J. M. (2021). *The doctor of nursing practice essentials: A new model for advanced nursing practice* (4th ed.). Jones & Bartlett Learning.

CHAPTER 9

Clinical Education: The Role of the Student, Faculty, and Preceptor

Susan M. DeNisco

The most exciting part of any nurse practitioner (NP) program is when the time comes to start clinical experiences. At minimum, 500 hours spent in supervised practice in the clinical setting are required for graduation and the certification examination. The American Nursing Credentialing Center (ANCC, 2021) requires 500 faculty-supervised clinical hours to take the certification exam, whereas the American Association of Colleges of Nursing (AACN, 2006) requires a total of 1,000 faculty-supervised clinical/practice hours for the nurse practitioner student graduating Doctorate of Nursing Practice (DNP). Therefore, students in a DNP program that are postmasters and are already certified as an NP still must complete 500 faculty-supervised clinical/practice hours. This chapter will first discuss traditional clinical education in a nurse practitioner program (master's NP program and post-BSN DNP program). Later, clinical education for the NP in a DNP program will be discussed.

Depending on the program track, clinical experiences could be in private medical offices, clinics, hospitals, or perhaps even national or global healthcare missions where the underserved are in great need of healthcare services. It is vital that the student, as well as the preceptor, is prepared for the experience, to avoid unnecessary frustration and possible negative outcomes. In particular, the experience needs to be focused on the goals and objectives for the clinical course, the skill level of the NP student, and the practice expectations of the preceptor. Specific goals are formulated and assessed for both the student and the preceptor throughout the clinical courses.

Each type of clinical setting has both general and site-specific planning requirements. For example, planning with the preceptor can help the student better understand how the practice functions on a daily basis, and identify the types of patients the student is able to see to meet course objectives, and in what capacity the student will see patients. Often, the first day is spent with the student observing the preceptor's interactions with patients and learning about the clinical site in general. In some practices, there may be patients who do not want to have a student do any portion of the history or physical; however, explaining that the patient's own provider (be it an NP, MD, DO, CNM, or PA) will always be aware of the patient's status and direct the assessment and treatment plan frequently allays any fears the patient may have. It is crucial the preceptor be aware of the role of the student NP and that the clinical setting should not consist of the student merely "shadowing" the provider for the entire clinical rotation. This rarely meets the expectations of the experience; preceptors (whether or not they have had a NP student in the past) need to be ready to assist the student in developing good interviewing, physical assessment, and diagnostic skills. This is especially important in the first clinical rotation, because a positive experience can give the student the confidence necessary to prevail in subsequent clinical arenas.

If the student has a clinical rotation in an outpatient clinic setting, whether it be a nurse-led clinic, community health center, federally funded health center, or an extension of a hospital-based clinic, these can be very worthwhile experiences. Although clinics tend to be very busy, and the healthcare providers often have a heavy patient load, it is a rich and rewarding opportunity for helping needy patients, in addition to honing clinical skills. Multiple languages may be spoken, so the NP student must be aware of what translation services the clinic provides. In addition, there are many culturally unique approaches to care that the NP student should be prepared for by reading and learning how to approach and provide culturally sensitive care. This topic is addressed in a separate chapter. Patients in clinic settings often have comorbid and complex healthcare issues in addition to psychosocial and financial difficulties. The clinical experience in this type of setting has multiple challenges as well as rewards.

An acute care site has a unique set of issues to be addressed prior to starting. The faculty and preceptor need to make sure the student is aware of the privileges awarded to the preceptor and to NPs in the setting through the credentialing process. The acute care setting may have additional policies about how much NP students are allowed to do with patients. Often, the student may be spending time shadowing the preceptor and performing portions of the history and physical together, then working collaboratively to develop a treatment plan. Faculty will need to determine if a greater scope of practice (e.g., skills or communicating with other disciplines involved in the patient's care) is needed if the scope is very narrow.

One method for gaining clinical experience is to be able to accompany faculty and other students on healthcare missions to provide care to a population needing assistance. Being prepared for the types of patients to be seen, the ability to dispense or prescribe medications, order diagnostic testing, and follow-up should be understood prior to embarking on this type of clinical immersion. Planning should be done to have local support wherever the group is going to ensure proper lodging, transportation, safety, and, importantly, to have identified specific needs of that population. It is vital that the host population dictate what the healthcare mission staff can and cannot do. Visiting mission groups are guests of the host community. NP students can learn much on these types of immersion experiences, and in particular, will discover how much they can offer patients by providing education about health and wellness, and disease management. The students may venture to a location where medications are not a viable option; therefore, diet and basic public health principles can be reviewed. It is important to remember that students may see and be exposed to infectious diseases rarely seen in the United States. This means the student must be sure to have had all appropriate travel vaccinations and bring emergency items such as Tylenol, bandages, and ointments on the trip.

Whatever the clinical site and patient population, clinical learning is a complex process for NP students. An option for the NP program and/or the individual student may consider is journaling. The ability to take the time for reflection can assist the student to process the patient interactions of the day, and help the student develop a deeper awareness of their own performance. Students can also consider concepts beyond the actual physical experience to write about, such as social and cultural issues that arise in most patient encounters (Wedgeworth, Carter, & Ford, 2017). It is important for the faculty to give direction on what reflective journaling could include. Some introductory "prompting" questions are offered here (Watson, 2016).

Daily Reflective Questions

Date/Location:

1. The images that remain with me from today are...
2. The best moment or part of today was...
3. The hardest or lowest point of today was...
4. Other thoughts, feelings, or learning from today:

The Role of Faculty

Nurse practitioner faculty are responsible for ensuring the NP student has adequate didactic knowledge prior to beginning clinical rotations. Nurse practitioner faculty who provide direct supervision of nurse practitioner students' clinical education should be nationally certified in the same population-focused area of practice (National Task Force on Quality Nurse Practitioner Education, 2016). Preparing students for clinical by reviewing course expectations, goals, and necessary forms, in addition to whatever the clinical site requires, needs to be accomplished prior to the start date. Leaving plenty of time for unexpected delays helps to avoid both a late start and the inability of the student to complete the necessary clinical hours for that course. Whenever possible, matching students and preceptors by the type of practice and physical location should be done. Many programs are fortunate to have clinical coordinators who are able to develop professional relationships with various practices and institutions, and they understand exactly what types of experiences will be best suited for specific student needs. The clinical coordinator is able to meet individually with students to get to know them on a more personal level, and then with the input of the responsible faculty, is apprised of the skill level of the student in order to try to match them to appropriate clinical sites.

The faculty and staff share in educating and communicating with preceptors regarding course objectives and program policies, keeping them current with expectations. Clinical advisors are either full-time faculty or adjunct faculty who are NPs responsible for overseeing the clinical experiences of up to six NP students. The clinical advisor is the link for the student and the preceptor, visiting the student on-site to determine that the student is progressing in a supportive learning environment, in addition to getting to know the preceptor. This role provides the student and preceptor with someone knowledgeable about the course objectives and someone who can troubleshoot any issues that may arise. One method for the clinical advisor to keep track of the types of experiences the student is getting, as well as how the student is evolving, is having the student submit nonidentifiable focused notes, with at least two per day being reasonable. The clinical advisor should also be given one to two comprehensive SOAP notes per semester, to be able to sit down with the student and give feedback and instruction in an environment outside of the clinical setting. This may also help the student to be more relaxed and able to bring up questions or comments pertinent to the role transition. At the end of the clinical rotation, the clinical advisor should be sure to obtain the student's evaluation of the clinical site and preceptor so the faculty and clinical coordinator are able to review students' evaluations of various clinical sites to maintain an up-to-date list of supportive environments.

Another option for evaluating the clinical skills of the NP student is by direct observation in a setting using actors as patients. This type of evaluation usually consists of a 20-minute direct observation assessment or "snapshot" of a trainee–patient interaction. This evaluation is based on the Mini-CEX or Objective Structured Clinical Examination (OSCE), which have been used as an evaluation of medical students or medical residents who perform the same types of patient experiences (American Board of Internal Medicine, 2021) and have become standard in most NP programs. Patient interviewing, focused physical examination, informed decision making or counseling, and clinical judgment and reasoning are evaluated by the faculty with input from the trained actors. Faculty provide timely and specific feedback to the trainee after each assessment of a trainee–patient encounter.

Another method gaining popularity among NP programs is the use of simulation. In the acute care tracks, simulation scenarios for cardiac arrest, complex procedures, and managing urgent care health problems is a safe method for allowing the student to perform these activities with no risk to an actual patient (Pittman, 2012). In addition, primary care NP tracks can use simulation or hybrid clinical scenarios for the students to evaluate abnormal heart and/or lung sounds to simulate congestive heart failure or asthma, for example. Being able to adequately assess students and provide feedback to help them learn how to improve skills in a productive manner will improve the students' abilities in real-life clinical situations.

There are over 500 accredited simulation centers in the United States (Society for Simulation in Health Care, 2021). So, in addition to students having the availability of mannequins and anatomical models, full simulation centers often include complete surgical suites, patient examination rooms fully equipped to mimic real examination rooms, and delivery rooms, in which scenarios can be played out. These simulation centers are often places where multiple disciplines can share space and work together.

The clinical instructor should also supervise students via site visits. This increases communication between the faculty and student, as well as the faculty and preceptor. Student and faculty should have open lines of communication that facilitate the student–faculty relationship. Students should be encouraged to discuss concerns, desires, and any issues that may have arisen during the clinical rotation. When visiting the clinical site, the advisor should use the opportunity to observe the student seeing a patient (with appropriate permissions). This is an excellent method for the clinical advisor, who is well aware of the level of competency the individual student should be functioning at, to assess the interaction and discuss the evaluation with the student as well as the preceptor. These site visits are also a time when not only the student performing skills can be observed, but when a face-to-face discussion related to the student's progress can be done. Brooks and Niederhauser (2010) found that preceptors expect at least two visits per semester. They further recommended that faculty be present for at least two to three patient visits and that a site visit should occur in the first four weeks of the clinical rotation.

The faculty should have a clear set of objectives for their site visits. Brooks and Niederhauser (2010) found that verifying that both the environment and the patients are suitable for the students to meet their learning objectives were of high priority during a site visit. In addition, answering the preceptor's questions and giving the preceptors support was imperative.

The Role of the Student

The NP student has tremendous responsibilities regarding the clinical experience. A few of the reminders may seem obvious; however, any experienced preceptor will verify that not all students adhere to these basic rules. These include being on time, being prepared, wearing appropriate dress, bringing reference materials, and coming to the clinical site with self-awareness of knowledge and skill level. The student needs to be in touch with the preceptor prior to starting the rotation to find out what time the preceptor expects the student to arrive and what time the day typically ends. Various practice sites have different policies regarding dress—some require professional attire with or without lab coats, some prefer scrubs, and so forth. Professional attire and manner is not always obvious to all students; therefore, what constitutes appropriate attire should be reviewed. Students should understand that appearing professional assists in gaining the trust of patients, as well as promoting professional communication among staff and colleagues.

Students should be aware of course goals, in order to discuss these with the preceptor, and should understand that each preceptor has a different style of teaching, as well as approach to patients. A good preceptor can teach the student through formal and informal methods. Being an engaged learner means that the student will seek out experiences that will help expand knowledge and relationship-building skills in whatever opportunities arise. It may be beneficial to expect that the first day will be spent following the preceptor as patients are being seen, to get a better feel for how the preceptor and practice setting work. As the student asks appropriate questions at the appropriate time, the preceptor will gain trust in the abilities of the student and begin to allow the student to perform the history, and then the physical examination, with less and less oversight. Setting mutual goals from the beginning of the experience helps to decrease misunderstandings and avoids frustration for both the student and preceptor. Having a realistic patient load is imperative. The student must remember that the goal is not to help see as many patients as possible—it is to engage in learning how to provide safe, high-quality care with the supervision and collaboration of a competent healthcare provider. Also, one of the best ways for the student to gain clinical experience and confidence is to care for patients with diverse diagnoses with increasing acuity as time goes on.

The role transition that occurs from RN to NP is often an uncomfortable one, in particular for the expert nurse who now becomes a novice as a student NP.

Numerous issues must be discussed to ease this transition. Issues include understanding the role of the NP, the expanded level of autonomy, leadership, clinical skills, and decision making (Spoelstra & Robbins, 2010). It is challenging for the student NP to fully comprehend the role of the NP, because it remains an abstract concept that is slowly coming into focus during the transition. Although numerous studies have been published on the transition from student to RN, not as many studies have investigated the transition from RN to NP. Some of these studies are discussed in the following paragraphs. They should be reviewed and discussed by student NPs in clinical seminar settings to increase awareness of the transition process and to encourage cohesion among the group.

Identity crisis and role confusion were identified in nurse practitioner students well over 30 years ago (Brown & Olshansky, 1997; Cusson & Strange, 2008; Roberts, Tabloski, & Bova, 1997). A period of resocialization was observed by Anderson, Leonard, and Yates in 1974, and was validated by NP faculty at the University of Minnesota in the late 1990s. While focusing on learning the skills of physical assessment and medical diagnosing, the NP students appeared to lose their expert nursing skills in the areas of psychosocial and developmental assessment. This return to a novice status was disconcerting and took months of guidance by the faculty to assist them in progressing through the stages of anxiety and anger to begin feeling competent and have a better understanding of the new role of nurse practitioner. Nurse practitioners' transition from novice to expert is the same as the novice RN's transition to expert as described by Benner (1984).

Imposter Syndrome

The phrase "imposter syndrome"' was coined in 1978 by two clinical psychologists to describe the sometimes draining emotions that can arise when, despite external evidence of success, you believe you are a phony and not worthy of the success you have achieved (Dalla-Camina, 2018). Individuals who experience this phenomenon have a deep feeling that they are fooling everyone. The nurse practitioner student may never feel as smart or accomplished as their peers. Even if they have done well on an exam or presentation, the "imposter" will pass it off as "luck."

Often individuals who are high achievers suffer from this syndrome. When you sit in class with other nurses who have years of clinical experience, it is hard not to compare yourself to them. Despite being a competent nurse and graduate student, you practice critical self-thought and doubt and waste enormous amounts of emotional energy trying to cover up your insecurities.

It is important to understand that up to 70% of people may experience varying degrees of this phenomenon sometime in their lives. It is essential to remember that we all have strengths and weaknesses. Practicing self-reflection and self-acceptance can help to alleviate these negative emotions. Discussing your feelings with other colleagues, especially those who are more experienced, may provide you with support and mentorship. Continue to develop your knowledge base through education and research, and seek expert assistance on topics that you are less familiar with.

Overcoming Imposter Syndrome In My OB/GYN Rotation

A few weeks ago I finished my OB/GYN rotation at a correctional institution—a women's prison in Connecticut. The good women of this correctional institution should have their sentences reduced for allowing me the privilege of performing my first gynecological assessments, Pap smears, and OB assessments on them. OB/GYN is not my strong suit, and I was definitely operating out of my comfort zone there. When I started, the thought of ever doing this independently was not on my radar.

On my final day, we had a quiet moment amid our cases. My preceptor went to the copy machine and left me in the clinic room. One of our patients arrived and was sitting in the hallway waiting. The least I could do was get her height, weight, and vital signs. My preceptor did not return. So, I continued to get a history: She was a 27-year-old woman, there for an annual gyn exam, and she was very nice, very eager to work with a newbie like myself. I got a really long history, because my preceptor still did not return. So, she put her gown on, and I continued to make conversation with her, noting that she had a package of contraband Jolly Ranchers in her bra—I did not confiscate it. My preceptor returned long before she had to "scoot to the end of the table" thank goodness, but I really felt, at that point, that I could have done her exam by myself. It was a pretty good feeling that I can function in that setting—and it isn't even in my comfort area. Things just started to click. —*Julie G. Stewart (deceased)*

In a grounded theory study that looked at the role transition from expert critical care nurse to advanced nurse practitioner in the critical care setting, researchers uncovered themes and categories that explained the linked processes that occur during this time frame (Fleming & Carberry, 2011). The first set of themes included the students' doubting their ability to become advanced practice nurses (APNs) after being expert critical care RNs, and issues revolving around role uncertainty and feelings of isolation and needing to fit in with other members of the healthcare team in the critical care unit (CCU). The first group of student APNs had to deal with conflict regarding boundaries between their role and the junior doctors' (residents') roles in the CCU. Peer support was identified as helpful for reducing conflict issues in a productive manner.

As the APN students started to correlate the medical knowledge to patient care, their confidence improved. As their confidence rose, so did their understanding of the new role. As this new role was internalized, the student APNs began to provide a more holistic approach to patient care, using their solid nursing base to formulate a unique role as critical care APNs. The researchers identify this uniqueness, describing it as embracing both medical and nursing knowledge, which provides patients with many benefits. Researchers caution that the processes and categories/themes are not isolated points in the role transition, but that they are more complex and are interrelated. These situational, developmental, and conceptual processes are the terms used by the researchers to describe these interrelated concepts.

An ethnographical study of student NPs analyzed data from two sets of interviews: one at the beginning of the educational program, and one at the conclusion of the training or education (Barton, 2007). All of the student NP participants were experienced RNs prior to attending the program. In the first phase of the training, the participants were worried about identity loss: having been expert nurses who were now novice NP students that had to disengage from their previous professional role to develop into the new role of NP. This was uncomfortable for the student NPs and was the source of much anxiety. As they moved into the transition phase, the participants remarked on the difficulty and ambiguity felt when not in the role of a nurse, nor in the role of a physician, but feeling inept in the newer role of nurse practitioner. The role boundaries that were well-defined were now crossing with medical professionals in the workplace, and this increased stress levels. The students identified needing to increase group cohesion at this stressful portion of their educational program and role transition. As they progressed through their program, there was an increase in clinical skills and knowledge—called the incorporation phase. At this time, the student NPs began to look for role models from medical and nursing colleagues and to begin to merge into their new professional role identity. This also had a positive impact on the student NPs' relationships with medical staff. These social, cultural, and professional transitions were believed to closely model the rites of passage as identified by Van Gannep (1960).

Spoelstra and Robbins (2010) ran a qualitative study that sought to describe the role transition from RN to APN as it related to a role development course. This online course was based on Hamric's Model of Advanced Practice Nursing competencies (Hamric, Spross, & Hanson, 2009). These competencies are direct clinical practice, expert coaching and guidance, consultation, research, clinical/professional/ systems leadership, collaboration, and ethical decision making. The overarching theme uncovered in this study was the "essence of nursing." The students integrated this theme throughout the core competencies as the basis of the APN role. The authors suggest methods to facilitate and strengthen the role transition process. Students are influenced by their preceptors, and a good preceptor and a good mentor can assist the student to enhance critical thinking skills and improve self-efficacy. Using reflective journaling is a useful tool for helping facilitate role integration.

Students must use some form of tracking method to record numbers and types of patients seen in the clinical experience, in addition to charting in the paper or electronic medical record. Keeping track of hours and procedures performed is a requirement for graduation and certification. Many NP programs have adopted clinical tracking systems for this purpose. Giving an honest evaluation of the clinical site and preceptor is also important so future students can be matched up with sites that will provide supportive learning environments.

The Role of the Preceptor

There exist many benefits of being a preceptor for an NP student. Although it may be difficult related to the need for productivity, limited physical space to accommodate students, concerns about access to electronic medical records, and cost-effectiveness related to precepting students, there are personal and professional rewards when a positive clinical experience with a student occurs (Barker & Pittman, 2010; Brooks & Niederhauser, 2010; Brykczynski, 2012; Burns, Beauchesne, Ryan-Krause, & Sawin, 2006). Motivation for becoming a preceptor varies from person to person; however, many NPs choose to precept NP students because it provides personal satisfaction, and many recall what their own student clinical experiences were like (Barker & Pittman, 2010). Qualities of a good preceptor from the students' view include the ability to be accessible, empathetic, have a good sense of humor, be flexible and fair, have enthusiasm for the role, and be consistent (Burns et al., 2006). The preceptor also needs to have a self-awareness of clinical skills and knowledge level, knowing that a recent graduate is not in the best position to be in the preceptor role. The new graduate has transitions to go through and needs time to settle into the role of a practicing NP.

It is important for the preceptor to have access to the course syllabus and thus the course and clinical objectives prior to the first face-to-face meeting with the student. The preceptor should have a contact number for both the student and the faculty for the course. In addition to having an affiliation agreement with the facility, there should be a written agreement between the preceptor, student, and faculty. The agreement should simply state what the basic expectations are of the preceptor, student, and faculty.

Once the NP has agreed to be a preceptor, the student should contact the preceptor to go over the start date and essential topics that need to be covered prior to the first day of clinical. Topics for discussion during the preclinical meeting, whether face-to-face or by phone, include the expectations of the student and mutual goal setting based on the student's current knowledge level and course objectives. The student also needs to know what the appropriate dress code is, what paperwork needs to be completed, any specific requirements about employee health, how to obtain a name badge, electronic health recording access, and the typical work schedule the student will be following.

When possible, the student and preceptor should meet 30 minutes before patients begin arriving on the first day of clinical so there is time for orienting the student to the facility (schedule, role of assistive personnel, etc.). Letting the student know the style of precepting that can be expected is beneficial for the student and helps to reduce anxiety from the unknown. Previous authors have suggested that preceptors encourage strategies that improve critical thinking skills of the student NP (Burns et al., 2006; Thompson, Kershbaumer, & Krisman-Scott, 2001). Thompson and colleagues (2001) describe the need for a comprehensive history as being a "detective," and that the student NP use reflection when considering the findings from the history and physical to develop an effective plan of care. Various approaches to teaching students have been described when working with adult learners such as graduate students. A successful approach is one where the student is given patients that are most appropriate for the individual student's previous experience and current skill level. As the student progresses, the patient load and the complexity of the patients increase. Each student may progress at varying rates, and the astute preceptor knows when to push the student to challenge his or her comfort level. Assisting the student NP with time management is necessary, particularly as the student nears graduation. Having a patient assignment reflective of what will be expected postgraduation is imperative during the final semester, with close oversight to ensure the student does not forego safe and comprehensive patient care to avoid getting behind. These are often great opportunities to discuss how to manage a situation such as this when they are out in practice.

Supplementary forms of clinical education can be used to help the students in addition to hours spent on-site. Some preceptors find it beneficial to assign students homework—researching a specific disease state or finding current treatment options for a patient seen during the clinical day. This is particularly beneficial when the student is rotating with a clinician who provides specialty care, such as pulmonary, cardiology, or infectious disease management. Having a student conduct this type of assignment can not only solidify his or her clinical judgment, but also assist the student in gaining new knowledge on a particular topic.

Two key components of precepting to be emphasized are discussing and using current evidence-based practice (EBP) guidelines for patient care, and, when the preceptor is an NP, role modeling. The NP preceptor has a valuable and unique opportunity to be a role model for the student. Discussing current scope of practice, legislative issues, collaborating and consulting with colleagues, and emphasizing the need to keep the "nurse" in "nurse practitioneering" is how the future NP can make a successful transition. Brykczynski (2012) investigated how student NPs are taught how to maintain the holistic approach to patient care that is the cornerstone of nursing practice. This qualitative study uncovered themes that reflected the role modeling that NP faculty perform when incorporating a mind–body–spirit approach to interviewing, listening, assessing, and devising plans of care for patients that address this holistic perspective. Brykczynski (2012) emphasized the importance of this approach, particularly when training students who do not come to NP programs with much nursing experience.

It is useful for the preceptor to be familiar with the evaluation tool used by the university and to go over each component with the student halfway through the clinical experience. Whether or not the preceptor is to complete a written evaluation should be established prior to the start of the clinical rotation. If the evaluation is complex, examples should be provided. This helps the student, as well as the preceptor, identify areas of strength and areas of weakness and then devise a plan to improve in those areas. One approach is to have the student also perform a self-evaluation at this point for comparison. The student may be reassured that certain areas are at the expected level for that point in time, or may need increased awareness that she or he needs to work harder in certain components. Pre- and post-student preceptor huddles can be useful in planning out goals for the day, as well as provide opportunities for the student to gain additional insight into how decision making occurs. The preceptor should discuss both what the student did well and what the student could have done differently/better, and how the student can improve. It is the preceptor's responsibility to alert the clinical advisor or faculty if there are any red flags regarding the student's performance. Keeping the lines of communication with the student and faculty open, and focusing on behaviors rather than personalities, will help to prevent potential problems from becoming serious issues leading to failure. Brooks and Niederhauser (2010) suggest a combined meeting with student, preceptor, and faculty if deficiency is observed.

Evaluation and Clinical Time Documentation

The National Task Force on Quality Nurse Practitioner Education (2016) recently published a report on criteria for the evaluation of nursing programs. Criterion III.E specifically relates to NP clinical hours. Required evidence of meeting the criterion includes "documentation of the process used to verify student learning experiences and clinical hours" (p. 26). Thus, there must be a procedure in place that documents both the student's learning experience and the clinical hours he or she has obtained. Various schools use different formats; however, any clinical evaluation form needs to document the skills the student has performed and the level of proficiency to which she or he has performed. Criteria need to relate to course objectives and expected outcomes detailed in the syllabus and at the onset of the class or clinical experience.

Furthermore, evaluations should be done by the preceptor and the faculty, and there should be a method for self-evaluation by the student. In addition, there should be an evaluation of the clinical site.

Pathways to the DNP

When planning clinical experiences, one must consider the student and individual level of experience. In addition, the student's path to the DNP must also be a factor. Currently there are several paths to the DNP; these include ADN to DNP, nonnursing baccalaureate degree to DNP, BSN to DNP, postmaster's DNP, and even postdoctorate DNP. Students may enter a program with experiences ranging from little to no nursing experience, several years of nursing experience, some years of nurse practitioner experience, to several years of nurse practitioner experience. Of course, those with less experience will have quite different clinical processes than those of experienced nurse practitioners. Not everyone will be a novice, according to Benner's (1984) novice to expert theory. Ideally, the preceptor should also be a DNP-prepared nurse practitioner. For students with less experience, early on in the clinical experience it is perfectly acceptable to pair them with MSN-prepared NPs so the students learn the overall role of a nurse practitioner. But, for later clinical experiences, and for more advanced students, preceptors should be doctorally prepared, assisting the students in learning the role of the doctorate-prepared nurse practitioner in a variety of roles.

Postmaster's NP Clinical Education in a DNP Program

It is essential that the curriculum of a DNP program extends beyond theory and contains structured clinical components. The AACN (2006) clearly requires a minimum of 1,000 hours of practice postbaccalaureate; however, how to achieve the additional hours for NPs who are already certified is not as clearly outlined. Thus, various programs have created varying models for students to achieve approximately 500 additional hours of clinical education. These clinical hours translate into roughly 11 credits with a ratio of 1 credit hour to 45 clinical hours.

An examination of several postmaster's DNP programs will reveal many similarities and differences. Some programs offer a "new specialty" option in which certified NPs obtain their clinical hours by becoming educated to be certified in a new area. Another option is to offer a specified subspecialty, where there would be a concentration of clinical hours in a specialty area such as cardiology or neurology, and the clinical education would be very specific to that specialty.

Many programs have an advance practice component. However, for the postmaster's student, these clinical experiences must go beyond the clinical educational experiences of their master's program. These clinical experiences must support integration of the DNP role into the complex circumstances of contemporary nursing practice.

An overarching theme that will emerge from examining varying programs is that many of the plans of study for postmaster's students will be highly individualized. Students' prior experience, program goals, individual goals, as well as final DNP project, must all be factors when determining how students will complete the remaining clinical hours.

The following are designated clinical tracks or courses that can be offered to assist students in obtaining the additional 500 clinical hours needed.

Teaching/Learning

Students with an expressed interest in teaching may choose to complete an established amount of clinical hours in a teaching capacity. These courses should include teaching/learning theory, and clinical hours can be achieved through student teaching as well as course and curriculum development at a collegiate level.

Clinical education should not only focus on basic teaching strategies but those of educational leadership as well. Students must be exposed to the multiple facets of nursing education including management in an academic setting, regulations and industry trends, curriculum development, and leadership skills.

Community Health and Population Focus

With the ever-increasing demand for skilled care outside of the hospital setting, there is a great need for advanced nursing practice in community health, as well as population focus care. Clinical hours can be achieved through examining advanced practice nursing roles in community health and public health.

Clinical education in this area should prepare the advanced practice nurse to evaluate major health issues in populations, use various public health approaches to reduce injury and improve health, and develop and implement key strategies to maintain and improve population health and safety at all levels.

Leadership and Management

Clinical hours with a healthcare leadership or management focus will ready the doctorate-prepared NP for executive leadership in healthcare settings. The focus of the clinical education should be centered on the following competencies: leadership, business intelligence, finance, health policy, and research. Ideally, preceptors will be DNP prepared, but MSN- or PhD-prepared nurses in executive positions, such as chief nurse officer (CNO), would be a good fit for the DNP student.

Final Project

A major clinical component to all DNP nurse practitioner programs is the development, implementation, and evaluation of a final doctoral project. Although there are multiple titles for the projects, including dissertation project and capstone project, many if not all clinical hours can be achieved in this process. There are multiple ways to complete such projects. According to the AACN (2006, p. 20):

> Unlike a dissertation, the work may take a number of forms. One example of a final DNP product is a practice change initiative. This may be represented by a pilot study, a program evaluation, a quality improvement project, an evaluation of a new practice model, a consulting project, or an integrated critical literature review. Improving patient outcomes is the ultimate goal for DNP projects and should be focused on systems and/or populations (AACN, 2015). Additional examples of a DNP final product

could include manuscripts submitted for publication, systematic review, research utilization project, practice topic dissemination, substantive involvement in a larger endeavor, or other practice project. The theme that links these forms of scholarly experiences is the use of evidence to improve either practice or patient outcomes.

Current Trends in NP Clinical Education

A growing trend in NP clinical education is to require institutions to pay preceptors for their services. Although providing one-on-one mentoring and direct patient care experiences for NP students by either nurse practitioners or physicians has been a time-honored tradition of service to the overall healthcare community, this is changing. With there being great competition for clinical sites, at times schools have few options and must place students at facilities where a few are required. "Some clinics are charging a minimum of $200 per week for a practicum experience. Which translates into $1,600–$2,000 for an eight to ten week session" (Brown, 2016, para. 4); and, at $1,000 per credit hour, depending on the course, this could be as much as $6,000 for a 15-week course. Institutions must then find ways to either absorb the cost or pass the cost on to the student, thus adding to the cost of tuition or lab fees.

Brown (2016) posed the question: Is it ethical for clinics to require payment for nursing practicums? Of course, there is no easy response. There have been requests for the Commission on Collegiate Nursing Education (CCNE), the accrediting body for many academic institutions, to regulate the guidelines for this practice (Graduate Nursing EDU, 2016).

Both the American Nurses Credentialing Center (ANCC) and the American Academy of Nurse Practitioners (AANP), through which NPs can be certified, offer precepting as a partial means to gain recertification. ANCC requires documentation of 120 hours of direct clinical supervision as one of the eligible categories, when combined with 75 hours of continuing education hours (of which 25 must be pharmacotherapeutics), the NP can gain recertification (ANCC, 2021). AANP allows 120 precepting hours to be converted to 25 nonpharmacology credits, of which 100 are required (AANP, 2017). In line with ANCC and AANP, there are states that allow precepting to be a component of renewal for state APRN licensing. North Carolina credits 30 of the required 50 contact hours for APRN license renewal for 30 hours of precepting (Nursing Center, 2017). Beginning in 2018, the state of Hawaii will allow 120 hours of precepting hours to be used as a component for renewal of APRN licensing (Department of Commerce and Consumer Affairs, 2017).

The state of Maryland has taken a unique approach to the preceptor shortage—providing an incentive, beyond that of direct pay, for nurse practitioners who serve as preceptors. In 2016, the state passed a bill that will allow a tax waiver for NP preceptors. It is called The Nurse Practitioner Preceptorship Tax Credit Fund. Preceptors are eligible for up to a $1,000 annual tax waiver subject to meeting certain requirements (Maryland Board of Nursing, 2016).

The Future of NP Clinical Education

Looking ahead, finding innovative approaches to providing effective, high-quality clinical education for NPs is challenging. Multiple issues have been identified, along with several strategies for seeking solutions (Fitzgerald, Kantrowitz-Gordon,

Katz, & Hirsch, 2012). The authors identified internal challenges such as issues related to lack of diversity in the workforce, the increased workload demands on faculty, noncompetitive salaries for NP faculty, and the challenges associated with access to education for those residing in rural areas. External challenges that were identified included the difficulty of finding adequate clinical sites and preceptors, NPs whose responsibilities include teaching medical residents instead of NP students, the numerous regulatory and specialty certification requirements, and the political and control issues associated with gender relationships (p. 2).

The Pandemic's Impact on Clinical Education

The multilayered effects of COVID-19's impact on the clinical education of nurse practitioner students has added major challenges for clinical training sites, NP faculty, and students, as well as preceptors. Nationwide, the pandemic caused disruption for colleges and universities in all aspects of teaching. As academic institutions explored alternative methods of classroom delivery, such as online instruction, NP faculty also had to reconceptualize the clinical experience of the NP student. While healthcare organizations closed themselves to students temporarily, innovative strategies have been incorporated to help students achieve clinical competencies. The use of simulated case studies, standardized patients, and interprofessional learning spaces add value to evaluating students' learning (Wynne, 2020).

As more practice sites engage in telehealth with their patients, students and preceptors must adapt to new communication technologies. Faculty must provide content that prepares students to meet a recommended set of telehealth competencies. These competencies are based on the knowledge and skills required to effectively deliver health care utilizing telehealth technologies. For example, students must become proficient in taking a history, performing a focused physical examination, and developing a diagnosis and treatment plan using a telehealth platform. Telehealth etiquette and skills in using peripherals, such as otoscope, stethoscope, and ophthalmoscope must be taught (NONPF, 2018). Chapter 13 will provide a detailed overview of telehealth competencies. It is vital to advocate for federal funding for telehealth training for the future workforce of NPs in order to increase access to health care for the entire population during this global pandemic.

Seminar Discussion Questions

1. Reflect on your past experiences in nursing, and consider how the role change to NP may challenge your knowledge and skills.
2. What strategies for using support in the clinical experiences are available?
3. Use the process of reflective journaling as you progress through the NP program. During each semester, take the time to review what you have written and consider the advances made to the current time. Reflective journaling is something to consider continuing beyond the educational program.

♀ CASE STUDY

Joe is an NP student entering his second clinical rotation. He received positive feedback and evaluation from his first preceptor who was a physician very experienced in clinical education of NPs, PAs, and medical residents. For the current clinical experience, he is at a busy federally qualified health center with a large immigrant population that are mainly Spanish-speaking. Joe does not speak Spanish but has started taking a medical Spanish course to help him communicate with these patients and to use Spanish in his future work as an NP.

It has been a very different experience thus far, although it has only been two full clinical days. The preceptor is a fairly new NP who has only been practicing for 2 years. Her schedule is always overloaded and there are multiple issues to address with the complex patients on her panel. The first day, Joe followed the preceptor and did not see any patients on his own. The second day, he was directed to see a patient but was told to be done in 10 minutes so the preceptor could come in and go over the history and physical herself before they made a plan of care. The patient was a 62-year-old male with a history of diabetes, hypertension, and depression. He did not speak much English and so Joe had to use the translation services phone line. Joe had barely gotten the translator on the phone when the preceptor entered, frustrated he had not completed the history and physical, so she took over and saw the patient with Joe shadowing once again. The next patient he was sent to see was a 21-year-old female who was at the clinic for a discussion about contraceptive options. Joe had not covered this topic yet in didactic education, so he went to his preceptor and explained this problem. The preceptor was visibly frustrated and said they would have to talk later, that this did not seem to be going well as a clinical experience for him and she was too busy to have such an "inexperienced student."

Discussion Questions
1. How could this situation have been avoided?
2. Are there steps to prepare a preceptor for what to expect with different students at different levels of experience?
3. Who should Joe reach out to?
4. Who should the preceptor reach out to? Can this clinical experience work for Joe?

References

American Academy of Nurse Practitioners. (2010). *Quality of nurse practitioner practice*. Austin, TX: Author.

American Academy of Nurse Practitioners. (2017). *Renewal requirements*. Retrieved from https://www.aanpcert.org/recert

American Association of Colleges of Nursing. (2006). *The essentials of doctoral education for advanced nursing practice*. Washington, DC: Author.

American Association of Colleges of Nursing. (2015). *The Doctoral of Nursing Practice: Current issues and clarifying recommendations*. Washington, DC: Author.

American Board of Internal Medicine. (2021). *The Mini-CEX*. Retrieved from https://www.abim.org/program-directors-administrators/assessment-tools/mini-cex.aspx

American Nursing Credentialing Center. (2021). *Family nurse practitioner certification eligibility criteria*. Retrieved from https://www.nursingworld.org/our-certifications/family-nurse-practitioner/

Anderson, E. M., Leonard, B., & Yates, J. A. (1974). Epigenesis of the nurse practitioner role. *American Journal of Nursing*, 10(18), 12–16.

Barker, E., & Pittman, O. (2010). Becoming a super preceptor: A practical guide to preceptorship in today's clinical climate. *Journal of the American Academy of Nurse Practitioners, 22,* 144–149.

Barton, T. D. (2007). Student nurse practitioners—A rite of passage? The universality of Van Gennep's model of social transition. *Nurse Education in Practice, 7,* 338–347.

Benner, P. (1984). *From novice to expert: Excellence and power in clinical nursing practice.* Menlo Park, CA: Addison-Wesley.

Brooks, M. V., & Niederhauser, V. P. (2010). Preceptor expectations and issues with nurse practitioner clinical rotations. *Journal of the American Academy of Nurse Practitioners, 22,* 573–579.

Brown, M., & Olshansky, E. F. (1997). From limbo to legitimacy: A theoretical model of the transition to the primary care nurse practitioner role. *Nursing Research, 46*(1), 46–51.

Brown, P. (2016). A new normal: Graduate nursing students paying for clinical rotations. *Minority Nurse.* Retrieved from http://minoritynurse.com/a-new-normal-graduate-nursing-students-paying-for-clinical-rotations/

Brykczynski, K. (2012). Clarifying, affirming, and preserving the nurse in nurse practitioner education and practice. *Journal of the American Academy of Nurse Practitioners, 24,* 554–564.

Buppert, C. (2011). *Nurse practitioner's business practice and legal guide* (4th ed.). Sudbury, MA: Jones and Bartlett.

Burns, C., Beauchesne, M., Ryan-Krause, P., & Sawin, K. (2006). Mastering the preceptor role: Challenges of clinical teaching. *Journal of Pediatric Health Care, 20*(3), 172–183. doi:10.1016/j.pedhc.2005.10.012

Cusson, R. M., & Strange, S. N. (2008). Neonatal nurse practitioner role transition: The process of re-attaining expert status. *Journal of Perinatal and Neonatal Nursing, 22*(4), 329–337.

Dalla-Camina, M. (2018). The reality of the imposter syndrome. *Psychology Today.* https://www.psychologytoday.com/us/blog/real-women/201809/the-reality-imposter-syndrome

Department of Commerce and Consumer Affairs. (2017). *Licensing area: Nursing.* Retrieved from http://cca.hawaii.gov/pvl/boards/nursing/

Fitzgerald, C., Kantrowitz-Gordon, I., Katz, J., & Hirsch, A. (2012). Advanced practice nursing education: Challenges and strategies. *Nursing Research and Practice.* doi:10.1155/2012/854918

Fleming, E., & Carberry, M. (2011). Steering a course towards advanced nurse practitioner: A critical care perspective. *Nursing in Critical Care, 16*(2), 67–76.

Graduate Nursing EDU (2016). *Fee-based practicums for nursing students raise ethical concerns.* Retrieved from https://www.graduatenursingedu.org/2016/07/fee-based-practicums-for-nursing-students-raise-ethical-concerns/

Hamric, A. B., Spross, J. A., & Hanson, C. M. (2009). *Advanced practice nursing: An integrative approach* (4th ed.). Philadelphia, PA: W. B. Saunders.

Institute of Medicine. (2010). *The future of nursing: Leading change, advancing health (consensus report).* Washington, DC: The National Academies Press. Retrieved from http://www.iom.edu/Reports/2010/The-Future-of-Nursing-Leading-Change-Advancing-Health.aspx

Krupa, C. (2010). Physician shortage projected to soar to more than 91,000 in a decade. *American Medical News.* Retrieved from http://www.ama-assn.org/amednews/2010/10/11/prsb1011.htm

Maryland Board of Nursing. (2016). *Advanced Practice Registered Nursing: Tax benefit for nurse practitioner preceptors.* Retrieved from http://mbon.maryland.gov/Pages/advanced-practice-tax-benefit-np-preceptors.aspx

Maylone, M. M., Ranieri, L., Quinn Griffin, M. T., McNulty, R., & Fitzpatrick, J. J. (2011). Collaboration and autonomy: Perceptions among nurses. *Journal of the American Academy of Nurse Practitioners, 23*(11), 51–57.

National Organization of Nurse Practitioner Faculties. (2018). NONPF supports telehealth competencies in nurse practitioner education. Washington, DC: Author. Retrieved from https://cdn.ymaws.com/www.nonpf.org/resource/resmgr/2018_Slate/Telehealth_Paper_2018.pdf

National Task Force on Quality Nurse Practitioner Education. (2016). *Criteria for evaluation of nurse practitioner programs.* Washington, DC: National Organization of Nurse Practitioner Faculties. Retrieved from https://cdn.ymaws.com/www.nonpf.org/resource/resmgr/Docs/EvalCriteria2016Final.pdf

Naylor, M. K. (2012). The role of nurse practitioners in reinventing primary care. *Health Affairs, 31*(11), 893–899.

Nursing Center. (2017). *Continuing education requirements for nurses by state.* Retrieved from http://www.nursingcenter.com/ceconnection/ce-state-requirements

O'Brien, J. L., Martin, D. R., Heyworth, J. A., & Meyer, N. R. (2009). A phenomenological perspective on advanced practice. *Journal of the American Academy of Nurse Practitioners, 21*(8), 444–453.

Pittman, O. (2012). The use of simulation with advanced practice nursing students. *Journal of the American Academy of Nurse Practitioners, 24,* 516–529. doi:10.1111/j.1745-7599.2012.00760.x

Roberts, S. J., Tabloski, P., & Bova, C. (1997). Epigenesis of the nurse practitioner role revisited. *Journal of Nursing Education, 36,* 67–73.

Society for Simulation in Health Care. (2021). *Sim Center Directory.* Retrieved from https://www.ssih.org/Home/SIM-Center-Directory/Area/US

Spoelstra, S. L., & Robbins, L. B. (2010). A qualitative study of role transition for RN to APN. *International Journal of Nursing Education Scholarship, 7*(1), 1–14. doi:10.2202/1548-923X.2020

Thompson, J., Kershbaumer, R., & Krisman-Scott, M. A. (2001). *Educating advanced practice nurses and midwives: From practice to teaching.* New York, NY: Springer.

Van Gannep, A. (1960). *The rites of passage.* London, England: Routledge.

Wagner, E. (2004). Effective team work and quality of care. *Medical Care, 42*(11), 1037–1039.

Watson, S. (2016). *International reflective journaling guidelines.* Unpublished paper.

Wedgeworth, M., Carter, S., & Ford, C. (2017). Clinical faculty preceptors and mental health reflections: Learning through journaling. *Journal for Nurse Practitioners, 13*(6), 411–417.

Wynne, P. (2020). Using virtual standardized patients in behavioral health interprofessional education. *Journal of Nursing Education, 59*(10), 599–600.

CHAPTER 10

Case Presentation, Consultation, and Collaboration in Primary Care

Susan M. DeNisco and Sylvie Rosenbloom

Introduction to the Case Presentation

Preparing an oral case study presentation is an essential part of the education of nurse practitioners (NPs), but because of the burden of an overly prescribed curriculum and use of nonfaculty clinical preceptors, the art of the formal "oral presentation" is often a skill requirement that is neglected. According to the National Organization of Nurse Practitioner Faculties (NONPF), there are nine core competencies that outline specific guidelines for educational programs preparing NPs to implement the full scope of practice as licensed independent practitioners (NONPF, 2017). Several of the practice domains state the following goals should be achieved during the education of the nurse practitioner:

- Critically analyzes data and evidence for improving advanced nursing practice
- Communicates practice knowledge effectively both orally and in writing
- Uses advanced health assessment skills to differentiate between normal, variations of normal, and abnormal findings

NONPF also purports that these competencies are acquired through mentored patient care experiences, with an emphasis on independent and interprofessional practice; providing evidence-based, patient-centered care across settings; and acquiring advanced knowledge of the healthcare delivery system (NONPF, 2017). Efforts to construct frameworks to help both medical and nursing students create (and teachers evaluate) oral case presentations presume that nursing and medical educators share mutual expectations for presentations (Green, 2011).

The oral case presentation skill is at the heart of interprofessional communication. It allows the nurse practitioner to succinctly convey a clear, organized analysis of a patient's health problem(s) to another provider in order to develop an effective management plan. The case presentation also serves as a method for clinical preceptors and peers to assess the level of expertise a practitioner has regarding a particular problem and to evaluate the assessment and management portion of that patient's care. Lastly, a clearly communicated case presentation enables the nurse practitioner to get a more experienced clinician's opinion about a patient in an efficient, cost-effective manner (Coralli, 2006).

The case presentation typically presented in the SOAP (subjective, objective, assessment, and plan) format is a sequential way of arranging the facts, thereby drawing the listener down a path of critical reasoning. Building the "argument" by clearly outlining the patient's history and physical examination findings helps make linkages to define the differential diagnosis and outline a treatment plan (Hinson Brown, 2006). Much of the clinical teaching involves the nurse practitioner student interviewing and examining a patient, and then presenting the information to the clinical preceptor. This approach is common in both inpatient and outpatient primary care settings. Studies involving third-year medical students indicated that, on average, these interactions take approximately 10 minutes, and the time is divided into several different activities. Much of the time is taken up by the presentation of the patient by the learner. Additional time is spent in questioning and clarifying the content of the presentation. As a result, only about 1 minute of time is actually spent in discussion and teaching (Rollins, 2012). To do this, the nurse practitioner must learn to present in the format accepted by the medical profession and include only the most relevant information—the pertinent positives and negatives.

Physicians, over the course of their training, spend a number of years not only presenting cases to other house staff and attending physicians, but also listening to such presentations from their peers and faculty. During their residencies, it is safe to say that most house staff develop skill in case presentations. This is accomplished in three ways: (1) by repeatedly being in the position of having to present cases "off the top of the head," (2) by having their case presentations critiqued frequently, and (3) by hearing excellent case presentations from others, which they then use as models for their own presentations (Coralli, 2006). In a study of 136 internal medicine clinician teachers from five U.S. medical schools, it was found that faculty share common expectations for oral case presentation (OCP) experiences, while students often report that clinical faculty fail to share common expectations for the OCP, frustrating their attempts to use the "rules" they have learned to create an OCP (Green, 2011).

With the passage of the Affordable Care Act (ACA) and the anticipated shortage of primary care physicians, nurse practitioners will be providing medical care in a variety of interdisciplinary settings, increasing the need for excellent case presentation skills to stay on par with our physician colleagues. The nurse practitioner who presents a clear, comprehensive summary of the patient's problem to a physician or other healthcare colleague may be able to expedite that patient's care to enhance positive patient outcomes.

Organizing the Oral Case Study Presentation

Prior to the presentation, it is important for the nurse practitioner student to consider the message, the purpose, and the appropriate depth of the case in relation to the audience being addressed (Paauw, Migeon, & Burkholder, 2003). The standard outline follows the format of the written history and physical exam with several important differences. Verbal case presentations are typically 5–7 minutes in length, which makes it imperative to prioritize essential data; organizing the facts into pertinent positive findings and pertinent negative findings make for an efficient delivery of information. In addition, the review of systems that directly relate to the patient problem should be included in the history of present illness (HPI). By leaving out unnecessary information, the presenter will avoid the pitfalls of too much information that may distract the listener (Hinson Brown, 2006). It is important to note that the oral case presentation should not be a verbatim recital of the history and physical condition of the patient. Novice clinicians often have a difficult time preparing a case as they learn to distinguish how much information is enough and what is too much or nonessential information. The goal of case presentation is to establish an argument for a differential diagnosis for the patient. Important data can argue in favor of the differential diagnosis or refute the diagnosis. The nurse practitioner must recognize that leaving out relevant information can misinform the diagnosis (Paauw et al., 2003).

Components of an Effective Case Presentation

Many nurse practitioner students approach case presentations as part of their student evaluation process. As previously mentioned, the main objective of the presentation is to convey the aspects of the patient's illness to the preceptor, collaborating physician, or other team members in order to participate in the patient's plan of care. The nurse practitioner student must avoid verbatim reciting of what the patient verbalized. Rather, the NP student should deliver a critical analysis of the information gathered to develop a clear and accurate plan. Brevity, organization, eye contact, and anticipation of questions are integral to an excellent presentation. On completion of the presentation, the other clinician should understand the priority issues for the patient and what your management plan is to address those issues. **Box 10-1** displays tips for an effective case study presentation, and **Boxes 10-2** and **10-3** represent the components of a case presentation.

Introduction or Chief Complaint

Your "opening statement" should be designed to focus the listener's attention and thinking on the patient's major concern. In general, the case study will begin with demographic information about the patient, such as age, marital status, ethnicity,

---

Box 10-1 Tips for an Effective Oral Case Presentation

Brevity: Do not ramble, but do not be too brief.
Organization: Present in SOAP format and avoid jumping back and forth between different problems.
Eye contact: Engage your audience and keep your presentation lively. Avoid reading directly from the chart.
Anticipate and expect questions: Be ready to answer any questions relevant to your patient.
Use clinical reasoning: Your listener should be able to consider a differential diagnosis.
Present the *patient* as well as the *problem*: Remember personal, family, and social factors.

Box 10-2 Components of an Oral Case Presentation

Introduction or chief complaint
History of present illness
Physical examination
Diagnostic tests
Differential diagnosis
Management plan
Summary

Box 10-3 Expanded Components of a Case Presentation

Chief Complaint

____ is a ____-year-old ____	____	____
(initials)　　(age)　(race)	(sex)	(gender preference)

who presented to the family health center with a chief complaint of
_____.

The chief complaint is a brief statement of why the patient sought medical attention, stated in the patient's own words. No medical term or diagnosis is used.

History of Present Illness (HPI)

The HPI is a more complete description of the patient's symptom(s). General features included in the HPI are:

- Date of onset
- Precise location and radiation if pertinent
- Nature of onset, severity, and duration
- Effect of any treatment
  - Associated symptoms
- Degree of interference with daily activities

Past Medical History (PMH)

The PMH includes serious illness, chronic diseases, surgical procedures, and injuries the patient has experienced. Minor complaints may be omitted.

Family History (FH)

The FH includes the age and health of parents, siblings, and children. Ages and cause of death should be recorded for deceased relatives. Only include data that is pertinent to the patient case.

Social History (SH)

The SH includes not only the social characteristics of the patient, but also the environmental factors and behaviors that may contribute to the development of disease. Items included are marital status, number of children, educational background, occupation, dietary habits, and use of tobacco, alcohol, or other drugs.

Medication History (MH)
The MH should include current medications prior to the office visit or admission. This includes prescription and nonprescription medications, as well as vitamins and herbal products. Include the name and dosing information for each.

Allergies
Allergies to drugs, foods, pets, and environmental factors should be included. An accurate description of the reaction that occurred should be presented.

Review of Systems and Physical Exam
In the ROS, the examiner questions the patient about the presence of symptoms that are pertinent to each body system. Only the pertinent positive and negative findings may be recorded.

The general sections for the PE are listed next. It is only necessary to list the findings that are "remarkable."

General appearance
Vital signs
Skin
HEENT
Lungs
Cardiovascular
Abdomen
Genital/rectal
Extremities
Neurological
Psychiatric

Diagnostic Tests
The results of laboratory and diagnostic tests should be recorded. List all laboratory results but comment only on those that are abnormal or pertinent to the case.

Differential Diagnosis
Based on the preceding information, what are the impressions, problems, or diseases? Develop a problem list according to the acuity and significance of the patient's conditions.

Management
For each problem, discuss your plan and rationale for it.
Present your plan in the following format:
Diagnostics (what tests, if any, will be ordered)
Therapeutics (what pharmacologic agents, if any, will be ordered)
Patient education
Follow-up plans: Next appointment, consultation, referral

Case Summary
Provide a brief summary of the chief complaint and the treatment provided. List other problems associated with current or past treatments.

sex, and occupation. The patient's chief complaint, while important to document in the medical record, should be presented as the clinician's view of the reason for the visit or patient encounter. If the reliability of the patient is in question, this should be stated early in your presentation and the reason, such as poor historian, confused, psychotic, or intoxicated.

History of the Present Illness

Following the introduction, the history of the present illness is given. It is well-known that obtaining an accurate history will provide the clinician with the differential diagnosis 90% of the time (Davenport, 2008). This is the most essential piece of your presentation, and if presented well, it should take up at least 50% of your presentation time. In this section, you will want to describe the development of the most important problem or "present illness" as you interpret the information the patient told you. In the outpatient setting, the typical patient will present with several issues for you to address in a limited amount of time (e.g., 15–30 minutes) depending on where you are practicing. You most likely will not have time to address each issue in a single visit and must become skilled at determining which problem is the priority for the visit and setting the goals without overlooking potentially serious problems.

The other ongoing major medical problems should be reported, but you will need to condense the information about these problems and select information that is most relevant to the main issue. The seven attributes of a symptom will provide you with a framework upon which to present your information. These variables are (Bickley, 2020):

1. Timing or chronology
2. Location
3. Quality
4. Quantity or severity
5. Progression
6. Aggravating or alleviating factors
7. Associated manifestations

Do not mention any of the attributes that are not important to the diagnosis. Information from the past medical history, surgical history, social history, medication, allergies, family history, and the review of other systems should be reported only if it is directly relevant to the current problem in order to keep your presentation focused and brief. Keep the report of the review of systems to pertinent positive and negative findings.

Physical Examination

As with the history, the explanation of the physical examination should be reported in a succinct format emphasizing the body systems associated with the presenting problems. A standard format for reporting the physical examination should include pertinent vital signs and the general appearance of the patient. Address all significant pertinent and abnormal findings. An accurate reporting of the pertinent physical examination should tie into your history, resulting in a critical analysis of what the differential diagnosis is for the patient. A standard format for describing the physical examination findings would be done systematically, as demonstrated in Box 10-3.

Diagnostic Studies

Presentation of diagnostic studies should follow the physical examination. Serum laboratory studies such as complete blood count and chemistries are generally presented first, followed by radiologic findings such as x-rays, ultrasounds, CT scans, and MRI results, followed by electrocardiograms and other diagnostic studies. Unless directly relevant to the case, normal findings can be presented as "normal," but if important to the diagnosis, the exact result should be reported. For example, in a patient with poorly controlled diabetes and chronic renal failure, although the creatinine level was "normal," it would be important to report the result of 1.2mg/dL for this case, as opposed to a result of the creatinine level for a healthy 28-year-old visiting for a general physical examination. If the patient is presenting with a new complaint and you are considering ordering diagnostic tests, be prepared to have a rationale of the importance and reliability of the tests, as well as their risks and their cost–benefit ratio. You must present an argument to order diagnostic tests based on the facts and if they will affect management of the patient.

Differential Diagnosis

Now that the clinician has gathered all the information by asking, listening, examining, and investigating diagnostic results as applicable, it is at this point in the case presentation that you identify the differential diagnoses or the list of possibilities for the symptoms. You must narrow to the most important one or two problems and discuss the differential diagnoses. The emphasis should be on the data that support or disprove various diagnoses and relate why the diagnosis you arrived at was made over others that were considered. Remember that the differential diagnosis should address the possible causes in the case at hand, not for the problem in general. For example, in a patient with sudden onset of fever, productive cough, rhonchi, and pulmonary infiltrate, discuss pneumonia, not the problem "cough." In your discussion, each abnormal or significant symptom or physical finding and each abnormal diagnostic study must be accounted for. If no follow-up or further study was done for some abnormal finding, provide a rationale for the decision. In addition, there is no shame in admitting that we cannot explain a particular finding or symptom. In fact, knowing what something is not has as much value as providing a specific label for a complaint or condition.

Management Plan

Lastly, the case presentation requires the nurse practitioner to discuss the management plan, being prepared to offer a strong rationale for taking proposed actions. Actions might include further diagnostics and pharmacologic or educational interventions. There are many suggested ways of developing and presenting a management plan for the clinical problem or differential diagnosis. You might find it helpful, especially if dealing with more than one or several complex clinical issues, to separate each problem into its most basic elements, with a separate plan noted for each one. By identifying the most basic components of each problem, you will be less likely to miss important issues and be better able to formulate the most complete plan possible (Coralli, 2006). Your ability to do this will obviously vary with your prior experience and knowledge base. However, this general approach applies to most clinical situations. Take, for example, a patient who presents with new dyspnea on exertion who also has known heart failure, hypertension, and hyperlipidemia. Each one of these problems is related to the patient's cardiovascular system. However, if you were to address all of them under a single "cardiovascular" heading, there is a good chance that the assessment and plan would become muddled and confusing. Describe any treatment and the patient's responses to date if known. If the patient has been followed over a period of time for the problem identified, convey some sense of the course of the illness or progression of the disease. A sample case study with a management plan is presented in **Box 10-4**.

Box 10-4 Case Presentation Example

Chief Complaint: Blair Daniels is a 51-year-old white female administrative assistant who presents to the family health center complaining of a recent episode of rectal pain and bleeding with defecation.

HPI: The blood was bright red and was present both on the wiping paper and in the toilet bowl but was mixed with stool. The rectal pain was most severe with the passage of stool but sometimes persisted for hours after defecation. The bleeding occurred last week for 3 to 4 days and has now stopped. She reports a history of a similar but more severe episode of rectal pain and bleeding 1 year ago, which responded to dietary changes and sitz baths. A dietary inventory reveals she has been avoiding food intake to prevent bouts of pain. The patient states that she has daily loose bowel movements the past 2–3 weeks and has lost a "few pounds."

PMH:
Iron deficiency anemia secondary to heavy menses
Obesity
Irritable bowel syndrome

Surgical History:
Gallbladder surgery at 19 years old

GYN: Menarche G1 P1 A0 L1, NSVD no complications age 25; history of fibroid uterus

Family History:
Mother: 72 years old, irritable bowel syndrome, diverticulitis, hypertension
Father: 75 years old, type 2 diabetes, hypertension

Allergies:
Sulfa—rash

Medications:
Imodium tablets prn diarrhea

Physical Exam Findings:
Gen: Moderately obese white female, appears comfortable. BMI: 36 VS 140/92
    P-76 R-12 T-101.2
Lungs: CTA. No wheeze.
CV: Normal S1 S2, no murmur, no rubs, no bruits
Abdominal exam: Hypoactive bowel sounds and diffuse RLQ tenderness. No
    rebound. No guarding. No rigidity. No organomegaly.
Rectal exam: External skin tags at the rectal verge. These are neither inflamed
    nor tender. A digital exam finds no masses or palpable hemorrhoids, but
    there is moderate tenderness at 6 o'clock. Stool in the vault is firm, brown,
    and negative for occult blood.

Diagnostic Tests: No diagnostic tests available
Differential Diagnosis:
Rectal bleeding: Anal fissure, diverticulitis, colon cancer, peptic ulcer disease
Elevated blood pressure
Obesity
Management Plan:
- **Rectal bleeding**

Diagnostics: CBC, CT scan abdomen with contrast
Therapeutics: None
Patient education: Educate regards need for CT scan, refer to GI
- Elevated blood pressure

Diagnostics: Chemistries, lipid panel, TSH
Therapeutics: Consider oral agent if BP elevated next visit in light of risk factors and family history of hypertension
Patient education: DASH diet
- **Obesity:** Deferred to next visit

Follow-up in 3 weeks following colonoscopy and GI consult
Summary: I am uncertain why she is having rectal bleeding, which warrants a complete work-up by a gastroenterologist. There may be an infectious process going on, given the patient is febrile and has a history of diverticulitis. We will send the patient to the hospital for a CT scan today and have her seen by GI. We didn't address her elevated blood pressure or obesity today, but I would like to see the patient in 3 weeks to review her lab work and discuss the consultant's findings.

Summary

Whether a 1–2 minute "hallway" consult or a formal oral presentation to your preceptor or your class, conclude by summarizing the key points of the entire case in several sentences. In formal presentations, after the concluding summary, it is routine to ask if anyone has any comments or questions. Always consider the patient's personal factors that may influence his or her response to the management plan.

Collaboration, Consultation, and Referral in Primary Care

According to the American Association of Nurse Practitioners (2021), nurse practitioners (NPs) practice autonomously and in collaboration with other healthcare professionals to assess, diagnose, treat, and manage the patient's health problems and needs. Consultation, referral, and collaboration are key roles in which the primary care NP is adept at as both direct care provider and coordinator of care. Regulations vary by state dictating NPs' scope of practice and prescribing privileges. Certifying bodies and professional nursing societies have accepted certain tasks, protocols, and decisions as part of NP scope of practice, which may be in direct conflict with organizational constraints and public perceptions of NP scope of practice. NPs acknowledge that they thrive on the ability to consult with others, and that they occasionally encounter clinical circumstances outside of their scope of practice, necessitating a request for direction or guidance from a physician or other healthcare provider with additional expertise. With the predicted shortage of between 21,400–55,200 primary care physicians in the United States by 2033 and the expansion of health coverage to the 32 million uninsured Americans by 2028, the Association of American Medical Colleges also acknowledges the need for physicians to find ways of effectively collaborating with other healthcare professionals including NPs (AAMC, 2020). Collaboration between healthcare providers is essential to provide safe, cost-effective, high-quality healthcare services with positive patient outcomes (Maylone, Ranieri, Quinn Griffin, McNulty, & Fitzpatrick, 2011).

Defining Collaboration

Collaboration can be defined as a joint communication and decision-making process between healthcare professionals working toward a mutual goal of addressing a patient and family's medical, social, and ethical problems (Green & Johnson, 2015). It is essential that the collaborative relationship be vetted with mutual respect and trust for one another's unique abilities. Other elements of a collaborative team are regular and open dialogue, like-minded practice philosophies, continuing education, shared decision making, and a willingness to learn from other's clinical expertise (Makowsky, 2009; IPEC, 2016). Such a relationship has the potential to improve patient care outcomes, enhance patient safety, and reduce the workload for the individual team member. Collaboration can also help to decrease burnout and enhance workplace satisfaction.

Collaboration Defined by State Statute

States define scope of practice in statutes enacted by the state legislature, or the state legislature giving the board of nursing the authority to define the scope of practice for the advanced practice nurse (Buppert, 2021). For example, according to the Connecticut General Statutes (20-87a), the term:

> *collaboration* means a mutually agreed upon relationship between an advanced practice registered nurse and a physician who is educated, trained, or has relevant experience that is related to the work of such advanced practice registered nurse. The collaboration shall address a reasonable and appropriate level of consultation and referral, coverage for the patient in the absence of the advanced practice registered nurse, a method to review patient outcomes, and a method of disclosure of the relationship with the patient.

The preceding example not only defines collaboration but subsumes the terminology of consultation and referral. Some states describe the NP's scope of practice in abbreviated formats, while other states have unclear language that can be become confusing to physician colleagues as well as the consumer. Many variables play a role as to when a NP should collaborate with, consult with, or refer a patient to another care provider. For example, the place of employment may dictate to the NP the exact consultation process depending on whether it is a specialty site, large institution, small private practice, or the geographic location, such as an urban, suburban, or rural setting. The terms *consultation* and *referral* are often used interchangeably, but there are distinct differences.

Defining Consultation

All clinicians engage in clinical decision making and need to manage clinical uncertainty and understand the consequences of delaying an appropriate treatment plan

> **Box 10-5** Mechanisms for Consultations
>
> **Informal Consultation**
> - Patient care rounds
> - Professional meetings
> - Telephone consultation
> - E-mail consultation
> - Video-based medical consultation
>
> **Formal Consultation**
> - Formal process of sending the patient to another provider for a comprehensive evaluation

for a patient. Nurse practitioners are faced with complex patients and need to exercise sound judgment regarding making a diagnosis, selecting an appropriate diagnostic test, observing patient care outcomes, and making a final decision on patient management. Managing clinical uncertainty is a skill that needs to be developed. Consultation can be defined as a request for direction or assistance on a diagnosis or treatment plan from another provider (Goolsby, 2002). Consultation can be either formal or informal, as depicted in **Box 10-5**.

Defining Referral

Referral can be defined as another provider accepting the ongoing treatment of a patient for a specific problem and often for a limited amount of time (Goolsby, 2002). For example, you may refer a patient to a cardiologist to assume care for the patient's heart failure. That patient may continue to visit the cardiologist for evaluation and treatment of heart failure but will remain with her primary care provider for treatment of her other medical problems (e.g., diabetes, osteoarthritis). Consultation does not suggest continued treatment as is implied in the referral process. Although the terms are used interchangeably, there are distinct differences in regard to overall responsibility for the patient's care for specific health issues.

When Should Nurse Practitioners Seek a Consultation or Referral?

There may be multiple variables that cause the NP to initiate the consultation or referral process. The NP should consult with another healthcare provider when there is a question or uncertainty about the patient's care. The NP may have a specific question regarding the treatment plan or may need "another set of eyes" to visually assess a portion of the physical exam to confirm diagnoses. Often, in the subsequent days following the patient visit, when either laboratory results or imaging results are received and reviewed, next steps may be to include additional consultation. Under all circumstances, the NP should clearly document the consultative discussion within the patient's medical record, as well as the interventions that the NP ordered. This is important both from a legal standpoint and in an effort to provide seamless care for the patient. Another situation that should prompt a consultation or referral is when patients express doubt in the NP's diagnosis and treatment plan.

Patients are increasingly looking up their symptoms on the internet, and it is common for patients to seek second opinions. The primary care NP is responsible for the coordination of care, which can become complex in particular when multiple healthcare providers are involved. Close coordination is essential to provide timely care, avoid morbidity, and decrease risk of litigation (Goolsby, 2002). The following is an example of a common patient scenario where, based on clinical experience and comfort level, the NP asks for a point-of-care consultation with a physician partner:

Miss P is a 25-year-old Caucasian female with a recent presentation of a skin lesion to her right posterior calf. She has no history of skin cancer but has a positive family history of melanoma. The NP involved in this scenario is a recent graduate with little experience in dermatological conditions. She asks a physician colleague to visually inspect the skin lesion.

Referrals are an integral part of the NP–patient experience. It is no different from physicians who refer their patients to specialists for reasons such as exhausting treatment options or receiving abnormal test results out of the physician's scope of practice. **Box 10-6** gives a list of common reasons to seek a consultation or referral.

Another important aspect within the referral process is the need for insurance verification and the specific procedure that needs to be followed for each carrier and plan. The patient and NP have combined ownership of the referral process and what it entails. If it has been predetermined that the insurance plan needs no formal referral, a letter of referral should be made. Also, accompanying the documentation should be any pertinent testing or ancillary information that would be helpful to the specialist/referral provider. We can take the earlier case presentation a bit further as follows:

Miss P is a 25-year-old Caucasian female with a recent presentation of a skin lesion to her right posterior calf. She has no history of skin cancer but has a positive family history of melanoma. The NP involved in this scenario is a recent graduate with little experience in dermatological conditions. The NP is unable to access the collaborating physician. The NP would then make a direct referral to dermatology for further evaluation of this lesion. The NP needs to make sure that the proper referral procedure is in place and that this process is documented and the appointment is secured with the other provider.

The Referral and Consultation Process

There is no one set procedure or format for initiating a referral. It is often dependent upon the setting the NP works in or the institution where the referral is being

---

Box 10-6 Common Reasons for Consultation and Referral

- Advice on diagnosis
- Advice on treatment plan
- Advice on prognosis
- Mental health counseling
- Specialized procedure (surgical and nonsurgical)
- Patient request (second opinion)
- Insurance company guidelines
- Failure of treatment plan

> **Box 10-7** Formal Consultation: Pertinent Information
>
> - Demographics
> - Summary of current problem
> - Past medical history
> - Medications
> - Allergies
> - Pertinent family history
> - Pertinent social history
> - Diagnostic test results
> - Previous consultation results
> - Clear outline of the problem you evaluated/treated
> - Urgency of the request

generated to. Many primary care offices have ancillary staff to facilitate the acquisition of the patient's information for the specialist, understand insurance company requirements, and set up the appointment when needed. If the institution does not have a formal process or policy, the NP should write the formal referral with the relevant patient information to give the consultant a guide for approaching the patient and to avoid duplicative services. **Box 10-7** gives an overview of the pertinent information for a formal consultation.

Tracking Referrals

Following the transmission of the patient information to the consulting physician, the patient needs to take ownership and responsibility for the overall process. Very often, patients do not believe they need to see the consultant and are nonadherent in attending the appointment. Giving the patient information to hand carry to the specialist may increase adherence to follow through with the consultation. The procedure to track referrals is dependent on the size of the practice and policies instituted, but regardless of the setting, all consultations should be documented appropriately within the patient's record. Some practices may have a referral book or field in the electronic medical record that can be referenced to make sure the appointment was booked, proper authorization was received, the patient made the appointment, and the consultant's report was received.

Consultant's Responsibilities

One of the most important areas regarding consultations and referrals is follow-up by the NP referral originator after the patient has had the visit. A source of frustration for many primary care providers is the failure of the consulting physician to provide adequate detail and feedback regarding patient findings and treatment plans. Depending on the severity of the patient issue, the NP may hear directly back from the specialist or receive documentation electronically or via mail. That is why it is extremely important that the NP know the exact date of the specialist visit, if possible. This is also another internally based tracking mechanism to ensure the patient kept the appointment as scheduled. Alerts can be instituted if using an electronic medical record. It is necessary to have this information in order to reduce liability or untoward patient outcomes. Maintaining referral records is a quality initiative that can be used by nursing, medical assistants, or whoever is in control of the referral procedure.

At the end of the day, the patient should be in control of his or her own health care and visits, but NPs need to ensure that the process in place is effective, with quality measures for further follow-up after the visit has been made. A direct patient follow-up visit should occur, if appropriate, following the specialist visit. This too would be a checkpoint to ensure proper follow-up with all parties is occurring and patient satisfaction is at a high level.

Interprofessional Collaboration

Interprofessional collaboration (IPC) is essential to optimize patient outcomes. Additionally, IPC has been shown to increase patient safety (Wen et al., 2019; Banks et al., 2019). Healthcare professionals need to be knowledgeable about their roles, as well as those of other healthcare workers when collaborating with one another. Interprofessional education (IPE) is a vital component for students pursuing careers as healthcare professionals. Communication, collaboration, and cooperation across professional boundaries are essential for patients and families to receive the individualized care they deserve and need to maximize their quality of life (Haas, 2009). The shortage of nurses and other healthcare professionals is well documented, particularly in rural and urban low-income areas. The shortages are expected to worsen as the current workforce retires and the demand for health care grows. The NP is a highly skilled clinician who collaborates with other members of the healthcare team to deliver high-quality, evidenced-based care to improve patient care outcomes and population health. Addressing these challenges requires a transformation of our educational system and healthcare workforce. Healthcare professionals need to be able to deliver care to the fullest extent of their education and training. Nurses represent the largest healthcare profession, armed with the scientific knowledge and adaptive capacity to lead the changes in the healthcare system. The nursing profession must reconceptualize its roles in coaching, advocacy, chronic disease management, transitional care, prevention activities, and quality improvement to ensure safe and optimal patient care.

The Institute of Medicine (IOM), in partnership with the Robert Wood Johnson Foundation (RWJF), published a landmark report called *The Future of Nursing: Leading Change, Advancing Health* (Institute of Medicine, 2010). This report is the nonpartisan work of 18 experts in nursing, medicine, economics, business, hospital administration, health policy, consumer issues, workforce policy, and health plan administration. Based on evidence from an extensive review of the research, the report outlines a blueprint for transforming the nursing profession, particularly NPs, to enhance the quality and value of U.S. health care in ways that meet the future needs of diverse populations. In launching the initiative, RWJF's president, Dr. Risa Lavizzo-Mourey, noted that "nursing is at the heart of patient care" and is therefore crucial to changing the way health care is delivered so that "patients receive better care at a cost we can afford."

One of the most viewed online reports in the IOM's history, this groundbreaking report calls on the nation's leaders and stakeholders to act on its recommendations, including changes in public and institutional policies at the federal, state, and local levels. These facts spurred the need for IPC and diversity across the continuum of care. Studies have demonstrated how effective coordination and communication among health professionals can enhance the quality and safety of patient care. Health professionals working collaboratively as integrated teams draw on individual and collective skills and experience across disciplines. They seek input and respect the contributions of everyone involved, allowing each person to practice at a higher level. The result is inevitably better patient outcomes, including higher levels of patient satisfaction and improved overall population health.

The passage of the Recovery and Reinvestment Act of 2009 and the Patient Protection and Affordable Care Act of 2010 has stimulated new approaches, such as the "medical home" concept, to achieving better outcomes in primary care, especially for high-risk chronically ill and other at-risk populations (Kaiser Family Foundation, 2021). Improved interprofessional teamwork and team-based care play core roles in many of the new primary care approaches.

NPs play an integral role in the foundations of the primary care model. The idea of primary care and its relationship to the broader context of health is itself being reconsidered. First, in primary care there is a focus on expanded accountability for population management of chronic diseases that links to a community context. Second, healthcare professionals and public health professionals jointly share roles and responsibilities for addressing health promotion and primary prevention needs related to behavioral change. Third, healthcare professionals and public health professionals work in collaboration with others on behalf of persons, families, and communities in maintaining healthy environments, including responding to public health emergencies.

D'Amour and Oandasan (2005) defined interprofessionality as:

> the process by which professionals reflect on and develop ways of practicing that provides an integrated and cohesive answer to the needs of the client/family/population....[I]t involves continuous interaction and knowledge sharing between professionals, organized to solve or explore a variety of education and care issues all while seeking to optimize the patient's participation.... Interprofessionality requires a paradigm shift, since interprofessional practice has unique characteristics in terms of values, codes of conduct, and ways of working. These characteristics must be elucidated. (p. 9)

The World Health Organization (WHO) developed a global Framework for Action on Interprofessional Education and Collaborative Practice (WHO, 2021). This illustrated the overall goal of interprofessional education as setting the stage for the preparation of a "collaborative practice-ready" workforce, which has underpinnings that are driven by the local community health needs and local community health systems designed in response and readiness for those needs.

The Interprofessional Education Collaborative (IPEC) was developed in 2009 with the purpose of ensuring that all healthcare curricula develop core competencies ensuring the provision of optimal IPC (IPEC, 2016). In 2016, IPEC amended its original 2011 IPEC report with 21 healthcare professional agencies, including the

> **Box 10-8** Core Competencies for Interprofessional Collaborative Practice (IPEC, 2016)
>
> Competency 1: Values and Ethics for Interprofessional Practice
> Competency 2: Roles and Responsibilities
> Competency 3: Interprofessional Communication
> Competency 4: Teams and Teamwork

Commission on Collegiate Nursing Education (CCNE) now part of the collaborative (IPEC, 2016). Studies have shown that many health professionals, at the time of graduation, feel ill prepared communicating with other members of the healthcare team and may be unsure of the exact roles of other health professionals (Wen et al., 2019; Banks et al., 2019). It has been shown that including IPE in the curriculum of NPs can improve attitudes toward IPE (Rosenbloom & Nemec, 2020).

The Interprofessional Education Collaborative (2016) defines four domains essential to interprofessional practice, which are discussed in the following sections (see **Box 10-8**).

Competency Domain 1: Values and Ethics for Interprofessional Practice

Collaborative care models are based on the ability of two or more distinct and separate healthcare disciplines to respect and trust each other's clinical judgment, skills, and expertise. There is a moral obligation of all healthcare professions with respect to the care of the patient and positive valuable outcomes. This domain's goal is to provide equitable health care to all.

Competency Domain 2: Roles and Responsibilities

Each profession has core competencies that define roles and responsibilities, as well as the scope of practice. Each member of a healthcare discipline should be able to articulate their unique role and patient care delivery methods to other members of the healthcare team and understand the roles of other healthcare providers. Diverse expertise builds effective teams. Through shared learning experiences, IPC will blossom. A diverse expertise helps build effective teams. Collaborative practice depends on maintaining this expertise through continued learning experiences and through refining, revising, and improving the roles and responsibilities of each profession involved in the collaborative effort.

Competency Domain 3: Interprofessional Communication

Effective communication is a core competency for every profession. This is especially true in the healthcare arena, where critical thinking coupled with the ability to disseminate findings in a concise manner is crucial. Transparency of information coupled with an effective communication style within professions is necessary to manage any sensitive patient information.

Competency Domain 4: Teams and Teamwork

Teamwork cannot take place without a good leader. Leadership qualities are essential to building patient-centered teams where care is carefully coordinated. NPs possess the leadership skills to develop effective teams. Teamwork will enhance patient care outcomes, decrease error, and increase satisfaction among patients and team members. Understanding the functionality of the team and its influence on individual team members, daily operations, and patient care outcomes is an important part of being an effective team member.

These important steps illustrate how in the reality of practice, different disciplines can come together for the greater good of the patient, family, community, and larger health system interplay. Also, many positive benefits of effective collaboration can be shared across disciplines to illustrate a team effort to patient care. We know that the core of the NP competencies specifically set by NONPF (2017) are acquired through mentored patient care experiences with emphasis on independent and interprofessional practice; analytical skills for evaluating and providing evidence-based, patient-centered care across settings; and advanced knowledge of the healthcare delivery system. This illustrates how NPs can be champions for their patients within the discipline of nursing, as well as across disciplines in a collaborative effort approach.

Collaboration within each discipline is also a necessity for a successful treatment plan and initiatives. NPs collaborate and partner with their registered nurse workforce continuously to improve patient outcomes. This team-based approach with multiple levels of knowledge and expertise is what separates nursing from other disciplines. It really demonstrates the evolution of the care plan model that has been utilized for many years in some facilities. Each profession within health care can contribute to the care of the patient and the quality of his or her experience.

Collaborative Health Management Model

With escalating healthcare costs and an aging population with complex chronic diseases, economists, administrators, and clinicians are exploring a variety of interprofessional and team-based care models to deliver cost-effective quality care. In our current standard primary care delivery system, patients with chronic healthcare conditions are not receiving all recommended interventions and are failing to meet targeted treatment goals. The literature discusses six collaborative primary care models that have had a positive impact on mental health services and the management of chronic health conditions, such as end-stage renal failure, diabetes, and heart failure (Wagner, 2004). One such care model, the Collaborative Health Management Model (CHMM), fosters teamwork between nurse practitioners and physicians based on an equal partnership. It serves to operationalize the call from the IOM report on the future of nursing for advanced practice registered nurses to deliver high-quality chronic disease management within their scope of practice and with a focus on team-based care and patient partnerships (Brown & Matthews, 2013). Nurse practitioners are poised to be at the forefront of this shift in activity and to engage in the philosophy of the CHMM. The Patient Centered Medical Home (PCMH) is a primary care collaborative model that is endorsed by the Agency for

Health Care Research and Quality. This model is patient-centered, comprehensive, team-based, coordinated, accessible, and focused on quality and safety. More information about PCMHs is discussed in Chapter 8.

The need for a CHMM can be justified by several elements: NPs have expertise in health prevention and promotion activities, which is lacking in medical education; volume-driven practices leave little time to provide comprehensive care by one clinician; and NPs are experts in facilitating effective patient self-management (Brown & Matthews, 2013). NPs in collaboration with physician partners can help streamline patient care, engage patients in the decision-making process, and provide patients with the tools needed to manage their conditions. This care model has been shown to be cost-effective because the patient receives care on a timely basis with early intervention, resulting in no unnecessary duplication of services and preventing medical error.

Aside from enjoying better patient outcomes, healthcare providers working in a CHMM also experience increased job satisfaction through a structure of collegial relationships. Collaboration among healthcare providers is based on a relationship of mutual trust, shared goals and decision making, and using the collective knowledge of all the healthcare providers involved in the care of the patient. Effective CHMMs will help the patient navigate seamlessly between providers based on his or her preferences and individual healthcare needs (Naylor, 2012).

Collaborative health management models align with the educational expertise that NPs gain. The curriculum in NP education immerses graduate students in population health management with a focus on healthcare trends and communities; health promotion and preventive measures; consultation, collaboration, and referral; and use of evidence-based medicine guidelines (NONPF, 2017). The NP educational focus on patient-centered and holistic care prepares them to care for individuals with chronic health conditions, such as diabetes, hypertension, and heart failure. The educational competencies outlined by NONPF and the American Association of Colleges of Nursing, support efforts to enhance NP scope of practice, regulation, and licensure across the country.

The framework for the CHMM is designed around the following concepts (Brown & Matthews, 2013):

- Delivery system design—including goals and team member roles (families, patients, NP, MD, RN, medical assistant, pharmacist, social worker, psychologist, specialist consultants)
- Clinical information systems—including risk stratification tools, acuity tools, electronic health records, and evidenced-based practice guidelines
- Decision support—including prompts for patient preferences
- Self-management support—directed by the NP
- Organizational support—aimed at improvements and leadership at all levels of the organization
- Community resources—to assist the patient and family in using community and cultural resources to support their needs

This comprehensive framework engages all the participants in an evidenced-based, patient-focused process that will drive accountable care through meaningful patient engagement and improved relationships within the multidisciplinary team. It is based on the premise that engagement and patient empowerment is essential to driving positive health outcomes. The future success of healthcare outcomes will be determined by how NPs and their physician counterparts and other specialty providers work collaboratively to ensure the positive patient experience that demonstrates quality and cost containment.

Barriers and Benefits to Effective Interprofessional Collaboration

Barriers to implementing effective collaborative teams can be based on the individual professions' isolated evidence base, which results in a foundation of decision making and distinct communication patterns that can result in role confusion and turf battles. Each discipline perceives itself as having sole expertise, power, and leadership in one care aspect over the discipline. To adequately prepare NP students, educators must recognize a blurring of the boundaries between nursing and medicine and must acknowledge that clinical practice demands not only similar competencies but also shared language and communication. Studies show that the way to effective collaboration is through communication that results in patient-centered care.

The astute NP must be cognizant of other barriers he or she may encounter when consulting with members of the medical or allied health team. Some examples of this include scheduling/timing conflicts, in-person versus telephone consults, and documentation and diagnostic reviews on a per-case basis. As previously mentioned, consultation and collaboration may be site specific and directly related to the individual state statutes on scope of practice, the NP's level of experience, and access to the provider that will be providing the consultation.

Many benefits exist for effective collaboration. The creation of a bridge among professions to provide evidence-based and patient-centered care to the patient, family, community, and overall population is of utmost importance. This type of collaborative experience can create major changes in how health care is perceived and provided across local, state, and federal arenas. This allows each person to practice at a higher level. This will ultimately improve patient outcomes and satisfaction, as well as professional and personal contentment, knowing that the care provided is evidence-based best practice.

Seminar Discussion Questions

1. Describe a clinical experience where the assessment and plan for treatment was not according to clinical guidelines. What would you have done differently and why?
2. Identify and discuss two patients seen in clinical practice, where one was referred to see a specialist and the other was sent for a consultation. What is the difference between these two appointments? How will you follow up on these patients?
3. Who are the different members of the healthcare team where you are doing clinical rotations? Does everyone tend to work collaboratively or do there appear to be any "turf wars"?

References

American Association of Medical Colleges. (2020). *New AAMC report confirms growing physician shortage*. Retrieved from https://www.aamc.org/news-insights/press-releases/new-aamc-report-confirms-growing-physician-shortage

American Association of Nurse Practitioners. (2021). *What's a nurse practitioner (NP)? Discover why Americans make more than 1.06 billion visits to NPs each year*. Austin, TX: Author. Retrieved from https://www.aanp.org/about/all-about-nps/whats-a-nurse-practitioner

American Board of Internal Medicine. (2021). *The Mini-CEX*. Retrieved from https://www.abim.org/program-directors-administrators/assessment-tools/mini-cex.aspx

American Nurses Credentialing Center. (2017). *ANCC 2021 certification renewal requirements*. Retrieved from https://www.nursingworld.org/~4ac164/globalassets/certification/renewals/RenewalRequirements

Anderson, E. M., Leonard, B., & Yates, J. A. (1974). Epigenesis of the nurse practitioner role. *American Journal of Nursing, 10*(18), 12–16.

Banks, S., Stanley, M. J., Brown, S., & Matthew, W. (2019). Simulation-based interprofessional education: A nursing and social work collaboration. *Journal of Nursing Education, 58,* 110–113. doi:10.3928/01484834-20190122-09

Bickley, L. (2020). *Bates' guide to physical examination* (13th ed.). Philadelphia, PA: Wolters Kluwer/Lippincott Williams & Wilkins.

Brown, M. A., & Matthews, S. W. (2013). APRN expertise: The collaborative health management model. *Nurse Practitioner: The American Journal of Primary Healthcare, 38*(1), 43–48.

Brown, M., & Olshansky, E. F. (1997). From limbo to legitimacy: A theoretical model of the transition to the primary care nurse practitioner role. *Nursing Research, 46*(1), 46–51.

Buppert, C. (2021). *Nurse practitioner's business practice and legal guide* (7th ed.). Sudbury, MA: Jones and Bartlett.

Connecticut State Department of Public Health. (2016). *Sec. 20-87a Definitions: Scope of practice*. Retrieved from https://www.cga.ct.gov/current/pub/Chap_378.htm#sec_20-87a

Coralli, C. (2006). Effective case presentations—An important clinical skill. *Journal of the American Academy of Nurse Practitioners, 18,* 216–220.

D'Amour, D. O., & Oandasan, I. (2005). Interprofessionality as the field of interprofessional practice and interprofessional education: An emerging concept. *Journal of Interprofessional Care, 19*(1), 80–20.

Davenport, C. H. (2008). The 3-minute emergency medicine medical student presentation: A variation on the theme. *Society for Academic Emergency Medicine, 15*(7), 683–687.

Goolsby, M. (2002). *Nurse practitioner secrets: Questions and answers to reveal the secrets to successful NP practice*. Philadelphia, PA: Hanley & Belfus.

Green, B. N., & Johnson, C. D. (2015). Interprofessional collaboration in research, education and clinical practice: Working together for a better future. *The Journal of Chiropractic Education.* doi:10.7899/JCE-14-36

Green, H. D. (2011). The oral case presentation: What internal medicine clinician–teachers expect from clinical clerks. *Teaching and Learning in Medicine, 23*(1), 58–61.

Haas, B. S.-B. (2009). Application of the Newell Liberal Arts Model for interdisciplinary course design and implementation. *Journal of Nursing Education, 48*(10), 579–582.

Hinson Brown, L. (2006). The case presentation as argument. *Journal of the American Academy of Nurse Practitioners, 18*(9), 395–396.

Institute of Medicine. (2010). *The future of nursing: Leading change, advancing health (consensus report)*. Washington, DC: The National Academies Press. Retrieved from http://www.iom.edu/Reports/2010/The-Future-of-Nursing-Leading-Change-Advancing-Health.aspx

Interprofessional Education Collaborative (IPEC). (2016). Core competencies for interprofessional collaborative practice: 2016 update. *Interprofessional Education Collaborative.* Washington, DC. Retrieved from https://nebula.wsimg.com/2f68a39520b03336b41038c370497473?AccessKeyId=DC06780E69ED19E2B3A5&disposition=0&alloworigin=1

Kaiser Family Foundation. (2021). *Health reform source*. Retrieved from https://www.kff.org/health-reform/issue-brief/health-homes-for-medicaid-beneficiaries-with-chronic/

Makowsky, M. C. (2009). Collaboration between pharmacists, physicians and nurse practitioners: A qualitative investigation of working. *Journal of Interprofessional Care, 23*(2), 169–184.

Maylone, M. M., Ranieri, L., Quinn Griffin, M. T., McNulty, R., & Fitzpatrick, J. J. (2011). Collaboration and autonomy: Perceptions among nurses. *Journal of the American Academy of Nurse Practitioners, 23*(11), 51–57.

National Organization of Nurse Practitioner Faculties. (2017). *Nurse practitioner core competencies.* Retrieved from https://cdn.ymaws.com/nonpf.site-ym.com/resource/resmgr/competencies/20170516_NPCoreCompsContentF.pdf

Naylor, M. K. (2012). The role of nurse practitioners in reinventing primary care. *Health Affairs, 31*(11), 893–899.

O'Brien, J. L., Martin, D. R., Heyworth, J. A., & Meyer, N. R. (2009). A phenomenological perspective on advanced practice. *Journal of the American Academy of Nurse Practitioners, 21*(8), 444–453.

Paauw, D., Migeon, M. B., & Burkholder, L. R. (2003). *Internal medicine clerkship guide.* St. Louis, MO: Mosby.

Rollins, L. G. (2012). *The one-minute preceptor.* University of Virginia Health System. Retrieved from http://www.med-ed.virginia.edu/courses/fm/precept/module5/m5p2.htm

Rosenbloom, S., & Nemec, E. C. (2020). Problem-based learning and case scenarios. *Nursing Education Perspectives.* doi:10.1097/01.NEP.0000000000000638

Steinemann, S., Kurosawa, G., Wei, A., Ho, N., Lim, E., Suares, G., Berg, B., et al. (2016). Role confusion and self-assessment in interprofessional trauma teams. *American Journal of Surgery, 211,* 482–488. doi:10.1016/j.amjsurg.2015.11.001

Wagner, E. (2004). Effective team work and quality of care. *Medical Care, 42*(11), 1037–1039.

Wen, A., Wong, L., Ma, C., Arndt, R., Katz, A., Richardson, K., Deutsch, M., & Masaki, K. (2019). An interprofessional team simulation exercise about a complex geriatric patient. *Gerontology & Geriatrics Education, 40,* 16–29. doi:10.1080/02701960.2018.1554568

World Health Organization. (2021). *Framework for action on interprofessional education and collaborative practice.* Retrieved from http://www.who.int/hrh/resources/framework_action/en

CHAPTER 11

Clinical Prevention/ Community and Population Health

Anna Goddard and Dorothea Esposito

Lillian Wald coined the term *public health nursing* in 1893 stating that the focus of public health nursing was prevention of disease (Fee, 2010). Throughout history, nurses and nurse practitioners have provided primary and acute care to a variety of patient populations, often rooted in health prevention and health promotion work. Of late, nurses initiate and manage nurse-managed health centers (NMHCs) often providing care to underserved and vulnerable populations (Bongiorno & deChesnay, 2020). Nurses also contribute to providing health care to populations across the globe. As part of master and doctoral nurse education, NPs are trained in the physical, psychosocial, and lifestyle considerations that influence of social determinants of health (AACN, 2021; AACN, 2006).

Nurses are well-known for their role in the public health sector and in providing health care to populations around the world. The Institute of Medicine (IOM) emphasizes the need to link primary care and public health as a means to improve population health for all (IOM, 2012). The NP needs to understand the intersection of social determinants of health, as well as how to incorporate physical, psychosocial, and lifestyle assessments, with prevention strategies, screenings, immunizations, and health promotion for all clients. In public health, performing data analysis and applying population health principles become critical when viewing health at a macrosystems level of care (Fos, 2011).

Principles of Epidemiology

The American Association of Colleges of Nursing (AACN) designated clinical prevention and population health as a core essential for Doctor of Nursing Practice (DNP) programs (AACN, 2021). Essential VII of the DNP essentials specifically outlines the parameters of clinical prevention and defines population health, to be addressed in DNP programs of study. Furthermore, according to AACN, DNP graduates should have a foundation in clinical prevention and population health

(AACN, 2021). Courses typically introduce students to epidemiology and methods used by epidemiologists to assess factors associated with the distribution and determinants of health and disease in populations and to read, interpret, and apply literature using epidemiological and statistical methods.

Clinical prevention is defined as health promotion and risk reduction/illness prevention for individuals and families. *Population health* includes aggregate, community, environmental/occupational, and cultural/socioeconomic dimensions of health. Aggregates are groups of individuals defined by a shared characteristic such as gender, diagnosis, or age. These framing definitions are endorsed by representatives of multiple disciplines, including nursing (AACN, 2006, p. 15).

According to the Centers for Disease Control and Prevention (CDC) (2021b), the definition of epidemiology correlates with the inherent fundamentals and "the spirit of public health" as "the study of the distribution and determinants of health-related states or events (including disease), and the application of this study to the control of diseases and other health problems." *Epidemiology* is derived from the Greek words *epi,* meaning "on"; *demos,* meaning "the people"; and *logos,* "the study of" (CDC, 2012). An understanding of the historical background, as well as the practical applications of epidemiology, methods for identifying and evaluating sources of health information, calculation of critical epidemiological measures, and investigation techniques are essential elements for nurse practitioners (NPs) who practice in population health. Further, an evaluation of the strengths and weaknesses of different study designs is a necessary component for evidence-based practice.

Current concepts of public health, health promotion, evidence-based recommendations, determinants of health, environmental and occupational health, and cultural diversity and sensitivity are interrelated concepts that provide the foundation for practice as a nurse practitioner for both a local and a global worldview. Core components of epidemiological concepts for the NP should include investigating methods for describing disease rates and other vital statistics; cohort, case-control, and cross-sectional studies; odds ratios, relative risks, their confidence intervals, and tests of significance; and concepts of confounding, effect modification, and bias (Vitale & Curley, 2020).

From the exceptional work of Jenner in developing the smallpox vaccination in 1798 to the groundbreaking work of Snow uncovering the transmission of cholera in the Soho area of London in 1854, the world of epidemiology can be captivating. In the 19th century, it was believed that the cause of most illnesses was related to infectious diseases. More than 100 years later, we have insight into the myriad factors that contribute to illness and disease, including infectious agents, elements within the environment, nutrition, and effects from trauma. Surveillance and research continue to uncover emerging factors (Macha & McDonough, 2012).

In 2021, the COVID-19 pandemic has shown real-world epidemiological principles and practices, including the unique challenges that epidemiologists have faced in identification, monitoring, tracking, and even studying this ever-changing coronavirus. This has directly led to the ongoing shifts in guidance for ways to both prevent and slow the spread of this virus (CDC, 2021a, 2021b). At the time of this writing, the COVID-19 pandemic had taken the lives of more than 500,000+ Americans and 2.6M+ worldwide (CDC, 2021c). As epidemiologists continue to explore the COVID-19 virus, they discover new information related to transmission and treatment.

The record-breaking speed surrounding the creation, testing, and approval of the COVID-19 vaccine is nothing short of miraculous and with roots in epidemiological principles. To date, there are three FDA authorized vaccines available for administration in the United States. These are Pfizer-BioTech COVID-19 vaccine, Moderna COVID-19 vaccine, and Johnson & Johnson's Janssen COVID-19 vaccine (CDC, 2021b). Phase three clinical trials are in effect for the AstraZeneca COVID-19 vaccine and Novavax COVID-19 vaccine (CDC, 2021b). Thus, we see how the study of the epidemiology of the virus produced vaccines that will prevent the future spread of the COVID-19 virus.

One example of a disease that has plagued public health and direct healthcare providers for hundreds of years is tuberculosis (TB). In 2019, despite medications to treat and cure tuberculosis, this disease caused 1.4 million deaths globally (WHO, 2021a). Experts in the topic attribute the inability to contain this epidemic to numerous factors, including the fact that the associated social determinants are most often "extreme poverty, severe malnutrition, and overcrowded living conditions" (Keshavjee & Farmer, 2012, p. 932). The countries that continue to suffer most from tuberculosis are the countries where incomes are low. In 2019, the countries responsible for two-thirds of the recent cases of TB were India, Indonesia, China, Philippines, Pakistan, Nigeria, Bangladesh, and South Africa (WHO, 2021a). Despite multifaceted efforts by global agencies such as the World Bank and the WHO to control tuberculosis, we now face multidrug-resistant strains of tuberculosis that have been fueled by HIV and inadequate funding to treat tuberculosis properly. Patients living with HIV are 15 to 21 times more likely to develop active TB than their counterparts without HIV (WHO, 2021b). Reasons for drug resistance are associated with incorrect prescriptions by providers, poor quality drugs, and patients stopping treatment prematurely (WHO, 2021a). Succinctly summarized, Keshavjee and Farmer (2012) state:

> The contours of global efforts against tuberculosis have always been mediated by both biologic and social determinants, and the reasons for the divergence in the rates of tuberculosis and drug resistance between rich and poor countries are biosocial. (p. 934)

Much has been completed recently to create a plan that will combat the TB epidemic. Presently, global commitments to treat TB have been made. An example of this is the first global ministerial conference hosted by the WHO and the Russian government in 2017, followed by the United Nations holding its first-ever high-level meeting on TB in September 2018 (WHO, 2021a). These discussions focused upon ways to end the TB epidemic worldwide with goals of ending the epidemic of TB by 2030.

NPs must stay informed regarding global and national trends in all diseases. It is critical for the practicing NP to be on the lookout for patients with any forms of infectious diseases; appropriately assess, treat, and report patients who need treatment; and through the development of trusted patient–NP relationships, see patients complete appropriate treatment regimens. This fosters the beginning of the important process of reducing the spread of disease and infection within the communities in which NPs practice.

Terminology in Epidemiology

Understanding public health and epidemiological research terminology is critical for the NP. Demographic and social data often refer to, and include, age and gender distribution, socioeconomic status, family structure (marital status, single parent, etc.), race and ethnicity, and religious affiliation. Community infrastructure variables include availability of social and health services (hospitals, community providers, emergency departments, etc.), housing quality (lead, asbestos, mold, etc.), social stability, safety and community policing, and employment opportunities.

Health-related outcomes often refer to interrelated attributes describing the consequences of disease for an individual, such as impairments, symptoms, and functioning (Ward, 2009). Common examples of health outcomes in epidemiology include access to health care, interpersonal violence (homicide and suicide rates), infant mortality rates, mortality from selected conditions, the prevalence of chronic and infectious diseases, alcohol and substance abuse rates, teenage pregnancy rates, the occurrence of sexually transmitted diseases (STDs), and birth rates. Environmental variables include air pollution (from both stationary and mobile sources), access to parks and recreation, clean water availability, radon and lead levels in soil, food access (including the availability of markets with healthy groceries, number of liquor stores, fast-food services, and the nutritional quality of foods and beverages at school).

The Framingham Heart Study, the surgeon general's report on smoking and health, and The Nurses' Health Study (2021) all demonstrate the use of health statistics in epidemiological research. The Nurses' Health Studies, led by Harvard Medical School, are the largest prospective investigation into risk factors for chronic diseases, specifically in women. Originating in 1976 and now in their third generation (with Nurses' Health Study 3 in 2020), the Nurses' Health Studies have more than 275,000 participants, with ongoing follow-up of study participants for assessments in health and lifestyle factors (such as diet and exercise). These studies played an instrumental role in shaping larger public health recommendations. Furthermore, these studies have been recognized as influential in developing and evaluating questionnaire-based methods to assess a variety of factors (The Nurses' Health Study, 2021).

Morbidity and *mortality* are often used in discussions of population health. Morbidity rates refer to how fast a disease is occurring in a population, the proportion is what fraction of the population is affected by the disease, and the incidence rate is the number of new cases of the disease in a specific time period. **Box 11-1** provides a mathematical method to calculate an incidence rate per 1,000 people. Mortality rates are most often used for the overall population and can be cause or age specific. Typically, mortality rates increase as age increases. **Box 11-2** provides calculations of a mortality (death) rate for deaths in a population during a specific time period.

Box 11-1 Incidence Rate per 1,000

$$\frac{\text{\# of new cases of a disease occuring in the population during a specific time period}}{\text{\# of persons who are at risk of developing the disease during that time period}} \times 1{,}000$$

Box 11-2 Mortality Rate for a Population

$$\frac{\text{\# of deaths in the population during a specified time period}}{\text{\# of persons in the population during the specified time period}} \times 1{,}000$$

Illness and disease are often studied through review of the natural history of disease and use of the *epidemiological triangle,* which considers the interaction of agent, host, and environment. The triangle has three vertices (corners): (1) agent/microbe ("what" causes the disease); (2) host ("who" is harboring the disease); and (3) the environment (external factors of "where" the disease is transmitted). See **Figure 11-1**. This triad of the infectious disease course allows consideration for transmission. *Transmission* occurs when the disease agent leaves its reservoir or host through a portal of exit, and enters through a portal of entry to the susceptible host. Humans serve as reservoirs for many infection diseases such as sexually transmitted diseases, measles, mumps, streptococcal infection, and respiratory viruses. Carriers may or may not have symptoms and, therefore, are not acutely aware they are transmitting infection. This process is known as the *chain of infection*, as depicted in **Figure 11-2**.

For example, using the epidemiological triangle with the agent anthrax, a single-celled bacillus bacterium called *Bacillus anthracis,* transmission most commonly occurs through the skin, when spores enter the body through a scrape or cut.

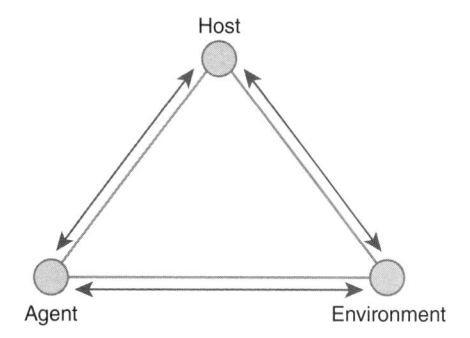

Figure 11-1 Epidemiological Triangle

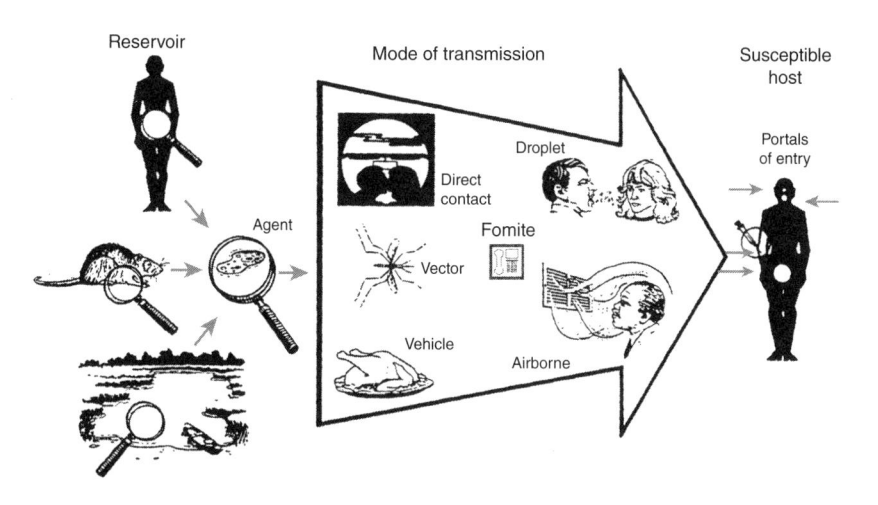

Figure 11-2 Chain of Infection
CDC. (1992). *Principles of epidemiology* (2nd ed.). Atlanta, GA: Author.

However, spores can also be inhaled or ingested by eating contaminated meat. This bacterium most often causes illness in cows and sheep as the host animal; however, it can also infect humans and veterinarians, and farm, wool, and tannery workers are most at risk. Anthrax has also been used as a biological weapon (Macha & McDonough, 2012).

Diseases are often discussed in terms of the impact of the outbreak as either an *epidemic, pandemic,* or *endemic*. An *epidemic* refers to a limited outbreak in both time and location. For example, in 2003 the severe acute respiratory syndrome (SARS) epidemic caused the death of nearly 800 people worldwide. A *pandemic* is an epidemic extending to an entire country or a large part of the world. Prior to the Coronavirus-19 pandemic, HIV/AIDS was often used as an example of a global pandemic disease. In history, influenza pandemics have killed millions: the Spanish influenza of 1918 (40–50 million people), the 1957 Asian influenza (2 million people), and the 1968 Hong Kong influenza (1 million people) (Fos, 2011). A disease is said to be *endemic* if it remains present in an area for a long period of time. For example, malaria is endemic in tropical climates, and hepatitis B (HBV) is endemic in China and many Asian countries. Vietnam is hyperendemic for HBV, meaning it is found in excessively high rates within a host population.

Understanding epidemiological terminology is important for myriad reasons. Portal exit and entry, modes of transmission, and the chain of infection guides clinicians and scientists in determining the appropriate control measures and treatment interventions, such as eliminating agents at the source of transmission, protecting portals of entry, and increasing a host's defenses (CDC, 2021a). For example, mosquito bed nets are often used to protect a sleeping individual from being bitten by malaria-carrying mosquitos: protecting the portal of entry. Long pants and insect repellants are used to prevent potential tick-borne illnesses such as Lyme disease when hiking. However, other methods such as vaccination and prophylactic antimalarial pharmaceuticals do not *prevent* mosquito or tick bites, but intervene at preventing infection from taking root (Fos, 2011).

Finally, when discussing disease prevention through the chain of infection, *herd immunity* is the concept that if enough individuals in a population are resistant to an agent, then those who are susceptible will be protected by the resistant majority. This indirect form of protection can occur from vaccination or previous infections. Individuals who then become immune protect those who cannot become immune, such as those with immunodeficiency or immunosuppression. Not everyone in a community requires immunity (or resistance) in order to prevent disease outbreak. However, when herd immunity reaches a certain threshold, disease gradually disappears from a population, which, if eliminated to infections of zero, is called *eradication*.

Population Health

Public health professionals are often responsible for population health, with expertise in epidemiology and biostatistics contributing to that larger domain. *Population health* is defined as the "health outcomes of a group of individuals, including distribution of such outcomes within the group" (Kindig & Stoddard, 2003). However, population health has now become an approach to health aimed at patterns of health determinants, outcomes, and interventions for the entire human population.

What constitutes a population? A population consists of a group of people who have some common characteristics (Fos, 2011; Friis & Sellers, 2012; Shi & Singh, 2021). Populations range from a large entity (an entire nation) to small subpopulations (a neighborhood, a common disease category, marital categories, same-sex marriages, people at risk for heart disease, racial/ethnic groups etc.). As one can see from the subpopulations listed, characteristics are not solely related to the physical boundaries of where one may reside (Friis & Sellers, 2021; Shi & Singh, 2021). A community may include members who share interpersonal and intrapersonal connections, known as a *phenomenological community* (Maurer & Smith, 2013). The types of characteristics held in common for a population subset or community can include age, gender, health behaviors, and exposure to a virus, among others.

The concept of vulnerability as it relates to healthy and unhealthy communities must be noted. "Vulnerability occurs at the individual, community, and systems levels" (Anderson, 2020, p. 363). One method for identifying an unhealthy community is by determining the lack of support for vulnerable populations that exists within the community. This premise includes all members of the community in addressing poverty and providing adequate housing, healthy food, job opportunities, and proper air, water, and sanitation for all its community members and is vital to the health and development of resilience within a population. One method to build a healthy community is to focus on the strengths within the community and its vulnerable populations (Anderson, 2020). Conversely, one may approach a specific population and identify problems within a community.

Nurse practitioners provide health care to many populations as part of their professional practice. Population-based programs increase access to available resources, and this access supports a stronger healthcare system (Bongiorno & deChesnay, 2020). Therefore, it is imperative that the NP remain current in issues contributing to health and be actively engaged in health promotion and disease prevention efforts.

Further, nurse practitioners (NPs) must feel at ease with people who are different from themselves. Examining their cultural awareness is one helpful step in this process. Knowledge of the social determinants of health (SDOH) and how these disparities affect the health of populations is key to understanding and serving the health needs of the populations that NPs serve. Having a concrete knowledge base from which to connect concepts of epidemiology with clinical prevention and population health is vital to being a successful NP or DNP.

Prevention Levels

Disease progresses through phases from a "preclinical state," which is the time when there are no symptoms, to the "clinical state," which is the time when symptoms first appear (Vitale & Curley, 2020, p. 54). Understanding the progression of disease is essential to the nurse practitioner because it helps develop programs and interventions that are valuable to those populations threatened by disease. The principal goal of disease prevention is to prevent the disease before it appears. Prevention is discussed in terms of the three levels of prevention: (1) primary prevention or avoiding disease altogether, (2) secondary prevention or early diagnosis of disease, and (3) tertiary prevention or measures taken to prevent or limit disease progression.

Primary Prevention

Primary prevention interventions are aimed at preventing disease. This step may be arguably the most important of the prevention levels, considering that half of all deaths are considered preventable. Handwashing is often mentioned as the most recognizable primary preventative effort to prevent the spread of infectious diseases. Lifestyle management, health promotion, proper nutrition, school health, immunizations, handwashing, and proper waste disposal are additional forms of primary prevention.

For instance, an estimated 16 million people (about the population of New York) in the United States suffer from preventable illness due to smoking (U.S. Department of Health and Human Services ODPHP, 2021). Further, smoking causes approximately 500,000 premature deaths per year. One of the primary prevention goals of Healthy People 2030 is to "reduce illness, disability, and death related to tobacco and secondhand smoke" (U.S. Department of Health and Human Services ODPHP, 2021, *Tobacco use,* para. 1). Smoking cessation is the chief way to prevent morbidity and mortality from tobacco use; however, it is incredibly difficult to execute due to the addictive properties of smoking (Vitale & Curley, 2020).

As of this writing, the current COVID-19 pandemic is the largest public health threat worldwide, and concerns over it continue to increase. Protecting populations from the spread of COVID-19 ranks as one of the top initiatives among the major worldwide health-related organizations. The CDC continues to emphasize the role of handwashing, social distancing, and the proper use of face masks as principal ways to prevent the spread of COVID-19 (CDC, 2021c).

Through examination of infectious disease trends, up until 1900, pneumonia, tuberculosis, and diarrheal diseases were the top three causes of death in the United States (CDC, 2021d). Largely due to primary preventative efforts to reduce morbidity and mortality, they are no longer the leading causes of death in the United States. See **BOX 11-3**.

Vaccinations, or immunizations, are perhaps one of the most noted primary preventative scientific revelations and are used to prevent pneumococcal pneumonia, influenza, tetanus, varicella, human papilloma virus, and now COVID-19. Of no surprise, the recommendation and promotion of vaccinations are core NP health

---

Box 11-3 Leading Causes of Death in the United States, 2019

- Heart disease: 659,041
- Cancer: 599,601
- Accidents (unintentional injuries): 173,040
- Chronic lower respiratory diseases: 156,979
- Stroke (cerebrovascular diseases): 150,005
- Alzheimer's disease: 121,499
- Diabetes: 87,647
- Nephritis, nephrotic syndrome, and nephrosis: 51,565
- Influenza and pneumonia: 49,783
- Intentional self-harm (suicide): 47,511

CDC. (2021d). *Leading causes of death.* Retrieved from https://www.cdc.gov/nchs/fastats/leading-causes-of-death.htm

management strategies. A variety of vaccination administration records are available for both adults and children. In fact, most if not all electronic health records include immunization records as part of the core functionality of the medical record. The Advisory Committee on Immunization Practices (ACIP, 2021), a committee within the CDC, governs dispensed advice and guidance on effective control of vaccine-preventable disease. The ACIP has met regularly since its creation in 1964 by the U.S. Surgeon General in order to assist in preventing communicable diseases. Both private and government insurance payers base their determination on which vaccines will be paid for according to ACIP recommendations (ACIP, 2021). ACIP also determines the vaccination schedules in regard to timing, dose, and contraindications, which are then published by the CDC (CDC, 2021b). The CDC regularly updates the recommended adult and pediatric vaccine schedules based on the available evidence from the ACIP, which can be found at https://www.cdc.gov/vaccines/schedules.

Over the last decade, the leading causes of death worldwide have changed. Ischemic heart disease currently tops this list. While HIV/AIDS at one time was more prevalent and in the top 10 causes of death, HIV/AIDS mortality has fallen 51% during the past 20 years, due to anti-viral treatments and increased awareness of the disease. While diarrheal diseases remain eighth, tuberculosis has been removed from the global list altogether. Cancers (specifically trachea, bronchus, and lung cancers) have shifted to the sixth leading cause of death globally. This provides an example of how the NP needs to think and reflect globally on changes in the distribution of disease, especially when caring for an aging population. Bearing this in mind, it is important for the NP to think globally when diagnosing and treating infectious diseases throughout the community. It's especially important in relation to both undocumented and documented citizens in a very transient society (WHO, 2021c).

Secondary Prevention

Secondary prevention includes actions that lead to early identification, diagnosis, and treatment of disease. The aim is to detect the disease earlier than it would have been detected with routine follow-up and care (Gordis, 2009). Health screenings and various detection activities are used in secondary prevention efforts. Collection and analysis of clinical data provide a starting point for identifying, selecting, and implementing interventions that target specific populations at risk. Early diagnosis and treatment prevent progression of the disease or spread of an infectious disease among a given population. For example, diagnosing community acquired pneumonia (CAP) in a nursing home resident involves isolating the resident and treating them with antibiotics. Simple measures, such as isolation, additionally prevent the spread of CAP to other residents. Another example of secondary prevention measures are breast self-exams and mammography for patients, starting at 40 years of age, because early diagnosis can accelerate treatment and prevent death.

The United States Preventive Services Task Force (USPSTF, 2021) is a source of evidence-based information in improving population health. Their website can be accessed at https://uspreventiveservicestaskforce.org/uspstf/home to review recommendations for all levels of preventive care. The USPSTF offers advice on preventive services that focuses on primary prevention efforts, supported by evidence-based expert review and recommendations. The task force performs a rigorous review of research on specific health topics prior to making recommendations on the merits of preventive measures. This includes screening tests, counseling, immunizations, and medications given for the prevention of diseases. Topics include type 2 diabetes mellitus, lipids, breast and colorectal cancer, depression, tobacco use, and many more. Further, NPs are encouraged to visit the CDC website for preventative screening recommendations at https://www.cdc.gov/publichealthgateway/didyouknow/topic/phs.html.

Tertiary Prevention

The primary aim at the tertiary level of prevention is to limit the progression of disability related to disease. Approaches used at this level of prevention are physical therapy, rehabilitation, and patient education to promote lifestyle changes. These approaches are all necessary components of treatment that decrease further disability caused by disease (Merrill, 2021). Probably the most crucial factor affecting tertiary prevention is an aging population. Current predictions estimate a 60% increase in people over the age of 65 years by the year 2030 (He et al., 2016). Many factors have played a part in this phenomenon of an increase in aging. One reason is increased lifespan related to medical advancements. Other factors include public health efforts to improve sanitation and the availability of clean water, as well as the impact of prevention efforts aimed at reducing risk factors for cardiovascular disease (Van Leuven, 2012). This change in population demographics has an enormous impact on NPs as "baby boomers" continue to age and pass away. As a result, NPs will be caring for an aging population with increased focus on diagnosing and treating chronic comorbid diseases, such as cardiovascular disease, diabetes, cancer, dementia, depression, osteoarthritis, and lung disease (Van Leuven, 2012).

HIV and Prevention Levels

Acquisition of the HIV virus is through a portal for transmission, which includes ingesting infected breastmilk, blood exposure (e.g., by sharing infected needles), or exposure to HIV-infected seminal or vaginal fluids during unprotected sex. HIV may also be perinatally transmitted in utero or during the birth process. Primary infection begins with an acute retroviral syndrome occurring early in the new HIV infection. More than half of individuals infected with HIV experience an influenza-like illness with fever, rash, pharyngitis, lymphadenopathy, and myalgia. About 3 to 6 weeks after acquiring an HIV infection, the CD4 cell count in the peripheral blood drops dramatically as the virus replicates rapidly and is widely disseminated throughout the body, where it is predominantly trapped in lymph nodes. During this time (usually 2–3 months), the amount of virus in the serum (viral load) is very high and can be detected by measuring viral copies in the serum; however, the HIV antibody test may be negative at this time. The *seroconversion period* is the time it takes an infected person's body to make antibodies to HIV. This can take 3 months (more common) to 6 months (less common) after infection. The asymptomatic period of HIV infection lasts anywhere from a few months to many years (up to 15 years). Varying from person to person, asymptomatic periods depend on the HIV viral load. Individuals with higher viral loads worsen faster than those with lower viral loads. As CD4 cells decline, opportunistic infections and diseases cause symptoms. If left untreated, the

HIV infection develops into AIDS. The rapid replication of HIV eventually depletes the immune system, and in most people, this causes immunosuppression where the body succumbs to infections, cancers, and ultimately death (Henry Kaiser Family Foundation, 2012; U.S. Department of Health and Human Services, 2016).

To reduce HIV infection worldwide, primary, secondary, and tertiary prevention must be sought. Following a 2006 CDC recommendation for HIV testing in healthcare settings, routine voluntary testing for patients aged 13 to 64 years was not to be based solely on patient risk for acquiring HIV, as in the past (Branson et al., 2006). The goal of primary HIV prevention is to reduce the incidence of transmission, whereas secondary HIV prevention aims to reduce the prevalence and severity of the disease through early detection and prompt treatment. This approach was based on the following CDC guidelines:

1. To catch "late testers," or patients who were diagnosed with AIDS within 12 months of a diagnosis of HIV, representing about 40% of all HIV diagnoses, and get them care sooner, thereby extending their lives.
2. To reduce unsafe practices that spread HIV by having people who are HIV positive know their status and take measures to reduce transmission.
3. To include HIV testing as part of routine medical screenings, helping reduce the stigma associated with being offered an HIV test.

Primary HIV prevention efforts include the following:

- Community and peer-based prevention and intervention programs
- School-based skills education and prevention
- The use of needleless technologies in healthcare settings to reduce injury and risk of blood-borne virus transmission
- Post-exposure prophylaxis, including nonoccupational post-exposure prophylaxis
- Pre-exposure prophylaxis

One of the advancements in **primary prevention of HIV** was approved by the Centers for Disease Control and Prevention in 2014. Pre-exposure prophylaxis (PrEP) using Truvada (tenofovir/emtricitabine) has been shown to reduce sexual transmission of HIV by 90% and transmission by injection drug use by 70% (US-DHHS, 2017). Primary care providers must perform thorough histories of every patient and identify those who may be at high risk for acquiring HIV, offering PrEP when applicable. This includes anyone in a relationship with a partner who is HIV positive, or anyone who has unprotected sex with partners of unknown HIV status, and/or injection drug users who share needles or drug paraphernalia. Baseline laboratory assessment and education about adherence to taking the once-daily medication is critical in avoiding adverse events, including HIV infection (Branson et al., 2006; USDHHS, 2017).

Secondary HIV prevention includes erasing barriers to HIV testing and detection by removing the requirement for pretest counseling and permission forms. Secondary prevention also includes increasing healthcare providers' knowledge about HIV and testing, the signs of acute antiretroviral infection, and what to do when a patient tests positive for HIV. Clinical setting barriers include insufficient time, the consent process, lack of knowledge or training, lack of patient acceptance, pretest counseling requirements, competing priorities, and inadequate reimbursement (Burke et al., 2007). In the emergency department, barriers also include the need to inform an HIV-positive patient, institutional costs, the availability of testing, administrative barriers, and provider belief that testing should only be offered at the patient's request. Other identified barriers include a lack of trust with the patient, gender differences between the provider and patient, differences in sexual orientation, the concept that HIV and sexually transmitted diseases were not an issue in the community, and a lack of institutional policies for testing (Burke et al., 2007).

Tertiary HIV prevention is aimed at reducing the disability and complications of HIV infection. Decades of ongoing research led to frequent updates of these guidelines, due to evidence-based practice recommendations. In addition to the CDC's HIV testing recommendations, standard guidelines for the treatment of HIV infection, as well as guidelines for preventing and treating opportunistic infections in children, adolescents, and adults can be found on the CDC website (USDHHS, 2016, 2017). These evidence-based guidelines allow all providers to offer the most current high-quality care to their patients.

COVID-19 and Prevention Levels

In early January 2020, coronavirus disease 2019 (COVID-19) was identified as a novel SARS-CoV-2 coronavirus, causing nationwide shutdowns and a global pandemic, with more than 3.4M deaths worldwide and 164 million infections, as of this writing. December 2019 marks the first reports of cluster cases of pneumonia associated with the Huanan Seafood Wholesale Market in Wuhan, China (Chen et al., 2020). In January 2020, the coronavirus spread quickly through New York, infecting more than a quarter of a million people in a matter of weeks, and replacing China as the epicenter of the virus transmission. COVID-19 quickly met all three pandemic criteria: (1) caused by an illness, and fatalities related to said illness; (2) person-to-person spread sustainability; and (3) worldwide spread (Munster et al., 2020).

COVID-19 is affiliated with severe infection and includes fever, headache, malaise, arthralgia, shortness of breath, and pneumonia. Older adults over 65 years of age and those with severe underlying medication conditions (heart disease, lung disease, and diabetes) are most at risk for developing serious complications and possibly dying from COVID-19 illness. While more than half of affected people have underlying chronic disease, risk factors for severe disease are only partially understood. Symptomatic patients usually present with fever, cough, and myalgia/fatigue (Holstein, 2020). Common laboratory findings include leukopenia, lymphopenia, and mild hepatic enzyme elevations. Pneumonia is the most common resulting pathology, with bilateral multilobe and segmental consolidation on imaging results. Atypical presentations in older adults and those with medical comorbidities include a delayed presentation of fever and respiratory symptoms. Other symptoms include headache, confusion, rhinorrhea, sore throat, hemoptysis, emesis, diarrhea, and anosmia or ageusia. Some patients with SARS-CoV-2 infection never develop any symptoms and remain asymptomatic throughout infection (Holstein, 2020; Gandhi et al., 2020).

Coronaviruses (*Coronaviriade*) are single-stranded RNA viruses with a nucleocapsid (a long, folded strand prone to spontaneous mutations and frequent recombination of the genome, accounting for difficulty in transmissibility), found in mammals, including humans (CDC, 2021a; Chen et al., 2020). The COVID-19 outbreak has been traced to a viral genome with an 85% match with SARS-CoV-2, which was previously named severe acute respiratory syndrome (SARS). This particular betacoronavirus has been linked to a bat as its possible origin, and has been labeled a zoonotic infection, with humans as the intermediate host (CDC, 2021a; Holstein, 2020). Transmission occurs through respiratory droplets from the coughing and sneezing of an infected person to those in close contact (i.e., people less than 6 feet from each other) (CDC, 2021a). While transmission may theoretically occur through contact with infected surfaces of objects, and then by subsequent contact with the eyes, nose, or mouth, this has been found as a less frequent route of transmission for COVID-19. While most transmissions have occurred while an individual is at the peak of symptom presentation, asymptomatic persons have also been found to transmit COVID-19. With a 12- to 14-day incubation period, the recommendation for quarantine for a minimum of 14 days by the CDC was made for more than a year during the virus outbreak (CDC, 2021a).

Individuals who suffered more severe pathology and mortalities, often in the intensive care unit (ICU) for care, are older adults with comorbid conditions such as obesity, preexisting cardiovascular or respiratory illness, high blood pressure, and diabetes (Holstein, 2020). Older age and showing signs of sepsis on admission, as well as prolonged use of noninvasive ventilation, are strongly correlated with death from COVID-19. Non-survivors are more likely to have had respiratory failure (98% vs. 36%), sepsis (100% vs. 42%), and secondary infections (50% vs. 1%) (Huang et al., 2020; Guan et al., 2020).

All practicing healthcare providers were called to the "front-lines" for early detection of the virus, as well as frequent and ongoing awareness and education of COVID-19 characteristics and cause recognition. While nationwide U.S. public health system coordination was needed, individual state public health departments led the preparedness and emerging infection protocols, which differed among the 50 states. The WHO and CDC universally promoted **primary prevention efforts** to avoid disease, which include:

- Wash hands frequently (for at least 20 seconds), especially after coughing, sneezing, or blowing the nose;
- Avoid touching the eyes, nose, and mouth with unwashed hands;
- Avoid any contact with people who exhibit any symptoms;
- Stay at home as much as possible (a.k.a., quarantining);
- Keep at least 6 feet of distance from yourself and others that do not live in the same home (a.k.a., "social distancing");
- Use masks that cover the mouth and nose for all people, with the exception of those under the age of 2 years old or those who cannot remove a mask unassisted or have breathing difficulties;
- Frequently clean and disinfect high-touch surfaces such as tables, doorknobs, light switches, handles, desks, phones, keyboards, toilets, faucets, and sinks;
- Self-monitor daily for individual symptoms, such as fever, cough, shortness of breath, and other symptoms.

Public health primary prevention strategies were delivered through awareness campaigns and ongoing health education aimed at the public regarding the risk of infection, symptoms, protective measures, and adoption of these aforementioned behaviors to reduce the likelihood of infection (CDC, 2021a). Worldwide countermeasures to transmission were particularly challenging due to the lack of knowledge related to COVID-19, especially at the advent of the outbreak, as there was no-known natural history of the disease upon the initial outbreak. Epidemiological responses were driven by location and context, which varied across more than 50 countries.

The foremost primary prevention strategy is the ongoing vaccination efforts. Several COVID-19 vaccinations rapidly emerged on the market, all of them contributing toward a hopeful herd immunity across the globe. Pfizer-BioNTech, Moderna, and then Johnson & Johnson received emergency use authorization (EUA) in the United States from the Food and Drug Administration (FDA) for the COVID-19 vaccines (CDC, 2021b). Other vaccines have been approved in other countries, such as Sinopharm (2021) in China, and Sputnik-V (2021) from the Gamaleya Research Institute of Epidemiology and Microbiology in Russia. Availability of the vaccines continues to fluctuate wildly, with variability on the strict requirements needed for vaccine storage, in order to maintain the vaccines' efficacy and availability. **Table 11-1** summarizes the current overview of the COVID-19 vaccines. To

Table 11-1 Overview of COVID-19 Vaccines

COVID-19 Vaccine	Mechanism of Action	Efficacy	Storage	Approved for (Age)	Common Side Effects
Gamaleya (Sputnik-V) 2 doses, 3 weeks apart	Viral vector is engineered to contain the gene for the SARS-CoV-2 spike protein	91.4%	−20°C	> 18 yrs	Headache, redness at injection site
Johnson & Johnson 1 dose	Carrier vaccine: Viral vector is engineered to contain the gene for the SARS-CoV-2 spike protein	72%	2–8°C (up to 3 months)	> 18 yrs	Fatigue, fever, headache, pain at injection site, myalgia
Moderna 2 doses, 28 days apart	mRNA instructs cells to produce SARS-CoV-2 spike protein to trigger immune response	94.1%	−20°C (up to 6 months); 30 days in normal refrigeration	> 18 yrs	Chills, headache, pain, tiredness, redness/swelling at injection site
Novavax	Protein adjuvant: contains the spike protein as a nanoparticle, which cannot cause disease and stimulates the immune system to produce antibodies and T-cell immune responses	89.3%	4–8°C	18–84 yrs	None reported

COVID-19 Vaccine	Mechanism of Action	Efficacy	Storage	Approved for (Age)	Common Side Effects
Oxford-AstraZeneca 2 doses, 4 weeks apart	Carrier vaccine: Viral vector is engineered to contain the gene for the SARS-CoV-2 spike protein	70%	2–8°C	> 18 yrs.	Tenderness, pain, warmth, redness, itching, swelling, or bruising at injection site
Pfizer-BioNTech 2 doses, 21 days apart	mRNA template for the spike protein to trigger immune response	95%	−70°C	> 16 yrs	Chills, headache, pain, tiredness, redness/swelling at injection site
Sinopharm 2 doses, 3 weeks apart	Inactivated SARS-CoV-2 virus is inert in a chemical process that preserves virus structure	79.34%	−20°C	> 18 yrs	Fever, itching and redness at injection site

Data from: CDC, 2021b; Livingston et al., 2021; Moderna, 2021; Novavax, 2021; AstraZeneca, 2021; Pfizer, 2021; Sputnik, 2021; Sinopharm, 2021.

note, both Pfizer and Moderna created new vaccine technology for the COVID-19 vaccine, called an mRNA vaccine (messenger RNA). These types of vaccines signal the body to make copies of spike proteins (such as the "spikes" sticking out in coronavirus pictorials) through a genetic code from the SARS-CoV-2 virus to host cells in the body, stimulating an immune response to produce antibodies.

Secondary prevention for COVID-19 is aimed at early disease detection through screening, as well as early intervention, before onset of symptoms if possible. Viral testing (nucleic acid or antigen testing) from the respiratory system using nasal, oral, or saliva swabs were developed to determine whether SARS-CoV-2 infection was present in an individual at the date of testing. Reliability of surveillance screening varied widely in early screening mechanisms. Authorized viral assay testing is recommended to diagnose acute infection for both symptomatic and asymptomatic individuals. These antigen tests are used to diagnose acute infections and guide contact testing including possible isolation requirements. Some tests are point-of-care tests with results in less than an hour available on-site, while other antigen tests are sent to a laboratory and results are processed between 1–2 days (CDC, 2020).

Contract tracing refers to the process of identifying, monitoring, and supporting individuals who tested positive for COVID-19, aimed at rapid identification and containment of other potential human vectors. This involves working backward from individuals infected with the virus to contact said individual and then isolate the person through quarantine, essentially separating those who might have been exposed to COVID-19 from others.

Epidemiologists are currently continuing to study emerging concerns, as well as analyze available data in real time, with most focused around the adequacy of the quarantine period for COVID-19, quality assurance for diagnostics, post-treatment monitoring guidelines, and convalescent carriers (individuals who recovered from COVID-19 but are still capable of transmission). Transmission-based precautions include the use of contact and droplet precautions on top of standard precautions. In some cases, airborne precautions are additionally recommended in cases of aerosol-generated procedures, especially by healthcare workers caring for suspected or confirmed COVID-19 individuals (CDC, 2021a, 2021b). Guidelines include disposable or patient-dedicated care equipment (blood pressure cuffs, stethoscopes, etc.), adequately ventilated single rooms (of at least 60L/s/patient), disinfection with at least 70% ethyl alcohol for any equipment used between patients, restricting visitors to healthcare facilities, and increased disinfection of said facilities (Harvard Health, 2021). Healthcare worker personal protective equipment (PPE) (e.g., masks, gowns, gloves) are especially important, specifically when caring for confirmed COVID-19 patients (Holstein, 2020). At the height of the pandemic, worldwide PPE shortages, including masks and gowns, caused hundreds of thousands of preventable deaths.

Tertiary prevention strategies were aimed at treating the clinical disease by reducing sequelae and complications, as well as improving quality of life post-disease. Treatment of COVID-19 remains supportive through the management of symptoms and treatment, and the prevention of complications. Dexamethasone, as well as other corticosteroids (prednisone, methylprednisolone), are recommended for individuals with moderate to severe cases of the disease, who require supplemental oxygen or mechanical ventilation. Clinical investigation treatments continue with antiviral therapy (remdesivir) and passive immunization (SARS-CoV-2 immune globulin from transfused plasma) (Harvard Health, 2021; Cao et al., 2020). Baricitinib, in combination with remdesivir, was approved for hospitalized adults and children 2 years and older who required respiratory support; however, this therapy was not recommended over dexamethasone with remdesivir. Monoclonal antibody treatments (bamlanivimab, and a combination of casirivimab and imdevimag) received emergency use authorization from the FDA for non-hospitalized adults and children over 12 years old with mild to moderate COVID-19 symptoms who are at risk for hospitalization or more severe infection. Receiving plenty of rest, maintaining hydration, and reducing fever and aches continue to be recommended for generalized management of COVID-19. While antimalarial drugs were used early in trial treatments of COVID-19, the National Institute of Health treatment guidelines currently recommend against the use of chloroquine and hydroxychloroquine as monotherapy or in combination with azithromycin (NIH, 2020; Harvard Health, 2021; Geleris et al., 2020).

Convalescent plasma has been used for more than 100 years, including in previous treatments of SARS, measles, polio, and chickenpox. Convalescent plasma containing antibodies from individuals who recovered from COVID-19 have continued to show mounting evidence on improving symptoms with COVID-19 infection, with 48% of people less likely to develop severe COVID (NIH, 2020).

While the development of primary and tertiary prevention strategies through vaccination and treatment development have caused a turnaround in the COVID-19 outbreaks, the pandemic is not playing out in the same way from place to place. While some countries such as China and New Zealand have reached a low level of cases after lengthy lockdowns and are slowly easing restrictions and watching for increases, countries such as the United States and Brazil had surges of cases after governments lifted lockdowns.

Population Health and *Healthy People 2030*

In 1979, the Surgeon General Julius Richmond delivered a groundbreaking report entitled *Healthy People: The Surgeon General's Report on Health Promotion and Disease Prevention*. In 1980, the Office of Disease Prevention and Health promotion (ODPHP), as a result of this report, released *Healthy People 1990*. This initiative was aimed at improving U.S. population health over a 10-year period (U.S. Department of Health and Human Services ODPHP, 2020). It was the beginning of the first aspiring and quantifiable objectives for improving the health of the U.S. population. This initiative focused on lessening mortality rates over lifespans and increasing the independence of older adults. Further, this initiative marked the beginning of four later versions of *Healthy People*: *Healthy People 2000, Healthy People 2010, Healthy People 2020,* and currently, *Healthy People 2030.*

Each *Healthy People* release builds upon prior versions from the previous decades. For example, *Healthy People 2000* built on the prior initiative and established three comprehensive goals of increasing the duration of a healthy life, decreasing health disparities, and attaining access to preventive services for all. *Healthy People 2010* continued to build upon its predecessor initiative by increasing the focus on quality of life and by eliminating, as opposed to reducing, health disparities. Moving forward, *Healthy People 2020* had four overarching goals: (1) achieve high-quality and longer lives unrestricted by disease, disability, injury, and premature death; (2) attain health justice and abolish disparities, thereby improving the health of all populations; (3) generate social and physical settings that support good health for everyone; and (4) foster quality life, health improvement, and health behaviors through all life phases. *Healthy People 2030,* launched in August 2020, is the fifth version of this initiative and builds on this knowledge and data, as well as the successes and failures of the previous initiatives. The current version has a greater emphasis on health equity, the social determinants of health (SDOH), and health literacy, adding a new concentration of well-being (U.S. Department of Health and Human Services ODPHP, 2020). As part of the health care for a nation, the NP must incorporate these goals as part of the practice, and as a result, create an enormous impact on the health of the populations they serve and ultimately the health of the nation. **Box 11-4** outlines the leading health indicators as defined by *Healthy People 2030.*

The Clinical Prevention and Population Health (CPPH) Curriculum Framework was developed by the Healthy People Curriculum Task Force and assembled by the Association for Prevention Teaching and Research (APTR) in 2002 (APTR, 2020). This task force includes representatives from eight health professional education associations, including allopathic and osteopathic medicine, nursing and nurse practitioners, allied health, dentistry, pharmacy, and physician assistants (APTR, 2020). The CPPH Curriculum Framework was developed to assist educators in teaching about health promotion to meet the goals identified by *Healthy People* initiatives. The CPPH task force believes that in order to achieve the *Healthy People 2030* objectives, population health should be incorporated into the education of practitioners and providers, as well as their clinical practices. The framework comprises four

Box 11-4 *Healthy People 2030* Leading Health Indicators (LHI)

Topics	Leading Health Indicators
Health Conditions	Addiction Arthritis Blood Disorders Cancer Chronic Kidney Disease Chronic Pain Dementias Diabetes Foodborne Illness Healthcare-Associated Infections Heart Disease and Stroke Infectious Disease Mental Health and Mental Disorders Oral Conditions Osteoporosis Overweight and Obesity Pregnancy and Childbirth Respiratory Disease Sensory or Communication Disorders Sexually Transmitted Diseases
Health Behaviors	Child and Adolescent Development Drug and Alcohol Use Emergency Preparedness Family Planning Health Communication Injury Prevention Nutrition and Healthy Eating Physical Activity Preventive Care Safe Food Handling Sleep Tobacco Use Vaccination Violence Prevention
Populations	Adolescents Children Infants LGBT Men Older Adults Parents or Caregivers People with Disabilities Women Workforce

Topics	Leading Health Indicators
Settings and Systems	Community Environmental Health Global Health Health Care Health Insurance Health Information Technology (IT) Health Policy Hospital and Emergency Systems Housing and Homes Public Health Infrastructure Schools Transportation Workplace
Social Determinants of Health (SDOH)	Economic Stability Education Access and Quality Health Care Access and Quality Neighborhood and Built Environment Social and Community Context

U.S. Department of Health and Human Services ODPHP. (2021). *Healthy People 2030: Browse Objectives*. Retrieved from https://health.gov/healthypeople/objectives-and-data/browse-objectives

---

components that include population health, clinical preventive services and health promotion, health systems and health policy, and population health and clinical aspects based in community health (APTR, 2020). Revised every five years, the current fourth revision focuses on the social determinants of health (SDOH) and health parity as clinical emphasis, and includes the introduction of a new domain addressing mental and behavioral health. Version four also includes updated illustrative models and the topic areas of: (1) biologic factors and health; (2) discrimination including sexism and racism on health; (3) data analytics; (4) integrating diverse perspectives on behavior change; (5) access to mental, behavioral, and addiction health services; (6) risk reduction; (7) mental and behavioral health screening; (8) provider health; (9) thoughts for the usage of preventive medication; (10) unfavorable drug events; (11) systems thinking related to populations health; (12) principles of successful partnering; and (13) the impact of health systems organizations on health outcomes (APTR, 2020). APTR offers further details by listing 23 domains based on the four main components of the framework (2020).

Component one, the foundations of population health, requires that evidence-based practice (EBP) be part of the curriculum, providing information regarding descriptive epidemiology and the etiology of disease. Health promotion and disease preventing interventions are discussed relative to the types of prevention and the role of the clinician in disease prevention, coupled with the impact of a population health focus on individual and family health. The SDOH and their impact on health, along with population health informatics, are examined, and evaluation of the process and outcomes are also recommended segments of the curriculum.

Component two addresses clinical preventive services and health promotion, including prevention-related practice screenings and screening tests, mental and behavioral health, immunizations, and the use of preventive medication. Component three examines clinical practice and population health, including population health management, along with recommendations, implementation, and evaluation of interventions aimed at improving population health. Further, partnering with the public to create community health assessments, research, using evidence-based recommendations for community preventive services, along with environmental, global, and occupational health and examination of the cultural dimensions of practice are listed as part of the curriculum in component three. Component three also examines and outlines emergency preparedness and response systems in conjunction with preparing the health system workforce in this regard. Component four relates to health systems and health policy as being part of the curriculum. This includes the clinical and public workforce and health systems, health services financing (especially as this relates to the medically underserved populations), the development of health policy, and its impact on population health.

As public health NPs treat different populations, it becomes necessary to develop and evaluate programs that will service/treat/change a particular population's needs. Benchmarking and evaluation of these programs is key to providing evidence for practice. There are a variety of tools available for evaluating population health, and there are also tools for developing targeted programs. An example of one such tool is the monitoring and evaluation to assess and use results (MEASURE) evaluation (MEASURE Evaluation, 2021). The MEASURE evaluation website offers tools for a variety of areas such as HIV/AIDS, child health, reproductive health, and gender and poverty issues. The following is a helpful matrix for developing a program targeted to improve a population's health. It can be found at the MEASURE evaluation website https://www.measureevaluation.org/resources/tools/population-health-and-environment/population-health-and-environment-training-materials.

This matrix can be useful to the NP involved in public health as they evaluate key populations they serve, as well as design a targeted and benchmarked approach to developing a proposal to assist this population toward better outcomes. The key components for a program development matrix are (MEASURE Evaluation, 2021):

- **Objective:** Statements of desired, specific, realistic, and measurable program results
- **Intermediate result:** Benchmark progress result measured along the way to achieving the objectives.
- **Outcome:** Indicator of changes in knowledge, attitudes, and practices that help demonstrate achievement of objectives
- **Output:** Indicator of activity or immediate result of program process
- **Indicator:** A variable that measures one aspect of a program, project, or outcome
- **Data source:** Where will you get this data? Will you collect it? Will your partner?
- **Frequency:** How often will this information be collected or reported?
- **Baseline:** What is the current level of this knowledge, attitude, or practice in the target area?
- **End-of-project target:** What level or change do you expect to see at the conclusion of the program?

- **Discussion points:** What issues, thoughts, concerns, and suggestions do you have about collecting this indicator information?
- **Information user comments:** Who needs this information? Where will it be reported? What decision makers have asked for it?

Another tool designed for planning and evaluating population health programs is the **PRECEDE-PROCEED** model (Rural Health Information [RHI] Hub, 2021). This model can be used by NPs working in public health to create and evaluate programs designed to improve population health. **PRECEDE** stands for Predisposing, Reinforcing, and Enabling Constructs in Educational/Environmental Diagnosis and Evaluation. **PROCEED** stands for Policy, Regulatory, and Organizational Constructs in Educational and Environmental Development. Although this may seem overwhelming and complex, it is more easily understood as a roadmap for health promotion that includes the social, epidemiological, and ecological environment, as well as people's beliefs, abilities, skills, and behaviors. Simply put, using this approach, the following information is gathered during the PRECEDE steps/phases.

There are four steps/phases of identification that take place in the PRECEDE part of the model: (1) identification of the concluding result; (2) identifying the actions, routines, and/or ecological factors that affect the creation of health or community priorities; (3) identifying the predisposing, enabling, and reinforcing factors that can affect the behaviors, lifestyles, and/or ecological factors identified in step two; and finally (4) identifying the organizational or policy influences that can influence the change being implemented (The Community Toolbox, 2021). This information is then used as the framework for the PROCEED steps, which involve implementation, process evaluation, impact evaluation, and outcome evaluation (RHI HUB, 2021). This model can be used for a one-time intervention, as well as in a continuing evaluation process, because the evaluation portion of PROCEED helps to inform and revise the steps in the PRECEDE portion of this model and covers the actual execution of the model. The steps of the PROCEED portion of the model are outlined as follows: (1) Implementation (the plan and actual guiding of the intervention), (2) Process Evaluation (Is the plan doing what it set out to do?), (3) Impact Evaluation (Is the desired effect that was planned for the population occurring?), and Outcome Evaluation (Is the planned intervention leading to the outcome anticipated in Phase 1?) (The Community Toolbox, 2021). See **Figure 11-3**.

Emergency Preparedness and the Nurse Practitioner

Emergency preparedness refers to the management of resources and responsibilities in order to reduce the harmful effects of hazards. The WHO (2021c) defines an emergency as the "state in which normal procedures are interrupted, and immediate management measures need to be taken to prevent a disaster." The most common disasters are often meteorological (weather) or geological events, with outcomes ranging from localized to widespread. Threats of natural forces (thunderstorms, floods, tornadoes, hurricanes, winter storms, droughts, wildfires, landslides, earthquakes, tsunamis, volcanos, and dam failures) can also range from predictable to unpredictable. Man-made hazards include hazardous material spills, acts of terrorism, and nuclear accidents (WHO, 2021c). Man-made disasters are caused by

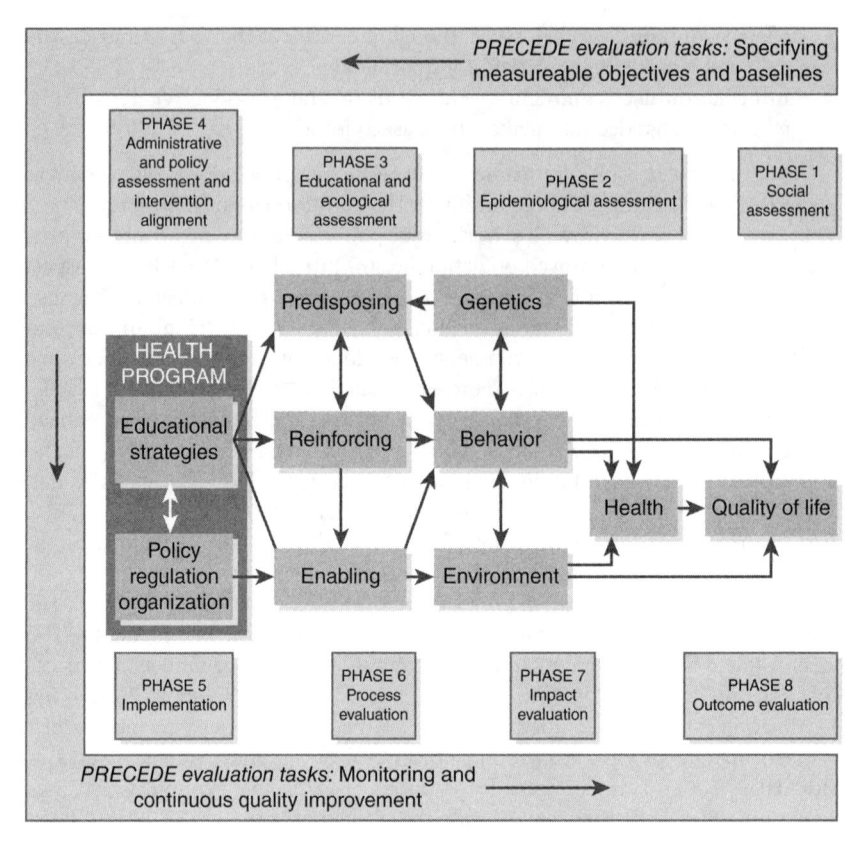

Figure 11-3 PRECEDE-PROCEED Model

Green, L., & Kreuter, M. (2005). *Health promotion planning: an educational and ecological approach* (4th ed.). Mayfield Publishers.

human actions, deliberate or otherwise, and include biological or biochemical terrorism, chemical spills, transportation accidents, and armed conflicts (WHO, 2021c). Complex emergencies occur when populations suffer significant casualties as the result of war and either civil or political conflict. Technological disasters are the result of industrial accidents, the release of nuclear energy, and fire or explosion from hazardous substances.

Since the tragedy of September 11th, 2001 (9/11), a new set of expectations has emerged for healthcare providers. However, the emergence of diseases such as Zika virus, Ebola virus, SARS, avian flu, hantavirus, West Nile virus, HIV/AIDS, influenza, and now COVID-19 add additional expectations for the NP (WHO, 2021c; Vitale & Curley, 2020; Fos, 2011). Emergency preparedness addresses not only being prepared for the event of biological, chemical, or nuclear/radiological terrorism, it also relates to emergent infectious diseases and conditions or events such as earthquakes, floods, tornadoes, blizzards, or hurricanes that place the health of families and communities at risk. The NP as a primary care provider is on the front lines of detecting emergent illness. Routine surveillance measures, such as the use of health indicator data, serve as baseline data. Hospitals routinely collect statistics on emergency room visits and volume, nosocomial infections, and unexplained or untimely deaths. Healthcare providers, hospitals, clinics, and public health departments must submit reports on specific communicable diseases. As NPs, you will be expected to file these reports pending assessment findings.

Syndromic surveillance can be used to detect uncommon and unusual health occurrences (CDC, 2021d). Based on an epidemiologic perspective, this approach relies on the recognition of unusual patterns of illness. For example, biological terrorism can be expected if a set of health patterns appear that are out of the ordinary, as in the following:

- A cluster of diseases with similar clinical presentations and at a similar stage of illness
- A cluster of unexplained illness in a well-defined population
- Unusually severe disease or higher mortality than expected for a given agent
- A cluster of cases with an unusual mode of transmission
- Multiple or serial outbreaks
- A disease not typical for a specific age group
- A disease unusual for a season or region of the country
- Clusters of the same illness in various locations
- Clusters of morbidity or mortality in animals or livestock similar to humans

One of the most important resources available to all practitioners is the CDC website. Visit www.cdc.gov or www.bt.cdc.gov, where an emergency preparedness/terrorism link can be found and is frequently updated. This website should be saved as a bookmark or on a favorites list for quick referencing.

COVID-19 has created worldwide, simultaneous, massive suffering. As NPs of today are entering a "different world" from one collectively known before, this has not been the only disaster of our times. Events such as Hurricane Katrina, tsunamis in Japan and Indonesia, earthquakes, and pandemic influenza, as well as the terrorist acts of 9/11 have increased the demand for human and financial resources needed to answer the pleas for relief of human suffering (L. Strong, personal communication, February 1, 2012). After 9/11, there has been an increased call for volunteers to become part of the resources available to respond to such events. A corps of volunteers is essential during these types of events, and volunteers can also be a valuable resource to promote the health and wellness of communities. Consider this short excerpt from Shery, a nurse volunteering to leave her own family and help others in need:

> After volunteering as a nurse in a small northeastern town of Sri Lanka a month after the devastating 2004 tsunami and volunteering a week after Hurricane Katrina in Biloxi, Mississippi, the similarities were striking and all too uncomfortable. The undercurrent of hopelessness and despondency was overwhelming, but the spirit in the response by the healthcare providers community was illuminating. Although the supplies were limited and communication was fragmented, it was the simplest words from another nurse who said, "You mean I can go see my family now?" that eliminated all other concerns and frustrations. The relief that crossed her face spoke volumes; my small team and I were able to cover shifts to provide much needed relief for the regular healthcare staff who were trying to care for their families and friends. The healthcare community response was unmistakable after such devastation. It is one community to help each other and patients, putting others first during their time of need.

Priority setting is the initial stage of planning in a disaster, as well as in any approach to improving a population's health. Volunteers may end up doing more than merely providing health care. The needs are far greater in most cases. Consider this reflection:

> Upon arriving a week after a devastating natural disaster, our team took pause on what is the priority. The makeshift "emergency departments" were set up each day to treat nonlife-threatening injuries and wounds and caring for the acute illnesses. Through the second week, the prioritization shifted to treating patients for their chronic illnesses, realizing that when their house was left in rubble and the local pharmacy was only a cement foundation, the people needed their everyday medications. Our team looked out to a sea of faces, each person sharing the same story, "I don't know the name of my medicine." The temporary ED then turned into more than caring for injuries, rather a primary care clinic and a place for someone to share their story.

Nurse practitioners might want to consider volunteer service in times of local, state, or national disasters by joining a medical reserve corps (MRC). The MRC units are composed of licensed healthcare professionals or students and support staff to assist and "strengthen the public health infrastructure of their communities. . . work towards increasing disease prevention, eliminating health disparities, and improving public health preparedness" (Office of the Surgeon General, 2013). The Division of the Civilian Volunteer Medical Reserve Corps (DCVMRC) takes the lead in organizing and training volunteers of the MRC, which was initiated post-9/11 by President Bush in 2002. Housed in the U.S. Surgeon General's Office and directed by members of the U.S. Public Health Service, MRCs are designed to be prepared to assist and respond to public health, medical, and emergency events (Office of the Surgeon General, 2013):

1. Public health and medical
   - Surgeon general priorities (disease prevention, elimination of health disparities, health literacy)
   - Disease detection
   - Health promotion
   - Health education
   - Health clinic support and staffing
2. Emergency preparedness and response
   - Mass dispensing and vaccinations
   - Pandemic flu planning
   - Preparedness campaigns
   - Shelter operations and support
   - First-responder rehab
   - Mass casualty incident/emergency response

The NP/DNP is poised as a future leader in assessing population health, designing interventions to improve community and population health, evaluating health outcomes of those interventions and programs, and implementing changes to improve programs. Health promotion and disease prevention topics for individual patients, families, and communities, as well as national and even global communities, are part of the NP/DNP charge for population health and care of the future of the nation.

Nurse practitioners like Julie have participated in global health experiences, demonstrating improved comprehensive physical assessment, the ability to recognize and diagnose infectious disease processes while demonstrating sensitivity to cultural norms. After participating in global experiences, NPs report an improved ability to work as a health care team, solving problems without the use of technology or laboratory equipment, and depending on their own knowledge and the expertise of their healthcare team. In these settings, health professions must work closely in order to broaden their assessment skills, because many health problems may not have been previously encountered in their own practice at "home."

Diverse populations are found throughout the world in both urban and rural locations. Global experiences in population health are not limited to "far-away" locations. As Julie's story concludes, "caring for patients in the environment in which they live is a 'global experience.' As members of the global community, it is our duty to care for each other."

♀ JULIE'S STORY

For over 12 years, Julie Stewart, DNP, APRN fostered relationships with communities in inner cities of Kingston, Jamaica, an area known for poverty and violence. Physician and nurse practitioner teams worked together to deliver care to this population, becoming the source of primary care for many of these communities. The healthcare professionals who serve on these mission trips work in makeshift clinics, upwards of 12 hours a day, often under a tent or in a small community building or church, treating over 100 patients a day. Diabetes and hypertension are common diagnoses but create challenges in education and prevention work due to confounding economic and dietary challenges. Other common ailments are skin diseases, parasites, and acute medical emergencies including gynecological and surgical interventions. Julie described her mission trips as being a member of a "global interdependent community" where her work as a DNP allowed her to share with unique cultures and societies abroad, but she was also able to assess and treat diseases in her patients' own environment, under unique social, economic, and political variables in which different populations reside. She would often remind her students that we become "comfortable" in the care environments in which we most often work: an office, hospital, or clinic. However, it is not until you integrate the care model into individual patient's lives that you understand the individual variables that affect health.

Seminar Discussion Questions

1. Identify three priority issues for improving health in your community.
2. Describe the incidence and prevalence of a disease monitored in your state.
3. Discuss each of the three prevention levels as it pertains to the disease you chose.
4. Why does identifying populations in practice help improve health outcomes?
5. How does *Healthy People 2030* assist in creating population health? How can you promote the goals of *Healthy People 2030*?
6. Using the PRECEDE-PROCEED model, draft a program plan and an evaluation of a health need.

References

Advisory Committee on Immunization Practices (ACIP). (2021). *Vaccines.* https://www.cdc.gov/vaccines/acip/index.html

American Association of Colleges of Nursing (AACN). (2006). *The essentials of master's education in nursing.* https://www.aacnnursing.org/Portals/42/Publications/DNPEssentials.pdf

American Association of Colleges of Nursing (AACN). (2021). *DNP essentials.* https://www.aacnnursing.org/DNP/DNP-Essentials

Anderson, B. A. (2020). Facing the nursing workforce shortage: Policies and initiatives to promote a resilient healthcare system. In deChesnay, M., & Anderson, B. A., *Caring for the vulnerable: Perspectives in nursing theory, practice, and research* (5th ed., pp. 363–372). Jones and Bartlett Learning.

Association for Prevention Teaching and Research (APTR). (2020). *Clinical Prevention and Population Health (CPPH) curriculum framework.* https://www.teachpopulationhealth.org/

AstraZeneca. (2021). *COVID-19 vaccine authorized for emergency use.* https://www.astrazeneca.com/media-centre/press-releases/2021/astrazeneca-covid-19-vaccine-authorised-for-emergency-use-by-the-world-health-organization.html

Bongiorno, A. W., & deChesnay, M. (2020). Developing population-based programs for the vulnerable. In deChesnay, M., & Anderson, B. A. (Eds.), *Caring for the vulnerable: Perspectives in nursing theory, practice, and research* (5th ed., pp. 229–237). Jones & Bartlett Learning.

Branson, B. M., Handsfield, H. H., Lampe, M. A., Janssen, R. S., Taylor, A. W., Lyss, S. B., & Clark, J. E. (2006). Revised recommendations for HIV testing of adults, adolescents, and pregnant women in health-care settings. *MMWR Recommendations and Reports, 55*(RR-14), 1–17.

Burke, R. C., Sepkowitz, K. A., Bernstein, K. T., Karpati, A. M., Myers, J. E., Tsoi, B. W., & Beiger, E. M. (2007). Why don't physicians test for HIV? A review of the US literature. *AIDS, 21,* 1617–1624.

Cao, B., Wang, Y., Wen, D., et al. (2020). A trial of lopinavir-ritonavir in adults hospitalized with severe COVID-19. *New England Journal of Medicine.* [Epub ahead of print].

Centers for Disease Control and Prevention. (2020). *Coronavirus: Resources and references.* https://www.cdc.gov/coronavirus/resources.html

Centers for Disease Control and Prevention. (2021a). *Principles of epidemiology in public health practice* (3rd ed.). http://www.cdc.gov/osels/scientific_edu/SS1978/Lesson1/Section10.html

Centers for Disease Control and Prevention. (2021b). *Different COVID-19 vaccines.* https://www.cdc.gov/coronavirus/2019-ncov/vaccines/different-vaccines.html

Centers for Disease Control and Prevention. (2021c). *Cases in the U.S.* https://www.cdc.gov/coronavirus/2019-ncov/cases-in-us.html.

Centers for Disease Control and Prevention. (2021d). *Syndromic surveillance.* https://www.cdc.gov/ehrmeaningfuluse/Syndromic.html

Chen, N., Min, Z., Dong, et al. (2020). Epidemiological and clinical characteristics of 99 cases of novel coronavirus in Wuhan, China: A retrospective study. *Lancet, 395,* 507–513. https://doi.10.1016/S0140-6736(20)30211-7

Fee, E., & Bu, L. (2010). The origins of public health nursing: the Henry Street Visiting Nurse Service. *American Journal of Public Health, 100*(7), 1206–1207. https://doi.org/10.2105/AJPH.2009.186049

Fos, P. (2011). *Epidemiology foundations: The science of public health.* Jossey-Bass.

Friis, R. H., & Sellers, A. T. (2004). *Epidemiology for public health practice* (3rd ed.). Jones and Bartlett.

Gandhi, M., Yokie, D. S., & Havlir, D. V. (2020). Asymptomatic transmission, the Achilles' heel of current strategies to control Covid-19. *New England Journal of Medicine.* [Epub ahead of print].

Geleris, J., Sun, Y., Platt, J., et al. (2020). Observational study of hydroxychloroquine in hospitalized patients with Covid-19. *New England Journal of Medicine.* [Epub ahead of print].

Gordis, L. (2009). *Epidemiology* (4th ed.). Saunders Elsevier.

Green, L., & Kreuter, M. K. (2005). *Health program planning: An educational and ecological approach* (4th ed.). McGraw-Hill.

Guan, W.-J., Ni, Z.-Y., Hu, Y., et al. (2020). Clinical characteristics of coronavirus disease 2019 in China. *New England Journal of Medicine.* [Epub ahead of print].

Harvard Health. (2021). *Treatments for COVID-19.* https://www.health.harvard.edu/diseases-and-conditions/treatments-for-covid-19

He, W., Goodkind, D., & Kowal, P. (2016). *An aging world: 2015.* U.S. Census Bureau, International Population Reports, P95/16-1, U.S. Government Publishing Office, Washington, DC.

Henry J. Kaiser Family Foundation. (2012). *The HIV/AIDS epidemic in the United States* (fact sheet). Author.

Holstein, B. (2020). Coronavirus 101. *The Journal for Nurse Practitioners, 16,* 416–419. https://doi.org/10.1016/j.nurpra.2020.02.021

Huang, C., Wang, Y., Li, X., et al. (2020). Clinical features of patients infected with 2019 novel coronavirus in Wuhan, China. *Lancet, 395*(10223), 497–506.

Institute of Medicine. (2012). *Primary care and public health: Exploring integration to improve population health.* Washington, DC: National Academies Press. http://www.iom.edu/Reports/2012/Primary-Care-and-Public-Health.aspx

Keshavjee, S., & Farmer, P. (2012). Tuberculosis, drug resistance, and the history of modern medicine. *New England Journal of Medicine, 67*(10), 931–936. https://doi.org/10.1056/NEJMra1205429

Kindig, D., & Stoddard, G. (2003). What is population health? *American Journal of Public Health, 93*(3), 380–383. https://doi.org/10.2105/ajph.93.3.380

Livingston, E. H., Malani, P., & Creech, C. (2021). The Johnson & Johnson Vaccine for COVID-19. *JAMA.* https://doi.org/10.1001/jama.2021.2927

Macha, K., & McDonough, J. (2012). *Epidemiology for advanced nursing practice.* Jones & Bartlett Learning.

Maurer, F. A., & Smith, C. M. (2013). Community/public health nursing practice: Health for families and populations (5th ed.). Elsevier/Saunders.

Measure Evaluation. (2021). *Population, health, and environment: M & E training tool kit.* https://www.measureevaluation.org/resources/tools/population-health-and-environment/population-health-and-environment-training-materials/

Merrill, R. M. (2021). *Introduction to epidemiology* (8th ed.). Jones & Bartlett Learning.

Moderna. (2021). *Moderna COVID-19 vaccine for providers.* https://www.modernatx.com/covid19vaccine-eua/providers/about-vaccine

Munster, V.J., Koopmans, M., van Doremalen, N., et al. (2020). A novel coronavirus emerging in China: Key questions for impact assessment. *New England Journal of Medicine, 382,* 692–694.

National Institute of Health. (2020). *COVID-19 treatment guidelines.* https://www.covid19treatmentguidelines.nih.gov/

Novavax. (2021). *COVID-19 vaccine updates.* https://www.novavax.com/covid-19-coronavirus-vaccine-candidate-updates

Office of the Surgeon General. (2013). *Strategic plan DCVMRC (2011–2013).* Retrieved from https://medicalreservecorps.gov/pageViewFldr/About/StrategicPlan1113

Pfizer. (2021). *All COVID vaccine updates.* https://www.pfizer.com/health/coronavirus/updates

Rural Health Information (RHI) Hub. (2021). *PRECEDE/PROCEED.* https://www.ruralhealthinfo.org/toolkits/health-promotion/2/program-models/precede-proceed

Shi, L., & Singh, D. A. (2021). The role of race, culture, ethics, and advocacy in advanced practice. In DeNisco, S. M. (Ed.) *Advanced practice nursing: Essential knowledge for the profession* (4th ed., pp. 667–705). Jones & Bartlett Learning.

Sinopharm. (2021). *Chinese COVID-19 vaccine efficacy better than expected.* http://www.sinopharm.com/en/s/1395-4173-38923.html

Sputnik. (2021). *The first registered COVID-19 vaccine: Proved human adenoviral vaccine technology.* https://sputnikvaccine.com/about-vaccine/

The Community Toolbox. (2021). *Chapter 2: Section 2. PRECEDE/PROCEED.* https://ctb.ku.edu/en/table-contents/overview/other-models-promoting-community-health-and-development/preceder-proceder/main

The Nurses' Health Study. (2021). *About NHS.* https://www.nurseshealthstudy.org/about-nhs

U.S. Department of Health and Human Services. (2016). *Guidelines for the use of prevention and treatment of opportunistic infections in HIV-infected adults and adolescents.* https://aidsinfo.nih.gov/contentfiles/lvguidelines/adult_oi.pdf

U.S. Department of Health and Human Services. (2017). *Guidelines for the use of antiretroviral agents in pediatric HIV infection.* https://aidsinfo.nih.gov/guidelines/html/2/pediatric-arv-guidelines/0

U.S. Department of Health and Human Services ODPHP. (2020). *History of the Healthy People Initiative.* https://health.gov/our-work/healthy-people/about-healthy-people/history-healthy-people

U.S. Department of Health and Human Services ODPHP. (2021). *Healthy People 2030: Tobacco use.* https://health.gov/healthypeople/objectives-and-data/browse-objectives/tobacco-use

U.S. Preventive Services Task Force (USPSTF). (2021). *Recommendation Topics.* https://uspreventiveservicestaskforce.org/uspstf/recommendation-topics

Van Leuven, K. (2012). Population aging: Implications for nurse practitioners. *Journal for Nurse Practitioners, 8*(7), 554–559.

Vitale, P. A., & Curley, A. L. (2020). Epidemiological methods and measurements: Part I. In Curley, A. L. (Ed.), *Population-based nursing: Concepts and competencies for advanced practice* (3rd ed., pp. 53–86). Springer Publishing Company.

Ward, M. (2009). Physical function. In Hochberg, M., Silman, A., Smolen, J., Weinblatt, & Weisman, M. (Eds.), *Rheumatoid Arthritis*, 231–236. https://www.sciencedirect.com/book/9780323054751/rheumatoid-arthritis

World Health Organization. (2021a). *Tuberculosis.* https://www.who.int/news-room/fact-sheets/detail/tuberculosis

World Health Organization. (2021b). *HIV/AIDS.* http://www.who.int/hiv/en

World Health Organization. (2021c). *Emergency preparedness.* https://www.who.int/environmental_health_emergencies/preparedness/en/

CHAPTER 12

Electronic Health Record and Impact on Healthcare Outcomes

Stephen C. Burrows

Moving to Electronic Documentation/ Electronic Health Record: Reasons for Doing So

The implementation of electronic health records (EHRs) has great potential to improve the quality of patient care compared to the use of paper medical records. An EHR offers many benefits for clinicians and their patients and provides functions unavailable without this technology.

Greater Access to More Complete and Accurate Patient Information

An EHR gives clinicians access to the information necessary to deliver quality health care that ensures the "right care to the right patient at the right time" (Clancy, 2009, p. 11; Collinsworth et al., 2014, p. 2).

King, Patel, Jamoom, and Furukawa (2014) examined the clinical benefits provided by EHRs to physicians by reviewing data from two large surveys of office-based physicians in the United States. With over 3,000 physician responses, King et al. concluded that "over three-quarters of EHR adopters reported that EHR use enhanced patient care overall" (2014, p. 400). Specifically, "EHR adopters reported benefits of EHR use for specific measures of clinical quality, patient safety, and efficiency" (King et al., 2014, p. 400).

Bae et al. (2017) examined the use of an EHR as part of the management of chronic conditions for primary care. Focusing on the effect of the EHR in regard to health behavior counseling in the primary care setting, the authors "examined 34,315 adult patient visits to 1,425 primary care physicians during 2007–2010" (Bae et al., 2017, p. 260). Utilizing the Institute of Medicine's (IOM) eight key functionalities, they focused on the Office of the National Coordinator for Health Information Technology's (ONC) four "core" functionalities of an EHR: (a) health information and data, (b) decision support, (c) order entry and management, and (d) result management of an EHR system (Blumenthal et al., 2006). Their analysis demonstrated a "significant increase in the probability of health behavior counseling services" with the use of an EHR "with seven of the eight components (excluding the availability of imaging results) increased the probability that counseling occurred at a primary care visit by 24.9%" (Bae et al., 2017, p. 265). Their study provided "empirical evidence that EHR systems with key functionalities can support the provision of effective primary care improved documentation" (Bae et al., 2017, p. 265).

Access to more complete information from evaluation and treatment strengthens a provider's clinical decision-making process by presenting a more complete picture of the patient's clinical information. Legibility of handwriting is not an issue when information is entered into and accessed from an EHR.

Increased Care Coordination

EHRs provide better access to data than their paper counterparts. Sharing of patient information among providers, therapists, other healthcare providers, hospitals, and health systems is greatly facilitated and enhances the coordination of care. A number of studies have looked at the effectiveness of EHRs in the coordination of care (Elfrink, 2009; Goldzweig et al., 2005; Merchant et al., 2014; O'Malley et al., 2010; Ribeiro & Cavalcanti, 2020; Watterson et al., 2020; Youngblut, 1998). O'Malley et al. (2010) found "that commercial ambulatory care EMRs facilitate care coordination within a practice by making data available at the point of care" (2010, p. 183). Goetz Goldberg et al. (2012) reported the greatest value and benefit to clinicians using EHRs as "increased organization, accessibility, and accuracy of patient documentation" (2012, p. e50). This was further evidenced by their findings regarding improvement in the quality of care performance measures "such as mammography screening and diabetes care, as demonstrated through performance reports shared with our research team" (p. e51).

Watterson et al. (2020) focused on the key role EHRs play in regard to communication among providers. Utilizing "relational coordination (RC), a measure of team communication and coordination" with the use of an EHR, they found that "EHR use facilitates improved RC among primary care team members" (Watterson et al., 2020, p. 271). Their findings "provide support for the hypothesis that EHRs contribute to better RC (team communication and task coordination), which, in turn, could lead to the observed improvements to care)" (Watterson et al., 2020, p. 272).

Greater Efficiency

Paper charts no longer need to be located and transported to the clinician. Electronic charts are more easily located and often allow more than one person to work within a chart at the same time. Walker et al. (2005) examined the value of electronic exchange of healthcare information between providers, including the bidirectional exchange with laboratories, imaging centers, pharmacies, and others. With full national exchange in place, they estimated a net savings of "$77.8 billion annually, or approximately 5 percent of the projected $1.661 trillion spent on U.S. health care in 2003" (2005, pp. W5-16). More modest savings can be seen in the ambulatory sector through a reduction in transcription costs, as well as the cost for chart pull, storage, and refiling. Improved documentation can support more accurate reimbursement coding (Office of the National Coordinator for Health Information Technology, 2018).

Patient Participation and Empowerment

Providers and patients sharing access to electronic health information supports a collaborative environment of informed decision making and promotes patient participation in the management of chronic conditions. Providers can give patients "full and accurate information about all of their medical evaluations" and "create an avenue for communication with their patients" (Office of the National Coordinator for Health Information Technology [ONC], 2018, para. 3,4). Included with this more active role in their care, patients can receive electronic copies of their medical records after a clinical visit or hospital stay, along with improved instructions, information, and education.

Influencing Forces

Over the past number of years, the implementation and use of EHRs has been one of the highest priorities for healthcare providers, organizations, and government agencies in the United States (Webster, 2010). In April 2004, then-President George W. Bush signed Executive Order 13335 (Bush, 2004). This provided for the establishment of the Office of the National Coordinator for Health Information Technology (ONCHIT) and created the "leadership," as well as a national vision, for the "development and nationwide implementation of an interoperable health information technology infrastructure to improve the quality and efficiency of health care" (Bush, 2004, p. 160). Over the ensuing years, several strategies, committees, and contracts were created and awarded. While the expectation was that many clinicians would move toward EHR implementation, very few did. In 2008, DesRoches et al. (2008) stated only "4% of physicians reported" were using a "fully functional electronic records system, and 13% reported having a basic system" (2008, p. 54). Decker, Jamoom, and Sisk (2012) found, as of 2011, only "24.2% of physicians in solo or two-physician practices had adopted a basic EHR, compared with 37.1% of groups of three to nine physicians and 60% of physicians in groups of 10 or more" (p. 1111). Shamus and Stern (2011) reported among physical therapists "anecdotal evidence suggests only 13–15% of physical therapists" and "most of these cases appear to be in the inpatient environment" (p. 196). These rates of adoption suggest "that EHRs will reach maximum penetration by the year 2024," 10 years beyond President Bush's original goal of 2104 (Zandieh et al., 2008, p. 755). Recognizing this lag, Meaningful Use (MU) was created as "we have not moved significantly to extend the availability of EHRs from a few large institutions to the smaller clinics and practices where most Americans receive their health care" (Blumenthal & Tavenner, 2010).

In February 2009, then-President Barack Obama signed into law the American Recovery and Reinvestment Act (ARRA). Often called the "The Stimulus Act," it appropriated federal expenditures toward a variety of national projects across differing sectors of the U.S. economy. Included within the ARRA was the Health Information Technology for Economic and Clinical Health Act (HITECH) providing $17.2 billion for incentives and $2 billion for grants toward "supporting the adoption and use of EHRs" which will "support [the] liftoff for the creation of a nationwide system of EHRs" (Blumenthal & Tavenner, 2010, p. 501). Equally important, HITECH's goal is not adoption alone but "meaningful use" of EHRs (Blumenthal & Tavenner, 2010, p. 501; Spicer, 2009; Wright et al., 2014).

Meaningful Use

Although the Meaningful Use Program has concluded, its impact on increased and widespread implementation of EHRs cannot be overlooked. The program's Eligible Professionals (EPs) and Eligible Hospitals (EHs) participated to receive incentive monies through the "Medicare and Medicaid EHR Incentive Programs" by using certified EHR technology and demonstrating "that they are meaningfully using their EHRs by meeting thresholds for a number of objectives" (Centers for Medicare and Medicaid Services, 2014, p. 28).

The final rule establishing the three stages of Meaningful Use was announced by the Centers of Medicare and Medicaid Services (CMS) in July 2010 and is designed to support EPs and EHs with implementing and using EHRs in a "meaningful" way with the ultimate goal of improving the quality and safety of health care in the United States. Each of the three stages has specific goals, priorities, and increasing requirements (**Figure 12-1**).

Stage 1

Stage 1 began in 2011 and includes the basic functionalities for EHRs. The requirements are focused on providers capturing patient data and sharing that data either with the patient or with other healthcare professionals.

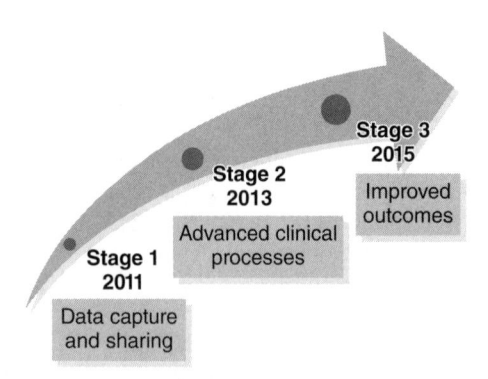

Figure 12-1 A Conceptual Approach to Meaningful Use

Centers for Medicare & Medicaid Services. (2010). Medicare & Medicaid EHR Incentive Program: Meaningful Use Stage 1 Requirements Overview. Retrieved from https://www.cms.gov/Regulations-and-Guidance/Legislation/EHRIncentivePrograms/downloads/MU_Stage1_ReqOverview.pdf

"Data capture and sharing"
- Electronically capturing health information in a standardized format
- Using that information to track key clinical conditions
- Communicating that information for care coordination processes
- Initiating the reporting of clinical quality measures and public health information
- Using information to engage patients and their families in their care

Stage 2
Stage 2 began in 2014 and looks toward the use of advanced clinical processes. The requirements in this stage are focused on health information exchange between providers and promotes patient engagement by giving patients secure online access to their health information.

"Advanced clinical processes"
- More rigorous health information exchange (HIE)
- Increased requirements for e-prescribing and incorporating lab results
- Electronic transmission of patient care summaries across multiple settings
- More patient-controlled data

Stage 3
"Improved outcomes"
- Improving quality, safety, and efficiency, leading to improved health outcomes
- Decision support for national high-priority conditions
- Patient access to self-management tools
- Access to comprehensive patient data through patient-centered HIE
- Improving population health (Centers for Medicare and Medicaid Services, 2010; Reisman, 2017, p. 572)

Each of the Meaningful Use stages has multiple clinically related measures with which EPs and EHs must meet to receive the bonus payments. By focusing not only on the implementation of certified EHRs but also on their meaningful use through the submission of the measures, the EHR Incentive Program is about "the effective use of EHRs to achieve health and efficiency" and to "improve the quality, safety, and efficiency of care while reducing disparities" (Centers for Medicare and Medicaid Services, 2010, p. 2).

In 2018, the Centers for Medicare and Medicaid Services transitioned the Meaningful Use program to "Promoting Interoperability" to "focus on interoperability, improve flexibility, relieve burden and place emphasis on measures that require the electronic exchange of health information between providers and patients" (Bresnick, 2018; Centers for Medicare and Medicaid Services, 2018, para. 16). In many ways similar to "Meaningful Use," this new program is also divided into three stages to "encourage eligible professionals (EPs), eligible hospitals and critical access hospitals (CAHs) to adopt, implement, upgrade and successfully demonstrate meaningful use of certified electronic health record technology (CEHRT)" (Centers for Medicare and Medicaid Services, 2017, p. 1).

The Electronic Health Record

Numerous terms are used to describe the concept of an EHR. However, basically it can be defined as providing "real-time, patient-centered records . . . available instantly and securely to authorized users" (Office of the National Coordinator for Health Information Technology, 2019a, para. 1). Additionally, EHRs are thought of as a "longitudinal electronic record of patient health information generated by one or more encounters in any care delivery setting" (Electronic Clinical Quality Measures, 2021, para. 1).

Often, the terms *electronic medical record (EMR)* and *electronic health record (EHR)* are used interchangeably. It is important to note that these terms describe completely different concepts, albeit dependent on each other. Electronic medical records are often thought of as simply the digital version of the paper medical record from a single clinician's office. It is the "legal record created in hospitals and ambulatory environments" (Garets & Davis, 2006, p. 2) and contains important pieces of the patient's medical history, including medical diagnoses, prescribed medication, provider-generated treatment plans, immunization records, medication and food or environmental allergies, radiology imaging, and laboratory results (Garrett & Seidman, 2011). An EHR contains all of the items in an EMR plus others that focus on the patient's entire health by "going beyond standard clinical data collected in the provider's office and inclusive of a broader view on a patient's care" by sharing "information with other health care providers, such as laboratories and specialists" (Garrett & Seidman, 2011, para. 5). The National Alliance for Health Information Technology adds that EHRs contain functions that "conform to nationally recognized interoperability standards and that can be created, managed, and consulted by authorized clinicians and staff across more than one health care organization" (The National Alliance for Health Information Technology, 2008, p. 6).

Benefits of Using an EHR

1. Improved quality of patient care
   Kern, Barrón, Dhopeshwarkar, Edwards, and Kaushal (2013) looked at data from 4,403 ambulatory providers and the effect using an EHR might have on several quality indicators—hemoglobin A1c testing for diabetic patients, breast cancer screening, chlamydia screening, and colorectal cancer screening. They found the physicians who were using an EHR "provided significantly higher rates of recommended care than physicians using paper for [the] four quality measures.... The magnitude of the differences between EHR use and paper for these measures ranged from approximately 3 to 13 percentage points" (p. 500).

   In a retrospective study of a 431 bed urban hospital, researchers examined the impact of the adoption of an integrated EHR on quality of nursing care, nursing care cost and nursing attrition rates (Walker-Czyz, 2016). The following data was extracted: fall rates, pressure ulcers, ventilator-associated pneumonia (VAP), central line associated bloodstream infections (CLABSIs), catheter-associated urinary tract infections (CAUTIs), and costs measured in nursing hours. It was found that the EHR did positively impact several quality outcomes including a 15% reduction in hospital fall rates and a decline in decreased catheter-associated urinary tract infections and central line-associated blood infections (Walker-Czyz, 2016).

Electronic health records also have the potential to improve quality of care by providing rapid access to more complete patient records and by providing enhanced decision support, clinical alerts, reminders, and medical information.

2. Reduction in medical errors
Zlabek, Wickus, and Mathiason (2011) reported a 14% decrease in medication errors and a 38.9% decrease in near misses per 1,000 hospital days after computerized provider order entry (CPOE) was implemented in their hospital.

Examining the occurrence of medication errors in emergency departments (ED) currently utilizing EHRs with two different departments using conventional handwritten records, Vaidotas et al. (2019) found "the use of electronic medical record(s) at emergency departments units was associated with lower rates of medication errors in this study" (Vaidotas et al., 2019, p. 5). The authors attributed this to "safety warnings at different steps of the prescription, separation, and administration of the medication" as part of the functions of EHRs (Vaidotas et al., 2019, p. 4).

3. Improved care coordination and communication
A number of studies have looked at the effectiveness of EHRs in the coordination of care (Goetz Goldberg et al., 2012; Goldzweig et al., 2005; O'Malley et al., 2010). O'Malley et al. (2010) found "that commercial ambulatory care EMRs facilitate care coordination within a practice by making data available at the point of care" (p. 183). Goetz Goldberg et al. (2012) reported the greatest value and benefit to clinicians using EHRs as "increased organization, accessibility, and accuracy of patient documentation" (p. e50). This was further evidenced by their findings regarding improvement in the quality of care performance measures "such as mammography screening and diabetes care, as demonstrated through performance reports shared with our research team" (2012, p. e51).

4. Enhanced patient safety
EHRs are ideal for alerting providers to allergies, drug interactions, abnormal laboratory test findings, and redundant test orders. As an EHR becomes more comprehensive and "intelligent," it can trigger provider-alerts to health safety issues such as newly identified medication side effects, product recalls, and new strategies for disease management and preventive care. Such a system would allow a provider to "preemptively" notify patients of important health issues based on a continual automated process of cross-referencing of their medical histories with the latest medical findings. That could change health care from an encounter- and patient-complaint-driven system of care to a more proactive approach to complete health management.

5. Increased efficiencies and cost savings
Kazley et al. (2014) looked at national data representing individuals 18 years or older who were admitted for inpatient care (Kazley et al., 2014). Examining data of over 5 million patients from 550 hospitals, they found a 9.66% reduction in the average cost per patient when treated in a hospital with advanced EHRs.

Zlabek, Wickus, and Mathiason (2009) investigated the cost savings impact of EHR implementation. They examined data over a 2-year period (1-year pre-EHR and 1-year post-EHR implementation). Among a number of other factors, they found a 74.6% drop in monthly transcription costs for a total yearly reduction of $667,896 and a 26.6% reduction in the cost of copy paper for an annual savings of $11,815.

In the ambulatory sector, Adler-Milstein, et al. (2013) found an average reduction of "$41.60 per member per month among Medicare beneficiaries when using an EHR" (Adler-Milstein et al., 2013, p. E8). Due to their very nature, EHRs provide the time-saving efficiency of "collect [data] once, [then] use many times" (Barton et al., 2011, p. 99).

Highfill (2020) conducted a literature review examining the association of EHR implementation with lower cost of care in hospitals (Highfill, 2020). Findings showed "hospitals with EHRs had lower costs than comparable hospitals by more than 7%, on average" with reductions in cost attributed to "the prevention of adverse drug events, shorter lengths of stay, and efficiencies arising from features unique to the EHR" (Highfill, 2020, p. 68).

6. Increased population health
   Electronic health records have great potential for public and population health through their ability to allow the aggregation of multiple sets of patient data and by "improving the reporting and investigation of diseases and conditions that are mandated for reporting to state and local public health agencies" (Friedman et al., 2013, p. 1561). Electronic health records also have the potential to provide estimates of "disease burden and its distribution in the population and population subgroups. Such estimates could facilitate program planning, targeting, implementation, and monitoring (Friedman et al., 2013, p. 1561).

   Lu et al. (2020) examined the EHR records of "373,861 patients aged 18 to 85 years" seen in an outpatient setting and having at least one blood pressure measurement on record (p. 4). They found over 15% of these patients to have markedly elevated blood pressure and "suggest that there are immense opportunities to improve care by prioritizing patients with markedly elevated blood pressure" and "partnering with them to efficiently and effectively control their blood pressure" (Lu et al., 2020, p. 7). Recognizing the important and growing role in the management of patient populations, the authors recognize how EHRs are "increasingly used to improve quality of care, support the design and conduct of intervention, and enhance public health efforts (Lu et al., 2020, p. 9).

Health Information Exchange

One of the ways in which full advantage of EHRs can be taken is through the electronic exchange of patient data. The goal of Meaningful Use is not to simply create isolated islands of clinical data but to form interconnected databases capable of leveraging each other's strengths. A health information exchange (HIE) allows "health care providers and patients to appropriately access and securely share a patient's vital medical information electronically—improving the speed, quality, safety and cost of patient care," and provides for "timely sharing of vital patient information [which] can better inform decision making at the point of care" (Office of the National Coordinator for Health Information Technology, 2019b, para. 1,2). It is the vision of the U.S. federal government to create "an interoperable health IT ecosystem (that) makes the right data available to the right people at the right time across products and organizations in a way that can be relied upon and meaningfully used by recipients" (ONCHIT, 2014, p. 9).

Barriers and Challenges to EHR Adoption

There are many obstacles to adoption of an EHR. These obstacles can be divided into a number of categories.

1. Financial
   The initial purchase cost of an EHR can be expensive. Estimates for the initial purchase of an EHR vary from $15,000 to $70,000 per provider, with most averaging about $30,000 (Office of the National Coordinator for Health Information Technology, 2014). Costs for larger institutions (multiple-hospital health systems) can reach over $600 million when all costs are considered (software licensing purchase, software/hardware upgrades, staffing, etc.). Costs that haven't been completely considered can also provide a financial drain: "Hospital boards and managers too frequently consider only the initial cost of acquisition plus initial annual maintenance fees when considering EHR bids" (Eastaugh, 2013, p. 36).

   In addition to these costs, there is inevitably a loss of productivity during the initial phases of implementation. Wang et al. (2003) estimate this to be a "temporary loss of productivity . . . of 20% in the first month, 10% in the second month, and 5% in the third month, with a subsequent return to baseline productivity levels" (p. 398).

2. Technical
   a. Electronic health records are complex systems and require a certain level of computer skills by those who may be using the software. Many clinicians have "insufficient technical knowledge and skills to deal with EMRs, and . . . this results in resistance" (Boonstra & Broekhuis, 2010, p. 4). It is imperative that all users receive "proper technical training and support" prior to any EHR implementation (Boonstra & Broekhuis, 2010, p. 8).
   b. To overcome some of this fear, training is highly recommended. Bredfeldt, Awad, Joseph, and Snyder (2013) surveyed providers who were undergoing implementation and found "the providers valued advanced training on EHR tools and workflows, to the extent that they were willing to participate on Saturdays and return for additional content" (p. 8).

3. Complexity of selection and implementation process
   Selecting the most appropriate EHR can be a daunting task. It is estimated there are over 400 software vendors from whom to select a product. Most clinicians are uncertain where to begin.

4. Organizational change barriers
   Implementation of a system as large and complex as an EHR represents tremendous change for any organization. There is bound to be moderate to significant disruption of workflow and processes (Carayon et al., 2009; Pugh, 2019). Lin, Lin, and Roan (2012) pinpoint the attitude toward change: "Change, after all, causes people concern and is closely followed by a sense of anxiety, insecurity, inequity and threat" (p. 1967). Implementation of an EHR typically involves approaches to "change management" and having a "good change management process established that creates reasonable expectations, anticipates changes, and sets a strong foundation for success process established that creates reasonable expectations, anticipates changes, and sets a strong foundation for success" (Cohen, 2015, p. 113; Giniat et al., 2012; Henderson et al., 2013).

Converting to Electronic Health Record

When converting to electronic documentation, a number of imperative steps can be taken to ensure a successful implementation. Preparing for a successful conversion requires both the right approach and mindset, as much as the right technology selection.

Preparation

Setting Goal and Vision

First and perhaps foremost is having a clear vision of the end state being pursued. A few simple questions can help this process: What is it we are trying to achieve? Why are we implementing an EHR? What are the reasons to do so?

Having a shared vision means "goals and benefits are clearly defined, meaningful and measurable . . . [the] organization knows what success looks like and how to achieve it. Once the goals are set, it is essential to communicate that vision with all of those who will be involved in the process. Keep the vision visible; once it has been created, share it with various people and revisit it often" (Merrill, 2010, para. 5).

After gaining an understanding of the organization's vision, an EHR selection committee should be formed. This group consists of individuals from cross-institutional settings and brings "differing perspectives on how the EHR will be used . . . possess[es] a wide array of skills and knowledge . . . [and] consist[s] of true end users and not just personnel who make IT purchasing decisions" (Office of the National Coordinator for Health Information Technology [ONC], 2019a, para. 4).

Readiness Assessment

Evaluating an organization's readiness to adopt an EHR provides a window into the areas that need attending. This step helps clarify the state of readiness of all members of an organization for EHR adoption, how an organization is using current resources, and what steps you need to take for successful adoption of an EHR.

Available Resources

Understand resources available for the EHR implementation. This includes funding for purchase, upgrades to current technology infrastructure, and personnel. This applies to both the current size and needs, as well as any potential or future growth. Determine your facility's current number of sites and users.

Workflow Documentation

Although this step is too often overlooked or not completed fully, understanding the current processes and how they will be completed in an EHR is prerequisite to a successful implementation. Documenting current workflow consists of recording (in written or graphical form) who is involved in each step of how business occurs. This will also assist in identifying changes that could occur with implementation and with use.

Request for Proposal

Once these factors have been assessed, vendor seeking may begin. From the list of required functionality, current resources, and the organization's vision, potential vendors can be narrowed down. To better understand how each may fulfill the needs of an organization, a request for proposal (RFP) can be prepared. This document is provided to selected vendors and solicits responses to specific information about their product and what their specific approach is to EHR implementation. A thorough RFP is typically a lengthy document and asks the vendor to provide general company information (length of time in business, number of employees, number of implementations), current EHR functionality (in response to organizations' specific needs as identified during the readiness assessment), how the vendor's system will follow the organization's current workflow, how much customization is necessary and what is the cost, timeline for implementation and personnel involved, and the technologic requirements of the vendor's EHR. It is solid practice to request a vendor to provide a reference list of current customers who may be contacted, and with whom a site visit may be scheduled. Vendor response to the RFP aids in narrowing the vendor candidates.

Communication Plan

Implementation of technology almost always entails change. Communicating the vision, plan, and expectations to all of the organization's members can ensure a successful outcome.

System/Product Selection

Choosing an EHR system that is "best" for an organization or facility can be an extremely daunting and overwhelming process. Ensuring a system will meet everyone's needs now and in the future is crucial. Often, users of an EHR will have one understanding of their "needs" and EHR capability will be different. Before choosing, understanding the users' requirements, as well as the capability of different EHRs, helps bring these two together. Key functionality needs to be identified and will be used to evaluate specific areas of the EHR. This step essentially assesses an EHR system's "fit" for an organization.

Vendor Demonstration

Once the RFP process has been completed and the potential EHRs have been narrowed to three or four options, onsite demonstrations of product functionality should be conducted. Potential vendors are invited to the organization to meet with the EHR selection committee and other key members of the organization. This is a vital step in understanding the functionality and capabilities of a potential EHR. Vendors should be asked to demonstrate how their product fulfills the organization's needs as set forth in the vision and goals, as well as conforming to the current workflow and crucial needs in the RFP. It is most advantageous to use a standard set of scenarios that each vendor completes. In addition, having an objective scoring tool such as the American Academy of Family Physicians "Vendor Rating Tool" can provide subjective assessment of the EHR system being evaluated, to aid in the final decision (American Academy of Family Physicians, 2005).

Contracting

Once the product has been selected, contracting can begin. It is advisable to have vendor contracts reviewed by legal counsel. These documents list areas of vendor and provider accountability. Involvement of legal representation for contract review may seem like a burden to the process, especially when both parties seem to be in complete agreement. However, "there are great benefits to a well-conceived contractual relationship. These may include robust and meaningful standards of performance. They may also include reasonable provisions and limitations on indemnification, liability, and damages, or even a plan for what happens when the relationship is terminated"...therefore each contract needs to be "tailored to meet the parties' needs and should be a help, rather than a hindrance" (Medical Association of the State of Alabama, 2020, para. 10). With attention from both parties on the front end of the contract, "a carefully negotiated contract can minimize future problems with the vendors and create an equally beneficial relationship for the vendor and provider" (Hartley, 2017, p. 50).

Implementation

Implementation involves the installation of the EHR system and other preparatory activities. The final project team is identified and an installation schedule developed. This stage comprises all of the necessary activities from contract signing until the actual "go-live."

Configuration

Prior to the EHR being used, the software must be installed and configured. The technology on which the EHR runs may need to be purchased or upgraded. This step includes the "creation and maintenance of the physical environment in which the system will operate" (Office of the National Coordinator for Health Information Technology, 2016, p. 2). Often, newer servers or other technology will need to be purchased and installed. Tasks may include setting up documentation templates for common types of visits or procedures; configuring data lists for diagnoses, medications, allegories, orders, etc.; and adding other customized items as identified during workflow analysis.

Training

Once the system is configured for the organization's needs, staff need to learn to use it. Depending on the size of the implementation, vendors may provide onsite classroom-based training. Other options include web-based training led by an instructor and self-guided scenarios. Training usually involves identifying a select number of "super users" who receive intense training and are then expected to train and assist others.

Testing

Ensuring that the EHR is configured correctly is essential prior to go-live. Testing of the EHR is "the process of executing a program or system with the intent of finding errors" (Pan, J, 1999, para.2) and ideally should be accomplished in a systemic manner. Testing plans are standard scenarios that, when followed, provide expected outcomes. Many vendors will provide high-level testing plans. Customized plans based on the organization's configuration are also necessary to fully test the system.

Paper Chart Migration

Patient information recorded on paper needs to be transitioned to the EHR. This can seem like an overwhelming task given the amount of information contained in the paper charts; however, there are different methods to managing this task. Most organizations opt for an abstracting approach, whereby only pertinent pieces of the patient's record are entered into the EHR (diagnosis, medications, allergies, procedures, etc.) and only for a finite period of time in the past (~7 years, depending on state laws). It is not recommended to create an electronic image of the entire patient record by scanning all of the paper pages because this can be extremely time consuming and uses significant technology resources (Adler, 2007). It is thus advised to only pull paper charts for a visit or two after go-live (Adler, 2007).

Go-Live

After all preparations have been completed, the EHR software will become "active" at the time of go-live. This can be a stressful time but can be minimized with some preparations. A smooth go-live requires that a number of details are addressed. Supporting the organization is key to a successful go-live. Many organizations designate a room or space as the "command center" and house support personnel in this one location to best support the end users on go-live day. In smaller organizations, this could be a corner of the staff lunch room. It is best to also provide "at the elbow" support of all users on the initial days or weeks. Many software vendors can provide onsite support but the cost may be a burden for small organizations. The previously identified "super users" can be utilized for this capacity.

Many organizations find it helpful to reduce patient schedules and load during a go-live. This will allow the organization to focus on a successful rollout. An alternative is to go live with a portion of providers or all providers using limited functionality.

Part of the aforementioned communication plan should include other key individuals and third parties such as other vendors (e.g., billing company) of the intended go-live date.

Post-Go-Live

Once the hard work of implementing the EHR has been completed, there are additional steps to be taken to ensure its continued use and smooth operation.

- Ensure system backups are occurring and have been tested and validated. EHR data need to be backed up on a regular basis and the data's integrity ensured in the rare event of a system failure.
- Downtime procedures should be established should the EHR not be available. Most organizations become highly dependent on EHRs but still need to function should the system be unavailable. Paper copies of all patient forms, templates, etc., need to be available in the event of a system failure.

- Upgrades are handled differently by different EHR vendors. It is vital to understand your vendor's approach. Upgrades may occur in the background without affecting any users and therefore do not affect daily performance. Others may require downtime, causing the system to be unavailable.

Electronic Health Records Features and Functionality

In 2003, the Institute of Medicine released "Key Capabilities of an Electronic Health Record System" and determined there were eight core functions of an EHR:

1. Health information and data
   Essentially, the EHR should "contain certain data about patients" in order that clinicians "make sound clinical decisions" (Committee on Data Standards for Patient Safety, 2003, p. 7).
2. Result management
   Electronically available test results provide distinctive advantages over those that are reported on paper. Once electronic, these results can be more easily accessed when they are needed, thereby reducing lag time. Having searchable data also reduces redundant testing and provides better interpretation and easier detection of abnormalities.
3. Order management
   There has been much written regarding the benefits of computerized provider order entry (CPOE) (Bates & Gawande, 2003; Kron et al., 2018; Martin, 2004; O'Connor, 2004). CPOE provides medication dose and frequency, allergy checking, and other clinical decision support functions.
4. Decision support
   Discussed further in another part of this chapter, clinical decision support (CDS) provides clinicians, staff, patients, or other individuals with person-specific, actionable knowledge that is "intelligently filtered or presented at appropriate times, to enhance health and health care" (Osheroff et al., 2007, p. 141). Clinical decision support utilizes alerts and reminders to providers and patients based on clinical guidelines that "improve health and healthcare delivery" (Miliard, 2015, para. 27).
5. Electronic communication and connectivity
   Coordination of care, as detailed earlier in this chapter, can only be accomplished if all parties are connected electronically (Burton et al., 2004).
6. Patient support
   Evidence has shown that patients engaged in their care have "better outcomes... and, some evidence suggests, lower costs" (James, 2013, p. 1). This is believed to be "shared decision making, in which patients and providers together consider the patient's condition, treatment options, the medical evidence behind the treatment options, the benefits and risks of treatment, and patients' preferences, and then arrive at and execute a treatment plan" (James, 2013, p. 2).
7. Administrative processes
   EHRs can assist with many of the nonclinical functions such as billing and claims, inpatient census, outpatient procedures, etc., to improve the efficiency of healthcare organizations (Mishuris & Linder, 2013; Vanderpool, 2015).

8. Reporting and population health
   As compared to patient health, population health is "the health outcomes of a group of individuals, including the distribution of such outcomes within the group" (Kindig & Stoddart, 2003, p. 381). With the availability of electronic clinical data, organizations can improve populations of patients with "increase[d] . . . accuracy of the data reported" (Committee on Data Standards for Patient Safety, 2003, p. 11).

Technical Considerations

When adopting technology, there are a number of technical details to consider and concepts to keep in mind. This section will discuss architectural approaches to an EHR, as well as the implementations options.

Architecture

Electronic health records will often be available via one of two methods: "cloud"-based systems or those locally installed.

With the "cloud"-based configuration, there is "on-demand network access to a shared pool of configurable computing resources (e.g., networks, servers, storage, applications, and services) that can be rapidly provisioned and released with minimal management effort or service provider interaction" (Mell & Grance, 2012, p. 2). As the computing resources are shared, this model can provide a more economically feasible option. The "cloud"-based solutions "don't require that users make upfront capital investments in new hardware or in-house storage systems" (Monica, 2018, para. 19). In this model, the EHR is "hosted" by the vendor, and customers access it via a connection to the internet. Also known as "software as a service" (SaaS), the organization must have a robust connection to the internet to access the software. The vendor/host is responsible for all software updates, hardware maintenance and upgrades, and system availability. This can represent a significant reduction in cost for a smaller organization. Alternatively, with the client-server option, the organization hosts the EHR software on an in-house computer system (called a server). This can require large capital expenditures and internal IT staffing to ensure that the system is properly supported and maintained. Servers are typically out of date within 3 to 4 years and thus need replacing. This model is used in larger organizations that can afford the initial financial outlay and ongoing costs to update, maintain, and repair the internal network as needed (Monica, 2018).

Best-of-Breed Versus Integrated Systems

With the complexity of EHRs and other clinical information systems, coupled with the intricate needs and size of many larger organizations, not all EHR products are able to meet their customers' needs. Best-of-breed involves purchasing different software systems from more than one vendor to obtain the best "fit" for each function or department. For instance, healthcare organizations may purchase the clinical documentation system from one vendor, a human resources module from another, and radiology from a third. This approach is followed when organizations have very specific needs and one vendor is unable to fulfill them. In order for information to be exchanged between these disparate systems, electronic interfaces need to be created. This can be a costly (both in time and resources) undertaking and often creates a discordant environment where information may not always be exchanged as expected.

Contrary to the best-of-breed system is an integrated system. With this model, all software is purchased from a single vendor and configures such that the complication of an interface is not necessary. Some refer to this as a "single database" or source of data. It can also simplify support in that a single vendor provides the convenience of a single point of contact for support and technical concerns.

Hardware Options

Selecting the correct hardware on which the EHR will run is an important decision in the success of the project. Many options are available, so choosing the one that fits best takes some research. Factors such as cost, current infrastructure (Will a hardware upgrade be necessary for an option to be implemented?), available support, the level of comfort with technology, and how the hardware fits into the current processes are all considered. Part of this decision centers on the workflow analysis (described earlier) and how the practitioners will be using the hardware. Will the clinicians prefer to use the EHR in a stationary location? Do they prefer mobility? Will they need to complete their work offsite? These are the types of questions that factor into the decision of hardware purchase. If mobility isn't a factor, fixed computer workstations can be the best option. However, it is important to consider the effect of a computer in the exam room because "many clinicians are concerned about how having a computer in the exam room will change their interaction with the patient" (Underwood, 2011, para. 3). Placement of the hardware is a key factor in minimizing this effect. If the workstation is placed such that the clinician must face away from the patient, many patients feel this presents a barrier to their relationship and interaction with the clinician: "The computer can act as a barrier and it can be disconcerting for patients to be looking at the back of a computer monitor wondering what it is that you are writing" (Brookstone, 2011, para. 7).

If the clinicians prefer mobility, the use of laptops or tablets can assist them in moving around the clinical areas. With the growth of wireless networks, these options provide much flexibility when using the EHR. Tablets have become particularly appealing because of their size and weight. Many vendors are customizing their software to run easily on a tablet. "Just like a paper chart, this device can be used to input data using a [touch] pen to select items from a checklist or to enter information using handwriting recognition" (Brookstone, 2011, para. 9).

Electronic Health Records and Clinician Burnout

While the value of an EHR as a tool to better care for patients seems quite evident, there are associated challenges. Much has been documented in recent years in regard to EHR-related clinician burnout (Ehrenfeld & Wanderer, 2018; Harris et al., 2018; Murphy, Giardina, et al., 2019; Murphy, Satterly, et al., 2019; Saag et al., 2019; Starren et al., 2021; Tai-Seale et al., 2019; Tate, 2020).

In a survey of 87 clinicians, Adler-Milstein et al. (2020) investigated five factors which could contribute to clinical burnout including: 1) minutes active after hours, 2) minutes active any time on days with no clinic sessions scheduled, 3) volume of EHR inbox messages received, 4) use of available EHR tools, and 5) Efficiency of clinicians use of the EHR related to time spent with patients. Empirically the researchers found two of the factors "time spent after hours on the EHR" and "volume of inbox messages," where related to clinician burnout and exhaustion (Adler-Milstein et al., 2020). The volume and timing (after hours) of messaging was cited by several others as a large contributing factor to clinical burnout related to EHR usage (Hilliard et al., 2020; Murphy, Satterly, et al., 2019). Kroth et al. (2019) examined clinicians' EHR usage from "282 ambulatory primary care and subspecialty clinicians from 3 institutions [which] measured stress and burnout, opinions on EHR design and use factors, and helpful coping strategies" (Kroth et al., 2019, p. 1). They identified a multi-factorial cause to this issue, including "information overload, slow system response times, excessive data entry, inability to navigate the system quickly, note bloat, interference with the patient-clinician relationship, fear of missing something, and notes geared toward billing" (Kroth et al., 2019, p. 10).

Recognizing this growing issue, ONCHIT published the "Strategy on Reducing Regulatory and Administrative Burden Relating to the Use of Health IT and EHRs" as part of the 21st Century Cures Act to address "specific sources of clinician burden that will require coordinated action on the part of a variety of stakeholders across the health care system" (Office of the National Coordinator for Health Information Technology, 2020, p. 3). Among their "Strategies and Recommendations," the authors call for a reduction in the "overall regulatory burden around documentation of patient encounters," as well as the use of "data already present in the EHR to reduce re-documentation in the clinical note" (Office of the National Coordinator for Health Information Technology, 2020, p. 44).

Seminar Discussion Questions

1. As a new student gathering information about your assigned patients via an EHR, what advantages can this approach provide you over traditional paper records?
2. Describe the ways in which electronic health records can eliminate redundant efforts. Provide detailed rationales.
3. When selecting an EHR system, why is it so vital to create and communicate a vision for its use? Which individuals should be involved in this process?
4. What are the ethical considerations related to interoperability and a shared EHR?
5. Discuss the advantages and disadvantages associated with implementing and using a regional and/or national EHR.

References

Adler, K. G. (2007). How to Successfully Navigate Your EHR Implementation. In *Family Practice Management* (Vol. 14, Issue 2). www.aafp.org/fpm

Adler-Milstein, J., Salzberg, C., Franz, C., Orav, E. J., & Bates, D. W. (2013). The impact of electronic health records on ambulatory costs among Medicaid beneficiaries. *Medicare & Medicaid Research Review*, 3(2), 1–16. https://doi.org/10.5600/mmrr.003.02.a03

Adler-Milstein, J., Zhao, W., Willard-Grace, R., Knox, M., & Grumbach, K. (2020). Electronic health records and burnout: Time spent on the electronic health record after hours and message volume associated with exhaustion but not with cynicism among primary care clinicians. *Journal of the American Medical Informatics Association*, 27(4), 531–538. http://10.0.4.69/jamia/ocz220

American Academy of Family Physicians. (2005). *EHR vendor rating tool.* Electronic Health Records FPM Toolbox. http://www.ncbi.nlm.nih.gov/pubmed/15813302

Bae, J., Hockenberry, J. M., Rask, K. J., & Becker, E. R. (2017). Evidence that electronic health records can promote physician counseling for healthy behaviors. *Health Care Management Review*, 42(3), 258–268. https://doi.org/10.1097/HMR.0000000000000108

Barton, C., Kallem, C., Van Dyke, P., Mon, D., & Richesson, R. (2011). Demonstrating "collect once, use many"—Assimilating public health secondary data use requirements into an existing Domain Analysis Model. *AMIA... Annual Symposium Proceedings/AMIA Symposium. AMIA Symposium, 2011*, 98–107.

Bates, D. W., & Gawande, A. A. (2003). Improving safety with information technology. *New England Journal of Medicine*, 348(25), 2526–2534. http://search.ebscohost.com/login.aspx?direct=true&db=cmedm&AN=12815139&cpidlogin.asp?custid=s6328807&site=ehost-live&scope=site

Blumenthal, D., DesRoches, C., Donelan, K., Ferris, T., Jha, A., Kaushal, R., Rao, S., & Rosenbaum, S. (2006). Health Information Technology in the United States: The Information Base for Progress. *Information and Communication Technologies in Healthcare*, 1–84. https://doi.org/10.1201/b11696-6

Blumenthal, D., & Tavenner, M. (2010). *The "Meaningful Use" Regulation for Electronic Health Records.* 501–504.

Boonstra, A., & Broekhuis, M. (2010). Barriers to the acceptance of electronic medical records by physicians from systematic review to taxonomy and interventions. *BMC Health Services Research*, 10, 231. https://doi.org/10.1186/1472-6963-10-231

Bredfeldt, C. E., Awad, E. B., Joseph, K., & Snyder, M. H. (2013). Training providers: Beyond the basics of electronic health records. *BMC Health Services Research*, 13, 503. https://doi.org/10.1186/1472-6963-13-503

Bresnick, J. (2018). CMS renames "meaningful use" to "promoting interoperability" and changes ensue. *HealthITAnalytics.* https://healthitanalytics.com/news/cms-renames-meaningful-use-to-highlight-interoperability-goals

Brookstone, A. (2011). *How to integrate computers into your practice for maximum patient benefit.* http://www.americanehr.com/blog/2011/04/how-to-integrate-computers-into-your-office-for-maximum-patient-benefit/

Burton, L. C., Anderson, G. F., & Kues, I. W. (2004). Using electronic health records to help coordinate care. *The Milbank Quarterly*, 82(3), 457–481, table of contents. https://doi.org/10.1111/j.0887-378X.2004.00318.x

Bush, G. W. (2004). *Presidential Documents: Executive Order 13335 of April 27, 2004 Incentives for the Use of Health Information Technology and Establishing the Position of the National Health Information Technology Coordinator* (Vol. 69, Issue 84, pp. 24059–24061).

Carayon, P., Smith, P., Hundt, A. S., Kuruchittham, V., & Li, Q. (2009). Implementation of an electronic health records system in a small clinic: The viewpoint of clinic staff. *Behaviour & Information Technology*, 28(1), 5–20. https://doi.org/10.1080/01449290701628178

Centers for Medicare and Medicaid Services. (2010). *Medicare & Medicaid EHR incentive program: What is meaningful use?*

Centers for Medicare and Medicaid Services. (2014). *An introduction to: Medicaid EHR incentive program* (Issue April).

Centers for Medicare and Medicaid Services. (2017). *Stages of promoting interoperability programs: First year demonstrating meaningful use*. 1–2. https://www.cms.gov/Regulations-and-Guidance/Legislation/EHRIncentivePrograms/Downloads/Stages_ofMeaningfulUseTable.pdf

Centers for Medicare and Medicaid Services. (2018). Fiscal Year (FY) 2019 Medicare Hospital Inpatient Prospective Payment System (IPPS) and Long Term Acute Care Hospital (LTCH) prospective payment system proposed rule, and request for information. *Fact Sheet*. https://www.cms.gov/newsroom/fact-sheets/fiscal-year-fy-2019-medicare-hospital-inpatient-prospective-payment-system-ipps-and-long-term-acute

Clancy, C. M. (2009). *What is health care quality, and who decides? 1633*(801), 1–91.

Cohen, M. (2015). The challenge of EHR acceptance by physicians. *Journal of Medical Practice Management*, *31*(2), 117–120.

Collinsworth, A. W., Masica, A. L., Priest, E. L., Berryman, C. D., Kouznetsova, M., Glorioso, O., & Montgomery, D. (2014). Modifying the Electronic Health Record to Facilitate the Implementation and Evaluation of a Bundled Care Program for Intensive Care Unit Delirium. *EGEMs (Generating Evidence & Methods to Improve Patient Outcomes)*, *2*(1), 20. https://doi.org/10.13063/2327-9214.1121

Committee on Data Standards for Patient Safety. (2003). *Key capabilities of an electronic health record system letter report*.

Decker, S. L., Jamoom, E. W., & Sisk, J. E. (2012). Physicians in nonprimary care and small practices and those age 55 and older lag in adopting electronic health record systems. *Health Affairs (Project Hope)*, *31*(5), 1108–1114. https://doi.org/10.1377/hlthaff.2011.1121

DesRoches, C. M., Campbell, E. G., Rao, S. R., Donelan, K., Ferris, T. G., Jha, A., Kaushal, R., Levy, D. E., Rosenbaum, S., Shields, A. E., & Blumenthal, D. (2008). Electronic health records in ambulatory care—A national survey of physicians. *New England Journal of Medicine*, *359*(1), 50–60. https://doi.org/10.1056/NEJMsa0802005

Eastaugh, S. R. (2013). Electronic health records lifecycle cost. *Journal of Health Care Finance*, *39*(4), 36–43. http://www.ncbi.nlm.nih.gov/pubmed/24003760

Ehrenfeld, J. M., & Wanderer, J. P. (2018). Technology as friend or foe? Do electronic health records increase burnout? *Current Opinion in Anaesthesiology*, *31*(3), 357–360. https://doi.org/10.1097/ACO.0000000000000588

Electronic Clinical Quality Measures. (2021). *eCQI Resource Center*. https://ecqi.healthit.gov/glossary/ehr

Elfrink, C. (2009). What I learned this summer. *Educational Leadership*. http://voicesblog.echovermont.org/2009/09/what-i-learned-this-summer.html

Friedman, D. J., Parrish, R. G., & Ross, D. A. (2013). Electronic health records and US public health: Current realities and future promise. *American Journal of Public Health*, *103*(9), 1560–1567. https://doi.org/10.2105/AJPH.2013.301220

Garets, D., & Davis, M. (2006). *Electronic medical records vs. electronic health records: Yes, there is a difference. A HIMSS analytics white paper*. https://www.himssanalytics.org/docs/WP_EMR_EHR.pdf

Garrett, P., & Seidman, J. (2011). EMR vs EHR – What is the difference? *Health IT Buzz*. http://www.healthit.gov/buzz-blog/electronic-health-and-medical-records/emr-vs-ehr-difference/

Giniat, E. J., Benton, B., Biegansky, E., & Grossman, R. (2012). People and change management in an uncertain environment. *Healthcare Financial Management: Journal of the Healthcare Financial Management Association*, *66*(10), 84–89. http://search.ebscohost.com/login.aspx?direct=true&db=mnh&AN=23088059&site=ehost-live&scope=site

Goetz Goldberg, D., Kuzel, A. J., Feng, L. B., DeShazo, J. P., & Love, L. E. (2012). EHRs in primary care practices: Benefits, challenges, and successful strategies. *The American Journal of Managed Care*, *18*(2), e48-54. http://www.ncbi.nlm.nih.gov/pubmed/22435884

Goldzweig, C. L., Towfigh, A., Maglione, M., & Shekelle, P. G. (2005). Costs and benefits of health information technology: New trends from the literature. *Health Affairs (Project Hope)*, *28*(2), w282-93. https://doi.org/10.1377/hlthaff.28.2.w282

Harris, D. A., Haskell, J., Cooper, E., Crouse, N., & Gardner, R. (2018). Estimating the association between burnout and electronic health record-related stress among advanced practice registered nurses. *Applied Nursing Research (ANR)*, *43*, 36–41. https://doi.org/10.1016/j.apnr.2018.06.014

Hartley, S. W. (ed.). (2017). Best practices: Improving contract management to strengthen your medical facility. *Healthcare Journal of New Orleans, 5*(April).

Henderson, A., Schoonbeek, S., & Auditore, A. (2013). Processes to engage and motivate staff. *Nursing Management - UK, 20*(8), 18–25. https://doi.org/10.7748/nm2013.12.20.8.18.e1150

Highfill, T. (2020). Do hospitals with electronic health records have lower costs? A systematic review and meta-analysis. *International Journal of Healthcare Management, 13*(1), 65–71. https://doi.org/10.1080/20479700.2019.1616895

Hilliard, R. W., Haskell, J., & Gardner, R. L. (2020). Are specific elements of electronic health record use associated with clinician burnout more than others? *Journal of the American Medical Informatics Association, 27*(9), 1401–1410. http://10.0.4.69/jamia/ocaa092

James, J. (2013). Health policy brief: Patient engagement. *Health Affairs.*

Kazley, A. S., Simpson, A. N., Simpson, K. N., & Teufel, R. (2014). Association of Electronic Health Records With, *20*(6), 183–191.

Kern, L. M., Barrón, Y., Dhopeshwarkar, R. V., Edwards, A., & Kaushal, R. (2013). Electronic health records and ambulatory quality of care. *Journal of General Internal Medicine, 28*(4), 496–503. https://doi.org/10.1007/s11606-012-2237-8

Kindig, D., & Stoddart, G. (2003). What is population health? *American Journal of Public Health, 93*(3), 380–383. https://doi.org/10.2105/AJPH.93.3.380

King, J., Patel, V., Jamoom, E. W., & Furukawa, M. F. (2014). Clinical benefits of electronic health record use: National findings. *Health Services Research, 49*(1 Pt 2), 392–404. https://doi.org/10.1111/1475-6773.12135

Kron, K., Myers, S., Volk, L., Nathan, A., Neri, P., Salazar, A., Amato, M. G., Wright, A., Karmiy, S., McCord, S., Seoane-Vazquez, E., Eguale, T., Rodriguez-Monguio, R., Bates, D. W., & Schiff, G. (2018). Incorporating medication indications into the prescribing process. *American Journal of Health-System Pharmacy, 75*(11), 774–783. https://doi.org/10.2146/ajhp170346

Kroth, P. J., Morioka-Douglas, N., Veres, S., Babbott, S., Poplau, S., Qeadan, F., Parshall, C., Corrigan, K., & Linzer, M. (2019). Association of electronic health record design and use factors with clinician stress and burnout. *JAMA Network Open, 2*(8), e199609. https://doi.org/10.1001/jamanetworkopen.2019.9609

Lin, C., Lin, I.-C., & Roan, J. (2012). Barriers to physicians' adoption of healthcare information technology: an empirical study on multiple hospitals. *Journal of Medical Systems, 36*(3), 1965–1977. https://doi.org/10.1007/s10916-011-9656-7

Lu, Y., Huang, C., Mahajan, S., Schulz, W. L., Nasir, K., Spatz, E. S., & Krumholz, H. M. (2020). Leveraging the electronic health records for population health: A case study of patients with markedly elevated blood pressure. *Journal of the American Heart Association, 9*(7), e015033. https://doi.org/10.1161/JAHA.119.015033

Martin, G. T. (2004). Leading up to CPOE. Benefits begin long before full implementation. *Healthcare Informatics, 21*(2), 96–98.

Medical Association of the State of Alabama. (2020). *Striking your best deal: Things to look at on the front end of negotiating an EHR vendor contract.* https://alabamamedicine.org/striking-your-best-deal-things-to-look-at-on-the-front-end-of-negotiating-an-ehr-vendor-contract/

Mell, P., & Grance, T. (2012). The NIST definition of cloud computing: Recommendations of the National Institute of Standards and Technology. In *Public Cloud Computing: Security and Privacy Guidelines* (pp. 97–101). https://doi.org/10.6028/NIST.SP.800-145

Merchant, Z., Goetz, E. T., Cifuentes, L., Keeney-Kennicutt, W., & Davis, T. J. (2014). Effectiveness of virtual reality-based instruction on students' learning outcomes in K-12 and higher education: A meta-analysis. *Computers and Education, 70,* 29–40. https://doi.org/10.1016/j.compedu.2013.07.033

Merrill, M. (2010). Top 10 factors for successful EHR implementation. *Healthcare IT News.* http://www.healthcareitnews.com/news/top-10-factors-successful-ehr-implementation?single-page=true

Miliard, M. (2015). Clinical decision support: No longer just a nice-to-have. *Healthcare IT News.* https://www.healthcareitnews.com/news/clinical-decision-support-no-longer-just-nice-have

Mishuris, R. G., & Linder, J. A. (2013). Electronic health records and the increasing complexity of medical practice: "It never gets easier, you just go faster." *Journal of General Internal Medicine, 28*(4), 490–492. https://doi.org/10.1007/s11606-012-2304-1

Monica, K. (2018). *Choosing an electronic health record: Cloud v. on premise EHRs.* https://ehrintelligence.com/features/choosing-an-electronic-health-record-cloud-vs.-on-premise-ehrs

Murphy, D. R., Giardina, T. D., Satterly, T., Sittig, D. F., & Singh, H. (2019). An exploration of barriers, facilitators, and suggestions for improving electronic health record inbox-related usability: A qualitative analysis. *JAMA Network Open, 2*(10), e1912638. https://doi.org/10.1001/jamanetworkopen.2019.12638

Murphy, D. R., Satterly, T., Giardina, T. D., Sittig, D. F., & Singh, H. (2019). Practicing clinicians' recommendations to reduce burden from the electronic health record inbox: A mixed-methods study. *Journal of General Internal Medicine, 34*(9), 1825–1832. https://doi.org/10.1007/s11606-019-05112-5

O'Connor, K. J. (2004). CPOE: Show me the benefits! *Journal of Healthcare Information Management, 18*(1), 11–12.

O'Malley, A. S., Grossman, J. M., Cohen, G. R., Kemper, N. M., & Pham, H. H. (2010). Are electronic medical records helpful for care coordination? Experiences of physician practices. *Journal of General Internal Medicine, 25*(3), 177–185. https://doi.org/10.1007/s11606-009-1195-2

Office of the National Coordinator for Health InTechnology (2014) How much is it going to cost me: the basics, Retrieved from: https://www.healthit.gov/faq/how-much-going-cost-me

Office of the National Coordinator for Health Information Technology. (2016). *System configuration general instructions for the SAFER Self-Assessment Guides. September*, 1–23.

Office of the National Coordinator for Health Information Technology. (2018). *Medical practice efficiencies & cost savings.* https://www.healthit.gov/topic/health-it-and-health-information-exchange-basics/medical-practice-efficiencies-cost-savings

Office of the National Coordinator for Health Information Technology. (2019a). *What is an electronic health record (EHR)?* http://www.healthit.gov/providers-professionals/faqs/what-electronic-health-record-ehr

Office of the National Coordinator for Health Information Technology. (2019b). *What is HIE?* https://www.healthit.gov/topic/health-it-and-health-information-exchange-basics/what-hie

ONCHIT. (2014). Connecting health and care for the nation a shared nationwide interoperability roadmap. *HealthIT.Gov.*

ONCHIT. (2018). Clinical Decision Support. *HealthIT.Gov.* https://www.healthit.gov/topic/safety/clinical-decision-support

Osheroff, J. A., Teich, J. M., Middleton, B., Steen, E. B., Wright, A., & Detmer, D. E. (2007). A roadmap for national action on clinical decision support. *Journal of the American Medical Informatics Association, 14*(2), 141–145. https://doi.org/10.1197/jamia.M2334

Pan, J. (1999). *Software testing.* http://users.ece.cmu.edu/~koopman/des_s99/sw_testing/

Pugh, C. M. (2019). Electronic health records, physician workflows and system change: Defining a pathway to better healthcare. *Annals of Translational Medicine, 7*(S1), S27–S27. https://doi.org/10.21037/atm.2019.01.83

Reisman, M. (2017). EHRs: The challenge of making electronic data usable and interoperable. *Pharmacy and Therapeutics, 42*(9), 572–575.

Ribeiro, S. P., & Cavalcanti, M. de L. T. (2020). Primary health care and coordination of care: Device to increase access and improve quality. *Ciencia e Saude Coletiva, 25*(5), 1799–1808. https://doi.org/10.1590/1413-81232020255.34122019

Saag, H. S., Shah, K., Jones, S. A., Testa, P. A., & Horwitz, L. I. (2019). Pajama time: Working After Work In The Electronic Health Record. *Journal of General Internal Medicine, 34*(9), 1695–1696. https://doi.org/10.1007/s11606-019-05055-x

Shamus, E., & Stern, D. (2011). *Effective documentation for physical therapy professionals* (2nd ed.). http://www.amazon.com/Effective-Documentation-Physical-Therapy-Professionals/dp/0071664041/ref=sr_1_1?ie=UTF8&qid=1406411230&sr=8-1&keywords=shamus+and+stern+physical+therapy

Spicer, S. S. (2009). HITECH stimulus for physicians. *North Carolina Medical Journal, 70*(4), 354–357. http://www.ncbi.nlm.nih.gov/pubmed/19835259

Starren, J. B., Tierney, W. M., Williams, M. S., Tang, P., Weir, C., Koppel, R., Payne, P., Hripcsak, G., & Detmer, D. E. (2021). A retrospective look at the predictions and recommendations from the 2009 AMIA policy meeting: Did we see EHR-related clinician burnout coming? *Journal of the American Medical Informatics Association, 00*(0), 1–7. https://doi.org/10.1093/jamia/ocaa320

Tai-Seale, M., Dillon, E. C., Yang, Y., Nordgren, R., Steinberg, R. L., Nauenberg, T., Lee, T. C., Meehan, A., Li, J., Solomon Chan, A., & Frosch, D. L. (2019). Physicians' well-being linked to in-basket messages generated by algorithms in electronic health records. *Health Affairs, 38*(7), 1073–1078. https://doi.org/10.1377/hlthaff.2018.05509

Tate, A. (2020). Avoiding clinical staff burnout during a rigorous EHR transition. *Medical Staff Briefing, 30*(3), 8–10. https://sacredheart.idm.oclc.org/login?url=https://search.ebscohost.com/login.aspx?direct=true&db=ccm&AN=142300949&site=eds-live&scope=site

The National Alliance for Health Information Technology. (2008). *Defining key health information technology terms.*

Underwood, W. S. (2011). *Choosing the right hardware for your practice.* http://www.americanehr.com/blog/2011/06/choosing-the-right-hardware-for-your-practice/

Vaidotas, M., Yokota, P. K. O., Negrini, N. M. M., Leiderman, D. B. D., Souza, V. P. de, Santos, O. F. P. Dos, & Wolosker, N. (2019). Medication errors in emergency departments: Is electronic medical record an effective barrier? *Einstein (Sao Paulo, Brazil), 17*(4), eGS4282. https://doi.org/10.31744/einstein_journal/2019GS4282

Vanderpool, D. (2015). EHR documentation: How to keep your patients safe, keep your hard-earned money, and stay out of court. *Innovations in Clinical Neuroscience, 12*(7–8), 34–38. https://pubmed.ncbi.nlm.nih.gov/26351623

Walker, J., Pan, E., Johnston, D., Adler-Milstein, J., Bates, D. W., & Middleton, B. (2005). The value of health care information exchange and interoperability. *Health Affairs (Project Hope), Suppl Web,* W5-10-W5-18. https://doi.org/10.1377/hlthaff.w5.10

Walker-Czyz, A. (2016). The impact of an integrated electronic health record adoption on nursing care quality. *Journal of Nursing Administration, 46*(7–8), 366–372. https://doi.org/10.1097/NNA.0000000000000360

Wang, S. J., Middleton, B., Prosser, L. A., Bardon, C. G., Spurr, C. D., Carchidi, P. J., Kittler, A. F., Goldszer, R. C., Fairchild, D. G., Sussman, A. J., Kuperman, G. J., & Bates, D. W. (2003). A cost-benefit analysis of electronic medical records in primary care. *The American Journal of Medicine, 114*(5), 397–403. https://doi.org/10.1016/S0002-9343(03)00057-3

Watterson, J. L., Rodriguez, H. P., Aguilera, A., & Shortell, S. M. (2020). Ease of use of electronic health records and relational coordination among primary care team members. *Health Care Management Review, 45*(3), 267–275. https://doi.org/10.1097/HMR.0000000000000222

Webster, P. C. (2010). Electronic health records a "strong priority" for US government. *CMAJ: Canadian Medical Association Journal = Journal de l'Association Medicale Canadienne, 182*(8), E315-6. https://doi.org/10.1503/cmaj.109-3218

Wright, A., Feblowitz, J., Samal, L., McCoy, A. B., & Sittig, D. F. (2014). The Medicare Electronic Health Record Incentive Program: Provider performance on core and menu measures. *Health Services Research, 49*(1 Pt 2), 325–346. https://doi.org/10.1111/1475-6773.12134

Youngblut, C. (1998). Educational uses of virtual reality technology. *IDA Document D-2128, January,* 131. http://www.hitl.washington.edu/scivw/youngblut-edvr/D2128.pdf

Zandieh, S. O., Yoon-Flannery, K., Kuperman, G. J., Langsam, D. J., Hyman, D., & Kaushal, R. (2008). Challenges to EHR implementation in electronic- versus paper-based office practices. *Journal of General Internal Medicine, 23*(6), 755–761. https://doi.org/10.1007/s11606-008-0573-5

Zlabek, J. A., Wickus, J. W., & Mathiason, M. A. (2011). Early cost and safety benefits of an inpatient electronic health record. Journal of the American Medical Informatics Association : JAMIA, 18(2), 169–172. https://doi.org/10.1136/jamia.2010.007229

CHAPTER 13

Telehealth: Increasing Access to Health Care

Donna F. McHaney and Nicole Kroll

"In an age where the average consumer manages nearly all aspects of life online, it's a no-brainer that health care should be just as convenient, accessible, and safe as online banking."

—Jonathan Linkous,
CEO of the American Telemedicine Association

Introduction to Telehealth

As one of the most disruptive healthcare innovations, telehealth has rapidly become a successful way to provide safe, cost-effective quality care to patients remotely. Nurse practitioners (NPs) who are the primary providers of care for populations that may be distant, underprivileged, or unable to easily get medical treatment need to develop the expertise, skills, and mindset to employ telehealth technologies (Finely & Shea, 2019). Current information and technology for example computers, the Internet, and smart phones have changed how people exchange information and how health care is provided (WHO, 2010). Telehealth was conceptualized early on but has evolved throughout the years to become an important way to deliver health care. It is important to define telehealth and how it is applicable for nurse practitioners in clinical practice.

Difference between Telehealth and Telemedicine

While many times the terms "telehealth" and "telemedicine" are used interchangeably, they have different meanings. Telehealth collectively can be defined as a conglomerate of health information methods or technology used to deliver healthcare service, including videoconferencing, the Internet, store and forward imaging, streaming media, and terrestrial and wireless communication (National Telehealth

Resource Centers, n.d.; National Coordinator for Health Information Technology, n.d.). In contrast, telemedicine is the actual remote clinical service. In Latin, it is literally translated as "healing at a distance" (National Coordinator for Health Information Technology, n.d.; WHO, 2010). Currently, the term *telehealth* covers an array of health disciplines, such as primary care, dentistry, mental health/counseling, home care services, and many others (National Telehealth Resource Centers, n.d.). It can refer to remote non-direct patient care services, such as training for providers, meeting forums, and continuing education opportunities (National Coordinator for Health Information Technology, n.d.). It includes provider-to-provider and provider-to-patient encounters (Wosik et al., 2020). Telehealth has developed well beyond its original intent to disseminate information, and to diagnose and monitor patient activities (National Telehealth Resource Centers, n.d.).

The History of Telehealth

Distance communication regarding health can be traced back to the 1600s when special flags were flown on ships to signal outbreaks of disease (Nesbitt 2021; Darkins & Cary, 2000). There are also reports in Australia of the Aborigines caring sticks to let others know of death and disease around this same time (Nesbitt & Katz-Bell, 2021). These communications evolved as technology became more readily available to telephone consultations and the broadcasting of surgeries via satellite (Nesbitt 2021; Darkins & Cary, 2000). In the late 1940s, pioneers of teleradiology developed protocols and used them to transfer images via phone lines for review (Nesbitt & Katz-Bell, 2021). By the 1980s, telemedicine was used in European countries frequently, but in the United States it was reserved mostly for the military, the space program, the incarcerated, and patients in remote areas (Darkins & Cary, 2000). Legislative and grant funding was set aside in the 1990s because video conferencing equipment was costly and typically used by academic health centers for healthcare education and specialty services. Much of this change developed as an answer to improving healthcare access to remote and medically underserved areas. As telehealth progressed to inpatient and outpatient settings in the new millennium, it began to be used in all 50 states. Advancements were made using telehealth in emergency medicine by remote video consults with stroke patients. This decreased response times and allowed patients to avoid traveling to rural hospitals to meet standards of care. During this time, remote monitoring was made available to ventilator-dependent, chronic disease and homecare patients, but insurance coverage and reimbursement were minimal if at all (Nesbitt & Katz-Bell, 2021). Telehealth still had many barriers, including compensation, across-state licensure complications, and confidentiality concerns related to the Health Insurance Portability and Accountability Act (HIPAA). There were also limitations related to provider proficiency and patient and staff perceptions (Smith & Raskin, 2021).

While telehealth visits were becoming more prevalent, the 2019 novel coronavirus disease (COVID-19) pandemic has altered our healthcare system to the tipping point for increased usage (Wosik et al., 2020). In 2020, the Centers for Medicaid and Medicare Services (CMS) recognized that delivering health care virtually can improve access to care, eliminate travel, and be cost-effective (Lam et al., 2020; CMS, 2020). CMS now reimburses telemedicine at the same rate as face-to-face visits as part of the Coronavirus Preparedness and Response Supplemental Appropriation Act, the Secretary of the U.S. Department of Health and Human Services enacted the Social Security Act Section 1135 (Waiver 1135) (CMS, 2020; Smith et al., 2020). Private insurers have slowly begun to follow in the footsteps of CMS and reimburse as if the patient had attended an in-person visit (Smith et al., 2021). During the COVID-19 "stay at home" and 6-foot spacing mandates, telehealth provided a way for patients to be seen while decreasing the spread of the disease (Smith et al., 2020; Wosik et al., 2020). At this time, when many routine patient visits were canceled, and countless clinics were closed, telehealth offered patients the opportunity to have health care without going to the emergency room and risking potential exposure (Smith et al., 2020). Telehealth visits were also an important contributor in conserving personal protective equipment that was in short supply (Smith et al., 2020; Wosik et al., 2020). COVID-19 increased hospital-related care, and many facilities were able to utilize telehealth to screen, triage, and determine which patients were in critical need of inpatient services versus those who were ambulatory and could be sent through an urgent care track. According to Wosik et al. (2020), with the increased use of hospital services, the need for providers to work inpatient facilities also increased. Telehealth bridged this gap by allowing providers to monitor patients remotely even if they were in quarantine, in a high-risk group (elderly or immunocompromised), or had childcare responsibilities that didn't permit them to report to work. Telehealth was also instrumental in connecting isolated hospitalized patients with their friends and families who could not visit due to visitor restrictions. COVID-19 has allowed telehealth to overcome much of the stigma associated with its use, and the American health system will be forever changed (Wosik et al., 2020).

Telehealth Modalities

Telehealth is comprised of live, store-and-forward, videoconferencing technologies utilizing tablets, cameras, smartphones, and peripheral medical devices to link patients with providers as well as remote patient monitoring and mobile health (Rutledge et al., 2017; National Telehealth Resource Center, n.d.). Telehealth can be divided into two fundamental categories: synchronous and asynchronous. *Synchronous* occurs in real time where the healthcare provider and the patient interact, whereas *asynchronous* occurs when the patient's health information is obtained and stored and the provider reviews it at a later time (Rutledge et al., 2018). It is imperative for advanced practice nurses to understand each of the modalities (Rutledge et al., 2017; National Telehealth Resource Center, n.d.). **Table 13-1** gives a list of modalities and examples.

Live Videoconferencing

Live videoconferencing (synchronous) is the connection of two or more individuals for the purpose of delivering health care or education in a live communication utilizing audiovisual telecommunications technology (Rutledge et al., 2018; National Telehealth Resource Center, n.d.). Videoconferencing can be as simple as a telephone call or can utilize specialized telemedicine equipment that has video capabilities with peripheral components such as an otoscope, ophthalmoscope, stethoscope, or vaginal probe.

Store-and-Forward

Store-and-Forward (asynchronous) technology collects, stores, and transmits a patient's healthcare data to the intended provider. This mode of care is most commonly

Table 13-1 Telehealth Modalities and Examples

Modality	Fundamental Category	Explanation	Examples
Live Videoconferencing	Synchronous	Uses audiovisual telecommunication technology (e.g., Zoom, Doximity, etc.). Live with face-to-face visual and person-to-person interaction.	Zoom, Doximity, WebEx, and other video technologies
Store-and-Forward	Asynchronous	Recorded health history is transmitted through electronic communications systems to a practitioner or specialist to evaluate a case and/or provide a service when live video or face-to-face contact is not necessary. Often used for medical consultations and to aid in diagnoses.	X-rays, MRIs, photos, patient data, and video-exam clips
Remote Patient Monitoring	RPM	Collection medical data and personal health information that is transmission via electronic communications systems or technologies from the patient in one location to a provider at another location. This information is used in care and other related support areas. It also allows for tracking healthcare data for a patient once released to home or a care facility, reducing readmission rates.	Any non-invasive device that can collect, store, process, and transmit patient data. Examples: Bluetooth-enabled devices such as scales, Fitbits, wearable heart monitors, glucose monitors, skin patches, shoes, belts, or maternity care trackers.
Mobile Health	mHealth/eHealth	Health care, public health practice and education that uses mobile communications (i.e., cell phones, tablets, smart watches, etc.). Applications vary. Could be used to promote healthy behaviors or notify public about disease outbreaks.	Smartphone, tablets, smart watches, or any other device that provides real-time monitoring, including some wearable devices.

engaged in by specialty providers such as radiologists, ophthalmologists, pathologists, and cardiologists who can review the images or diagnostic data and render a medical opinion without meeting with a patient (Rutledge et al., 2018; National Telehealth Resource Center, n.d.).

Remote Patient Monitoring

Remote Patient Monitoring (RPM) uses medical devices that obtain physiologic information remotely and transfer the data back to a central monitoring system to be evaluated by a provider. Examples of RPM systems include scales, pulse oximetry, stethoscopes, and pacemaker/defibrillators. These devices collect pertinent information such as weight, oxygen saturation, lung and heart sounds, and heart rate and rhythms (Rutledge et al., 2018; National Telehealth Resource Center, n.d.).

Mobile Health/eHealth

Mobile Health (mHealth) technology uses synchronous and asynchronous methods to disseminate health information. This form of telehealth is supported by mobile applications and utilize them in a variety of ways to spread health and medical information. Some examples include text messaging that encourages healthy lifestyle changes, alerts about infectious disease outbreaks, and healthcare-related presentations and podcasts (Rutledge et al., 2018; National Telehealth Resource Center, n.d.).

Guidelines for the Entry-Level Primary Provider

The National Organization of Nurse Practitioner Faculty (NONPF) has developed eight suggested telehealth competencies it considers important for an entry-level primary care nurse practitioner to be proficient in (Rutledge et al., 2018). Taking into account the NONPF competencies the authors suggest challenging yourself with the following skills consistent with telehealth vs. in-person provider visits:

1. Telehealth decorum and exercising skill with video conferencing
2. The use of peripheral assessment devices such as an otoscope, stethoscope, and ophthalmoscope
3. Understanding when a telehealth patient encounter should be conducted and when it is not appropriate given the patient's reason for visit
4. Provider abiding by privacy/protected health information (PHI) regulations
5. Ability to use synchronous and asynchronous technology platforms for patient encounters
6. Apply clinical documentation and bill appropriately for the telehealth visit
7. Collaborate intra and interprofessionally with other disciplines when using telehealth platforms
8. Develop expertise in obtaining the chief complaint, history, review of systems and performing a focused physical exam with the goal of formulating differential

Etiquette during a telehealth visit is imperative in order to have a successful remote encounter. This would include the proper camera angle, removal of distractions such as clutter or noise, and even proper clothing choices, since some non-professional clothing can be distracting. Communication skills may need to be subtly changed when utilizing telehealth, such as peering into the camera and not the client's face on the screen. This lets the patient feel eye contact is being made. In addition, limiting note-taking and looking away from the camera is suggested. Compassion and understanding may also look a little different in a telehealth visit. The nurse practitioner should be encouraged to lean into the camera and nod their head so clients feel they should continue sharing their medical information (Rutledge et al., 2017).

Training and practice utilizing telehealth equipment is encouraged prior to an NP's initial telehealth visit. This alleviates anxiety and allows the NP to gain the proper skills prior to speaking with actual patients.

State and federal regulations of telehealth change rapidly. During COVID-19, telehealth regulations lessened for providers, however it is vital to stay abreast of the changes. Each state is different, and as the body of knowledge changes, it is assumed they will continue to evolve to include telehealth practices. NPs in many states are governed by both the Board of Nursing and the Board of Medicine. Understanding their regulations will help guide your telehealth endeavors (Rutledge et al., 2017).

"Communication is the number one factor influencing the patient experience, and one interaction can change the course of someone's life."

—**Anthony Orsini**, DO

The Code of Ethics remains the same when using telehealth. There are several ethical hurdles that every NP should address when using telehealth: loss of the provider–patient relationship, compromising patient privacy, using an approach to care that is not individualized, and presuming effectiveness of the technology. NPs should be receptive to these barriers and approach telehealth visits with a positive attitude (Rutledge et al., 2017).

Collaboration with other providers via phone or video regarding patient care is also an important skill. NPs who practice in remote or underserved areas where specialists do not reside, often communicate using telehealth. This allows patients to gain access to care they might not otherwise have the means to obtain (Rutledge et al., 2017).

NPs can utilize telehealth in many ways in their practices. Common usages include remote monitoring of chronic diseases such as respiratory and cardiac ailments, diabetes, and subjects such as health education, patient, and family counseling. Other uses described in this text include consultation with colleagues, triage to determine the urgency of visits, and continuing education conferences.

The Role of the Advanced Practice Nurse Practitioner in Telehealth

Transmission of heart sounds over telephone lines was one of the earliest documented uses of telehealth. Because of this, approximately 27 years later an ECG was transmitted. Physicians began using telephone technology over 10 decades ago. Early on, a variety of technologies such as phones, cable TV, and slow-scan video equipment were used to connect nurses, nurse practitioners, and physicians to minimally trained individuals in rural areas (McKendrick, 1878; Ricon, 2019).

Telehealth technology use has been available for many years; however, its adoption by healthcare providers and patients, other than telephone use, was extremely slow before the coronavirus pandemic. The COVID-19 pandemic resulted in reduced barriers to healthcare access. Although some providers are still reluctant to engage in telehealth activities fully, there has been a significant increase in the adoption and use of telehealth as a way to deliver acute, chronic, primary, and specialty care (CDC, 2020).

Today, telehealth technology has paved the way for expanded access to many individuals across the globe. Although millions of people in the United States may not have access to technologies for health at home, a variety of options provides this capability. Many professionals, according to the Centers for Medicaid and Medicare (CMS, 2020), provide telehealth services today, and nurse practitioners, APRNs, certified mid-wives, clinical nurse specialists, physician assistants, and certified registered nurse anesthetists are no exception. Telehealth technologies can improve accessibility to care and provide affordable quality health care to those that have been outside the reachable areas. Nurse practitioners can play a major role in providing accessible care to those individuals in underserved communities and rural areas as expansion of telehealth technology advancement continues.

Healthcare Provider Shortages

The American Association of Medical Colleges (AAMC) reported in their 2020 report an estimated shortage of up to 139,000 physicians by 2033 in primary and specialty care in the United States (AAMC, 2020). The AAMC specifically noted three areas that play a role in physician shortages: demographics, physicians nearing retirement age, and less barriers to care such as access through telehealth. **Table 13-2** provides further information on the three areas.

In August 2020, the American Association of Nurse Practitioners (AANP.org) reported there are over 290,000 licensed NPs in the United States, and new NPs continue to complete academic programs each year. **Table 13-3** shows a breakdown of statistics related to NPs in the U.S. nurse practitioners have been in practice for an average of 10 years with low malpractice rates where only 1.1% have been

Table 13-2 Key Findings on Physician Shortages

Demographics	Population growth and aging; U.S. population projected to grow by 10.4%; under-age population growth by 3.9%; age 65 or older population growth by 45.1%.
Nearing Retirement Age	Burnout; shift in retirement patterns; more than 2 of 5 physicians over 65.
Increase Access to Care	Underserved populations may have an increase in healthcare demands as barriers to access continue to lessen with technology such as telehealth.

Data from Association of American Medical Colleges (AAMC). (2020). Report: The Complexities of Physician Supply and Demand: Projections from 2018 to 2033. https://www.aamc.org/media/45976/download

Table 13-3 Nurse Practitioner Facts (AANP, 2020)

Areas or Ways Nurse Practitioners Practice	Percentage
Certification in an area of primary care	89.7%
Total number delivering primary care	69.0%
Full time that accept Medicare patients	82.9%
Accept Medicaid patients	80.2%
Holding hospital privileges	41.7%
Long-term care privileges	11.7%
Prescriptive authority and prescribing an average of 20 prescriptions per day (full-time NPs)	95.7%
See three or more patients per hour	57.4%

Data from American Association of Nurse Practitioners (AANP). (2020). NP Fact Sheet. https://www.aanp.org/about/all-about-nps/np-fact-sheet

named as a primary defendant. Like physicians, NPs can have prescriptive authority, including controlled substances, in all 50 states and in the District of Columbia (DC). Nurse Practitioners must follow their State Boards of Nursing regulations and practice act (AANP, 2020).

With over 290,000 APRNs currently licensed in the United States (AANP, 2020; Bureau of Labor Statistics, 2021) and the predicted growth of the telehealth industry, it is likely that APRNs will engage in telehealth in one form or another, allowing care to expand beyond the walls of the traditional office or clinic. With the expanded use, more opportunities will be available for all healthcare providers, which will increase access to care for patients, especially those in rural and underserved areas (Garber & Chike-Harris, 2018).

Nurse practitioners are positioned to fill healthcare provider shortages in many areas, including the rural underserved areas, and acute and critical care settings. Nurse practitioners can fill shortages from both the originating site or the remote location with the use of telehealth technology. All telehealth modalities along with a variety of services can be provided to assist in healthcare provider shortages and the increasing demand for healthcare services as our population continues to increase and age.

Access to Care

For many years, APRNs have provided care in primary, acute, and specialized areas. Remote patient monitoring has been used for over two decades, and nurse practitioners have been involved in this telehealth modality providing valuable services such as surveillance, quality data collection and analysis for performance reporting, translation of evidence into practice, and expert care management and guidance (Ricon, 2019).

Although barriers to healthcare access still exist, telehealth technology and telemedicine offers an opportunity for nurse practitioners to extend services to those patients in rural or distant geographical areas and underserved communities where care is not easily available. It is important to maintain patient–provider contact for those patients requiring continuous care for long-term and preventive care. Patients can avoid negative healthcare consequences if continuity of care exists. Remote access to providers can help to eliminate any issues related to delayed care such as preventive, chronic, or even routine care. **Box 13-1** provides ways telemedicine can be used for remote patient care (CDC, 2020).

Preventive Education, Management of Complex and Chronic Diseases, and Improving Outcomes

As more and more patients adopt the use of telehealth, it will be important for nurse practitioners and other providers to consider options and solutions to educating and managing complex and chronic diseases through telehealth options (Rush et al., 2018). Virtual delivery of patient education to help promote management and care of complex and chronic disease can improve patient outcomes. Rush et al. (2018) conducted a systematic review to compare the efficacy of virtual education delivery on patient outcomes compared with traditional in-person care. In the systematic review, selected papers compared virtual education to traditional care and used designs that measured the influence of one event (virtual delivery) to traditional care (in-person delivery). A variety of telehealth modalities were used in 16 studies reviewed. In 11 of 16 studies, virtual delivery of education and management of diseases significantly improved patient outcomes. In the remaining five studies, comparable outcomes were shown in both virtual and traditional visits. Some studies found the web-based delivery of patient education significantly increased patients'

Box 13-1 Telemedicine Uses

- Screen patients who may have symptoms and refer as appropriate (i.e., infectious diseases)
- Access primary care providers and specialists
- Consultation among providers
- Provide education and support for patients (i.e., chronic health conditions, including weight management and nutrition counseling)
- Low-risk urgent care services
- Monitor clinical signs of chronic medical conditions
- Case management for patients who have difficulty accessing care
- Hospital discharge follow-up
- Advance care planning and counseling to patients and/or caregivers
- Non-emergent care to residents in long-term care facilities
- Education and training for healthcare providers

Data from Centers for Disease Control and Prevention (CDC). (June 2020). Using telehealth to expand access to essential health services during the COVID-19 pandemic. March 3, 2020. Retrieved from https://www.cdc.gov/coronavirus/2019-ncov/hcp/telehealth.html

self-care behaviors, including in the areas of diet education for chronic diseases (Fredericks et al., 2015; Kelly et al., 2016).

Telehealth Regulations

With an increased use of APRNs in provider roles, it is important that APRNs are familiar with their state telehealth regulations. APRNS should be aware of federal and state laws and regulations, credentialing and privileging, malpractice coverage, position statements by governing bodies, established guidelines, and reimbursement policies related to telehealth. Because telehealth policy is impacted by government laws, regulations, and policies, it is important that APRNs evaluate state laws in both their state of practice and where the provider is located. Some states have laws related to telehealth, whereas other states address things such as definitions and guidelines. Another consideration is that telehealth laws may pertain only to physicians and not APRNs, as in South Carolina (Garber & Chike-Harris, 2019).

Garber & Chike-Harris (2019) reported that only 9 states had advisory opinions in the practice acts, 14 had position statements related to telehealth, and only 2 of those addressed telenursing, but not specifically at APRNs. Nurse practitioners need to pay particular attention to language in practice acts, identify prior legislation, and focus on current legislation surrounding telehealth regulations. If a state definition refers to "practice of medicine," APRNs need to review the language in the state Nurse Practice Act for scope of practice regarding telehealth, because it may not refer to APRNs. As valuable healthcare providers, APRNs continue to provide quality health care in a variety of settings across the lifespan. With the primary care physician shortage and the growth of the telehealth industry, along with the shift toward value-based care, APRNs may need to expand their options for the availability of virtual health care to patients (Garber & Chike-Harris, 2019).

Opportunities exist for APRNs to contact their State Board of Nursing to get a clear understanding of regulatory guidelines for telehealth care and the APRN practice. Enacting the APRN Compact as suggested by the National Council of State Boards of Nursing (NCSBN) allows APRNS to practice across state lines and may increase opportunities for access to telehealth care. Currently, only Idaho, Wyoming, and North Dakota have joined the APRN Compact. According to the NCSBN, when 10 states have enacted legislation toward the APRN Compact, it will be implemented. Today, most states require a provider to be licensed in the state where the patient is located (Garber & Chike-Harris, 2019).

Privacy and Protective Health Information Requirements Relevant to Telehealth

In March 2020, the Office for Civil Rights (OCR), a part of the Department of Health & Human Services (HHS), announced that healthcare providers would not receive penalties if they were acting in good faith to provide telehealth technologies during the public health emergency of COVID-19 (HHS.gov, 2020). Some examples of bad faith provisions can be found in **Box 13-2**.

Box 13-2 Telehealth Services That Fall Under Bad Faith Provision

- Conducting criminal acts, such as fraud, identity theft, and intentional invasion of privacy
- Violation of use or disclosures of patient data transmitted during a telehealth communication that are in violation of the HIPAA Privacy Rule (e.g., sale of the data, or use of the data for marketing without authorization)
- Use of public-facing or open forum remote communication products, such as TikTok, Facebook Live, Twitch, or a public chat room, which is identified as unacceptable forms of remote communication for telehealth
- Violations of state licensing laws or professional ethical standards (i.e., based on documented findings of a healthcare licensing or professional ethics board)

The issued notification applies to all healthcare providers covered by HIPAA who provide telehealth services during the emergency, and it will remain in effect until the public health emergency no longer exists as declared by the secretary of HHS. A public announcement will be issued when the existing notification is no longer enforced (HHS.gov, 2020).

The current good faith provision does not exclude current HIPAA guidelines for protecting patient information. Typically, if you have provider-to-provider telehealth communication, both providers must ensure protection of patient data. However, when you have provider-to-patient communication via telehealth or even patient-to-provider, such as when data is being transmitted from a device to the provider, HIPAA regulations must be considered. Relevant threats exist during these types of transmissions that include but are not limited to breach of confidentiality during transmission and/or collection of data, unauthorized access to data, and untrusted distribution of the software and hardware being used. Technology can be vulnerable to a security breech, and telehealth technology is no different. Protection of PHI remains the first obligation of providers to patients in all healthcare environments, including telemedicine.

Integration of Telehealth into Clinical Practice

Integration of telehealth into clinical practice must be effective, efficient, and meet the healthcare needs of the patient population. There are several steps to integrating telehealth technology and processes in practice every day. All stakeholders involved should have an understanding of the laws and regulations, including NP practice act requirements surrounding the use of telehealth. Staff and patients need to be educated on the use of telehealth equipment. Accessory platforms that will facilitate video and audio communication need to be considered, as well as updates to EMR systems that support telehealth. This may include updates that build upon the original equipment or new equipment altogether. Considerations for the adoption of new billing codes will need to be implemented as well (Neville, 2018).

Telehealth Frameworks

Telehealth is experiencing an increase in growth, with little resources available to guide the adoption of telehealth services. Small care services are poorly integrated into current systems and some are not sustained and/or only temporary. Many practices and organizations need help with the infrastructure of telehealth systems, as well as the regulations, education, implementation, and evaluation of telehealth systems. Having a framework to guide decisions on telehealth may increase interest in providing virtual services. Three such frameworks are the Telehealth Service Implementation Model (TSIM™), the Tietz Telehealth Framework, and the B.E.L.T.™ Framework.

Telehealth Service Implementation Model (TSIM™)

TSIM™ was developed by the Medical University of South Carolina (MUSC) as an approach to telehealth service implementation (MUSChealth.org, 2019). The framework has five phases that include strategy, design, transition, operations, and continual quality improvement.

The strategy phase is where the scope of the telehealth service is defined. Key areas such as conditions, the location of patients, type of providers, and what problem is being solved by the implementation of services are discussed and determined during this phase. The design phase is when the system build begins. Clinical and operational protocols and procedures are drafted and performance metrics are determined. Workflow is considered for all aspects of patient care related to the telehealth process. The transition phase is the test and go-live phase. Training and education occur during this phase. Workflows and equipment are tested, mock calls are practiced, and the go-live date is established. The operations phase is when the services are being offered in full operation, issues are managed on an ongoing basis, and the focus is on improving patient and provider experiences. The last phase of continual quality improvement is ongoing throughout the life cycle. Continual assessment and evaluation of performance metrics are completed and evaluated for improvements (MUSChealth.org, 2019).

Tietze Telehealth Framework

The Tietze Telehealth Framework was developed to distinguish different component methods of care delivery (Tietze, Hawkins & McElreath, 2021). As **Figure 13-1** shows, the Tietz framework encompasses three board digital modalities of telehealth: telemedicine, remote management/monitoring/coaching, and mobile health.

Telemedicine

Tietze et al. (2021) developed the Tietze framework, which defines telemedicine as stationary scheduled remote diagnostic encounters for health status in settings such as clinical-based, ICU, MICU, and emergency department–based telemedicine (Tietze et al., 2021).

Remote Management/Monitoring/Coaching

The second modality is stationary telemedicine as well, and generally occurs in settings such as home- or facility-based environments. These interactions can be scheduled or as-needed remote transmissions (Tietze et al., 2021).

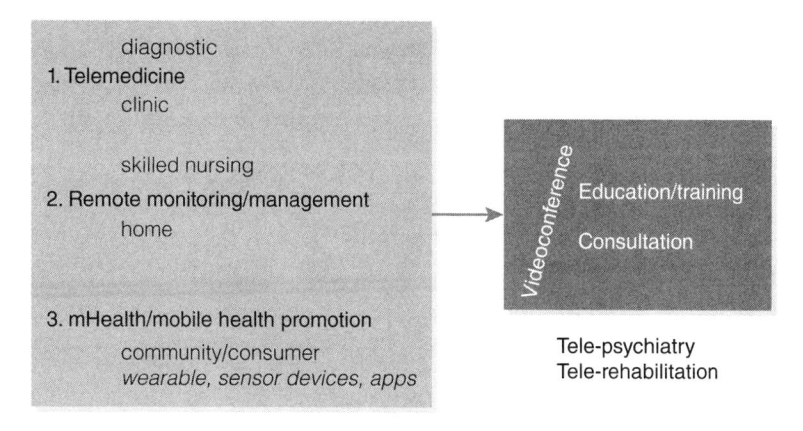

Figure 13-1 Tietze Telehealth Framework
Reproduced from McBride, S and Tietze, M: Nursing Informatics for the Advanced Practice Nurse, Second Edition, 2019, Springer Publishing Company.

Mobile Health (mHealth)

The third modality involves "community" groups and social media groups. This involves the use of wearable mobile patient–generated data that is collected over time or daily. These interactions can be scheduled or as-needed remote transmissions of data related to health issues (Tietze et al., 2021).

Videoconferencing

As shown in Figure 13-1, videoconferencing can occur as part of any of the three modalities and include education/training or consultation. This type of telemedicine may also be used in tele-psychiatry and tele-rehabilitation, as noted in Figure 13-1 (Tietze et al., 2021).

B.E.L.T.™ Framework

The B.EL.T.™ framework contains four key contextual elements. These elements are Bandwidth/Broadband, Education/Environment, Leadership and Technology. These four elements were identify by Arnaert and Debe (2019) as necessary for the provision, implementation, and sustainability of telehealth services. The B.E.L.T.™ framework represents a loop, as shown in **Figure 13-2**, showing interdependence. Any breach in the loop influences one's readiness for implementation.

Bandwidth/Broadband

Successful telehealth use requires an adequate internet connection and appropriate bandwidth capacity. Network bandwidth refers to the amount of data that can move across the connection over time. Broadband refers to the speed of access to the internet.

Over the last decade, highspeed data transmission has greatly enhanced the effectiveness and range of telehealth services. Telehealth services range in use and

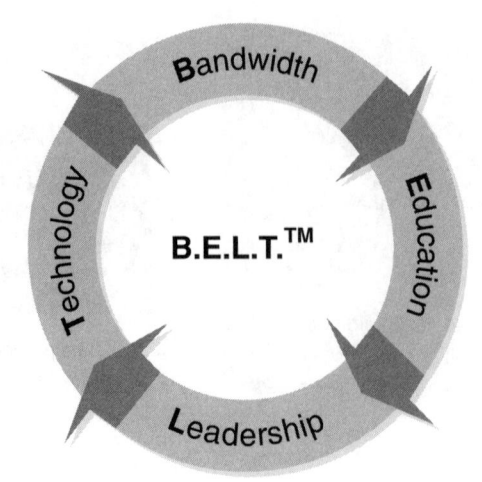

Figure 13-2 B.E.L.T.™ Framework

Antonia Arnaert, Zoumanan Debe. B.E.L.T.TM: Framework for Nurse Champions to Successful Implement Sustainable Telehealth Services Iris J of Nur & Car. 1(5): 2019. IJNC.MS.ID.000521. DOI: 10.33552/IJNC.2019.01.000521. Retrieved from https://irispublishers.com/ijnc/pdf/IJNC.MS.ID.000521.pdf.

needs and may require different bandwidths. Telecommunication infrastructure in geographical areas needs to be considered as well in regard to the reach of the services and where the patient population may live (Arnaert & Debe, 2019).

Education/Environment

Education, which includes raising awareness of the potential opportunities and benefits of telehealth to both staff, nurses, providers, and patients is critical to the success of the development and implementation phases. Many clinicians lack an understanding of software and hardware and will need training and education on using telehealth technology in order to deliver the services every day. Both patient and provider education will need to be developed and should continue throughout the process and after deployment of the telehealth services (Arnaert & Debe, 2019).

Leadership

Having leadership buy-in to telehealth services is important as a component of success. Many nurses take on the role of champion during the implementation process. These leaders should have experience with clinical and medical issues that will be addressed by the services, have the ability to navigate difficult change process, and have the ability to build relationships among stakeholders related to telehealth technology implementation and its processes (Arnaert & Debe, 2019).

Technology

Telehealth technology covers many aspects, including the hardware, software, communications, and general infrastructure of the technology. Interoperability needs to be considered, along with integration with the current technology and software. Evaluation of the current technology will need to be conducted and upgraded as needed to meet the needs of a new system telehealth program (Arnaert & Debe, 2019).

Steps When Implementing a Telehealth Program

The following seven steps should be considered when implementing a telehealth program in a practice.

1. Understand how HIPAA and state regulations apply to telehealth.
2. Determine how the practice will use telehealth.
3. Identify individuals or a team to lead the implementation of telehealth.
4. Find the right telehealth equipment and software.
5. Integrate telehealth workflow with the electronic medical record.
6. Train staff and providers to use the telehealth equipment, including how to troubleshoot issues that may arise.
7. Educate patients about telehealth services (Liezl van Dyk, 2014).

HIPAA and State Regulations

All healthcare technology must be HIPAA-compliant and telehealth technology is no different. Practices must ensure the security and privacy of all protected health information (PHI) even in the telehealth environment.

State regulations for telemedicine vary from state to state but many policies have begun to include some regulations that supplement traditional healthcare requirements. Federal entities such as HHS have announced broader use of telemedicine, and some regulatory and reimbursement barriers have been removed. The Centers for Medicare & Medicaid Services (CMS) has, and continues to add, various flexibilities to improve virtual care access (CMS, 2020; Hall & McGraw, 2014).

Telehealth Use in the Practice

Deciding on the type of telehealth services to provide may depend on the patient population seen in the practice. Having a clear vision and defining goals for how a practice will use telehealth services will be important to the overall implementation process. Understanding the goals will help to determine how to measure progress toward a successful telehealth launch.

A systematic review of telemedicine service frameworks conducted by Liezl van Dyk (2014) highlighted a feasibility study outlining the seven core principles of successful development of telehealth services. These principles include taking a pragmatic approach to selecting telehealth applications sites. Clinicians and telehealth users take ownership of the system, and management and support should start at the bottom and go up, technology should be user-friendly, users must be trained and supported in all aspects of the system, telehealth applications should be evaluated, and information about the development of telehealth must be shared (Liezl van Dyk, 2014). Practices should consider these core principles when determining the range of telemedicine healthcare services to deliver. A variety of telehealth services can be implemented across small practices and large health systems. For example, some practices may only offer video consultations where other practices may offer a full range of telehealth services from consultations to complete care virtual visits. Some practices may choose to only offer telehealth services on certain days at different times; others may transition to a virtual-only practice offering telehealth services.

Identify Individuals/Team to Lead the Telehealth Implementation

Involvement of staff, nurses, and providers is important to the overall success of telehealth in a practice. Working in collaboration with the IT department/person and administration of the practice or organization is also required. Involving personnel early in the process will help everyone feel invested in the implementation of telehealth services. This is where you may consider selecting a team that involves some staff, nurses, and providers that can lead the charge. This team should be individuals dedicated to the project that can delegate tasks, troubleshoot concerns, and coordinate communication.

Find the Equipment and Platform for Telehealth

After a team has been selected and decisions made on the types of telehealth services to offer, the equipment and software need to be considered. Partnering with a company that can meet the goals of the organization will be important. The following questions should be considered.

- Is the telehealth platform HIPAA-compliant?
- Is it a quick implementation and roll-out process?
- Are there options for customizing workflows?
- How are reimbursement requirements met?
- Does the telehealth system integrate with the current electronic health records system?
- Is the system easy to use and intuitive for staff, nurses, providers, and patients (Smith et al., 2020)?

Integrate Telehealth Workflow with the Electronic Medical Record

Developing and integrating custom workflows into the telehealth system and electronic medical records can help meet the needs of the patient population and practice. Having integrated systems allows a practice to have services beyond video sessions and helps them stay connected with patients throughout their care. A well-integrated system could send appointment reminders ahead of visits via text messaging and/or email. Reminders for preventive screenings and other healthcare services could also be sent to patients as needed. Ensuring a practice has selected a system that meets the needs of the organization and patients is important. With robust systems that are thoroughly integrated, practices and organizations can customize telehealth services in conjunction with the electronic health records. Systems can sync, allowing continuity of care, as the patient is seen during their healthcare visits (Neville, 2018).

Educating Staff and Providers

Educating staff and providers is an essential part of the success in providing telehealth services. Training should include, at minimum, equipment use, software training, how to troubleshoot issues that arise for both the provider and patient before and during the virtual visits, how to determine if patients have telehealth ready access, and best practices on how to conduct virtual appointments. Virtual appointments should remain personalized and done via an atmosphere of caring (Edirippulige & Armfield, 2016; Rutledge et al., 2017).

Patient-Centered Telehealth Practices

Providers and staff should be trained on how to conduct patient-centered telehealth practices. Staff should screen patients to determine telehealth suitability. Screening questions should identify patient factors that may eliminate a telehealth option, including their level of technology knowledge. Providers and staff should be trained in workflow processes involving telehealth visits, such as scheduling, documentation that meets billing requirements, compliance with regulations, and training on a backup plan if technology issues occur during the visit (Song et al., 2021).

Educate Patients About Telehealth Services

Once the telehealth system has been implemented and is ready to go, and education and training has been completed, patients will need to be notified of the telehealth services provided. The practice can promote telehealth and virtual visits through email, phone, social media, and in-office collateral. Be prepared to address frequently asked questions so patients understand the expectations of telehealth and virtual visits. Developing and providing frequently asked questions (FAQs) is valuable to patients in online environments. More and more patients are adopting telehealth services due to convenience and ease of access to care, so educating patients is important for a smooth transition.

Evaluation of Telehealth Systems

Telehealth systems should be evaluated for optimization and sustainability to maintain the level of care needed for the virtual care environment. As a result of the rapid deployment of telehealth systems due to the COVID-19 pandemic, many practices and organizations are facing how to evaluate the telehealth systems and services they have implemented. While measures are in place to evaluate the new implementation of technological systems, outcome information from telehealth systems implementation is mostly disorganized and dispersed. The Agency for Health Research and Quality (AHRQ)'s (2020) technical brief, emphasizes the critical nature of evaluating the impact on health outcomes in a telehealth evaluation. Several frameworks from current literature were identified, and each of them focused on many of the same measurement areas. The National Quality Forum (NQF) (2020) and the WHO (2016) looked at measurement concepts or domains for evaluating programs that include health outcomes, health delivery (quality and cost), experience, and program implementation and key performance indicators (Chuo et al., 2020). Agboola et al. (2014) describes the Re-Aim Framework that includes the five areas of evaluation, reach, effectiveness, adoption, implementation, and maintenance. To evaluate a telehealth program, each of these areas should be assessed and reviewed.

The Future of Telehealth

Although telemedicine has been in use for nearly 40 years, telehealth has created a wave across medical communities, transforming what we know in health care. This disruptive healthcare innovation continues to prompt providers to evaluate ways to implement telemedicine services in practice. In 2016, the American Medical Association surveyed 1,300 physicians in the AMA Digital Health Study and found that telehealth had doubled from 14% to 28% (Strazawski, 2020). The coronavirus pandemic was the tipping point for telehealth use in telemedicine, and it will continue to grow at an increased rate in the United States and internationally in the future. A comparison of the number of telehealth visits during the first quarter of 2019 and 2020 was conducted, showing a 50% increase in 2020 during January through March of 2020. By week 13 of 2020, there was an increase of 154% in telehealth visits compared to the same period in 2019 (Koonin et al., 2020). In 2020, the telehealth technology industry rushed to meet the increasing demand to use telemedicine technology and applications. As telehealth continues to accelerate, it will become more advanced over time and new devices, and applications and processes will continue to be available that can aid healthcare providers with the increasing demand of meeting the care needs of patients suffering from chronic and long-term diseases.

As one of the most disruptive healthcare innovations, telehealth has already changed the way providers are responding to their patients and in how they provide continuous care. Telehealth has the potential to reduce healthcare costs and improve patient outreach and health outcomes for many individuals, setting the stage for different patient healthcare experiences (Modern Healthcare, 2020). In the future, providers will need to consider ongoing options for ways to incorporate telemedicine into practice to meet the ever-growing needs of patients.

⚲ CASE STUDIES

Telemedicine Case Studies

LeadingAge's Center for Aging Services Technologies (CAST) offers a number of case studies related to telehealth and remote patient monitoring. See the following table for a list of relevant case studies and brief descriptions of technology implementations in real life. These case studies can be found online at https://leadingage.org/case-studies/cast-telehealth-case-studies.

Case Study	Examples of Real-Life Technology Implementation
Supporting Residents with Telehealth During COVID-19	The sixth-largest nonprofit senior living provider implemented telehealth when the coronavirus pandemic started.
Lexington Health Network and Curatess Open Telehealth Platform	Case study that demonstrates the use of open telemedicine that is integrated with a patient's medical records and medical peripherals. Resulted in better managed return-to-hospital rates, leave-of-absence rates, and operational inefficiencies.

Case Study	Examples of Real-Life Technology Implementation
Reducing Blood Pressure among Engaged Participants through Multi-User Telehealth, Gamification, and Engagement Platform	This case study examined the relationship between ambulatory blood pressure (ABP) and patient engagement with a kiosk platform placed in pharmacies, grocery stores, and other community centers. A statistically significant relationship between the frequency of engagement and the lowering of systolic blood pressure was shown in the study.
Telehealth Helps Great Plains Health Patients Manage Their Conditions Confidently in the Comfort of Their Home to Improve Outcomes	In this case study, a custom Ambulatory Care platform and Remote Patient Monitoring Program for Transitional Care was used to scale up their ambulatory program. Patient satisfaction scores were 98% and it showed reduced hospital readmissions. The technology also improved patient education, care coordination, and helped patients reconcile their medications. Patients also report that they liked being monitored.
Targeting the "Superusers" of Health Care with Telehealth	This case study describes how 135 clients who had at least 5 chronic health conditions were monitored. The project used a range of biometric sensors that involved emergency response systems with automatic fall detection. Participants were matched with a multidisciplinary care team that included health coaches, nurses, social workers, pharmacists, and primary care providers. Outcomes showed a 27% reduction in cost of care, a 32% reduction in acute and long-term care costs, and a 45% reduction in hospitalizations.

Seminar Discussion Questions

1. How does telehealth differ from face-to-face patient visits?
2. Describe the advantages and barriers of telehealth visits in your practice.
3. Discuss the different telehealth modalities and how they would be used in practice.
4. In recognizing that telehealth technology will continue to advance, what policies should be addressed to maintain the telehealth practice?
5. Discuss your state licensure and the Nurse Practice Act as it relates to telehealth.

References

Agboola, S., Hale, T. M., Masters, C., Kvedar, J., & Jethwani, K. (2014). "Real-world" practical evaluation strategies: A review of telehealth evaluation. *JMIR Res Protoc*, 3(4), e75. https://doi.org/10.2196/resprot.3459, PMID: 25524892, PMCID: 4275475

American Association of Nurse Practitioners (AANP). (2020). NP fact sheet. https://www.aanp.org/about/all-about-nps/np-fact-sheet

Arnaert, A., & Debe, Z. (2019). B.E.L.T.™: Framework for nurse champions to successfully implement sustainable telehealth services. *Iris Journal of Nursing and Care*. https://irispublishers.com/ijnc/pdf/IJNC.MS.ID.000521.pdf

Association of American Medical Colleges (AAMC). (2020). Report: The complexities of physician supply and demand: Projections from 2018 to 2033. https://www.aamc.org/media/45976/download

Bureau of Labor Statistics. (2021). *Occupational outlook handbook*. Department of Labor. https://www.bls.gov/ooh/healthcare/nurse-anesthetists-nurse-midwives-and-nurse-practitioners.htm

Centers for Disease Control and Prevention (CDC). (2020). Using telehealth to expand access to essential health services during the COVID-19 pandemic. Retrieved March 3, 2020 from https://www.cdc.gov/coronavirus/2019-ncov/hcp/telehealth.html

Centers for Medicare & Medicaid Services (CMS). (2020). Medicare telemedicine health care provider fact sheet: Telehealth. https://www.cms.gov/newsroom/fact-sheets/medicare-telemedicine-health-care-provider-fact-sheet

Chuo, J., Macy, M. L., & Lorch, S. A. (2020). Strategies for evaluating telehealth. *Pediatrics*. https://doi.org/10.1542/peds.2020-1781

Darkins, A. W., & Cary, M. A. (2000). Telemedicine and telehealth: Principles, policies, performance, and pitfalls. *American Journal of Public Health*, 90(8), 1322.

Edirippulige, S., & Armfield, N. R. (2016). Education and training to support the use of clinical telehealth: A review of the literature. *Journal of Telemedicine and Telecare*, 23(2). 10.1177/1357633X16632968

Fredericks S., Martorella, G., & Catallo, C. (2015). A systematic review of web-based educational interventions. *Clinical Nurse Research*, 24, 91–113.

Finely, B. A., & Shea, K. D. (2019). Telehealth: Disrupting time for health care quantity and quality. *Nursing Administration Quarterly*, 43(3), 256–262. https://doi.org/10.1097/NAQ.0000000000000357

Garber, K. M., & Chike-Harris, K. E. (2019). Nurse practitioners and virtual care: A 50-state review of APRN telehealth law and policy. *Telehealth and Medicine Today*. https://doi.org/10.30953/tmt.v4.136

Hall, J. L., & McGraw, D. (2014). For telehealth to succeed, privacy and security risks must be identified and addressed. *Health Affairs*, 33(2), 216–221. https://doi.org/10.1377/hlthaff.2013.0997

HHS.gov. (2020). *OCR issues guidance on telehealth remote communications following its notification of enforcement discretion*. Retrieved March 21, 2021 from https://www.hhs.gov/about/news/2020/03/20/ocr-issues-guidance-on-telehealth-remote-communications-following-its-notification-of-enforcement-discretion.html

InTouch Health. (n.d.). *The future of telehealth in the U.S. and across the globe*. Retrieved March 13, 2021 from https://intouchhealth.com/future-telehealth-us-across-globe/

Kelly, J., Reidlinger, D., Hoffmann, T., & Campbell, K. (2016). Telehealth methods to deliver dietary interventions in adults with chronic disease: A systematic review and meta-analysis. *American Journal of Clinical Nutrition*, 104, 1693–1702.

Koonin, L. M., Hoots B., Tsang C. A., Leroy, Z., Farris, K. Jolly, B., Antall, P., McCabe, B., Zelis, C. B., Tong, I., & Harris, A. M. (2020). Trends in the use of telehealth during the emergence of the COVID-19 pandemic—United States, January–March 2020. *Morbidity & Mortality Weekly Report (MMWR)*, 69, 1595–1599. http://dx.doi.org/10.15585/mmwr.mm6943a3

Lam K., Lu A. D., Shi Y., & Covinsky, K. E. (2020). Assessing telemedicine unreadiness among older adults in the United States during the COVID-19 pandemic. *JAMA Intern Medicine*. Advance online publication. 10.1001/jamainternmed.2020.2671

McKendrick, J. G. (1878). Note on the microphone and telephone in auscultation. *British Medical Journal*, 1(911), 856–857.

Medical University of South Carolina. (2019). Telehealth Service Implementation Model (TSIM™): A framework for telehealth service development, implementation, and sustainability. https://muschealth.org/-/sm/health/telehealth/f/tsim-summary.ashx?la=en

Modern Healthcare. (2020). *Predicting the future role of telemedicine*. Retrieved March 1, 2021 from https://www.modernhealthcare.com/technology/predicting-future-role-telemedicine

National Coordinator for Health Information Technology. (n.d.). *What is telehealth? How is telehealth different from telemedicine?* https://www.healthit.gov/faq/what-telehealth-how-telehealth-different-telemedicine

National Quality Forum. (2020). *National Quality Forum measures reports and tools*. Updated March 2020. http://www.qualityforum.org/Measures_Reports_Tools.aspx

National Telehealth Resource Centers. (n.d.). *A framework for defining telehealth: The center for connected health policy*. https://www.cchpca.org/sites/default/files/2018-10/Telehealth%20Definintion%20Framework%20for%20TRCs_0.pdf

Nesbitt, T. S., & Katz-Bell, J. (2021). *History of telehealth*. In Rheuban, K., Krupinski, E. A. Rheuban K, & Krupinski E. A. (Eds.), *Understanding Telehealth*. McGraw-Hill.

Neville, C. W. (2018). Telehealth: A balanced look at incorporating this technology into practice. *SAGE Open Nursing*, 4(1–5), 1–5. https://doi.org/10.1177/2377960818786504

Ontario Agency for Health Protection and Promotion (Public Health Ontario). (2015). *At a glance: The ten steps for conducting an evaluation*. Toronto, ON: Queen's Printer for Ontario. https://www.publichealthontario.ca/-/media/documents/A/2015/at-a-glance-10step-evaluation.pdf?la=en

Ricon, T. A. (2019). How NPs can help expand telehealth services. *The Nurse Practitioner*, 44(11), 30–35. https://doi.org/10.1097/01.NPR.0000586004.85303.05

Rush, K. L., Hatt, L., Janke, R., Burton, L., Ferrier, M., & Tetrault, M. (2018). *The efficacy of telehealth delivered educational approaches for patients with chronic diseases: A systematic review* [Article]. http://dx.doi.org/10.14288/1.0380468

Rutledge, C. M., Kott, K., Schweickert, P., Poston, R., Fowler, C., & Haney, T. (2017). Telehealth and eHealth in nurse practitioner training: Current perspectives. *Advances in Medical Educations and Practice*, 399–409.

Rutledge, C. M., Pitts, C., Poston, R., & Schweickert, P. (2018). *NONPF supports telehealth in nurse practitioner education 2018*. Telehealth_Paper_2018 (1).pdf

Smith, S., & Raskin, S. (2021). Achieving health equity: Examining telehealth in response to a pandemic. *The Journal for Nurse Practitioners*, 17(2), 214–217. htps://doi.org/10.1016/j.nurpra.2020.10.001

Smith, W. R., Atala, A. J., Terlecki, R. P., Kelly, E. E., & Matthews, C. A. (2020). Implementation guide for rapid integration of an outpatient telemedicine program during the COVID-19 pandemic. *Journal of American College of Surgeons*, 231(2), 216–222.e2. https://doi.org/10.1016/j.jamcollsurg.2020.04.030. Epub 2020 Apr 30. PMID: 32360960; PMCID: PMC7192116

Song, E. H., Milne, C., Mitchell, L., Hamm, T., Mize, J., Evans, K., Shah, J., Robinson, S. Lebedinskaya, N., & Tharalson, E. M. (2021). *Patient-centered telehealth best practices: What have we learned?* https://www.todayswoundclinic.com/articles/patient-centered-telehealth-best-practices-what-have-we-learned

Strazawski, L. (2020). *Telehealth's post-pandemic future: Where do we go from here?* Retrieved March 15, 2021 from https://www.ama-assn.org/practice-management/digital/telehealth-s-post-pandemic-future-where-do-we-go-here

Tietze, M., Hawkins, S., & McElreath, D. (2021). Telehealth and nursing education: Remote patient monitoring clinical site application. Texas Board of Nursing Bulletin. LII(I). https://www.bon.texas.gov/pdfs/newsletter_pdfs/2021/January%202021%20Bulletin%20web.pdf

Totten AM, McDonagh MS, Wagner JH. The Evidence Base for Telehealth: Reassurance in the Face of Rapid Expansion During the COVID-19 Pandemic. White Paper Commentary. (Pacific Northwest Evidence-based Practice Center, Oregon Health & Science University under Contract No. 290-2015-00009-I). AHRQ Publication No. 20-EHC015. Rockville, MD: Agency for Healthcare Research and Quality. May 2020. DOI: https://doi.org/10.23970/AHRQEPC COVIDTELEHEALTH. Posted final reports are located on the Effective Health Care Program

Totten, A. M., Womack, D. M., Eden, K. B., McDonagh, M. S., Griffin, J. C., Grusing, S., & Hersh, W. R. (2016). Telehealth: Mapping the evidence for patient outcomes from systematic Reviews. Technical Brief No. 26. (Prepared by the Pacific Northwest Evidence-based Practice Center under Contract No. 290-2015-00009-I.) AHRQ Publication No.16-EHC034-EF. Rockville, MD: Agency for Healthcare Research and Quality. https://www.ncbi.nlm.nih.gov/books/NBK379320/pdf/Bookshelf_NBK379320.pdf

van Dyk L. (2014). A review of telehealth service implementation frameworks. *International Journal of Environmental Research and Public Health*, 11(2), 1279–1298. https://doi.org/10.3390/ijerph110201279

World Health Organization (WHO). (2010). *Telemedicine: Opportunities and developments in Member States*. https://www.who.int/goe/publications/goe_telemedicine_2010.pdf

World Health Organization (WHO). (2016). *Monitoring and evaluating digital health interventions: a practical guide to conducting research and assessment*. https://apps.who.int/iris/handle/10665/252183

Wosik, J., Fudim, M., Cameron, B., Gellad, Z. F., Cho, A., Phinney, D., Curtis, S., Roman, M., Poon, E. G., Ferranti, J., Katz, J. N., & Tcheng, J. (2020). Telehealth transformation: COVID-19 and the rise of virtual care. *Journal of the American Medical Informatics Association*, 27(6), 957–962. https://doi.org/10.1093/jamia/ocaa067

PART 4

The Professional Nurse Practitioner

CHAPTER 14	Concepts and Challenges of the Professional Nurse Practitioner............ 351
CHAPTER 15	Health Policy and the Nurse Practitioner 367
CHAPTER 16	Mentoring and Lifelong Learning 389
CHAPTER 17	Reimbursement for Nurse Practitioner Services 403
CHAPTER 18	Professional Employment: Preparing for Licensure, Certification, and Credentialing 431
CHAPTER 19	Nurse Practitioner as a Business Owner: Entrepreneurship and Practice Management 449

CHAPTER 14

Concepts and Challenges of the Professional Nurse Practitioner

Constance H. Glenn and Geraldine Budd

As the student NP prepares for graduation, or the employed NP considers a workplace change, factors that can enhance the work environment can assist in choosing a successful practice setting. Having a supportive workplace environment has been shown to improve work efficiency, enhance the ability to provide high-quality patient care, contribute to cost effectiveness, and promote the retention of NPs in successful collaborative practices in a variety of healthcare settings. To prepare the graduate NP for professional practice, it is important to review the core concepts related to being a professional.

Professionalism

Historically, the title of *professional* has been reserved for lawyers, the clergy, and physicians. In broader terms, this title traditionally refers to occupational groups who have control over their own work, exercise governance and regulation over themselves and others, and consequently, play a civic role in protecting society (Evetts, 2013). In the early 1900s, Abraham Flexner (1910) wrote *The Flexner Report,* which was a critical assessment of medical education of that time. Many reformations were made in response to this assessment. After Flexner studied a wide variety of disciplines, he then became an expert on what constituted a profession. These characteristics have been revised and expanded by various disciplines; however, there are several attributes that define the core characteristics of professionalism. These are autonomy, ethics, specialized knowledge, and service and altruism (Black, 2019).

A study by Anderson (2017) developed a strategy to explore the relationship between professional identity and ANP practice in primary care. Her study strategy suggests it is helpful to look through the lens of professional identity being characterized at three different levels. These levels are micro (individual), meso (interactional/relational), and macro (group/societal) levels. This study aimed to explore how, and to what extent, each level impacts ANP practice. It is important to note that the study was specifically informed by two identity frameworks, the first being the social identity theory (SIT), and the second, professional identity theory (PIT), an extension of the SIT of Tajfel and Turner (1986). These identity frameworks consider identity a process of interaction between the three different levels and allow for exploration of the relationship between professional identity and ANP practice in primary care (Anderson, 2017).

In their book *The Making of Nurse Professionals,* Crigger and Godfrey (2011) focused on virtue ethics as the core framework for professionalism in nursing. In this view, an individual responds to specific situations in a manner that is appropriate to that particular situation. When performed in an admirable manner, the moral message that this was "good" is reinforced so the person will conduct the action similarly in future situations. This viewpoint emphasizes that the nurse has a choice in how to interact with patients and in society at large. This experiential development process is transformational and moves toward encompassing professional ideals and ethics when good choices are reinforced. Occasionally, "doing good" for the patient may not be what the patient believes is best, and this is when the integrity of the nurse professional, based on an ethical code, must prevail. For NPs, these types of situations occur fairly frequently in daily practice: patients who want narcotics for prolonged periods of time without a known etiology of pain, the neighbor who calls and asks for an antibiotic prescription without being evaluated as a patient of that practitioner's practice setting, and so forth. We can all come up with numerous examples of when the patient view and the NP view of "doing good" do not coincide.

More recently, a dissertation by Gilman (2018) regarding, *Relationships between APRN State Practice Authority, Perceived Autonomy, Professionalism, and Interprofessional Team Function Among a National Sample of APRNs in the US,* describes the development of professional identity in nursing. She includes the position that all professional identity begins with education and socialization, and continues to evolve and further develop throughout a professional career (Godfrey & Crigger, 2017). She describes that the beginning student nurse forms professional identity through the socialization process within academic programs, becoming familiar with the philosophy, ethics, expectations, mores, and associated values of the nursing profession and is shaped by didactic and clinical experiences. This professional identity for the student is generally well-formed by the time of entering the workforce.

New professional identity is formed by the APN however. Formation of this new professional identity begins upon entry into the program when the student is reintroduced to the foundations of nursing philosophy and association of self with the profession at a higher level, with the addition of new skills and new knowledge (Godfrey & Crigger, 2017). As the philosophical foundations of nursing are explored, professional identity matures, and the APRN enhances both individual identity (the beliefs, values, independent and critical-thinking decision making) and social identity, which grows with the development of social skills, collaboration, communication, and group skills. As the student experiences APN role transition, a new professional identity emerges while still retaining the original nursing identity. This tension point between the nurse and the APN role is a critical point, yielding the emergence of a new professional identity as the APN student develops further into the mature professional stage.

Godfrey and Crigger (2017) additionally state that the most significant virtues for nursing professionals are compassion, humility, integrity, and courage. It is hoped that nurse practitioner students have developed these virtues during their nursing education and career. It is imperative that these virtues are transferred and developed during the transformative process in the NP educational experience in order to make the best choices in the provision of excellent health care to patients, and to be responsive to the moral and ethical code of professionalism required to succeed.

Nurse practitioner behaviors indicative of professionalism were investigated by Adams and Miller (2001). Over 500 NPs were recruited to complete the Professionalism in Nursing Behaviors, Inventory questionnaire at the 1998 American Academy of Nurse Practitioners annual conference held in Arizona. The Professionalism in Nursing Behaviors' Inventory was adapted for NPs by the authors in 1998 and is composed of 48 items that cover demographic information and nine categories of behaviors:

1. Educational preparation
2. Autonomy
3. Adherence to the American Nurses Association (ANA) code of ethics
4. Theory
5. Competency maintenance
6. Participation in research
7. Participation in publication
8. Participation in community service
9. Participation in professional organizations

In their seminal article, the authors report findings in the self-regulation and autonomy category, including that 74% of the NPs regularly performed self-evaluation. Furthermore, the majority of NPs were making autonomous clinical decisions, were accountable for patient outcomes, and were independently determining what their job positions entailed. This is particularly noteworthy as the study was performed in 1998.

Interestingly, in the United Kingdom, professionalism for nurses describes skills, attitudes, values, and behaviors that are similar to those who practice medicine (UK Department of Health, 2006). It includes concepts such as the maintenance of competence for a unique body of knowledge and skill set, personal integrity, altruism, adherence to ethical codes of conduct, accountability, a dedication to self-regulation, and the exercise of discretionary judgment (UK Department of Health, 2006). Professionalism is also described as a moral understanding among health professionals when providing health care to individuals and the community as a whole. Healthcare professionals determine how to use medical knowledge, have the right to practice with considerable autonomy, and have the privilege of self-regulation.

In an ethnographic study, a researcher observed advanced practice nurses (APNs) who relocated to an area with high needs for healthcare services and then started the only partnership with general practitioners (MDs) in the country (McMurray, 2010). The study relates the accounts of the APNs' struggles to be accepted as professionals. The author's discussions are quite thought provoking and worth a short review here. McMurray provides a background on nurses struggling to be seen as more than the performers of "dirty" tasks—those directed to be done by the physician, but not esoteric enough for the physician to perform. In addition, there is reference to the hierarchical model of health care, with medicine being in charge of the division of labor and, indeed, even proclaiming its right to "challenge the legitimacy of other occupations" (McMurray, 2010, p. 805). The relationship of nurses and physicians is noted to have been one of subservience—the nurse being the "handmaiden"—and that the nurses' work was "women's work."

McMurray goes on to describe the vast amount of interpersonal and social expertise nurses need to deal with: "the messy and dirty work of emotions, bodies, fluids, relations, attending, nurturing, and being there" (2010, p. 806). As noted in an earlier chapter, the attributes of emotions, nurturing, and being there are part of the theoretical basis that gives meaning to what nurses and NPs do. The study uncovered what it meant to be an APN, and how difficult it was to combine "the nurturing skills of nursing with the curative knowledge of medicine" (p. 810). Upon graduation, finding an appropriate place for an APN to practice to the full scope of his or her knowledge was difficult; therefore, this unique small group of APNs went where they were needed most and hired general practitioners to work *with* them instead of the APNs working *for* them.

It is interesting to note how the objective observer collecting research material was able to clearly describe that the biggest issue causing the rift between professions was related to diagnosing. Diagnosing was noted to be the specialized knowledge of the physician group, and barriers to practice in the United Kingdom are the same as seen in the United States. These included limited prescribing rights, difficulties with signing progress notes, insurance reimbursement inequalities, difficulty admitting patients to the hospital, and having referrals and consults occasionally denied unless there was an attending physician in charge of the patient instead of an APN. The researcher found the process of APNs becoming accepted as professionals to be one that has not yet been fully embraced. McMurray uses the term "occupational equivalent" to sum up how the APNs worked with GPs on a similar level—with *equivalent* being the operative term. This is obviously not the same as *equal*.

In many states, the law dictating how NPs practice (state practice acts) use the word "collaboration" to describe the NP relationship with physicians. Typically, collaboration for NPs and physicians is usually a hierarchical relationship, with the physician as leader and decision maker who steps in or takes over when uncertainty arises. In contrast, Norful et al. (2018) used a systematic scientific approach built on their research to develop a theoretical model of NP-physician co-management. This model allows professional NPs to function at the independent role for which their education prepared them.

Qualities uncovered in research about NPs highlight the core values of professionalism. In a study conducted with NPs in New Zealand and Australia (Carryer et al., 2007), professionalism was identified as one of the core roles of the NP. In addition, dynamic practice and clinical leadership were also identified as core components of the role of the NP. When discussing the transition from nurse to nurse practitioner, the study findings cause the authors to dispute that nurses leave nursing behind when they learn medical aspects of patient care. Instead, Carryer et al. (2007) state that tasks are not the defining characteristics of a profession; rather, it is the "philosophical approach guiding practice that defines the nature of the discipline" (p. 1824).

APN professional identity is based on the longstanding principles, practice standards, and ethics of nursing (American Nurses Association [ANA], 2015a).

Professional identity development represents both the individual (self) and the collective (nursing profession) dimensions of the concept of identity and characterizes two stages of identity: the development and professional stages (Cardoso et al., 2014). Crigger and Godfrey (2011) emphasize that both psychological paradigms, referring to character-building and being, and social paradigms, referring to socialization and doing, must be present to establish an individual's professional identity.

Various models revolving around professionalism in nursing exist, all incorporating the basic tenets of the more generalized definitions of what constitutes a profession. Later in this section, Harriet Fields, EdD, RN, discusses professional behaviors that she developed while at Columbia University and that she articulates as she teaches: both nursing and health policy. Adams and Miller (2001) developed a wheel of professionalism that has, at its base, education in a university setting, with wheel spokes that include the following: publication and communication; adherence to a code of ethics for nurses; theory development, use, and evaluation; community service orientation; continuing education/competence; research development, use, and evaluation; self-regulation (autonomy); and professional organization participation.

A nurse leader who spent many years studying nursing as a profession, Lucie Kelly, RN, PhD, FAAN, developed eight characteristics of professional practitioners (Black, 2019).

Autonomy

Autonomy is the authority of an individual to make their own decisions without oversight or control by others (Goolsby et al., 2020). It is an attribute of all professions and is often discussed as a cornerstone to the professional practice of NPs (Weiland, 2015). Autonomy is often used synonymously with independence and can be seen as the ability to exercise full decision making in the care provided to patients (Weiland, 2008).

In 1967, Loretta Ford and a physician colleague conceptualized the NP role for public health nurses to provide pediatric well child–care. When conceiving the role, Dr. Ford recognized the new NPs would not function as physician extenders, but instead would act with autonomy and independence, using health promotion and disease prevention to promote self-care for individuals, families, and communities (Ford, 1997). It is interesting to note that NP autonomy has always been an uphill battle. A descriptive study of early NPs found that the study participants strongly desired to not only move beyond traditional nursing boundaries but to strive for autonomy (Brown & Draye, 2003).

In the early years of the profession, NPs were subjected to much resistance from physicians, other nurses, insurers, and pharmacists. Individual physicians often support NP autonomy, but the profession of medicine does not support legislative changes for NP independence (Choi & DeGagne, 2016). Early in the NP movement, even the nursing profession was not supportive of the autonomous NP role, perhaps indicating how deep-rooted the subservience to medicine concept of nursing was. Nonetheless, in subsequent years the nursing profession transitioned to wholeheartedly support the independence of NPs. Indeed, autonomy and independence for NPs has become entrenched in the APN role. The National Council of State Boards of Nursing (NCSBN) (2008, 2012, 2019) consistently and frequently clarifies independent practice as an expectation of all certified NPs, and in a position paper on NP practice, the American Association of Nurse Practitioners (AANP) (n.d.) insists that NPs must practice autonomously to deliver the highest quality of patient care.

Weiland (2015), in a qualitative study intended to understand NP autonomy, found a major theme was that autonomy is real and true when the NP practices independently and alone with the patient. An important subtheme of Weiland's study on autonomy was the NP–patient relationship. The NP and patient were viewed as reciprocal in that both take part in making healthcare decisions. NPs were found to have a moral obligation to advocate for patients and this increased their sense of autonomy as an NP.

In one concept analysis of autonomy, Peacock and Hernandez (2020) found the defining attributes of autonomy fell into two domains: personal and professional. Personal attributes included empowerment, accountability, and self-governance. Two of the professional attributes of autonomy relied on antecedents of NP education, training, and certification and included independent clinical decision making and voluntary collaboration with peers. Independent practice is one of the core NP Competencies (NONPF, 2011), along with professionalism, ethics, leadership, and other essential components necessary for delivering optimum care. The remaining three professional attributes discussed by Peacock and Hernandez found that legislative legitimacy as an independent healthcare provider, prescriptive authority, and direct reimbursement for services rely on health policy for attainment and are outside the direct purview of NPs. Moreover, the health policies governing these three professional attributes have extensive scope and layers. Fifty different state practice acts, federal and state regulations from many agencies of government regarding prescribing and payment for services, and institutional level policies are involved in determining if an NP can succeed in being autonomous, often leading to confusion.

Poghosyan and Liu (2016) conducted research with NPs working in primary care practices to see whether teamwork between NPs and physicians was affected by NP autonomy and independent practice and their relationship with administrative leadership. The results of this research suggested that when NPs working in primary care practices believed they had autonomy and had positive relationships with administrative leadership, the teamwork between physicians and NPs was enhanced. These findings demonstrate that if autonomy can be encouraged, teamwork among the healthcare team will be fostered and will lead to improved healthcare outcomes. The best hope for improving autonomy is for all states to have legislation that provides full practice authority and independence for NPs. As of this writing, 23 states and the District of Columbia have done this (Phillips, 2021).

Schirle and Norful (2020) compiled an integrative review of facilitators and barriers to optimal APN practice. Results of their review indicated most APNs believe they have either moderately high or high levels of autonomy. NPs working in primary care settings were found to have higher autonomy than those in hospital-based surgical or acute care settings. The lowest levels of autonomy were found in NPs who worked in hospital-based surgical specialty settings (Athey et al., 2016). Other factors were reported to increase a sense of autonomy: more experience as an APRN, less physician interaction, and working in a rural setting (Spetz et al., 2017). Multiple studies found that APNs were satisfied with the level of autonomy in their work settings (Brom et al., 2016; Faris et al., 2010; Poghosyan et al., 2017; Pron, 2013).

The importance of autonomy to NP practice has resulted in the development and testing of important research instruments to measure an APN's perceived levels of autonomy. The Dempster Practice Behavior Scale (DPBS) was developed in 1990 in order to understand and predict autonomy in practice (Goolsby et al., 2020). The DPBS is a 30-item questionnaire with a five-point response scale that has four dimensions signifying relatedness to autonomy: readiness, empowerment, actualization, and valuation. Over 20 publications have reported use of the DPB since it was first published in Dempster's dissertation (Dempster, 1990). These studies have related autonomy to increased job satisfaction, intent to remain in practice, ability to collaborate with other professionals, and/or management of ethical concerns. Unfortunately, small and nonrandom samples and limited studies in the United States minimized the generalizability of the findings (Goolsby et al., 2020).

As discussed earlier, Poghosyan and Liu's (2016) survey instrument, the *Nurse Practitioner Primary Care Organizational Climate (NPPCOC)*, was constructed with autonomy and independent practice as one of several factors. The autonomy and independent practice scale consists of five questions that can help identify if NPs believe they have autonomy at their practice site. These questions address whether the NP needs to discuss every patient detail with a physician: Is the NP free to apply one's knowledge and skills in patient care? Is the NP being restricted to practice within their own scope of practice? And is the NP in an organization that creates an environment to practice independently? Reliability and validity of this questionnaire was completed by Poghosyan et al. (2013). The questionnaire is useful for examining autonomy in relation to the organizational climate where NPs perform patient care. Reported findings have been telling. For example, when NPs received organizational support for their independent practice, they were more likely to serve as primary care providers and deliver ongoing continuous care to their own group of patients (Pohosyan et al., 2017). Carthon, et al. (2020) have continued to do research using the NPPCOC on a large group of NPs, recently finding that practice environments characterized by adequate resources and good relations between all members of the healthcare team enabled NPs to work more autonomously and provide care that was tailored to the individual, family, or community patient.

The need to discover and ensure autonomy for NPs is ongoing. The NPs' path for the future is in ensuring every state has a nurse practice act that states clearly that NPs have the authority to practice independently to the full scope of their education. The necessity of teamwork and collaboration with other healthcare professionals is inherent within the legislative scope. Through this, NPs will have the structure for autonomy that will lead to the best health outcomes for individuals, families, and the community.

Ethics

According to a reputable national poll by Gallup, nurses have been judged to be the most ethical and honest profession for 18 years in a row (Reinhart, 2020).

This might not have occurred without the *Nursing Code of Ethics*, which is fundamental in providing guidance to the nursing profession in ethical as well as legal situations. Ethics are "the moral principles that dictate how a person will conduct themselves" (Gaines, 2020). The code of ethics provides a social contract between nurses and patients. Updated in 2015, there are nine provisions listed in the Code of Ethics for Nurses developed by the American Nurses Association (ANA, 2015b). Every nursing student is expected to incorporate these obligations of the nursing profession, and all nurses have a moral obligation to act in accord with this code. The International Council of Nurses (ICN) also has a code of ethics, which was initially developed in 1953. The organization encourages all nurses to share the code as widely as possible. The preamble to the elements of the code states:

> Nurses have four fundamental responsibilities: to promote health, to prevent illness, to restore health and to alleviate suffering. The need for nursing is universal. Inherent in nursing is a respect for human rights, including cultural rights, the right to life and choice, to dignity and to be treated with respect. Nursing care is respectful of and unrestricted by considerations of age, colour, creed, culture, disability or illness, gender, sexual orientation, nationality, politics, race or social status. Nurses render health services to the individual, the family and the community and coordinate their services with those of related groups. (ICN, 2012)

An area that lacks significant study is related to applied ethics and nurse practitioners, particularly outside of the acute care setting. In daily interactions with patients, families, colleagues, institutions, and even our sociopolitical world, dilemmas are often presented to the NP who needs to respond in an ethical and culturally sensitive manner. Studies have identified issues that can cause moral distress and/or ethical dilemmas for NPs. These include conflicts of conscience in which an NP may be asked by an employer to do something that is contrary to their religious beliefs or moral convictions, such as issues related to abortion, other surgical procedures, and end-of-life matters (McMullen & Philipsen, 2017). There are also constraints that occur in the primary care of patients that foster injustice. For example, a patients' lack of adequate healthcare coverage, limited time to spend with patients due to scheduling pressures, and restrictive drug formularies (Fox & Chesla, 2008; Laabs, 2005) can lead to an inequity of health resources.

Over 20 years ago, a qualitative study by Viens titled "The Moral Reasoning of Nurse Practitioners" (1995) discussed the limitations of the biomedical ethics approach for NPs facing moral dilemmas in the outpatient setting. In addition, this insightful study pinpointed issues related to gender bias that critics identified in Kohlberg's model of moral development; in particular, Carol Gilligan as critic, whose model of moral development (Gilligan, 1982; Gilligan et al., 1988) suggests that females and males have differing approaches to moral reasoning. Often, NPs have difficult patient situations requiring the ability to make clinical decisions based on moral values held by the NPs. For most NPs, these types of decisions are faced daily in clinical practice. The NP participants in this study valued caring and the patient–NP relationship as essential components of successful practice. Another qualitative study found that forming a personal and caring relationship with patients is a foundation for a trusting patient–healthcare provider relationship, which leads to better health outcomes for patients (Fox & Chesla, 2008). Terms that were uncovered to describe this positive relationship included *partnership, mutual respect, empathetic attunement, negotiation, flexibility, patience, encouragement, personableness, authentic,* and *open*. This type of patient, or person-centered, care is now the standard expectation because it serves to foster the patient's individual choice in healthcare decisions. This type of care is achieved through dynamic and collaborative relationships among all healthcare providers and patients, the latter of which drive the decisions over care.

Service/Altruism

In an effort to explore and stimulate critical thinking and professional self-reflection at this author's university, family NP students who accompany faculty to developing countries to provide health care to underserved or unserved needy populations are required to write two comprehensive SOAP notes on at least two different patients focusing on the plan of care. One of the plans covers what was actually done while in the guest country; the other is a treatment plan that reflects what would have been done for the same patient if he or she were in the United States with good health insurance. The teaching "moment" is remarkable. In addition, students who take the opportunity to work in a community health clinic are also encouraged to share patient experiences they find frustrating: for instance, being unable to offer treatment plans per expert guidelines because the patient does not have adequate—or any—health insurance. Deciding what diagnostic testing is truly required, and at what expense, is frequently illuminating for NP students who have been working as RNs in an acute care setting, where most often care is provided without thought to the cost or absolute necessity, and students may find that care is sometimes provided as a proactive defense against malpractice claims.

Following is an example of using the qualities discussed thus far and how we, as faculty, try to instill these qualities in our students.

CASE STUDY

Faculty/Student Healthcare Mission (Julie Stewart)
We sat very tightly together in a cramped small bus that was took us to a Mayan village, which expected us to see about 150 children who were coming to the malnutrition center that day. The roads were quite bumpy and curvy as we headed up the mountain. Despite the trash on the sides of the road, the scenery was beautiful and amazing. Such a dichotomy . . . The nursing students and NP students were anxious that day because they didn't know what the clinic would be like. Would interpreters be there? Would the children be very sick? Would they even want to come see us? The other faculty member, two host mission workers, and I tried to

reassure them that we would be welcomed with open arms. We were going there by their request, and we would be their guests during our time there. I reminded my NP students that they were nurses—the skills they already possessed would take care of most of the needs that day. We only had a limited supply of medications: mostly vitamins, acetaminophen, topicals, a few antibiotics, and antiparasitics. As we arrived, we saw a long line of young children, dressed in the traditional colorful clothing of their Mayan village. Many of the children were obviously malnourished, but almost every face beamed at us with smiles.

As we got set up, I took a few students with me so we'd get a general idea of where everything was and how things would work for us. As our outdoor "tour" began, we saw a tiny area that contained brand new bathroom stalls (which were leaking water everywhere). Our village host was very proud of them, so we made sure to acknowledge the monies and effort this must have taken. However, this 5-foot-square area also housed chickens and a guard dog. One chicken was being plucked, another was being cooked, and yet another cooked chicken was being deboned—all on the ground next to the leaking toilets. After a very busy day taking care of small undernourished children with horribly decaying teeth and superficial burns, most of the children also having symptoms of parasites, our group learning discussion that evening revolved around basic public health principles and the education we could provide the villagers to help improve their health without complex medication regimens. Also part of the discussion was how to incorporate cultural considerations and professionalism, as well as kindness and understanding, when offering suggestions to our patients. Our patients were typically 10- to 12-year-old girls who were in charge of the younger children all day while their mother did household chores and their fathers worked out in the fields. These were the patients we were directing our educational efforts to. We needed them to understand how to take care of both themselves and the younger children in their charge. The most obvious answer to most of the problems we were seeing was clean water for drinking, cooking, bathing, and cleaning. It was the one thing we really could not provide.

Later that night, someone knocked on my bedroom door. I scurried outside to find out what was wrong. A student said someone needed me. Someone's niece in another village had been burned with hot water, and they wanted me to come see her. A jeep was waiting outside to take me there. A nonmedical friend offered to accompany me since it was dangerous to be out alone in the evenings. The two of us hopped into the car with only a first aid kit in hand, and off we went into the night, having no clue what we'd find. I asked our escort why they didn't bring the girl to a hospital ER. They said her family couldn't afford it; they hoped we could do something instead. When we arrived, we made our way along a tiny pathway to an open cooking area with two small rooms beside it. The shelter was made of tin. The girl turned out to be a teenager and was lying on a single bed with her thin nightgown falling off her. She was moaning, holding her ear, and pointing to her throat. Only one of us could fit in the tiny room, so I had to climb onto the bed and crawl up beside her using a flashlight. Although it didn't seem to be a bad burn, she told the translator she had a lot of pain in her ear and it ran down her throat to her chest. Apparently the hot liquid splashed into her ear and she felt it go down her throat. I was now faced with some difficult clinical decision making. Once the translator told us there was no 9-1-1 in the area if her throat started to swell, and that they had no medical equipment for me to look in her ear or down her throat, I told them she needed a more thorough assessment (her moaning was pitiful). We asked them to take us and the patient to the private hospital in the next town, and that we would pay for the visit and any medication she might need if the medicines were ones we didn't have it. They agreed, relieved, and we took the girl to this private hospital. It was tiny but clean. So tiny that the doctor also acted as the triage nurse and admitting person! After a thorough inspection, he gave her some pain medicine, a prescription for some ear drops, Silvadene cream for her skin burns, and a wonderful education on how to care for herself and what things to watch out for that might be concerning enough that she'd need to return to the ER. What a surprise to find out the entire visit and medications cost us about $40 U.S.!

Leadership

According to the National Organization of Nurse Practitioner Faculties, leadership is a core NP competency (Thomas et al., 2017). According to Joyce (2001), NPs perceived that those who displayed leadership qualities had the attribute of being a "professional." In addition, a professional leader had the characteristics of being competent and having integrity, accountability, resourceful, confident in their judgment, a good manager of time, and the ability to raise the bar for setting standards.

Practice models for NPs need to incorporate core values of professionalism and leadership. One example of a model of practice for acute care NPs was developed at Strong Memorial Hospital in Rochester, New York (Ackerman et al., 1996). Although the model was developed for the then-new role of acute care NP, the conceptual strands encompassed with it are still pertinent to all NP practice types today. The concepts of scholarship, collaboration, and empowerment are threaded throughout the domains of the model, which are direct, comprehensive care; support of systems, education, and research; and publication and professional leadership. The concept of scholarship integrates the need to maintain a high standard of clinical competence to provide excellent patient care. Collaboration encompasses the belief that the unique skills of a variety of healthcare providers are needed to provide excellence in patient care. Attributes that underscore the concept of collaboration for NPs in this model include cooperation, autonomy, assertiveness, responsibility, communication, and coordination. This framework is dependent on mutual regard and respect. The Strong model described empowerment as the atmosphere that sustains advanced practice. This concept is central to the model. The NP is responsible for, and has the authority to, identify and analyze patient problems, develop and implement a plan of action, as well as evaluate and be accountable for these decisions.

A key function of a leader is to maintain ties to one's profession and to use these to advance the agenda set forth by the profession. For most professions, this is done through being a member of one's professional organization. The American Association of Nurse Practitioners (AANP) is the national organization for NPs and represents approximately 120,000 student and licensed NP members. Local and state NP groups are part of the organization, organized by regions of the country. Each state organization has a representative that sits on the national AANP board so as to represent the NP interests of that state. The goal of AANP is to empower all NPs to advance quality health care through practice, education, advocacy, research, and leadership

(AANP, n.d.). The association offers continuing education, state and national policy development, research grants to members, and leadership opportunities. Of particular importance is that AANP makes a great effort in having a "seat at the table" when national health policy on issues such as education and research funding, medical reimbursement, and occupation regulation is developed. It is important for all NPs to be active members of their professional organization. This allows AANP to carry out the NP profession's agenda with one common voice of leadership.

Clearly, self reflection during didactic and clinical educational experiences is essential for strengthening one's own leadership traits. The AANP includes descriptors for integrity and professionalism, which are trust and transparency, accountability, ethical commitment, reliability, respect, personal and professional accountability, unity within the profession/discipline, and inclusivity.

That people trust nurses to provide ethically based care, be an integral part in improving patient outcomes, increase access to care, and help to reduce costs of health care puts nurses at the forefront of health care. Nurse practitioners are in a position to be an advanced practice role model, who continue to build on the characteristics of professionalism. Additionally, the NP/DNP has a responsibility to patients and to the profession to mature into leadership roles in nursing, the healthcare arena, and the broader community.

Barriers

Review of the literature provides acknowledgement of several potential barriers to practice. Awareness of these barriers can provide impetus to acknowledge important steps needed for change. Lack of role clarity, intra-professional tensions, differing legislation among states regarding full, reduced, or restricted practice authority, individual APN reluctance to perform autonomously, time management, reimbursement inequalities, and media presence have been identified as needing clarification so that NPs can assume more leadership in health care.

Lack of role clarity was the most frequently highlighted barrier to practice. Discussed by Gilman (2018), this was supported by a meta-ethnographic systematic review of 26 qualitative studies by Andregård and Jangland (2015), which was not primary care specific (Gilman, 2018). It identified that lack of information about ANP roles contributed to underutilization in relation to the scope of practice. It appears then that there is a growing body of evidence suggesting lack of role clarity limits the role of the ANP in primary care. Adding to this confusion is some APNs' reluctance to perform autonomously, and also reduced effectiveness (Gilman, 2018).

The lack of uniformity of state regulations and legislative bodies provides potential lack of access and sends an unclear message to the public and an interprofessional understanding of the nurse practitioner role as well. However, even in states that provide legislative language for full scope of practice, some organizations (healthcare institutions, systems, and insurers) reduce or restrict APRN practice authority (National Governor's Association, 2012). Restrictions to APRN practice authority applied at the organizational level prevent the APRN from fulfilling their professional role and have the potential for ambiguity and confusion.

Gilman (2018) also discussed the impact of intra-professional tensions within nursing, as well as other subordinate groups who resisted change in order to defend the status quo. As a result, nurses working in new roles were mistrusted and hindered by nursing colleagues.

Limitations of the NP to be directly reimbursed by both public and private insurers also may vary from state to state. While federal laws allow NPs to be recognized as primary care providers under Medicaid, states may vary in this recognition. It is important to note that The VA granted veterans direct access in a final ruling, an important recognition of NP value-ordered care (AANP, 2016).

Seminar Discussion Questions

1. What constitutes a "profession"? What are the most commonly referred to professional disciplines?
2. Discuss your personal beliefs of the three most important components or identifiers of autonomy as an NP.
3. What does leadership as a nurse practitioner mean to you?
4. Discuss examples of daily clinical situations that have posed moral dilemmas for you and/or your preceptor and how you approached these with patients and families.

References

AANP. (2016). *Nurse practitioners in primary care.* Retrieved from: https://www.aanp.org/advocacy/advocacy-resource/position-statements/nurse-practitioners-in-primary-care

American Association of Nurse Practitioners (2016). Recent Legislative Changes: U.S. Department of Veterans Affairs Final Rule Veterans Gain Better Access to Care. Retrieved from: https://www.aanp.org/advocacy/recent-legislative-changes/u-s-department-of-veterans-affairs-final-rule

Ackerman, M. H., Norsen, L., Martin, B., Wiedrich, J., & Kitzman, H. J. (1996). Development of a model of advanced practice. *American Journal of Critical Care, 5*(1), 68–73.

Adams, D., & Miller, B. K. (2001). Professionalism in nursing behaviors of nurse practitioners. *Journal of Professional Nursing, 17*(4), 203–210.

American Geriatrics Society Expert Panel on Person-Centered Care, Brummel-Smith, K., Butler, D., Frieder, M., Gibbs, N., Henry, M., Vladeck, B. C., et al. (2016). Person-centered care: A definition and essential elements. *Journal of the American Geriatrics Society, 64*(1), 15–18.

American Nurses Association. (2015a). Code of ethics for nurses with interpretive statements. doi:978-1-55810-600-0

American Nurses Association. (2015b). Nursing: Scope and standards of practice (3rd ed.). Silver Spring, MD: Author.

Anderson, H. (2017). *Professional identity and the advanced nurse practitioner in primary care: A qualitative study* (Doctoral dissertation, University of York). Available at: http://etheses.whiterose.ac.uk/17287/1/HELEN%20ANDERSON%20THESIS.pdf

Andregård, A., & Jangland, E. (2015). The tortuous journey of introducing the nurse practitioner as a new member of the healthcare team: a meta-synthesis. Scandinavian journal of caring sciences, 29 1, 3–14.

Athey, E. K., Leslie, M. S., Briggs, L. A., Park, J., Falk, N. L., Pericak, A., Greene, J., et al. (2016). How important are autonomy and work setting to nurse practitioners' job satisfaction? *Journal of the American Association of Nurse Practitioners, 28*(6), 320–326.

Black, B. P. (2019). *Professional nursing: Concepts and challenges* (9th ed.). Maryland Heights, MO: Saunders.

Brom, H. M., Melnyk, B. M., Szalacha, L. A., & Graham, M. (2016). Nurse practitioners' role perception, stress, satisfaction, and intent to stay at a Midwestern academic medical center. *Journal of the American Association of Nurse Practitioners, 28*(5), 269–276.

Brown, M. A., & Draye, M. A. (2003). Experiences of pioneer nurse practitioners in establishing advanced practice roles. *Journal of Nursing Scholarship, 35,* 391–397.

Cardoso, I., Batista, P., & Graca, A. (2014) Professional Identity in Analysis: A Systematic Review of the Literature. The Open Sports Science Journal, 2014, 7, (Suppl-2, M2) 83–97. Retrieved from: https://www.researchgate.net/publication/273481453_Professional_Identity_in_Analysis_A_Systematic_Review_of_the_Literature

Carryer, J., Gardner, G., Dunn, S., & Gardner, A. (2007). The core role of the nurse practitioner: Practice, professionalism and clinical leadership. *Journal of Clinical Nursing*, 16(10), 1818–1825. doi:10.1111/j.1365-2702.2006.01823.x

Carthon, J. M. B., Brom, H., Poghosyan, L., Daus, M., Todd, B., & Aiken, L. (2020). Supportive clinical practice environments associated with patient-centered care. *The Journal for Nurse Practitioners*, 16(4), 294–298. doi.org/10.1016/j.nurpra.2020.01.019

Choi, M., & De Gagne, J. C. (2016). Autonomy of nurse practitioners in primary care: An integrative review. *Journal of the American Association of Nurse Practitioners*, 28(3), 170–174.

Chumbler, N. R., Geller, J. M., & Weier, A. W. (2000). The effects of clinical decision making on nurse practitioners' clinical productivity. *Evaluation & the Health Professions*, 23(3), 284–304.

Crigger, N., & Godfrey, N. (2011). *The making of nurse professionals: A transtheoretical approach*. Sudbury, MA: Jones and Bartlett.

Dempster, J. (1990). Autonomy in practice: Conceptualization, construction, and psychometric evaluation of an empirical instrument (Doctoral dissertation). Retrieved from ProQuest Dissertations and Theses (ID 9030752).

Evetts, J. (2013). Professionalism: Value and ideology. *Current Sociology*, 61(5–6), 778–796.

Faris, J. A., Douglas, M. K., Maples, D. C., Berg, L. R., & Thrailkill, A. (2010). Job satisfaction of advanced practice nurses in the Veterans Health Administration. *Journal of the American Academy of Nurse Practitioners*, 22(1), 35–44.

Flexner, A. (1910). *Medical education in the U.S. and Canada*. The Carnegie Foundation.

Ford, L. C. (1997). A deviant comes of age. *Heart & Lung: The Journal of Critical Care*, 26(2), 87–91. https://doi.org/10.1016/s0147-9563(97)90067-4

Fox, S., & Chesla, C. (2008). Living with chronic illness: A phenomenological study of the health effects of the patient-provider relationship. *Journal of the American Academy of Nurse Practitioners*, 20(3), 109–117.

Gaines, K. (2020). *What is the nursing code of ethics?* Retrieved from https://nurse.org/education/nursing-code-of-ethics/

Gilligan, C. (1982). *In a different voice: Psychological theory and women's development*. Cambridge, MA: Harvard University Press.

Gilligan, C., Ward, J. V., & Taylor, J. M. (Eds.). (1988). *Mapping the moral domain*. Cambridge, MA: Harvard University Press.

Gilman, P. R. (2018). *Relationships between APRN state practice authority, perceived autonomy, professionalism, and interprofessional team function among a national sample of APRNs in the US*. Retrieved from https://digitalrepository.unm.edu/cgi/viewcontent.cgi?article=1049&context=nurs_etds

Godfrey, N., & Crigger, N. (2017). Professional identity. In J. F. Giddens (Ed.), *Concepts for nursing practice* (2nd ed., pp. 379–385). St. Louis, MO: Elsevier.

Goolsby, M. J., Pierson, C. A., & Sheer, B. (2020). Twenty-eight years of experience measuring autonomy using the Dempster Practice Behavior Scale. *Journal of the American Association of Nurse Practitioners*, 32(10), 696–702.

International Council of Nurses. (2012). *Code of ethics*. Geneva, Switzerland: Author.

Joyce, E. (2001). Leadership perceptions of nurse practitioners. *Lippincott's Case Management*, 6(1), 24–30.

Keenan, J. (1999). A concept analysis of autonomy. *Journal of Advanced Nursing*, 29(3), 556–562.

Kelly, L. (1981). *Dimensions of professional nursing* (4th ed.). New York, NY: Macmillan.

Laabs, C. (2005). Moral problems and distress among nurse practitioners in primary care. *Journal of the American Academy of Nurse Practitioners*, 17(2), 76–84.

McMullen, P. C., & Philipsen, N. (2017). Conscience clauses and refusal to treat: Implications for nurse practitioners. *The Journal for Nurse Practitioners*, 13(2), 138–144.

McMurray, R. (2010). The struggle to professionalize: An ethnographic account of the occupational position of advanced nurse practitioners. *Human Relations*, 64(6), 801–822. doi:10.1177/0018726710387949

National Council of State Boards of Nursing. (2008). *Consensus model for APRN regulation: Licensure, accreditation, certification & education.* Retrieved from https://www.ncsbn.org/Consensus_Model_Report.pdf

National Council of State Boards of Nursing. (2012). *APRN model act and rules.* Retrieved from https://www.ncsbn.org/2012_APRN_Model_and_Rules.pdf

National Council of State Boards of Nursing. (2019). *APRN model act: Rules and regulations.* Retrieved from https://www.ncsbn.org/2019AM_APRN-Consensus.pdf

National Governor's Association. (2012). *The role of nurse practitioners in meeting increasing demand for primary care.* Washington, DC: Author.

Norful, A. A., de Jacq, K., Carlino, R., & Poghosyan, L. (2018). Nurse practitioner-physician comanagement: A theoretical model to alleviate primary care strain. *Annals of family medicine, 16*(3), 250–256. https://doi.org/10.1370/afm.2230

Peacock, M., & Hernandez, S. (2020). A concept analysis of nurse practitioner autonomy. *Journal of the American Association of Nurse Practitioners, 32*(2), 113–119.

Peterson, M., & Potter, R. L. (2004). A proposal for a code of ethics for nurse practitioners. *Journal of the American Academy of Nurse Practitioners, 16*(3), 116–124.

Phillips, S. J. (2021). 33rd annual APRN legislative update: Unprecedented changes to APRN practice authority in unprecedented times. *The Nurse Practitioner, 46*(1), 27–55.

Poghosyan, L., & Liu, J. (2016). Nurse practitioner autonomy and relationships with leadership affect teamwork in primary care practices: A cross-sectional survey. *Journal of General Internal Medicine, 31*(7), 771–777. doi:10.1007/s11606-016-3652-z

Poghosyan, L., Liu, J., & Norful, A. A. (2017). Nurse practitioners as primary care providers with their own patient panels and organizational structures: A cross-sectional study. *International Journal of Nursing Studies, 74,* 1–7. doi.org/10.1016/j.ijnurstu.2017.05.004

Pron, A. L. (2013). Job satisfaction and perceived autonomy for nurse practitioners working in nurse-managed health centers. *Journal of the American Academy of Nurse Practitioners, 25*(4), 213–221.

Reinhart, R. J. (2020). *Nurses continue to rate highest in honesty, ethics.* Gallup. Retrieved from https://news.gallup.com/poll/274673/nurses-continue-rate-highest-honesty-ethics.aspx

Schirle, L., Norful, A. A., Rudner, N., & Poghosyan, L. (2020). Organizational facilitators and barriers to optimal APRN practice: An integrative review. *Health Care Management Review, 45*(4), 311–320.

Spetz, J., Skillman, S. M., & Andrilla, C. H. A. (2017). Nurse practitioner autonomy and satisfaction in rural settings. *Medical Care Research and Review, 74*(2), 227–235.

Tajfel, H., & Turner, J. C. (1986). An integrative theory of intergroup conflict. In W. G. Austin & S. Worchel (Eds.), *The social psychology of intergroup relations.* Monterey, CA: Brooks/Cole.

Thomas, A., Crabtree, M. K., Delaney, K., Dumas, M. A., Kleinpell, R., Marfell, J., & Wolf, A. (2017). *Nurse practitioner core competencies content. The National Organization of Nurse Practitioner Faculties.* Retrieved from: https://cdn.ymaws.com/www.nonpf.org/resource/resmgr/competencies/2017_NPCoreComps_with_Curric.pdf

UK Department of Health. (2006). *Professionalism—The big conversation by Karen Middleton. Voicepiece.* Retrieved from http://ahp.dh.gov.uk/2012/02/27/voicepiece-karen-middleton-chief-health-professions-officer

Viens, D. (1995). The moral reasoning of nurse practitioners. *Journal of the American Academy of Nurse Practitioners, 7*(6), 277–284.

Weiland, S. A. (2008). Reflections on independence in nurse practitioner practice. *Journal of the American Academy of Nurse Practitioners, 20*(7), 345–352.

Weiland, S. A. (2015). Understanding nurse practitioner autonomy. *Journal of the American Association of Nurse Practitioners, 27*(2), 95–104.

Additional Resources

Deming, W. E. (1994). *The new economics for industry, government, education* (2nd ed.). Cambridge, MA: The MIT Press.

DeNisco, S., & Barker, A. (2021). *Advanced practice nursing: Evolving roles for the transformation of the profession* (4th ed.). Burlington, MA: Jones & Bartlett Learning.

CHAPTER 15

Health Policy and the Nurse Practitioner

Julie A. Koch and Linda Washington-Brown

The need for political activism in the healthcare arena has never been greater. Since the 1960s, nurse practitioners (NPs) have been advocating for the profession and the improvement of social policies impacting health care. Over the past 50 years, NPs have gained ground in efforts to eliminate barriers in the delivery of care and to enhance patient access to their services, but additional work is needed. At the time of this writing, NPs within 23 states, the District of Columbia, and U.S. territories (Guam and Mariana Islands) had been granted full practice authority (American Association of Nurse Practitioners [AANP], 2021), the ability to practice to the full extent of training and education. Additional states had similar legislation in various stages of development or approval. Yet, those with full practice authority still may face barriers to providing optimal care for their patients, and a number of issues still warrant attention on an institutional, regional, or national level.

The push for practicing to the full extent of one's academic and experiential preparation is vitally important as the number of primary care physicians stagnates. The Association of American Medical Colleges (AAMC) reported that the United States could face a shortage of 21,400 to 55,200 primary care physicians by the year 2033 (AAMC, 2020). Three major factors may contribute to that shortage: growth and aging of the population, an aging physician workforce, and unmet needs of underserved populations. Although the overall population is expected to grow by more than 10% from 2018 to 2033, the population of adults aged 65 and older is projected to grow by more than 45% (AAMC, 2020). Based on existing data, it can be assumed that these older adults will face the challenges of living with chronic health conditions, adding to the healthcare economic burden and increasing the need for primary care providers. Currently, more than three-quarters of older Americans have multiple chronic conditions, and medical treatment for this population accounts for 75% of the country's healthcare budget (National Council on Aging [NCOA], n.d.). These data present a strong economic incentive for cost-effective health care; yet, an increasing number of thought leaders have recognized that physicians alone will not be able to meet the healthcare needs of older adults. Compounding the issue is the fact that physicians themselves are represented in this aging population, with more than 40% of currently active physicians reaching the age of 65 within the next decade (AAMC, 2020). In addition to the needs of our aging population, long-standing vulnerabilities in our nation's health care have been exposed by the COVID-19 pandemic. Currently, more than 75 million Americans (commonly individuals of differing races and ethnicities) live in communities without access to primary health care, while nearly 80% of rural America falls under the designation of *medically underserved* (AANP, 2020a). Addressing these health disparities will further highlight the need for primary care providers as physician shortages become more apparent. More importantly, the lack of access to primary care providers and the need to provide cost-effective quality care to the U.S. population can be addressed by the more than 290,000 NPs who have been educationally and experientially prepared to fill this gap (AANP, 2020e).

As NPs prepare to further meet the healthcare needs of the American population, it is paramount to recognize where we have come from in order to understand the ramifications of where we are going and where we need to be to meet the needs of the nation's health care. This chapter reviews the history of health policy related to nurse practitioners, examines the current regulatory structure impacting health care today, addresses current health policy issues (including a view of the quest for full practice authority), and identifies strategies to enhance the NP's role in political activism, meeting the healthcare needs of Americans nationwide.

History of the NP and Related Health Policy

The foundation of nurse practitioner healthcare advocacy can be linked to Florence Nightingale, a visionary of public policy on numerous healthcare issues: e.g., promoting clean water, good nutrition, decent lodging, and adequate ventilation to reduce infection rates (McDonald, 2006). Astutely political, as a woman living in the 1800s, Nightingale was unable to vote, yet she was able to move healthcare reform issues through leadership, innovative thought, and perseverance. She lobbied the British Parliament to educate nurses who would serve in public workhouses and was passionate in her opinion that individuals who were sick should avoid hospitalization, advocating for home health services provided by nurses and physicians. The fact that Nightingale was able to obtain the support of high-level medical experts, cabinet ministers, and senior governmental officials has been attributed to her careful preparation and attention to detail. The most prominent sanitarians of the time, statisticians, engineers, and water experts alike were willing to work with her to advance health policies because they shared her vision and respected her methods (McDonald, 2006).

Building upon Nightingale's legacy of using innovative thoughts and actions to improve health care, Loretta C. Ford developed the first NP program in 1965 at the University of Colorado Schools of Medicine and Nursing (National Women's Hall of Fame, 2017). Dr. Ford, along with pediatrician Henry K. Silver, recognized that a shortage of family care physicians and pediatricians was impacting the ability to provide health care in rural and underserved areas. The pair obtained a small grant from the University of Colorado and implemented the nation's first pediatric nurse practitioner program. The curriculum combined clinical practice, education, and research to address the social, psychological, environmental, and economic aspects of patient care. Through her innovative thought and actions, Dr. Ford transformed the nursing profession, enhanced access to care for the general public, and led the future movement for nurse practitioners (National Women's Hall of Fame, 2017).

By the early 1970s, more than 65 programs were preparing nurse practitioners across the nation, with approximately 10,000 NPs practicing (AANP, n.d.). As this was occurring, discussion began on standardizing nursing licensure, certification examinations, and national certification of NPs. Since national NP organizations were in their infancy at that time (the National Association of Pediatric Nurse Practitioners [NAPNAP] was established in 1973), grassroots movements were essential in the attainment of formal reimbursement of NP services. Momentum continued to build with support from nursing and the legal community to develop a model nurse practice law that could further expand the role of the NP. In 1974, the first federal legislation was introduced; the bill was intended to amend the Social Security Act so that NPs' services would be covered under Medicare and Medicaid (Bartol, 2015). Over the next 20 years, at least 10 pieces of federal legislation that gradually established the role of the NP and provided reimbursement for NP services were adopted (Bartol, 2015). In 1985, the American Academy of Nurse Practitioners (AANP) was established, and the organization quickly began a concerted effort to affect pertinent national legislation (AANP, n.d.). The ultimate culmination of these early health policy efforts was the Balanced Budget Act of 1997, signed by President Clinton, which granted provider status to NPs and authorized them to bill Medicare directly for providing services to its recipients, regardless of setting (Bartol, 2015).

These early grassroots movements, followed by structured advocacy set forth in part by national organizations, resulted in significant changes in the landscape of NP practice. Yet, additional policy changes are still needed. With education advancing to the doctoral level, NPs are now being prepared to position themselves as leaders who impact, guide, and develop health policies that address accessible, quality care for all Americans and in turn advance NPs' professional status.

Formal Health Policy Education for NPs

Consistent with the beliefs of the Advanced Practice Registered Nurse (APRN) Joint Dialogue Group (2008), today's doctorally prepared NPs need to have the knowledge and skills to respond to the increased need for healthcare providers and be positioned as leaders in the development of health policies affecting patients and professional practice. Instead of reacting to potentially detrimental policy proposals, the NP can and should be at the forefront contributing to the policy-making process. While the scope of health policy education is far more comprehensive than can be covered in this chapter, the intention is to cover essential elements of health policy as they pertain to NPs, with the goal of stimulating discussion and action plans for current issues.

Recognizing that practice-focused doctoral programs, designed to prepare experts in specialized, innovative, evidence-based advanced nursing practice, differ from traditional PhD programs, the American Association of Colleges of Nursing (AACN) created a task force to develop curricular expectations for DNP education. In October 2006, the AACN released *The Essentials of Doctoral Education for*

Advanced Nursing Practice, previously referred to as The DNP Essentials. In 2018, a taskforce was charged with the task of re-envisioning the Essentials, which delineate the expected competencies of graduates and identify essential curricular elements that need to be present within nursing programs (AACN, 2021b). In April 2021, *The Essentials: Core Competencies for Professional Nursing Education* was released. The updated essentials includes 10 domains and 8 concepts for nursing practice, which are outlined in Chapter 1 of this textbook. Health Policy is one of the eight concepts that are noted to be interrelated and interwoven within the domains and competencies (AACN, 2020). Health policy is noted to represent an important aspect of advocacy for both patients and the profession, with nurses being prepared to interpret, evaluate, and lead policy change (AACN, 2020). Below is a brief example of how health policy is threaded throughout the domains for nursing and can be found in select sub-competencies in which advanced-level nurses are prepared to (AACN, 2021a):

- Domain 2: Person-Centered Care contribute to the development of policies and processes that program transparency and accountability
- Domain 3: Population Health contribute to policy development at the system, local, regional, or national levels design policies to impact health equity and structural racism within systems, communities, and population

Please see Table 1-3 for a Comparison of the Essentials Major Domains, Select Nursing Education Competencies, Select Advanced Nursing Practice Sub-competencies, and NONPF Competencies.

Recognizing that today's nurse practitioners have the opportunity to address the scope of practice issues identified by the Institute of Medicine (IOM) and positively impact the nation's health, the National Organization for Nurse Practitioner Faculties (NONPF) developed a set of NP core competencies. The health policy competencies, which are reflective of the DNP Essentials, were published in 2014 and updated in 2017. The *Nurse Practitioner Core Competencies Content* includes suggestions for curricular content relative to the core competencies (NONPF, 2017). Under the policy competency area, NONPF has noted that the NP graduate:

1. Demonstrates an understanding of the interdependence of policy and practice.
2. Advocates for ethical policies that promote access, equity, quality, and cost.
3. Analyzes ethical, legal, and social factors influencing policy development.
4. Contributes in the development of health policy.
5. Analyzes the implications of health policy across disciplines.
6. Evaluates the impact of globalization on healthcare policy development.
7. Advocates for policies for safe and healthy practice environments.

   (*NONPF. Nurse Practitioner Core Competencies Content, 2017, pp. 9–10. Reprinted with permission from the National Organization of Nurse Practitioner Faculties*)

These outcomes and competencies reflect the DNP graduate's ability to assume broad leadership in political activism and policy development. The health policy objectives have been incorporated within DNP programs throughout the nation and are still being instituted today.

Advancing NP Practice Through Health Policy

In order to advance the profession, it is imperative that doctorally prepared NPs have a foundational knowledge of healthcare legislation and regulation. These two areas of health policy significantly impact the profession's movement toward full practice authority. Depending upon how healthcare legislation is written and implemented, regulations related to NPs' scope of practice can either enhance or limit patient access to care.

Healthcare Legislation

Understanding the key processes in the health policy arena can assist the doctorally prepared NP to keep abreast of current issues and take steps to initiate change that will further advance the profession. NPs can play a major role in leading health policy change, from the introduction of a policy issue through petitioning legislators for a vote to support a specific healthcare bill. More importantly, once legislation is enacted, NPs should exercise their practice authority to the full extent of their education, training, and competencies (LeBuhn & Swankin, 2010).

Policy issues warranting the NP's attention can range from patient-related issues (e.g., funding for immunizations and smoking cessation programs) to practice-specific issues (i.e., restrictions to scope of professional practice and reimbursement). Once an issue is identified that warrants legislative change, the doctorally prepared NP should prepare a brief synopsis, frequently called an "elevator speech" or "sound bite" that can be presented to others who share the same vision for moving the issue forward. Short messages that convey the key points succinctly are useful when communicating with other professionals, the media, and politicians. This process of agenda setting has the greatest chance for success when it is founded in statistics and pertinent factual information, yet provided in language that is easily understood by those not employed in health care.

Getting the appropriate organization to work on the bill will help to move it forward. Most NP organizations have lobbyists who know how and who to reach with the message. Lobbyists can advise the NP organization if there are other interests competing with their efforts or if the timing is right to introduce a specific bill, thus maximizing the potential for passage. This underscores the need for NPs to be involved with local, state, and national NP organizations. In addition to lobbying, these organizations can initiate grassroots advocacy movements, educating their members about pending legislation and asking them to contact their legislators and other government officials. NPs can participate in letter-writing campaigns or meet with their legislators on an individual basis or as part of a larger group. Legislators are often willing to meet with NP constituents who reside in their legislative districts during periods when they are not in session, and NP organizations can schedule session meetings as part of their grassroots advocacy. House session calendars are available on each state's general assembly website, and these sites also serve as a valuable resource for NPs, identifying legislators by district/region (which can be searched by constituent's zip code), specifying the committees that they serve on, and providing contact information. Websites of state and local NP organizations often include political action agenda items, and there is a wealth of federal and state legislative information on the AANP's website. NAPNAP also has resources available for its members that will be reviewed later in this chapter.

Although a bill can be drafted by an individual or an organization, the actual text is usually drafted by a legislative aide, and it can only be introduced once a legislator in the Senate or House of Representatives has sponsored it (National Human Genome Research Institute, 2020). Legislators usually sponsor bills that are important to them and their constituents, so it is integral for the individual NP or NP organization to convey the issue's impact on constituents to key legislators. Having previously established relationships with legislators provides an opportunity for NPs to further advocate for bill sponsorship.

Drafted bills are sent to the appropriate clerk who assigns a title and number. Once printed, the bill's legislative author will garner support for the bill as it is sent to the appropriate committee(s) to view and discuss. Legislators with a strong degree of political clout are more likely to gather significant support at the stage of committee review. During the committee review period, there may be public hearings where NPs and others with interest in the topic can provide short testimonials. If the bill is viewed favorably, it may be passed on to other involved committees and be discussed and approved. If the proposed bill does not fail along the way, the process moves on to the state assemblies, and the governor can sign it or veto the bill. The process is similar for federal bills and laws, with the president being the one to veto or approve a bill (**Figure 15-1**).

Healthcare Regulation

Once a federal bill has been signed into law, agencies create regulations or rules under the authority of Congress to help carry out public health policies. Proposed rules are published daily by the National Archives and Records Administration (NARA) in the *Federal Register* (https://www.federalregister.gov). Interested parties are invited to provide comments on the website and/or attend a scheduled hearing or public meeting to provide input into the regulatory process. Once the agency has reviewed and considered all related information and associated comments, an implementation plan is developed and the rule is published in the *Federal Register*; the rule becomes effective 30 days after publication.

For NPs across the nation, many policies related to practice are regulated by the U.S. Department of Health and Human Services (DHHS). The overall mission of DHHS is "to enhance the health and well-being of Americans by providing for effective health and human services and by fostering sound, sustained advances in the sciences underlying medicine, public health, and social services" (DHHS, 2018). The DHHS develops a strategic plan to further define its mission, goals, and the methods for evaluating progress in meeting selected goals for a 4-year period. Because the GPRA (Government Performance and Results Act) Modernization Act requires federal agencies to consult with Congress and to solicit and consider views of external parties, while developing its strategic plan, the DHHS engages the public through the DHHS Open Government website (http://www.hhs.gov/open),

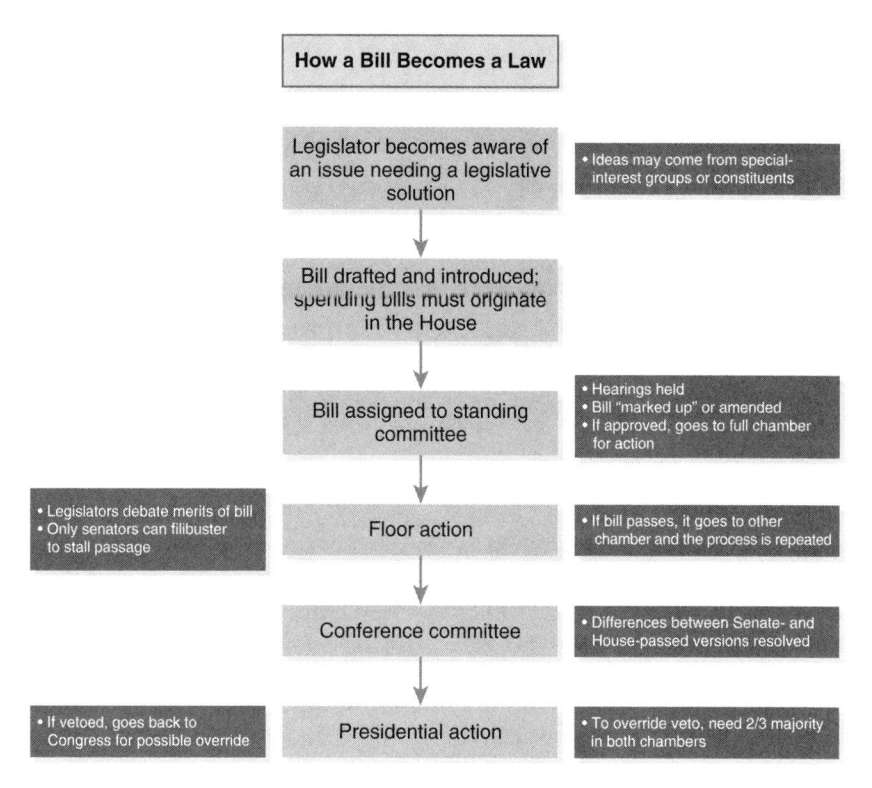

Advancing NP Practice Through Health Policy **373**

How a Bill Becomes a Law

- Legislator becomes aware of an issue needing a legislative solution
  - Ideas may come from special-interest groups or constituents
- Bill drafted and introduced; spending bills must originate in the House
- Bill assigned to standing committee
  - Hearings held
  - Bill "marked up" or amended
  - If approved, goes to full chamber for action
- Floor action
  - Legislators debate merits of bill
  - Only senators can filibuster to stall passage
  - If bill passes, it goes to other chamber and the process is repeated
- Conference committee
  - Differences between Senate- and House-passed versions resolved
- Presidential action
  - If vetoed, goes back to Congress for possible override
  - To override veto, need 2/3 majority in both chambers

Figure 15-1 How a bill passes through Congress

the *Federal Register*, conference calls or email notices to key stakeholders, and social media postings. Feedback from all sources is used to finalize the DHHS's strategic plan.

For fiscal years 2018–2022, DDHS has five overarching strategic goals that align with its mission (DHHS, 2018):

Goal 1: Reform, strengthen, and modernize the nation's healthcare system.

Goal 2: Protect the health of Americans where they live, learn, work, and play.

Goal 3: Strengthen the economic and social well-being of Americans across the lifespan.

Goal 4: Foster sound, sustained advances in the sciences.

Goal 5: Promote effective and efficient management and stewardship.

The DHHS includes 11 operating divisions (outlined in on the right side of the organizational chart; see **Figure 15-2**). These 11 divisions include 8 in the U.S. Public Health Service and 3 human service agencies that administer a wide array of health and human services and conduct life-saving research for the nation (USDHHS, 2018).

374 **Chapter 15** Health Policy and the Nurse Practitioner

```
                        ┌─────────────────────┐
                        │     Secretary       │
                        │  Deputy Secretary   │
                        │   Chief of Staff    │
                        └─────────────────────┘
```

- The Executive Secretariat (ES)
- Office of Intergovernmental and External Affairs (IEA)

Office of the Secretary
- Office of the Assistant Secretary for Administration (ASA)
- Office of the Assistant Secretary for Financial Resources (ASFR)
- Office of the Assistant Secretary for Health (OASH)
- Office of the Assistant Secretary for Legislation (ASL)
- Office of the Assistant Secretary for Planning and Evaluation (ASPE)
- Office of the Assistant Secretary for Preparedness and Response (ASPR)*
- Office of the Assistant Secretary for Public Affairs (ASPA)
- Office for Civil Rights (OCR)
- Departmental Appeals Board (DAB)
- Office of the General Counsel (OGC)
- Office of Global Affairs (OGA)*
- Office of Inspector General (OIG)
- Office of Medicare Hearings and Appeals (OMHA)
- Office of the National Coordinator for Health Information Technology (ONC)
- HHS Chief Information Officer

Operating Divisions
- Administration for Children and Families (ACF)
- Administration for Community Living (ACL)
- Agency for Healthcare Research and Quality (AHRQ)*
- Agency for Toxic Substances and Disease Registry (ATSDR)*
- Centers for Disease Control and Prevention (CDC)*
- Centers for Medicare & Medicaid Services (CMS)
- Food and Drug Administration (FDA)*
- Health Resources and Services Administration (HRSA)*
- Indian Health Service (IHS)*
- National Institutes of Health (NIH)*
- Substance Abuse and Mental Health Services Administration (SAMHSA)*

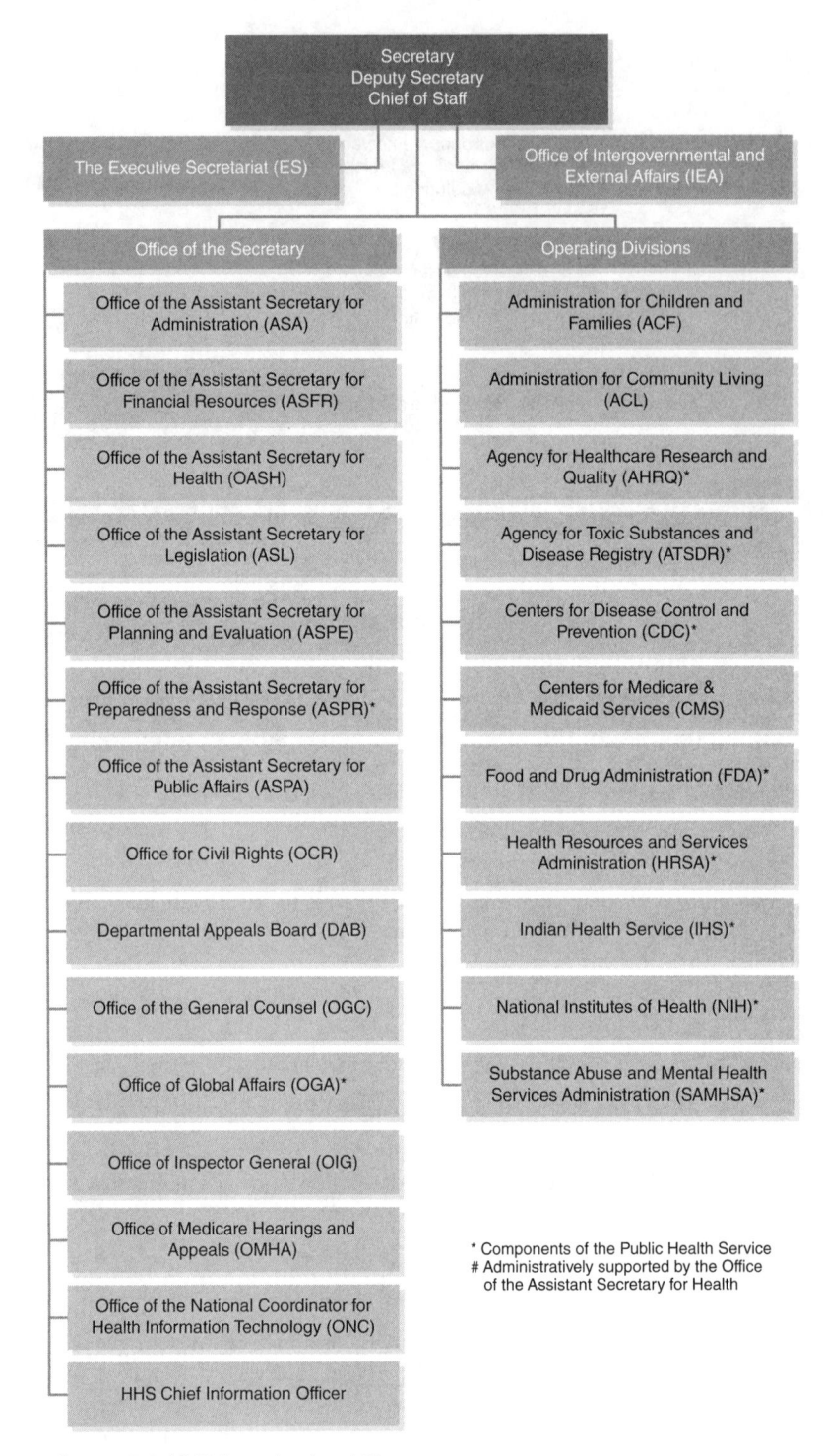

* Components of the Public Health Service
\# Administratively supported by the Office of the Assistant Secretary for Health

Figure 15-2 HHS Organizational Chart

U.S. Department of Health & Human Services. (2020). HHS Organizational Chart. Retrieved from https://www.hhs.gov/about/agencies/orgchart/index.html

Current Health Policy Issues

Keeping abreast of current health policy issues is essential to the advocacy initiatives of socially conscious healthcare providers. Topics that continue to generate interest among doctorally prepared NPs include scope of practice, healthcare reform, access to care, and healthcare "crises."

Defining Scope of Practice

Scope of practice issues continue to serve as barriers for NPs who strive to practice to the full extent of their educational and experiential preparation. In 1980, two nurse practitioners (NPs) were charged with practicing medicine without a license in the Missouri landmark case, *Smerchief v. Gonzales* (1983). The ruling was overturned by the Missouri Supreme Court concluding "that the scope of practice of advanced practice nurses (APNs) could evolve without statutory constraints" (Wolff, 1984). This court ruling provided the foundation for addressing issues related to expanding the NP role, practice, and functions. Twenty-eight years later, in 2008, The Robert Wood Johnson Foundation (RWJF) and the IOM launched a 2-year initiative to respond to the need to advance the nursing profession; a joint committee was charged with the task of producing a report outlining an action-oriented blueprint. As a result of this joint effort, in 2011, the IOM issued *The Future of Nursing: Leading Change, Advancing Health*, which called for the removal of policies, regulations, and laws that prevent APRNs, including NPs, from providing the full scope of services they have been trained and educated to provide (Institute of Medicine [IOM], 2011).

As a follow-up to the IOM's publication, in 2017, the RWJF published a brief outlining the barriers to APRN practice, including the patchwork of laws and regulations that restrict patients' access to APRN services and the cost of collaborative practice agreements. The authors of the RWJF brief noted that state practice acts, institutional policies, and federal statutes and regulations that require physician oversight or otherwise restrict APRN practice continue to limit access to care, create disruptions in care, increase the cost of care, and undermine efforts to improve the quality of care. The authors also cited that a growing body of research suggests that removing practice restrictions on NPs has the potential to actually reduce cost and improve access to care without compromising the quality of that care (RWJF, 2017). Within the brief, it was also noted that physician oversight in collaborative agreements can be financially burdensome for APRNs and confusing for policy makers and members of the public, who may mistakenly think that the agreements facilitate true collaborative care (RWJF, 2017).

The Consensus Model for APRN Regulation: Licensure, Accreditation, Certification, & Education (LACE), an APRN Joint Dialogue Group Report, was completed through work of the APRN Consensus Work Group and the National Council of State Boards of Nursing APRN Advisory Committee. The APRN Joint Dialogue Group described the APRN regulatory model; defined APRN practice, roles, and population foci; and presented strategies for implementation including the requisite education, certification, and licensure in terms of role and population foci (APRN Joint Dialogue Group, 2008). Although the authors determined that APRNs could specialize in a specific area (e.g., endocrinology or oncology), they must be licensed in one of the four roles (CRNA, CNM, CNS, or CNP) with a population focus (see **Figure 15-3**). Furthermore, certification must meet the standards provided within the LACE guidelines, ensuring entry-level competency of the APRN. The Joint Dialogue Group noted that the boards of nursing within individual states need to be the regulatory body that issues licenses and provides oversight of APRNs. The group's goal was to ultimately have consistency in licensure, accreditation, certification, and education in all states. When the COVID-19 pandemic prompted some state governors to temporarily remove restrictions on APRNS, the National Council of State Boards of Nursing (2021) noted that lifting the barriers that did not follow the Consensus Model allowed APRNs to practice across state lines to meet the healthcare needs in surge areas. The organization further noted that differing regulatory requirements from state to state continues to represent an obstacle to portability which potentially prevents access to APRNs and the high-quality health care they provide (NCSBN, 2021).

To date, each state has been able to define the APRN legal scope of practice, recognize APRN roles and titles, as well as define criteria for entry into practice and acceptable or approved certification examinations. The scope of practice for nurse practitioners across the nation, by state, can be found on the AANP website (https://aanp.org/practice-information-by-state). Because each state can define the scope of practice in statutes, some of which are detailed and others more general, it is essential that NPs review the most current scope of practice legislated by the state in which they practice. NPs have the authority to diagnose, treat, and prescribe medications without the requirement of physician collaboration or oversight in 23 states and the District of Columbia (Phillips, 2021). In the remaining 27 states, there is some form of physician collaboration or supervision required, despite the IOM's recommendations to allow APRNs to practice to the full extent of their education and training.

An exception to these scope of practice limitations can be found within the Veterans Affairs health system. In December 2016, the Department of Veterans Affairs

APRN REGULATORY MODEL

APRN Specialties
Focus of practice beyond role and population focus linked to healthcare needs.
Examples include but are not limited to: Oncology, Older Adults, Orthopedics, Nephrology and Palliative Care

POPULATION FOCI

Family/Individual Across Life Span | Adult-Gerontology | Neonatal | Pediatrics | Women's Health/Gender | Psychiatric-Mental Health

APRN ROLES

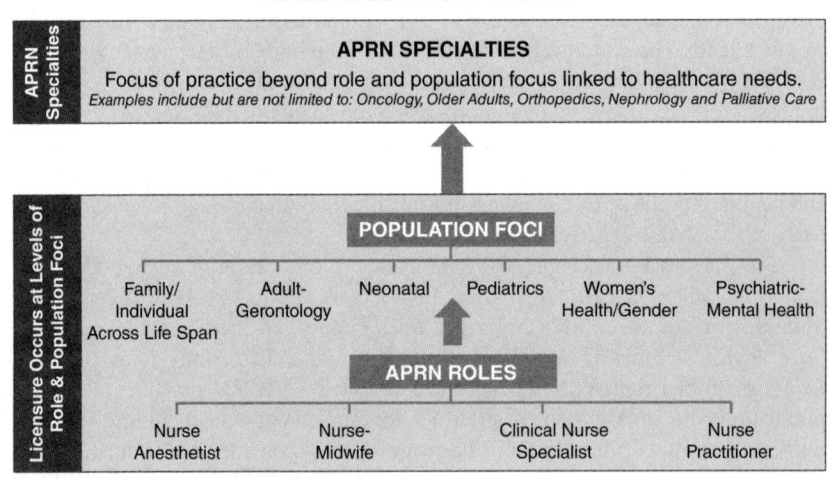

Nurse Anesthetist | Nurse-Midwife | Clinical Nurse Specialist | Nurse Practitioner

Licensure Occurs at Levels of Role & Population Foci

Figure 15-3 APRN Regulatory Model
Reproduced from APRN Joint Dialogue Group Report, July 7, 2008, p. 10. Reprinted by permission of American Association of Colleges of Nursing.

(VA) published a final rule (81 FR 90198) that granted veterans direct access to care from three of the four APRN specialties (CNMs, CNSs, and NPs) (Sofer, 2017). The final rule authorized NPs to practice to the full extent of their education and preparation without physician supervision in all states, with the exception of prescribing controlled medications (which are still subject to individual state restrictions under the Controlled Substances Act).

Expanding Scope of Practice During the Public Health Emergency

In March of 2020, Federal Health and Human Services Secretary Alex Azar recommended that all governors promptly relax scope of practice requirements for healthcare professionals. Governors in Kentucky, Louisiana, New Jersey, New York, and Wisconsin were among the first to suspend state regulatory barriers and served as a model for the nation (AANP, 2020c). AANP's President Sophia Thomas (featured in the Exemplar section of this chapter) called upon the remaining governors to take immediate action to waive restrictive barriers undermining access to NP-provided care. One month later, all but seven of the states that still limited NP practice, at the time had partially or fully waived the collaborative practice requirements, and state emergency responses were updated as information became available on the AANP website: https://www.aanp.org/advocacy/advocacy-resource/coronavirus-disease-2019-covid-19-policy-updates.

During the national health crisis, many nurses were able to cross states lines to assist in areas of greatest need, but the lack of multistate licensure of NPs and continued restrictions on scope of practice impeded mobilization of the APRN workforce. In August of 2020, the National Council of State Boards of Nursing (NCSBN) adopted a revised APRN Compact for multistate licensure. The APRN Compact will allow NPs to hold licensure which provides the privilege to practice in other compact states (NCSBN, 2021). The NCSBN has developed model legislation and rules for states to adopt the compact, noting that the compact will be implemented when seven states have enacted the legislation (NCSBN, 2021). At the time of this writing, the NCSBN reported that only two states (North Dakota [HB 1044] and Delaware [HB 21]) had APRN Compact legislation pending. Updates will be posted on their website at https://www.ncsbn.org/aprn-compact.htm. Although the adoption of the compact could be viewed as positive movement in supporting advancement of the profession, neither the AANP nor NAPNAP support the compact in its current state. Both organizations specifically oppose the inclusion of practice hours as a prerequisite of multistate licensure, noting that this requirement is in direct conflict with the *Consensus Model for APRN Regulation: Licensure, Accreditation, Certification, and Education* (introduced earlier in this chapter and depicted in Figure 15-3). These national NP organizations have noted that the inclusion of minimum practice hours creates costly and unnecessary regulations and impacts states that are currently working to retire these barriers to full practice authority (AANP, 2020b; NAPNAP, 2020). Furthermore, the AANP and NAPNAP reaffirmed their position that an APRN Compact must include an APRN advisory committee to provide resources and expertise needed to address complex practice issues.

Although the previously noted policy changes reflect movement toward expanding the NP's role in meeting the healthcare needs of Americans, there remains an underlying need to continue to address legislative barriers once the designated period of public health emergency has passed. The temporary expansion of scope of practice further highlights the need for persistent efforts advocating for full practice authority.

Challenging the Patient Protection and Affordable Care Act (ACA)

Few current issues incite as much passionate debate as healthcare reform. At the time of this writing, the nation was transitioning under new leadership and was at a major crossroad in health policy. A number of unfolding events were guiding the direction for U.S. health care for the short term and long term. Foremost among those events were actions within the judicial and executive branches of the government. In November 2020, the U.S. Supreme Court heard oral arguments on whether the Patient Protection and Affordable Care Act (commonly referred to as the Affordable Care Act [ACA]) was constitutional, in whole or in part. The case was brought by several state attorneys general, who argued that because Congress effectively eliminated the tax-based mandate (the fee or "penalty tax" for those who choose not to enroll in an insurance plan), the entire law was an unconstitutional intrusion into states' rights. The court is expected to rule on the matter before its term ends in June 2021. Although it is not anticipated that the majority of justices would vote to strike down the entire ACA, in the interim, the healthcare law will remain fully in effect, including all employer coverage obligations and reporting requirements.

Proponents of the law note that it has been especially beneficial during the pandemic. More than 3 million adults lost employer-sponsored health insurance during the COVID-19 pandemic, but bolstered by the ACA, a significant portion of these were able to retain some form of insurance (Karpman & Zuckerman, 2020). Recognizing the loss of job-based health insurance during the pandemic, in one of his first executive actions, President Biden signed an executive order directing the federal government to open a special enrollment period for individuals to obtain insurance through ACA exchanges. The move was reflective of key pillars of Biden's healthcare roadmap that includes fortifying the ACA and expanding the program for lower-income Americans in non-Medicaid expansion states (The White House, 2021).

Enhancing Access to Care Through Telehealth/Telemedicine

Noted to be a landmark publication within the past two decades, *Crossing the Quality Chasm*, addressed the benefit of the provision of healthcare services via technology, noting that information technology needed to be a central component in the redesign of the healthcare system to achieve a substantial improvement in quality (Institute of Medicine, 2001). Advances in technology have been noted to be essential in overcoming health disparities by redistributing knowledge and expertise to when and where it is needed, especially rural communities.

This need became more pronounced during the nation's public health emergency in 2020, when President Trump and a number of governors enacted swift, unprecedented regulatory change through executive orders to address the nation's healthcare crisis. These orders included expanding telehealth delivery, and policy changes regarding the use of technology in the provision of healthcare services ensued.

In February 2020, the Centers for Disease Control and Prevention (CDC) issued guidance advising individuals and healthcare providers in areas affected by the COVID-19 pandemic to adopt social distancing practices, specifically recommending that healthcare facilities and providers offer clinical services through virtual means (Koonin et al., 2020), commonly called telehealth or telemedicine. Another important use of telehealth or telemedicine was the decreased in-patient demand on healthcare facilities; thus, reducing the use of personal protective equipment, which was in short supply. Most importantly, these modalities allowed NPs to maintain continuity of care, avoiding the possible negative consequences associated with delays in routine, preventive, or chronic patient management.

Based on the expansion of the telehealth adoption, it became imperative for providers to be able to bill for these services. Shortly after the CDC's guidance, the Centers for Medicare and Medicare Services (CMS) announced a waiver removing the limitation of telehealth to rural areas, removing restrictions on telehealth originating sites (e.g., the patient's home could be an originating site), and allowing the use of phones with audio and video capabilities to furnish Medicare telehealth services (AANP, 2020d). The waiver applied broadly throughout the Medicare program and was not specific for treatment of patients with COVID-19. The waiver underwent additional review by the CMS and changes were included in a final rule near the end of 2020; updates included removing frequency limitations on visits to nursing facilities, providing payments for seven remote physiologic monitoring (RPM) codes, and revising the definition of direct supervision to include virtual presence of the supervising physician using interactive audio/video real-time communications technology to decrease infection exposure risk to all parties (CMS, 2020). CMS also allowed for billing of e-visits (communication between the patient and provider through an online patient portal). In response to the CMS policies, many commercial health plans broadened their coverage for telehealth (telemedicine) services and adopted frequently used Current Procedural Terminology (CPT®) codes for telehealth services.

For NPs, it is important to understand policies and procedures for properly conducting videoconference visits, as well as state and legal regulations required for informed consent. It is also imperative to recognize that telemedicine rules are subject to change as legislators reconsider the laws and policies impacting patient safety. Additionally, NPs are in a prime position to lobby Congress to support legislation that makes high-speed broadband internet service accessible and affordable to all Americans. The Federal Communication Commission has noted that "there were 18 million Americans without any broadband connectivity and another 25 million without adequate, reliable internet access" leading to an approximate 42 million to 162 million Americans unserved (FCC, 2020). Comprehensive efforts are needed by NPs to address the inequities due to this digital divide and to effectively implement telemedicine to underserved and economically deprived communities, throughout and beyond the pandemic. Furthermore, to provide quality telemedicine services, internet access is critical and requires effective broadband connectivity.

Addressing the Opioid Crisis

In the late 1990s, pharmaceutical companies reassured healthcare professionals that patients were unlikely to become addicted to opioids, and providers (including NPs) began to prescribe these medications at an increased rate. This increase in prescribing was attributed to the opioid epidemic, which gained public notoriety near 2010. While state laws continued to expand NP practice over the next decade, including the ability of NPs to *prescribe* opioids, in 2016 the U.S. Drug Enforcement Administration (US DEA, 2020) provided licensed non-physician mid-level practitioners the authority to *dispense* controlled substances (Title 21, Code of Federal Regulations, Section 1300.01). This presented unique timing, as in 2016, the United States saw more than 63,000 deaths from drug overdose, with more than 60% of those from opioids (Seth et al., 2018).

To address this national crisis, the first major federal addiction legislation in 40 years was signed into law by President Obama: The Comprehensive Addiction and Recovery Act (CARA). CARA (Public Law 114-198) was the most comprehensive effort undertaken to address the opioid epidemic and encompassed six pillars of coordinated response: prevention, treatment, recovery, law enforcement, criminal justice reform, and overdose reversal (Community Anti-Drug Coalitions of America, n.d.). Prior to CARA, only physicians could apply for Controlled Substances Act (CSA) waivers, allowing them to prescribe buprenorphine (an FDA-approved medication used to treat opioid addiction). CARA authorized NPs who underwent specific training to prescribe buprenorphine for patients with opioid use disorder, but the prescribing authorization was limited to a 5-year period, expiring in October 2021. Following adoption of CARA, the Substance Abuse and Mental Health Services Administration (SAMHSA) and the DEA issued relevant licenses to more than 500 NPs, but some states still have laws prohibiting NPs from prescribing buprenorphine, unless the NP is working with a physician who has a federal license to prescribe it. These state regulations have been especially problematic for rural America, as half of all counties in the United States do not have any physicians with a license to prescribe buprenorphine (Huhn & Dunn, 2017), and NPs are more likely to practice in rural and underserved regions, especially within states disproportionately impacted by opioid use and abuse (AANP, 2019). Recognizing that patient access to substance use-disorder treatment remains a significant barrier, The Substance Use-Disorder Prevention that Promotes Opioid Recovery and Treatment (SUPPORT) Act was signed into law in 2018, removing the 5-year limitation for NP prescribing. SUPPORT also initiated efforts by the CMS to eliminate "place bound" restriction requirements for patients to receive treatment. Authorized NPs are now able to manage patients with opioid use disorders at a patient's home through telemedicine (CMS, 2018).

Getting Involved

After gaining political competency within a DNP program, it is imperative that NPs remain politically engaged after graduation. Whether the DNP graduate opts to get involved in local activities or state and national NP organizations, it is the responsibility of the NP to remain aware of current issues that affect scope of practice, reimbursement, and patient and community health. Several options for political advocacy are available, but many NPs will benefit from the health policy resources available through membership in a national, state, or local NP organization.

National organizations offer a plethora of health policy information on their respective websites. The AANP's advocacy webpage (https://www.aanp.org/advocacy) includes position papers, policy briefs, NP and roundtable joint statements, and think tank and stakeholder policy statements. Government affairs updates are posted weekly, and the Advocacy Center has helpful links for finding one's elected officials and searching for legislation by topic or key words. The AANP's State Advocacy webpage includes state policy priorities, issue briefs, and policy maps, while their Federal Advocacy webpage contains an in-depth look into the regulatory process, issue briefs, and policy priorities. The National Association of Pediatric Nurse Practitioners (https://www.napnap.org/advocacy) has a Health Policy Agenda webpage that includes goals for focused advocacy and strategic partnerships designed to support their mission and aid in responding to health policy issues. NAPNAP's Advocacy Center mirrors that of AANP, but within their drop-down menu, members are linked to a number of additional resources and the online publication *Inside the Beltway*, which features legislative and regulatory news that impacts the profession.

It should be recognized that although proposed rules are published daily in the *Federal Register*, searching for and viewing pertinent topics can be a laborious, time-consuming process. Both AANP and NAPNAP have the personnel resources available to monitor legislation as it is being developed and send calls to action out to members. Calls to action include contact information for legislators and drafted letters that can be personalized.

Membership within a professional organization helps to support the development and maintenance of the previously noted health policy resources, but dues are also used to offset the cost of lobbyists who serve the political interests of the organization. In addition to membership funds, AANP also has a Political Action Committee (AANP-PAC) that provides members the opportunity to contribute support to candidates for national office whose actions or stated beliefs are congruent with the mission, principles, and purposes of the organization.

In addition to these national resources, the majority of state organizations can apprise the NP of current news, upcoming bills, and issues specific to NP practice within that state. Like federal legislation, state laws require processes that afford all interested parties reasonable opportunity to submit data, comments, or arguments, but many NPs do not take advantage of this opportunity. It would be appropriate for the NP to determine if the state organization has legislative committees in place to monitor and participate in the development of new or revised regulations that impact practice.

Professional organizations also offer experiences that directly connect members with their legislators. AANP holds their Annual Health Policy Conference in late winter. The conference includes an introduction to Capitol Hill, a government affairs update, presentations by the organization's health policy committee, interactions with NP-elected officials representing various states across the nation, presentations on key legislative issues, and a day-long visit to Capitol Hill. NAPNAP also hosts a Capitol Hill Day. This event, which is typically held in the fall of odd years, affords members the opportunity to learn about priority issues in child health and advanced practice nursing. All members are encouraged to participate and engage legislators. The organization also selects individuals for their Advocacy Scholars Program that fosters policy leadership skills, allowing members to better understand the legislative process, develop health policy advocacy skills, and apply the new skills when visiting members of Congress.

Although the previous paragraphs contain information about face-to-face experiences supported by national organizations, it is important to recognize that individual state NP organizations often coordinate similar services within state capitals. Therefore, NPs are once again encouraged to become active members of their state's NP organizations and to familiarize themselves with the resources available within these groups as well. Armed with the resources available to support political activism, the NP will be in an excellent position to contribute to policy-making processes. The following strategies can be used as part of an overall goal of moving forth legislation to advance the profession and/or enhance health care:

- Become an active member of local, state, and/or national NP organizations.
- Become familiar with the resources available on NP organization websites.
- Volunteer to serve on legislative committees within these organizations.
- Become familiar with processes for passing legislation.
- Identify state and federal legislators who represent their residence and place of employment.
- Review "do's and don'ts" of meeting with legislators.
- Establish collegial relationships with key legislators.
- Develop "elevator speeches" or "sound bites" for topics of interest.
- Garner support or identify other like-minded individuals through a variety of resources, including social media and NP organization meetings.
- Contact legislators to garner their support and recognize those who do.
- Recognize parties who may oppose a specific bill.
- Prepare to provide testimony to legislative committees when appropriate.

Ideally, politically competent NPs will assume prominent roles in political activism and policy development. Doctorally prepared NPs are also prime candidates for leadership positions in government agencies or powerful consumer groups. Those with an earnest desire to further serve the public should also consider running for political office.

Nurse Practitioner Health Policy Exemplars

Health policies affect every NP; therefore, it is imperative that NPs have the tools to stay current in what is happening in their own state as well as nationally. The NP can become a leader in helping to move issues regarding health disparities, disease prevention, and practice issues to actualize the IOM's recommendation to become "full partners, with physicians and other health care professionals, in redesigning health care in the United States" (IOM, 2011, p. 4). The following exemplars highlight the work of NPs who have made significant contributions through their healthcare policy actions.

Exemplar 1

Colleen Leners, DNP, APRN, FNP-BC, ENP, FAAN, FAANP is a distinguished leader in the national health policy arena. She currently serves as the director of policy at the American Association of Colleges of Nursing (AACN) in Washington, D.C. In addition to maintaining an active NP practice for more than 25 years, Dr. Leners has served our country in the U.S. Army Nurse Corps and was awarded the Bronze Star for her meritorious service in the Middle East. Back in the states, Dr. Leners created a nurse-managed primary care clinic for wounded warriors at Navy Medical Center San Diego (C5). She notes that her effective leadership in today's health policy arena stems from her distinguished military service as an NP.

In her current role, Dr. Leners focuses on advancing health policy and elevating nursing leadership, goals congruent with AACN's focus on excellence and innovation in nursing education, research, and practice. As the director of policy, Dr. Leners has cultivated strong relationships with Congress and the executive branch; these relationships serve as the foundation for collaborative partnerships that help advance policies reflecting the critical role advanced practice nurses play in delivering high-quality, cost-effective, team-based health care. Within her daily work at AACN, Dr. Leners keeps abreast of proposed rules published in the *Federal Register*. As outlined earlier in this chapter, Dr. Leners' work is an important component of the healthcare regulation processes. In her leadership role, she directs the AACN in submitting public comments on regulatory proposals, including those that directly impact the APRN scope of practice.

Dr. Leners has a unique ability and responsibility to liaison with the White House and the U.S. Department of Health and Human Services to build a united front with practice partners. As one example of her recent work, Dr. Leners participated in coalition-led efforts to recommend significant policy changes that were adopted by the Centers for Medicare and Medicaid Services (CMS): the revision of medical record documentation requirements that ultimately reduced the burden on APRNs who bill under CMS's Physician Fee Schedule. In coordination with CMS, she continues to work tirelessly to correct provider attestation to accurately document services billed, by removing "incident to" billing.

To improve the healthcare system for providers and patients, Dr. Leners emphasizes the importance of the military's "mission first" approach. She envisions APRNs working together in a more unified voice to achieve national recognition on boards, councils, and committees. Reflective of this perspective, Dr. Leners initiated the Nominations Consortium at AACN in 2018. Through this ad hoc consortium, AACN collaborates with other nursing organizations to nominate experts in the nursing field for membership on federal advisory committees. This unified voice has resulted in the nomination of more than 40 nursing professionals to high-level federal positions, organizations in which nursing leadership was not previously represented (e.g., the National Institute for Occupational Safety and Health, the Medicare Payment Advisory Commission, and the Patient-Centered Outcomes Research Institute).

Reflecting on her career, Dr. Leners is most proud of her military service and achievement in not losing one soldier, sailor, airman, or marine as the primary care manager for wounded warriors. Her advocacy for our servicemen and women continues to be manifested in her health policy initiatives. Selected as a Robert Wood Johnson Foundation Health Policy Fellow in the office of Senator John Thune (R-SD) of the Senate Finance Committee, she developed solutions to healthcare system deficits, resulting in improvements within the Department of Defense and the Department of Veterans Affairs. Regarding the future of advanced practice nursing, Dr. Leners envisions NPs more actively engaged in local, state, and federal legislation. She stresses the need for NPs to experience service-based volunteering (i.e., The Medical Corps) to gain practical knowledge of policy implications. She notes that to elevate the nursing voice, "nurses need to play a larger and more impactful role in interdisciplinary teams."

Exemplar 2

Sophia L. Thomas, DNP, APRN, MN, FNP-BC, PPCNP-BC, FNAP, FAANP, is a certified family and pediatric nurse practitioner dedicated to providing care to medically underserved families. Compassionate, with a single focus to treat all equally, she practices at a federally qualified health center in New Orleans. In addition to her clinical practice, Dr. Thomas has long-standing service in the American Association of Nurse Practitioners (AANP), impacting health policy initiatives within her home state of Louisiana, as well as other states in the organization's Region 6 (i.e., Arkansas, Oklahoma, and Texas). Emerging as a recognized and integral leader within the organization, Dr. Thomas received a prestigious AANP Leadership Fellowship. The knowledge and skills attained through the fellowship led to further development of her role within AANP; Dr. Thomas is currently serving a two-year term as the organization's president. Her leadership in health policy is enmeshed within this role, as she continues to maintain a focus on removing the barriers faced by many Americans as they seek quality health care.

As AANP president, Dr. Thomas oversees the organization's legislative initiatives at local, state, and national levels. These initiatives are strategically developed to advance health policy; promote excellence in practice, education, and research; and establish standards that best serve patients and other healthcare consumers. Through practice, education, advocacy, research, and leadership, AANP is dedicated to addressing the systemic causes of health disparities among vulnerable populations and encompassing a holistic approach to address the issues in marginalized communities; as the organization's president, Dr. Thomas' work embodies this mission. She concentrates her efforts on providing NPs with policy and clinical information, boosting direct member communications, enhancing continuing education offerings, and ensuring the organization is responsive to social and cultural needs. Like many early NP leaders, Dr. Thomas stays abreast of state issues as she believes in engaging NPs in grassroots advocacy movements to initiate change.

In her leadership role, Dr. Thomas has worked to enhance NP visibility in the media. As host of the newly launched *NP Pulse* podcast, she helps AANP provide an arena for NP thought leaders to address issues of interest to the NP population and a forum for clinical and regulatory matters. Reflective of her belief in the need for equality in health care, Dr. Thomas initiated AANP position statements against racial and health disparities. Her public communication during National NP Week in 2020 advocated for a coordinated national response to combat health disparities and called on state legislatures nationwide to expand healthcare access through passage of full practice authority (FPA).

Since the outbreak of the coronavirus, NP recognition as frontline providers has been pushed to the forefront in an "all-hands-on-deck" effort to treat patients stricken by this invisible enemy. With Dr. Thomas in her leadership role, AANP successfully urged governors of several states to remove restrictions to NP practice during the pandemic, allowing NPs to provide lifesaving health care without delays. As introduced earlier in this chapter, AANP advocated for passage of the Coronavirus Aid, Relief and Economic Security (CARES) Act, bolstering older adults' access to home healthcare services and funding for personal protective equipment for healthcare providers during the pandemic. In addition to the organization's work, Dr. Thomas served as a consultant for the U.S. Department of Health and Human Services Vaccine Consultation Panel: Operation Warp Speed.

Reflecting on her career, Dr. Thomas is most proud of her 25 years as an AANP member and her advocacy for the NP role. Her lifelong efforts against negative social determinants of health and her desire to improve access to care for all were factors in her being selected in 2020 as one of Modern Healthcare's 100 Most Influential People in Healthcare. "This honor reflects the selfless efforts of AANP members who have sacrificed so much, combating the COVID-19 pandemic and maintaining access to health care for patients during this difficult time," Dr. Thomas said.

Seminar Discussion Questions

1. What are the key legislative issues that your state NP organization is currently working on?
2. Identify a health policy issue that you feel passionate about. Develop a 30-second elevator speech/sound bite that clearly articulates your position.
3. What topic would you be most comfortable discussing with a federal legislator? Why?
4. In the Health Policy Exemplars section of this chapter, Dr. Thomas notes the importance of "grassroots advocacy." Do you think this is an effective way of initiating policy change? Why or why not?

References

American Association of Colleges of Nursing. (2006). *The essentials of doctoral education for advanced nursing practice*. https://www.aacnnursing.org/Portals/42/Publications/DNPEssentials.pdf

American Association of Colleges of Nursing. (2020). *Draft—The essentials: Core competencies for professional nursing education*. https://www.aacnnursing.org/Portals/42/Downloads/Essentials/Essentials-Draft-Document.pdf

American Association of Colleges for Nursing. (2021a). *The Essentials*. https://www.aacnnursing.org/Education-Resources/AACN-Essentials

American Association of Colleges of Nursing. (2021b). *Essentials task force*. https://www.aacnnursing.org/About-AACN/AACN-Governance/Committees-and-Task-Forces/Essentials

American Association of Nurse Practitioners. (n.d.). *Historical timeline*. https://www.aanp.org/all-about-nps/historical-timeline

American Association of Nurse Practitioners. (2019). *How nurse practitioners are key to expanding the opioid treatment workforce*. https://aanp.org/news-feed/how-nurse-practitioners-are-key-to-expanding-the-opioid-treatment-workforce

American Association of Nurse Practitioners. (2020a). *AANP calls for urgent action to combat COVID-19's disproportionate impact on minorities*. https://www.aanp.org/news-feed/aanp-calls-for-urgent-action-to-combat-covid-19s-disproportionate-impact-on-minorities

American Association of Nurse Practitioners. (2020b). *APRN compact licensure*. https://www.aanp.org/advocacy/advocacy-resource/position-statements/aprn-compact-licensure

American Association of Nurse Practitioners. (2020c). *Five states take action to expand access to care during COVID-19 pandemic*. https://www.aanp.org/news-feed/five-states-take-action-to-expand-access-to-care-during-covid-19-pandemic

American Association of Nurse Practitioners. (2020d). *Medicare telehealth waivers update*. https://www.aanp.org/news-feed/medicare-telehealth-waivers-update

American Association of Nurse Practitioners. (2020e). *NP fact sheet*. https://www.aanp.org/about/all-about-nps/np-fact-sheet

American Association of Nurse Practitioners. (2021). *State practice environment*. https://www.aanp.org/advocacy/state/state-practice-environment

APRN Joint Dialogue Group. (2008). *Consensus model for APRN regulation: Licensure, accreditation, certification, & education.* http://www.aacn.nche.edu/education-resources/APRNReport.pdf

Association of American Medical Colleges. (2020). *The complexities of physician supply and demand: Projections for 2018 to 2033.* https://www.aamc.org/media/45976/download

Bartol, T. (2015). Nurse practitioners: Enhancing healthcare for 50 years. *Nurse Practitioner, 40*(6), 14–15.

Centers for Medicare and Medicaid Services. (2018). *Information on Medicare telehealth.* https://www.cms.gov/About-CMS/Agency-Information/OMH/Downloads/Information-on-Medicare-Telehealth-Report.pdf

Centers for Medicare and Medicaid Services. (2020). *Final policy, payment, and quality provisions changes to the Medicare Physician Free Schedule for calendar year 2021.* https://www.cms.gov/newsroom/fact-sheets/final-policy-payment-and-quality-provisions-changes-medicare-physician-fee-schedule-calendar-year-1

Community Anti-Drug Coalitions of America. (n.d.). *The Comprehensive Addiction and Recovery Act (CARA).* https://www.cadca.org/comprehensive-addiction-and-recovery-act-cara

Federal Communications Commission. (2020). *Bridging the digital divide for all Americans.* https://www.fcc.gov/about-fcc/fcc-initiatives/bridging-digital-divide-all-americans

Huhn, A. S., & Dunn, K. E. (2017). Why aren't physicians prescribing more buprenorphine? *Journal of Substance Abuse Treatment, 78,* 1–7. https://doi.org/10.1016/j.jsat.2017.04.005

Institute of Medicine. (2001). *Crossing the quality chasm: A new health system for the 21st century.* National Academies Press.

Institute of Medicine of the National Academies. (2011). *The future of nursing: Leading change, advancing health.* National Academies Press. https://www.nap.edu/read/12956/chapter/1#ii

Karpman, M., & Zuckerman, S. (2020). *ACA offers protection as the COVID-19 pandemic erodes employer health insurance coverage.* https://www.rwjf.org/en/library/research/2020/11/aca-offers-protection-as-the-covid-19-pandemic-erodes-employer-health-insurance-coverage.html

Koonin, L. M., Hoots, B., Tsang, C. A., Leroy, Z., Farris, K., Jolly, B. T., Antall, P., McCabe, B., Zelis, C. B. R., Tong, I., & Harris, A. M. (2020). Trends in the use of telehealth during the emergence of the COVID-19 pandemic–United States, January–March 2020. *Morbidity and Mortality Weekly Report, 69*(43), 1595–1599.

LeBuhn, R., & Swankin, D. A. (2010). *Reforming scopes of practice: A white paper.* https://www.ncsbn.org/ReformingScopesofPractice-WhitePaper.pdf

McDonald, L. (2006). *Florence Nightingale as a social reformer.* http://www.historytoday.com/lynn-mcdonald/florence-nightingale-social-reformer

National Association of Pediatric Nurse Practitioners. (2020). *National Association of Pediatric Nurse Practitioners official statement opposing new APRN Compact requirements.* https://www.napnap.org/national-association-of-pediatric-nurse-practitioners-official-statement-opposing-new-aprn-compact-requirements/

National Council of State Boards of Nursing. (2021). *APRN Consensus Model.* https://www.ncsbn.org/aprn-consensus.htm

National Council on Aging. (n.d.). *Healthy aging facts.* https://www.ncoa.org/news/resources-for-reporters/get-the-facts/healthy-aging-facts/

National Human Genome Research Institute. (2020). *How a bill becomes law.* https://www.genome.gov/about-genomics/policy-issues/How-Bill-Becomes-Law

National Organization of Nurse Practitioner Faculties. (2017). *Nurse practitioner core competencies content.* https://www.nonpf.org/resource/resmgr/competencies/2017_NPCoreComps_with_Curric.pdf

National Women's Hall of Fame. (2017). *Loretta C. Ford.* https://www.womenofthehall.org/inductee/loretta-c-ford/

Phillips, S. J. (2021). 30th annual APRN legislative update. *Nurse Practitioner, 43*(1), 27–54.

Robert Wood Johnson Foundation. (2017). *Charting nursing's future: Reports that can inform policy and practice.* http://www.rwjf.org/content/dam/farm/reports/issue_briefs/2017/rwjf435543

Seth, P., Scholl, L., Rudd, R., & Bacon, S. (2018). Overdose deaths involving opioids, cocaine, and psychostimulants–United States, 2015–2016. *Morbidity and Mortality Weekly Report, 67*(12), 349–358. https://www.cdc.gov/mmwr/volumes/67/wr/mm6712a1.htm#:~:text=In%202016%2C%20there%20were%2063%2C632,urbanization%20levels%2C%20and%20multiple%20states.

Sofer, D. (2017). VA grants most APRNs full practice authority. *American Journal of Nursing, 117*(3), 14.
U.S. Department of Health and Human Services. (2018). *Introduction: About HHS.* https://www.hhs.gov/about/strategic-plan/introduction/index.html#:~:text=Cross%2DAgency%20Collaborations-,Mission%20Statement,public%20health%2C%20and%20social%20services.
U.S. Drug Enforcement Administration. (2020). *Title 21 United States Code (USC) Controlled Substances Act.* https://www.deadiversion.usdoj.gov/21cfr/21usc/811.htm
The White House. (2021). Executive order on strengthening Medicaid and the Affordable Care Act. https://www.whitehouse.gov/briefing-room/presidential-actions/2021/01/28/executive-order-on-strengthening-medicaid-and-the-affordable-care-act/
Wolff, M. A. (1984). Court upholds expanded practice roles for nurses. *Law, Medicine, and Health Care, 12*(1), 26–29. https://doi:10.1111/j.1748-720X.1984.tb01757.x

CHAPTER 16

Mentoring and Lifelong Learning

Susan M. DeNisco and Dori Taylor-Sullivan

Historically, there has been a lack of emphasis in the nursing profession on being mentored or on mentoring others. As the business world has known for years, the benefits of mentoring for mentees include having a definitive career plan, increased job satisfaction, improved socialization to the role, higher levels of self-esteem and confidence, higher salaries, and more opportunity for advancement (Grindell, 2003; Harrington, 2011; Tracy, 2012).

Although new nursing professionals are often "precepted" by a more experienced nurse, these novice providers are frequently expected to practice on their own after the specified orientation period is over. Nurse practitioner graduates may or may not have a period of orientation with a preceptor, depending on the practice site. Various terms have been used to describe those who assist others as they develop and learn professionally. Common terms are *preceptor*, *teacher*, *educator*, *guide*, *coach*, *manager*, *role model*, and *mentor*. Oftentimes, these terms are used interchangeably, which adds to confusion about the roles. What defines these roles will be reviewed in this chapter with the focus on the mentor.

Preceptor

A very common term in the nursing world is *preceptor*. The concept has been discussed in an earlier chapter; however, a short review is offered here. Prior to enrolling in a NP program, most nurses have been precepted by another nurse in a new clinical setting, and very often may have functioned in the preceptor role. A preceptor has been defined as "a teacher; in nursing, usually an experienced nurse who assumes responsibility for teaching a novice" (Chitty & Black, 2011, p. 460). Typically, NP students are assigned a preceptor for clinical experiences. In all of these scenarios, the preceptor has been assigned to the student or new graduate. The relationship is usually a prescribed length of time—typically a short duration—and the relationship is usually confined to the work environment.

Preceptors themselves should have at least 1 year of experience with a solid skill set in whatever clinical setting the experience will take place. Beyond their clinical expertise, the preceptor should have knowledge of the NP role in order to be a role model for the preceptee. For the NP student, the preceptor is not always another NP; the preceptor could be a physician's assistant, a certified nurse–midwife, or commonly, a physician.

The goals for the training period are prescribed by an organization such as the National Organization for Nurse Practitioner Faculty (NONPF) or an institution, such as an acute care hospital or university, and evaluation forms are used to ensure the preceptee has adequately met the goals upon completion of the predetermined time period. Obviously, the NP role cannot be role modeled by non-NP preceptors (i.e., physicians); however, they should be cognizant of what the role entails to provide some insight for direction and the skill set needed for practice. In addition, a non-NP preceptor most likely will have difficulty in discussing the scope of practice while training an NP student. However, the preceptor role is quite important, and a long-lasting relationship may occur with some preceptors and preceptees.

⚑ EXCERPT FROM A PRECEPTOR

Over the 18 years I have spent as an NP, I have precepted many students from a variety of universities, as well as precepted NPs new to the clinical practice I work in. Precepting NP students can be very challenging, as well as rewarding. I have learned it is imperative to be aware of where the student is in the program, and what didactic information has already been covered to avoid unrealistic expectations. In addition, I have usually not met the student in advance, so that once we start working together we may discover personality differences that make the relationship strained. Successful strategies have included being open and honest with the student, but never in front of a patient, nor in front of other staff. Instead, spending 10–15 minutes in the morning reviewing the schedule, and going over appropriate patients and goals for the day is very helpful.

Spending time during the lunch break to check in and identify what went well and what could have been handled differently is beneficial. At the end of clinic, we touch base in this regard as well. Occasionally I end with assigning a little homework regarding a patient for the student to do prior to returning the following week. This is a similar approach to precepting novice NPs to the practice setting. There have been a few students and novice NPs who have maintained their relationship with me and are colleagues that I have become a mentor for.

Role Model

The definition of a role model is "an individual who serves as an example of desirable behavior for another person" (Chitty & Black, 2011, p. 462). Role models include those people in whom we find qualities that are admirable or appealing. We can choose one or more role models. There may not be a direct contact or a relationship with a role model. The role model could be a person who is from the same discipline, such as a current NP leader or faculty member, or the role model may not be from the same profession. NP students can identify what qualities they feel are important and would like to emulate. For instance, an altruistic NP may say that Mother Theresa is a role model because her qualities of selflessness, and working with the poor and needy, are goals that the NP would like to work toward. Oftentimes students who spend clinical hours in a center providing health care for the indigent find a preceptor who goes above and beyond in caring about each patient, despite what his or her appearance or socioeconomic status may be. Having such a rewarding experience with a role model can set the NP student's professional self-expectations and goals.

Coach

Coaches, on the other hand, may be assigned, such as a sports team coach, or may be chosen, such as a writing or life coach. A coach is someone who helps move an individual forward to where he or she wants to be, whether this relates to a goal weight, becoming an expert swimmer, or writing an article for publication. Specific goals could be set by the coach, the individual, or mutually set depending on the context. Most often, the literature points to the individual's objectives and goals as the focus of the coaching relationship. The time limit of the relationship can be short term or long term, depending on the individual's desire to be coached and the setting. A preceptor can be viewed as a coach because he or she helps the NP student during the transition from RN to NP (Link, 2009). In this preceptor-as-coach role, NP students are coached to believe they are capable of meeting their goals.

Nurse practitioners are often taught during their role seminars that one of the functions of the NP is to be a coach for patients and families. In fact, coaching to assist the patient with positive behavior changes to improve health is a component of the standards set by NONPF (2017). A NP coach can be described as someone who encourages, inspires, and empowers patients to reach their maximum health potential. In this scenario, patients' desires and goals drive the coaching relationship. Many chronic diseases have shown improved health outcomes when NPs act as coaches. Today, there are NPs who are working as wellness coaches and holistic coaches. Two NPs who practice together as wellness coaches, Darlene Trandel, PhD, MSN, RN/FNP, and Eileen T. O'Grady, PhD, RN, NP, are very enthusiastic about this role. According to Trandel:

> The premise underlying health and wellness coaching is helping people define and design their personal health and wellness goals to create a lifestyle that is based on who they are. Many clients come to us to rev up their wellness status and live a more healthful lifestyle; some seek to prevent or reduce the risk of a chronic illness and to age with vitality; and still others want to better manage an existing condition. Wellness coaches help their clients develop a personal blueprint for their health and wellness, increase their awareness of barriers that impede their progress, and create strategies to overcome the impediments that prevent them from mastering and sustaining their goals in their everyday life. As wellness coaches, we leverage both the relationship and the process to raise self-confidence and self-esteem and encourage clients to feel empowered and in charge of their health. (Hanson, 2012)

Mentor

Although many people have written that the origin of the term *mentor* comes from Homer's *Odyssey*, written in approximately 700 BCE, the actual author and date of origin are debatable. In this epic poem, Odysseus provided Mentor, who was really the goddess of wisdom, Athena, as a protector for his son while he was away. In addition to protecting the prince, Mentor educated, coached, and guided Odysseus' son, Telemachus. Mentor was more than a teacher. He was half-god and half-human, half-male and half-female. Mentor was a representation of the merger of both goal and path, as well as the yin and yang of life. Mentors need to both push and pull their mentees at times, leading by guiding the interaction with the mentees—while always remaining supportive.

Grossman (2013) points out that a more modernized version has been identified, depicting the origination of the term as occurring in approximately 1699, by Fenelon. The definition of mentoring which is more applicable currently to NPs is a "voluntary, intense, committed, extended, dynamic, interactive, supportive, trusting relationship between two people, one experienced, and the other a newcomer, characterized by mutuality" (Hayes, 1998, p. 525).

A mentor may be a faculty person, a clinical preceptor, or a professional the graduate comes into contact with and identifies as a person that the graduate would like to engage in a supportive relationship for an extended period of time. Mentoring may be a formal relationship, where a mentor is assigned by an organization, or an informal agreement made between a mentor and mentee that have chosen each other; the relationship lasts for a mutually agreed upon time, typically long-lasting. In the ideal mentoring relationship, both parties "develop personally and professionally within the auspices of a caring, collaborative, and respectful environment" (Grossman, 2013, p. 186). The mentor, then, is different from a preceptor or a coach, yet may function in those roles in addition, but a mentor encompasses much more. The differences between these roles are summarized in **Table 16-1**.

Kram (1986), an authority on mentoring, identified two components of this type of relationship: career and psychosocial. Within the career mentoring portion are activities such as sponsorship, networking, and coaching, while psychosocial aspects include helping the mentee to move forward in professional development, role modeling, and friendship. Even within an informal mentorship, there may be a contract or agreement to clarify goals and timelines. Mentors are inspirers, supporters, envisioners, sponsors, coaches, and role models.

Often there are not enough opportunities for nursing professionals to benefit from a formal mentoring relationship. However, nursing literature does provide evidence about the benefits of mentor–mentee relationships. Nurses who have been mentored reported the capability to model positive traits of their mentors, such

Table 16-1 Differences Among Mentor, Preceptor, and Coach

	Mentor	**Preceptor**	**Coach**
Match	By desire	Assigned	Either
Time	Longer term	Shorter term	Either
Goals	Set mutually	Prescribed	Either
Setting	Work/other	Work	Either

Reproduced with permission of Dori Taylor Sullivan.

as persistence, job dedication, honesty, and discipline (Carey & Campbell, 1994; Dyer, 2008). The mentor–mentee relationship was found to help the socialization of the mentored nurse into a specific nursing unit or nursing position (Dyer, 2008). In addition, nurses who have been mentored noted career advice, role modeling, education, and emotional support to be benefits of the relationship (Dyer, 2008).

Few studies have been published regarding outcomes related to NPs and mentorship (Harrington, 2011). Hayes (1998) found a positive correlation between NP students' discernment of mentoring by their clinical preceptor and their own sense of self-efficacy. Brown and Olshansky (1997) found that productivity increased in the primary care setting when novice NPs had supportive work environments. Neal (2008) completed a study that examined NP students' perception of self-efficacy based upon whether the student had at least one preceptor identified as a mentor during clinical training. Neal found that predictors of self-efficacy included students' identification of a mentor and how the mentoring relationship facilitated the enhancement of skills needed to practice as an NP. In a survey seeking to identify the needs of APNs in a tertiary care center, findings were that both formal and informal mentoring would be useful, and that NPs should be matched with NPs (Doerksen, 2010). Also identified in this small survey were needs related to intellectual, financial, and administrative support, and that the needs for the mentee and mentor change over time.

For NP/DNP students, identifying a clinical mentor may be required by the university that encompasses more than the role of a clinical preceptor. Clinical mentors are academically and clinically qualified advanced practice nurses, physicians, faculty, nurse executives, and other healthcare professionals or health policy leaders who are able to facilitate and support the objectives of the student's clinical residency and DNP project.

Needs of the novice NP were identified in a think tank conducted by the American Academy of Nurse Practitioners (AANP, 2006). There were seven areas noted by these experienced NPs:

1. Caseload management
2. Time management and productivity
3. Developing clinical skills
4. Understanding the business component of practice
5. Overcoming fear and anxiety
6. Dealing with isolation
7. How to balance personal life and clinical practice effectively

The development of a career enrichment, formally called a mentorship program by the fellows of the AANP have identified the following important aspects of the relationship (AANP, 2021):

- Mutually benefit both the mentee and mentor
- Focus on helping and guiding toward professional goals
- Involve time, energy, initiative, and follow-through to be successful
- Involve mentors as generous learning brokers
- Involve mentees committed to achieving defined objectives

Various stages in the mentoring relationship are discussed, such as the ones listed in **Box 16-1**.

In stage 1, initiation, the mentee and mentor are becoming acquainted. The experienced person believes that the novice can be successful and is willing to mentor

> **Box 16-1** Stages of the Mentor Relationship
>
> 1. Initiation
> 2. Cultivation
> 3. Separation
> 4. Redefinition
>
> Data from Kram, K. E. (1983, December). Phases of the mentor relationship. *Academy of Management Journal, 26,* 608–625.

the novice. The novice finds the mentor admirable and is willing to be guided and coached by the mentor. Mutual goals should be set in the cultivation stage. A contract clearly identifying what achievements are desired, and how the mentor will guide the mentee to reach those achievements, a note articulating the frequency and mode of meetings, as well as confidentiality, and a clause written about openness and conflict resolution should be included (see **Figure 16-1**).

At this time, the mentee is becoming more confident that her or his professional and personal goals can be met. Dependence on the mentor can be strong during these early stages. In stage 4, the mentee has become self-confident and is not as dependent on the mentor, and will start the separation process. This time period can cause anxiety in the mentee (Grossman, 2013; Kram, 1986). As the relationship matures, the mentee and mentor have a more collegial relationship, and most likely, the mentee in turn has now become a mentor to a novice.

What should one look for when trying to find a mentor? In a study of 565 NPs, five aspects of a successful mentor were uncovered (Harrington 2011). Components of these five aspects included (Grossman, 2013):

- Having a personal commitment to mentoring
- Having expertise in the field the mentoring occurs in
- Having the necessary qualities of counselor and educator
- Being prepared to be a sponsor
- Having an effective communication style
- Being respected in the profession
- Having good self-esteem
- Balancing work and personal life
- Willing to take on new challenges
- Being open to change

Four core competencies for effective mentoring developed by Bell (2002) form the acronym SAGE:

- **S**urrendering—leveling the learning field
- **A**ccepting—creating a safe haven for risk taking
- **G**ifting—the main event
- **E**xtending—nurturing protégé independence

In the surrendering component, all attempts to rid the relationship of the anxiety that can occur from the mentor's power and authority are embraced. Accepting the mentee as she or he is and providing a safe environment for learning and growth are vital to success. The value of being generous with useful advice, feedback, and opportunities without expecting anything in return is called gifting. Although we

> We are voluntarily entering into a mentoring relationship from which we both expect to benefit. To this end, we have mutually agreed upon the terms and conditions of our relationship as outlined in this agreement.
>
> **Objectives/Goals**
> We hope to achieve:
> Goal 1: _____
> Goal 2: _____
> Goal 3: _____
>
> Responsibilities of Mentor:
> _____
>
> Responsibilities of Mentee:
> _____
>
> **Frequency of Meetings**
> We will attempt to meet at least _____ *[fill in amount]* times each month. If we cannot attend a scheduled meeting, we agree to be responsible and notify our partner, and make a specific plan to talk by phone, email, or text.
>
> **Duration**
> This mentoring relationship will continue as long as we both feel comfortable or until:
> _____
> _____
>
> **Confidentiality**
> Any sensitive issues that we discuss will be held in confidence. Issues that are off limits in this relationship include: _____
>
> **No-Fault Termination**
> We are committed to open and honest communication in our relationship. We will discuss and attempt to resolve any conflicts as they arise. If, however, one of us needs to terminate the relationship for any reason, we agree to abide by the decision of our partner.
>
> Mentor _____ Date _____
> Mentee _____ Date _____

Figure 16-1 Sample Mentor and Mentee Agreement

Reproduced from Brainard, S., Harkus, D., & George, M. (1998). *A Curriculum for Training Mentors and Mentees: Guide for Administration.* Seattle, WA: The Center for Workforce Development. (http://www.grad.washington.edu/mentoring/students/worksheet5.pdf). Reprinted by permission.

may think this is most beneficial to the mentee, anyone who has gifted in this manner knows that the equal, if not greater, gift is the satisfaction the mentor gets from watching the mentee flourish. Extending requires the mentor to be able to let go, to push the mentee beyond the boundaries of comfort, and to realize when to end the current relationship and allow the mentee to use alternate methods for future growth.

The Barker-Sullivan Model of Mentor Partnerships (DeNisco, 2021) begins with mutual attraction, which is based on congruency of values, and it is characterized by respect and trust. Honest, open, and discreet communications are emphasized in this model. The mentor, who has expertise that the mentee is seeking to learn from, has skills required by a mentor, and is a transformational leader in the role the mentee is involved with, or seeks to become expert in. The mentee needs to develop competence in the new role and in leadership skills. This type of mentoring relationship should encourage the mentee to be energized to engage in self-reflection, learn new skills and competencies, and take action to move forward.

Mentees can get the most of a mentoring relationship by recognizing that they have found someone who genuinely cares about them and their career. The following tips have been adapted for new NP/DNP graduates (Tracy, 2012; Zwilling, 2012):

- Set clear objectives for yourself in your career growth. Decide exactly what it is you need mentoring on before you start thinking of the ideal person to work with. This will help you to seek out the right person as mentor.
- Work to continually put the guidance into action. The best mentors are the most interested in helping someone who is willing to learn and grow; so take advantage by putting the suggestions and advice into action.
- Remember, the best mentors are busy people. When you meet, be prepared by having specific issues to discuss.
- Remember the difference between a mentor, a friend, and a coach. Expect a mentor to tell you what you need to hear, not like a friend who may tell you what you want to hear. A business coach is focused on helping you with generic skills, whereas a mentor's aim is to teach you based on specific situations.
- Send a note to communicate progress or touch base on a regular basis. A mentor is more likely to want to help you if you are making it clear you are following through, and the relationship is helping you to reach your objectives and goals.

The mentor should use the following guidelines when working with a mentee:

- Advise the mentee about the duration of the meeting.
- Discuss the mentee's achievements and give positive feedback.
- Be specific and kind when giving necessary constructive feedback that may not be what the mentee might want to hear.
- Be prepared to fill the meeting time with specific issues and objectives.
- Take every moment seriously.
- Reassure the mentee that trust, honesty, and confidentiality are of paramount importance to your relationship.

Peer mentoring is another format for a mentoring relationship that may be useful as the increased number of NP/DNP graduates seeking experienced NP/DNPs is mismatched. Identification of a peer mentor that can help in areas where she or he has expertise that the NP needs further growth in, and where the NP can offer her or his own expertise in an area the other person needs to grow in, can be a very rewarding experience. It can also be beneficial and practical to have a group of peer mentors who can offer a pool of expertise to help the NPs that form this group.

Prior to graduating from NP programs, students should consider identifying a mentor and prepare to discuss the relationship with the person so there is more of a formal relationship for supporting the novice NP. Mentees should be prepared that, down the road, they may consider becoming mentors to others, whether peer mentors, or the more familiar relationship with a novice NP. The rewards are many for both.

Nurse Practitioner Residency and Fellowship Programs

The rapid increase of nurse practitioner fellowships and residency programs over the past decade is an indication that our profession is growing and experiencing increased autonomy. The first primary care residency program was developed by Margret Flinter to support novice NPs who aspired to work with complex patients in a federally qualified health center (FQHC) in Connecticut (2005). Flinter posits that NPs should have the opportunity for training with the support of experienced healthcare providers in order to provide the comprehensive, complicated care that most patients who use those types of health centers need. In this model, however, it may not be an NP who is formally provided as a mentor; it may be a physician.

While not a requirement in order to practice, fellowships and residencies provide a newly graduated nurse practitioner the opportunity to smoothly transition into the practice setting by bridging their didactic education with semi-supervised clinical hours. There is some confusion with regard to the difference between a residency and a fellowship. Like the long-standing physician residency model, a NP residency is also a postgraduate program in a major practice area such as primary care. On the other hand, a fellowship program is a post-graduate program with didactic and clinical training in a subspecialty, such as emergency medicine, gastroenterology, cardiology, etc.

Choosing either a fellowship or residency or going directly into practice is a personal decision. It is important to keep in mind that these programs are paid positions and come with typical employee benefits, but sometimes the salaries may be lower than you would receive going directly into the workforce (Zbrog, 2021). Major universities and medical centers such as Johns Hopkins, the Mayo Clinic, Memorial Sloan Cancer Center, Columbia University, and New York University Langone Medical Center are just a few of the many renowned organizations offering these opportunities. It is becoming clear that nurse practitioners who complete fellowships and residencies will see their skill sets, as well as their career options, objectively improve.

Nurse Practitioners as Lifelong Learners

As you begin your career as a nurse practitioner, making lifelong learning a priority in your professional and personal life is essential. Lifelong learning is a dynamic and intentional process aimed at improving knowledge, skills, and approaches to life. Lifelong learning offers individuals the opportunity to maintain current knowledge in a rapidly changing world, acquire new skills, and pursue a wide variety of interests through intellectual growth and expansion. Whether formally or informally, being committed to lifelong learning in the healthcare arena provides benefits and welfare for everyone in society. As a novice nurse practitioner, you will continue to learn throughout your careers to gain knowledge to provide safe, competent care within your scope of practice (Beauvais, 2021). **Box 16-2** provides examples of ways to engage in lifelong learning opportunities to enhance your professional life.

As a professional NP, by engaging in learning activities following graduation you can improve patient outcomes, decrease mortality rates, and reduce the chance of harm.

Chapter 16 Mentoring and Lifelong Learning

Whereas some lifelong learning activities are formal and take place in the classroom, many are self-directed and can take many forms. **Box 16-3** displays the multiple benefits of being a lifelong learner whether you are a student, a practicing clinician, or nearing retirement.

While some lifelong learning activities are formal and take place in the classroom, many are self-directed and can take many forms. **Box 16-4** provides examples of personal lifelong learning activities.

Box 16-2 Lifelong Learning Activities for the Professional Nurse Practitioner

- Watching online webinars and videos.
- Attending conferences.
- Joining and becoming active in professional nursing associations.
- Obtaining specialty certification.
- Receiving on-the-job training.
- Researching and reading professional journals, articles, and evidence-based literature.
- Collaborating with other healthcare professionals.
- Volunteering on committees at work or in your community
- Learning a new clinical skill: suturing, splinting and casting, bedside ultrasound, etc.

Box 16-3 Benefits of Being a Lifelong Learner

- Assists in establishing valuable relationships
- Keeps you actively involved as a contributing member to society
- Helps you enrich your life and find meaning in it
- Opens your mind to improve the world
- Strengthens your abilities
- Provides you with options
- Prevents boredom
- Makes you a valuable employee
- Boosts your confidence and self-esteem
- Challenges your ideas and beliefs

Box 16-4 Personal Growth Lifelong Learning Activities

- Read books and professional journals
- Learn a second language
- Take continuing education classes
- Keep a "to learn" list
- Join a book or journal club
- Teach/mentor/precept others
- Keep a reflective journal

⚕ MY MENTOR

Feeling competent in my skills as a nurse practitioner, I realized that it was time to find a professional challenge in my career trajectory. I joined a few colleagues from a previous employment site who had contacted me to start a DNP cohort program that was going to begin in our area. Since I knew that my goal had never included a PhD in nursing because I did not want to focus solely on nursing research, I agreed the DNP was a great option.

We progressed through, sometimes loving the learning and networking this cohort afforded us, and sometimes moaning and groaning over the necessary research and writing of papers at such an advanced level. We were fortunate to have a senior faculty person discuss with us the need to seek mentors, and briefly cover the reason why we would need our own mentor. Another seasoned colleague spoke about her mentor, and how their relationship had been critical for her to meet the goals in her career. She also discussed how the time had come to part ways—when her mentor no longer seemed to be supporting her mentee's choices and current goals.

I realized I needed a mentor—but who? Who had been around a long enough time with a DNP and was an NP that could guide me? I also realized that I really wasn't sure what my goals were now. Accomplishing the completion of my research and publishing it were behind me now. What next?

After taking a full-time job in a university setting, having my clinical work each week, in addition to a full load of teaching and advising NP students, I quickly realized I needed a mentor to help me balance this juggling act. I was an expert clinician, and a good preceptor; however, my formal teaching abilities needed mentoring from someone who was doing both clinical and teaching, and had a family, and doing it all in a balanced manner. Not an easy bill to fill!

I am so fortunate to have found someone who is probably more of a peer mentor in some areas, but who has had many years of teaching and doing clinical, as well as an active family life. We both had obtained our DNPs doing classes and research together, so this new role was an area we agreed to work on together—finding ways to really help advance our careers and make a difference in our profession. Since these are early days for the NP/DNP, peer mentoring might be more accessible, and we suggest others consider that as an option. —Julie Stewart (deceased)

Seminar Discussion Questions

1. How does a preceptor differ from a mentor?
2. Write down three professional or career objectives or goals that you want to work on.
3. Identify one or two people you consider as possible mentors to help reach those goals.
4. How will you discuss forming a mentor relationship with the person you think best suited to your goals and personality?
5. What lifelong learning activities aside from your formal education do you already engage in and what drives you to do this?

References

American Academy of Nurse Practitioners. (2006). *Mentoring assessment*. Retrieved from http://www.aanp.org

American Academy of Nurse Practitioners. (2021). FAANP Career Enrichment Program: Preparing the Next Generation of Nurse Practitioner (NP) Leaders https://www.aanp.org/membership/fellows-program/fellows-workgroup-products-and-initiatives/faanp-career-enrichment-program

Beauvais, A. (2021). *Entering the job market and promoting your future success*, Chapter 31, in DeNisco, S. (2021) *Advanced practice nursing: Essential knowledge for the profession* (4th ed.). Burlington, MA: Jones & Bartlett Learning.

Bell, C. (2002). *Managers as mentors: Building partnerships for learning*. San Francisco, CA: Berrett Koehler.

Brainard, S., Harkus, D., & George, M. (1998). *A curriculum for training mentors and mentees: Guide for administration*. Seattle, WA: The Center for Workforce Development. Retrieved from http://www.grad.washington.edu/mentoring/students/worksheet5.pdf

Brown, M., & Olshansky, E. F. (1997). From limbo to legitimacy: A theoretical model of the transition to the primary care nurse practitioner role. *Nursing Research, 46*(1), 46–51.

Carey, S., & Campbell, S. (1994). Preceptor, mentor and sponsor roles: Creative strategies for nurse retention. *Journal of Nursing Administration, 24*(12), 39–48.

Chitty, K., & Black, B. (2011). *Professional nursing: Concepts and challenges*. Maryland Heights, MO: Saunders.

DeNisco, S. (2021). *Advanced practice nursing: Essential knowledge for the profession* (4th ed.). Burlington, MA: Jones & Bartlett Learning.

Doerksen, K. (2010). What are the professional and mentorship needs of advanced practice nurses? *Journal of Professional Nursing, 26*(3), 141–151.

Dyer, L. (2008). The continuing need for mentors in nursing. *Journal for Nurses in Staff Development, 24*(2), 86–90.

Flinter, M. (2005). Residency programs for primary care nurse practitioners in federally qualified health centers: A service perspective. *Online Journal of Issues in Nursing, 10*(3). doi:10.3912/OJIN.Vol10No03Man05

Grindell, C. (2003). Mentoring managers. *Nephrology Nursing Journal, 30*(5), 517–522.

Grossman S. (2013). *Mentoring in nursing: A dynamic and collaborative process* (2nd ed.). New York, NY: Springer.

Hanson, D. (2012). Interview with nurse practitioner wellness coaches. *WebNPOnline*. Retrieved from http://www.webnponline.com/articles/article_details/interview-with-nurse-practitioner-wellness-coaches/

Harrington, S. (2011). Mentoring new nurse practitioners to accelerate their development as primary care providers: A literature review. *Journal of the American Academy of Nurse Practitioners, 23*(4), 168–174.

Hayes, E. (1998). Mentoring and self-efficacy for advanced practice: A philosophical approach for nurse practitioner preceptors. *Journal of the American Academy of Nurse Practitioners, 10*(2), 1–5.

Kram, K. (1986). Mentoring in the workplace. In D. Hall (Ed.), *Career development in organizations*. San Francisco, CA: Jossey-Bass.

Kram, K. E. (1983). Phases of the mentor relationship. *The Academy of Management Journal, 26*(4), 608–625.

Link, D. (2009). The teaching-coaching role of the APN. *Journal of Perinatal and Neonatal Nursing, 23*(3), 279–283.

National Organization of Nurse Practitioner Faculties. (2017). *Nurse practitioner core competencies content*. Washington, DC: Author. Retrieved from https://cdn.ymaws.com/www.nonpf.org/resource/resmgr/competencies/2017_NPCoreComps_with_Curric.pdf

Neal, T. I. (2008). *Mentoring, self-efficacy, and nurse practitioner students: A modified replication*. Doctoral dissertation, Ball State University, Muncie, IN. Retrieved from Cumulative Index to Nursing and Allied Health Literature, 2010757741.

Tracy, B. (2012). *Earn what you're really worth: Maximize your income in any market at any time*. New York, NY: Vanguard Press.

Zbrog, M. (2021). *Guide to nurse practitioner fellowships & residencies*. Retrieved from https://www.npschools.com/blog/top-np-fellowships-and-residencies

Zwilling, M. (2012). How to make a business mentoring relationship work. *Forbes Online*. Retrieved from http://www.forbes.com/sites/martinzwilling/2012/03/20/effective-business-mentoring-is-a-relationship

CHAPTER 17

Reimbursement for Nurse Practitioner Services

Lynn Rapsilber

Introduction

Greater availability of primary and preventative healthcare services has been tied to cost savings and improved patient care outcomes. Nurse practitioners (NPs) have been shown to provide cost-effective care compared to their physician colleagues; therefore, reimbursement for healthcare services is the fiscal responsibility of every nurse practitioner. The 1997 Balanced Budget Act authorized specialists to bill directly for their professional services and be reimbursed at 85% of the physician rate for services provided to a patient (Department of Health and Human Services [DHHS], 2007). The rise in healthcare costs and the inability for the nursing profession to show cost savings has been an obstacle to obtaining direct payment for services (Stanley, 2010). The majority of patients, unless uninsured, will have a third-party insurance participant involved in setting fee schedules and reimbursement criteria.

    Understanding proper medical record documentation and billing procedures for an office visit can maximize reimbursement for services affecting both the practice and the nurse practitioner's bottom line. This chapter will inform the nurse practitioner of the tools for reimbursement and how to use the key components of evaluation and management to select the most appropriate code for the service provided based upon medical decision making or time and recognize audit triggers. Lastly, "incident to" billing will be reviewed so the nurse practitioner will be able to identify and protect him- or herself from unintentional fraudulent billing and legal issues, as the NP is accountable for all the services billed by a practice.

Important Steps in Reimbursement Eligibility

Nurse practitioners have been providing safe, cost-effective, quality health care for years and graduate with the competencies needed to provide excellent patient care at the point of service. While NPs are making strides in understanding the business of health care, they still lack the reimbursement knowledge and skills needed to be key players in the healthcare arena. Aside from the educational, board certification, and licensure requirements, the nurse practitioner must obtain several other identifiers to be eligible for reimbursement by a third-party payor. Obtaining a national provider number and employer number, and being credentialed by private and public insurers, will be described in the following sections.

National Provider Number

Nurse practitioners, physician assistants, and physicians can be reimbursed for the provision of healthcare services. For a nurse practitioner to be eligible for reimbursement, he or she must hold a minimum of a master's degree in nursing and successfully pass the national certification exam given by the American Association of Nurse Practitioners (AANP) or the American Nurses Credentialing Center (ANCC). The Health Insurance Portability and Accountability Act of 1996 (HIPAA) mandated the adoption of a standard unique identifier for healthcare providers. In 2004, the Centers for Medicare and Medicaid Services (CMS) adopted the national provider number as the standard unique identifier number for all healthcare providers to use when filing and processing healthcare claims (Stanley, 2010). All NPs are required to apply for a national provider number and be assigned only one number that will follow the NP wherever he or she practices. The application must be completed by the nurse practitioner to avoid any potential error that could delay billing and reimbursement National Plan and Provider Enumeration System. (2021).

Employer Provider Number

Whether employed by a practice or as a practice owner, a unique provider number will be assigned, reflecting where the services will be provided to a patient. If the medical practice has two office locations, there will be a different provider number for both practice settings. Before billing a third-party payor, whether Medicare, Medicaid, or private insurer, the patient service must have the national provider number of who provided the service and the provider number where the service occurred in order to bill.

Third-Party Credentialing

Lastly, the nurse practitioner must receive credentialing by the third-party payor in order to bill insurance companies for his or her services. While this is usually completed by the practice manager, the nurse practitioner should become familiar with the rules and policies of the third-party payor. A provider application form is filled out, which is also known as the "credentialing form." The nurse practitioner will be required to complete an attestation form to verify that the information submitted is correct. The nurse practitioner must make sure the information is correct. Any errors may delay the application process or compromise timely reimbursement. Once the nurse practitioner has obtained a national provider number, employer provider number, and third-party credentialing or insurance company membership, he or she is ready to begin billing for services.

Practice Authority

The nurse practitioner practice authority is determined by the state. The level of practice authority is defined by the American Association of Nurse Practitioners as full, reduced, or restricted practice, as determined by the ability to assess, diagnose, treat, and prescribe. Reduced practice authority requires a collaborative agreement with an outside "like-minded" healthcare discipline to provide patient care. Some states allow a physician or a nurse practitioner to be a collaborator. Restricted practice requires supervision, delegation, or team management by an outside health discipline in order for the nurse practitioner to provide patient care. Consult the AANP website (www.aanp.org) for the latest state practice map.

Coding and Billing Resources

Before billing for services rendered, the nurse practitioner needs to identify appropriate diagnoses for the patient, the type of patient encounter (for example, new or established visit), and what procedures were performed during the patient encounter. Other reportable, billable services would include medications administered, if any, and what supplies were used to provide care. Lastly, the nurse practitioner must provide clear and accurate documentation validating the reported diagnoses and procedural codes reported for billing purposes. An understanding of medical coding and resources to support these activities are the responsibility of the nurse practitioner.

Definition of Medical Coding

Medical coding is best defined as the translation of the original medical record documentation regarding patient diagnoses and procedures into a series of code numbers that describe the information in a standard manner. Coded medical information is used for patient care, research, reimbursement, and evaluation of services (Aalseth, 2006). International Classification of Diseases (ICD) codes, developed by the World Health Organization, are used to identify the patient's diagnoses or reasons for seeking care. These codes cover specific illnesses or diseases, as well as signs and symptoms resulting in the patient encounter (Centers for Disease Control and Prevention [CDC], 2021). ICD codes are also useful for classifying morbidity and mortality data from inpatient and outpatient records and most National Center for Health Statistics (NCHS) surveys.

Another component of medical billing is the *Current Procedural Terminology* (CPT), which describes the services and/or procedures for which reimbursement is sought. The American Medical Association publishes the CPT. This publication was initiated in 1966 as a way of standardizing terms for medical procedures used for documentation purposes (Phillipsen, 2008). CPT codes are used for specific types of patient encounters, innumerable procedures, and diagnostic studies that will be described in more detail later in this chapter Contexo Media. (2015).

The CPT and ICD-10 Books

There are several resources the nurse practitioner needs to be aware of regarding medical coding and billing for services. As previously mentioned, one such publication is the CPT. This book is updated annually providing coding additions and deletions. Only nurse practitioners, physician assistants, and physicians can use these codes. CPT reflects "what was done," such as types of visits, consultations, referrals, procedures, diagnostic studies, and treatment regimens. Obtaining a copy of the current CPT is very important, as the information presented in this chapter is found in the beginning sections of the book, and 2021 saw significant changes to new and established patient codes for office and outpatient services. An abridged version of the CPT changes is published annually (AMA, 2021).

Another necessary reference book is the *International Classification of Diseases, Tenth Edition*, or ICD-10. This reflects "why it was done." This book classifies diseases, symptoms, injuries, and accidents with numeric codes. The NP must select a code for the disease or symptom by "what you know," being as specific as possible. If you have not yet determined or confirmed the patient's diagnosis, you should list or code for the presenting symptoms. For example, if the patient has "heartburn" and you have not completed your evaluation, do not choose the ICD-10 code for gastroesophageal reflux with esophagitis (K 21.0). Instead, designate heartburn as the diagnostic code (R 12.0) until you have results of an endoscopic testing.

The ICD-10 classification system is widely used in Europe and was adapted in the United States on October 1, 2015 (National Center for Health Statistics, 2012).

Medical Necessity

When you have the "what was done" with the "why it was done," this equals medical necessity: CPT + ICD-10 = medical necessity. Medical necessity is defined as medical items and services that are "reasonable and necessary" for a variety of purposes. By statute, Medicare may only pay for items and services that are "reasonable and necessary for the diagnosis or treatment of illness or injury or to improve the functioning of a malformed body member," unless there is another statutory authorization for payment. Determination of medical necessity involves comparing the procedure being billed to the diagnosis being submitted. Determining medical necessity does not necessarily guarantee payment. If the NP receives a denial notification from the payor for a particular procedure, it means the payor does not think the procedure was justified for the diagnosis given (Aalseth, 2006).

There is an additional resource called the *Healthcare Common Procedure Coding System*, or HCPCS ("hicks-picks"). For Medicare and other health insurance programs to ensure that healthcare claims are processed in an orderly and consistent manner, standardized coding systems are essential. The HCPCS Level II code set is one of the standard code sets used by medical coders and billers for services such as medical supplies, durable medical goods, non-physician services, and services not represented in the Level I code set determined by the CPT (e.g., ambulance, prosthetics, orthotics) (American Association of Professional Coders [AAPC], 2021). With the utilization of the electronic health record, all these codes are recorded and the information is submitted electronically to the insurance payer for reimbursement (**Exhibit 17-1**).

Medical Record Documentation

The medical record is the most important document in the reimbursement process. Any information provided to the patient on a particular date of service must be recorded in the record. **If it was not documented, it was not done.** The medical

Exhibit 17-1 Sample Encounter Form

Date of service:	Insurance:	Account #:
Patient name:	Subscriber name:	Provider name:
Address:	Group #:	Provider signature:
Phone:	Copay:	
DOB:	Age:	Sex:

Procedure Codes

Labs	CPT	Office Procedures	CPT	Immunizations and Injections	CPT	Office Visit	CPT New	CPT Est
Blood draw	36415	Anoscopy	46600	Allergen, one	95115	Minimal		99211
CT/DNA probe	87490	Audiometry	92551	Allergen, multiple	95117	Problem focused		
GC/DNA probe	87590	Cerumen removal	69210	Imm admin, one	90471	Expanded problem focused		
Glucose	82948	Colposcopy	57452	Imm admin, each add'l	90472	Detailed		
Hem occult	82270	Colposcopy w/biopsy	57455	Imm admin, intranasal, one	90473	Comprehensive		

(continues)

Exhibit 17-1 Sample Encounter Form

Labs	CPT	Office Procedures	CPT	Immunizations and Injections	CPT	Office Visit	CPT New	CPT Est
HGB	83068	ECG, w/interpretation	93000	Imm admin, intranasal, each add'l	90474	Comprehensive (new pt.)		
KDH prep	87220	ECG, rhythm strip	93040	Injection, joint, small	20600	Significant, separate service		
Pap smear	88150	Endometrial biopsy	58100	Injection, joint, intermediate	20605	**Well Visit**	**New**	**Est**
Sed rate	85651	Flexible sigmoidoscopy	45330	Injection, joint, major	20610	< 1 y	99381	99391
Strep screen	86403	Flexible sigmoidoscopy w/biopsy	45331	Injection, ther/proph/ diag	90772	1–4 y	99382	99392
Urinalysis (dipstick)	81005	Fracture care, cast/splint Site: _____	29___	Injection, trigger point	20552	5–11 y	99383	99393
Urine pregnancy test	81025	Nebulizer	94640	**Vaccines**	**CPT**	12–17 y	99384	99394
Wet mount	87210	Nebulizer demo	94664	DT, < 7 y	90702	18–39 y	99385	99395

(continued)

Medical Record Documentation

Dressings	CPT							
Ace wrap/elastic		Spirometry	94010	DTP	90701	40–64 y	99386	99396
Bandage (amt ___)	A4460	Spirometry pre & post	94060	DTaP, < 7 y	90700	65 y +	99387	99397
		Tympanometry	92567	Flu, 6–35 mos	90657	**Medicare Preventive Services**		**CPT**
Casting tape	A4590	Vasectomy	55250	Flu, 3 y +	90658	Pap		Q0091
Foam dressing	A6209	**Skin Procedures**	**CPT**	Hep A, adult	90632	Pelvic & breast		G0101
Irrigation solution	A4323	Burn care, initial	16000	Hep A, ped/adol, 2 dose	90633	Prostate/PSA		G0103
Nonsterile gauze	A6216	Foreign body, skin, simple	10120	Hep B, adult	90746	Tobacco counseling/3–10 min		99406
Skin sealants	A6250	Foreign body, skin, complex		Hep B, ped/adol, 3 dose	90744	Tobacco counseling/> 10 min		99407
Tapes (all types)	A6265	I&D, abscess		Hep B-Hib	90748	Welcome to Medicare exam		G0344
Other Services	**CPT**	I&D, hematoma/seroma		Hib, 4 dose	90645	ECG w/Welcome to Medicare exam		G0366
After posted hours	99050	Laceration repair, simple Site: ___ Size: ___		HPV	90649	Flexible sigmoidoscopy		G0104

(continues)

Exhibit 17-1 Sample Encounter Form

Labs	CPT	Office Procedures	CPT	Immunizations and Injections	CPT	Office Visit	CPT New	CPT Est
Evening/weekend appointment	99051	Laceration repair, layered Site: ___ Size: ___		IPV	90713	Hemoccult, guaiac		G0107
Home health certification	G0180	Lesion, biopsy, one		MMR	90707	Flu shot		G0008
Home health recertification	G0179	Lesion, biopsy, each add'l		Pneumonia, > 2 y	90732	Pneumonia shot		G0009
Post-op follow-up	99024	Lesion, destruct., benign, 1–14		Pneumonia conjugate, < 5 y	90669	**Consultation/ Pre-op Clearance**		**CPT**
Prolonged/30–74 min	99354	Lesion, destruct., premal, single		Td, > 7 y	90718	Expanded problem focused		99242
Special reports/ forms	99080	Lesion, destruct., premal, each add'l		Varicella	90716	Detailed		99243
Disability/work-ers' comp	99455	Lesion, excision, benign Site: ___ Size: ___		**Misc. Procedures**	**CPT**	Comprehensive/mod complexity		99244

(continued)

Miscellaneous	CPT			Pulse oximetry	94762	Comprehensive/high complexity			99245
		Lesion, excision, malig. Site: ____ Size: ____							CPT
		Lesion, paring/cutting, one		Vision test	92583	**Radiology**			
		Lesion, paring/cutting, 2–4		O^2 treatment	94760				
		Lesion, shave Site: ____ Size: ____		Burn treatment	16020	**Diagnoses**			
		Nail removal, partial		Cast removal	29705				
		Nail removal, w/matrix		Peak flow	94735			1	
		Skin tag, 1–15		EKG				2	
		Current	30 Days	60 Days	90 Days	120+ Days			Total
Pt. balance									
Ins. balance									

> **CMS medical record documentation criteria**
> - The medical record should be complete and legible
> - Reason for the encounter and relevant history, physical examination findings, and prior diagnostic test results
> - Assessment, clinical impression, or diagnosis
> - Plan for care
> - If not documented, the rationale for ordering diagnostic and other ancillary services should be easily inferred
> - Past and present diagnoses should be accessible to the treating and/or consulting physician
> - Appropriate health risk factors should be identified
> - The patient's progress, response to and changes in treatment, and revision of diagnosis should be documented
> - The CPT and ICD-10 codes reported on the health insurance claim form or billing statement should be supported by the documentation in the medical record

Figure 17-1 CMS Medical Record Documentation Criteria.

record clearly should state what was done and why it was done. CMS has specific documentation criteria. The medical record should be complete and legible. It should include a chief complaint, why the patient presents to the office or management of chronic disease(s), relevant history, assessment, physical exam, diagnostic testing, and treatment plan. It must be signed by the provider of record (the one who performed the service). Rationale for testing must be apparent. Health risks must be identified. Responses to treatment and follow-up must be clear. CPT and ICD-10 must be supported in the documentation. The data must be sequential. If something is inadvertently omitted from a previous date of service (DOS), it can be entered using today's date and stated as an "addenda to DOS on date" and added as the omitted information. If something is erroneously entered, an addendum to the health record is made detailing the reason for the error and the correction. CMS recognizes the electronic health record should not replace the need for good documentation by the nurse practitioner. A summary of CMS documentation criteria is represented in **Figure 17-1**.

Payment for Services

The current system for reimbursement is based upon the resource-based relative value scale (RBRVS). This system replaced the fee for service. The system was developed based upon data acquired by Dr. Hsaio and a multidisciplinary team of researchers from Harvard University in 1988 (Goodson, 2007). Three separate factors were used to calculate physician value: (1) work effort (52%), (2) practice expense (44%), and (3) malpractice expense (4%). Provider work effort is defined by a relative value unit (see **Box 17-1**). The Geographic Practice Cost Index (GPCI) refers to the cost of service applied to geographic locations within the country. In New York and California, it costs more to deliver care than in Tennessee or Mississippi.

> **Box 17-1** Resource-Based Relative Value Scale (RBRVS)
>
> **Converting an RBRVS to a Dollar Amount**
> (Work RVU × Work GPCI) + (Practice Expense RVU × Practice Expense GPCI) + (Malpractice RVU × Malpractice GPCI) × Conversion Factor × Practitioner Payment Rate = Allowed Amount
>
> RVU = relative value unit
>
> GPCI = geographic practice cost indices

The conversion factor is the variable that changes from year to year. Medicare reimburses the nurse practitioner at 85% of the physician rate. Other insurance payors' reimbursement fees can and should be negotiated.

Evaluation and Management Documentation Guidelines

Evaluation and management documentation guidelines are the foundation of fiscal responsibility and were developed by the American Medical Association and the Health Care Financing Administration (HCFA) (Aalseth, 2006), which is now the Centers for Medicare and Medicaid Services (CMS). Understanding this system will ensure proper coding of visits and maximize reimbursement; these guidelines are used by Medicare and other third-party payors when making reimbursement decisions. There are three key components to evaluation and management documentation: (1) history, (2) examination, and (3) medical decision making or time. These variables get broken down into their own set of levels. This will be discussed further in the key components section of this chapter.

Additionally, the NP needs to identify who is a new patient versus an established patient. A new patient is defined as an individual new to the practice (seeing any provider in the practice for the first time) or has not been seen in 3 years. The new patient can also be a hospital patient who is being referred for care and not previously seen by any provider in the practice. An established patient is one who has an ongoing relationship with a practice. The hospital patient can be an established patient if a provider from the practice has seen the patient in the hospital and is returning for a follow-up visit. Contained within the CPT book is a decision tree that helps a provider identify the difference. A specialty provider for this discussion will be defined as a healthcare provider and as part of a group and is considered a specialist; the provider must have received special training and be board certified in that specialty.

General Coding Guidelines

The next step is to know which ICD-10 codes you will use to bill for the office visit. Coding takes the words the NP used as the diagnosis or symptom and converts them into a category code. Codes for valid diagnoses may have seven digits. Codes that describe symptoms as opposed to diagnoses are acceptable if the NP has not yet established a diagnosis responsible for the symptomatology of the patient.

Structure of the ICD-10 Diagnoses Codes

The diagnosis system is contained in three volumes: Tabular List, Instruction Manual, and Alphabetical Index accounting for 64,000 codes.

1. Tabular List: Diseases and health-related problems containing 22 chapters. Within each of these chapters are categories logically sequenced by body system, site, or etiology. Combination codes are available for certain diseases. The use of "other" NOS (not otherwise specified) or NEC (not elsewhere classified) codes are no longer permitted in ICD-10.
2. Instruction Manual provides data for morbidity (hospital statistics) and mortality (causes of death).
3. The Alphabetical Index contains diseases and nature of injury, external causes of injury, and a table of drugs and chemicals.

Submission electronically allows an unlimited number of diagnostic codes to be used, each is linked to a CPT or procedural code. A word of caution: Use only the codes you intend to do something about or that have a correlation to the patient's treatment plan, which is more specifically defined in the 2021 coding changes for new and established patients in office or outpatient locations, otherwise it can trigger an audit.

Structure of the CPT Procedure Codes

CPT codes are categorized into six main sections with five numbers representing a service:

1. Anesthesia (00100–01999)
2. Surgery (10021–69990)
3. Radiology (70010–79999)
4. Pathology and Laboratory (80300–8939)
5. Medicine (90281–99607)
6. Evaluation and Management (99201–99499)

The categories of the codes do not mean that a primary care provider cannot use a code in the surgery section. For example, CPT code 10060—Incision and Drainage of Abscess (cutaneous or subcutaneous abscess, cyst, or paronychia)—may be used by the NP in the outpatient setting. The categorization of the codes is set up for the expediency of the provider, and billing personnel may also use the index to look up specific items.

Location of Patient Encounter

Know where your feet are planted and that specific patient encounter locations will result in a different code for billing purposes. If the NP is in the office, the following CPT codes will be used: (1) new patient codes 99202–99205, and (2) established patient codes 99211–99215. Care may be provided in the inpatient or outpatient settings, or in the home or extended care facility. See **Box 17-2** for codes corresponding to the geographic location of care. Consult the CPT book for specific criteria for each code.

Box 17-2 Geographic Location of Care

Common Codes
Office or outpatient
New patient: 99201, 99202, 99203, 99204, 99205
Established patient: 99211, 99212, 99213, 99214, 99215
Hospital inpatient
Initial: 99221, 99222, 99223
Subsequent: 99231, 99232, 99233
Discharge: 99238, 99239
Nursing facility
Comprehensive assessment: 99301, 99302, 99303
Subsequent: 99311, 99312, 99313
Discharge: 99315, 99316
Home services
New patient: 99341, 99342, 99343, 99344, 99345
Established: 99347, 99348, 99349, 99350

Used with author permission.

Breaking News: Significant Changes to Outpatient and Office Visits

The most significant changes to evaluation and management in over 30 years have occurred for 2021. This was a project undertaken by CMS to put patients first and reduce unnecessary burdens, increase efficiencies, and improve the patient experience Centers for Medicare and Medicaid (2020). Listening sessions occurred with providers who offered suggestions on ways to reduce provider burden and streamline documentation. As a result, medical record documentation of history and physical examination can be entered into the medical record by the students, as long as the documentation is reviewed and verified (signed and dated) by the billing provider (NP).

Levels of Patient Encounter

The NP will bill for level of office visit based upon the amount of work involved with medical decision making or time. There is an expected level of history and physical examination appropriate for the visit. However, this is no longer factored into the level of service billed (CPT, 2021). There are five levels of codes to bill for new and established office patients. The level 1 visit code for an established patient is for a nurse visit and is not listed in the discussion. Level 1 visit code for a new patient was deleted for 2021. Problem focused is a level 2. Expanded problem focused is a level 3. Detailed is a level 4. Comprehensive is a level 5.

Key Components of Reimbursement

Medical decision making or time are the key components determining reimbursement for the patient encounter. There should be an appropriate level of history and physical exam; however, this does not factor into the level of billable for the visit.

The History and Reimbursement Decisions

The history is a component of the reimbursement process. With the new changes for 2021, history can be obtained by ancillary staff under the supervision of the NP (https://www.ama-assn.org/practice-management/medicare/ancillary-staff-who-can-document-components-em-services). There are four components of the history:

1. The chief complaint: what brought the patient to the office that day. It can also include chronic disease management and follow-up care.
2. History of present illness (HPI). This includes location, quality, severity and timing, context, modifying factors, and associated signs and symptoms.
3. The review of systems (ROS) is performed, which is conducted systematically to gather information, including constitutional signs such as weight loss and overall condition: ears, eyes, nose, mouth, throat, respiratory, cardiovascular, gastrointestinal, genitourinary, musculoskeletal, skin, neurological, psychiatric, hematologic and lymphatic, and immune and allergy.
4. Past family and social history (PFSH) is considered. Past medical history includes illnesses, surgeries, injuries, treatments, and current medications. Family history includes hereditary diseases that increase the patient's risk factors for those conditions. Social history should include military service. The components of history are documented in the medical record. For billing purposes, the level of history must be medically appropriate.

Services Provided Other Than Office or Outpatient Visits

If the NP is using other evaluation and management services such as hospital observation, hospital inpatient, consultations, emergency department, nursing home, domiciliary, rest home custodial care, home, then the level of history is a key component in reimbursement.

Problem focused is a level 2, which includes only a brief HPI. Expanded problem focused is a level 3, which includes a brief HPI, and problem focused ROS but no PFSH is done. Detailed visits are coded at level 4, which includes an extensive HPI, ROS, and pertinent PFSH. Comprehensive visits are coded at level 5 and include comprehensive histories, extended HPI, extended ROS, complete ROS, and complete PFHS (see **Table 17-1**).

The Physical Examination and Reimbursement Decisions

The next component is the physical examination. For the 2021 changes, the physical examination must be medically appropriate for the patient encounter. If the service is other than office or outpatient, the level of physical examination is factored into the reimbursement.

There are four levels of physical examination:

- Level 2 problem focused (brief or perform and document one to five elements identified by a bullet)

Key Components of Reimbursement

Table 17-1 Components of History

History of Present Illness (HPI)	Review of Systems (ROS)	Past, Family, and/or Social History (PFSH)	Type of History (number equals level of history)
Brief	n/a	n/a	Problem focused (2)
Brief	Problem pertinent	n/a	Expanded problem focused (3)
Extended	Extended	Pertinent	Detailed (4)
Extended	Complete	Complete	Comprehensive (5)

Used with author permission.

- Level 3 expanded problem (focused and brief or perform and document at least six elements identified by a bullet)
- Level 4 detailed (perform and document at least two elements identified by a bullet from six areas/systems or at least 12 elements identified by a bullet in two or more areas/systems)
- Level 5 comprehensive (perform all elements identified by a bullet and document at least two elements identified by a bullet from nine areas/systems)

There are specific documentation guidelines created by the American Medical Association and CMS. There are two sets of documentation guidelines: those published in 1995 and those published in 1997. The 1995 guidelines are body system focused, and the 1997 is system area focused (Medicare Learning Network, 2010).

The documentation guidelines determine the level of physical exam to be performed. There is a general multisystem examination and several specialty examination options. The specialty examinations include cardiology; hematology/oncology; musculoskeletal; neurology; ear, nose, and throat; genitourinary; psychiatry; respiratory; and skin. The NP should select the examination appropriate for the patient population. **Table 17-2** lists the differences between the 1995 and 1997 guidelines for physical examination.

If the provider documents an abnormal finding, an accompanying explanation is required. Normal and negative examination results must be listed by organ or body system. Subjective results without any documentation cannot be counted.

Medical Decision Making and Reimbursement

Medical decision making (MDM) is the last key component. It takes into account the diagnosis, the information required to make the diagnosis, and risks and complications associated with the diagnosis. This is where the NP obtains credit for the decision regarding diagnosing and treatment options. The evaluation and management documentation guidelines describe four levels of medical decision making:

- Level 2 straightforward
- Level 3 low complexity
- Level 4 moderate complexity
- Level 5 high complexity

Table 17-2 Documentation Guidelines for Physical Examinations

Exam Description	1995 Guidelines	1997 Guidelines	Type of Exam
Limited to affected body area of organ system	1 body area or organ system	1, 2, 3, 4, 5 bulleted items	Problem focused (2)
Affected body area/organ system and other symptomatic or related organ system	2, 3, 4, 5, 6, 7 body areas or organ systems	6, 7, 8, 9, 10, 11, or more bulleted areas	Expanded problem focused (3)
Extended exam of affected area/organ system and other related symptomatic or related organ systems	2, 3, 4, 5, 6, 7 body areas or organ systems	12, 13, 14, 15, 16, 17, or more for 2 or more systems	Detailed (4)
General multisystem	≥ 8 body areas or organ systems	18 or more for 9 or more systems	Comprehensive (5)
Complete single organ system	n/a	See the specific criteria for each	Comprehensive (5)

Used with author permission.

Factors such as number of diagnoses, comorbid conditions, data to be reviewed, number of management options, and risk of morbidity and mortality are considered in the level of medical decision making selected. The more risk involved in the patient's care, the greater the level of medical decision making. **Table 17-3** details what is included in a minimal, low, moderate, and high complexity level if services are other than office and outpatient.

Medical Decision Making for Office and Outpatient, 2021

Significant changes are made to medical decision making for office and outpatient services. The codes for new and established patients are treated the same for each level. The level of MDM is based upon two out of three elements of MDM: number and complexity of problems addressed, amount and/or complexity of data to be reviewed and analyzed, and risk of complication and/or morbidity or mortality of patient management. There are several new additions to the risk which can benefit the NP when considering a level of code. Social determinants of health are listed under moderate level. NPs often assess these when evaluating a patient and now there is a way to quantify for reimbursement. There are new terms the NP must be familiar with. Unique source: defined as a physician, NP, or other healthcare professional in a specialty or other entity. An example of a unique entity would be a PCP when a specialist is seeing the patient. Unique test: defined by a CPT code set. For example, a CBC with differential or complete metabolic profile has a CPT code and would be counted as one unique test. See **Table 17-4**.

Table 17-3 Risks Associated with Complexity Level of Visit

Level of Risk	Presenting Problem	Diagnostic Procedures Ordered	Management Options Selected
Minimal	One self-limited or minor problem (e.g., rash or oral ulcers, cold, insect bites)	Lab tests requiring venipuncture Chest X-rays EKG/ECG UA Ultrasound	Rest Splints Superficial dressings
Low	Two or more self-limited or minor problems or symptoms One stable chronic illness (e.g., well-controlled HTN or NIDDM, BPH) Acute uncomplicated illness (e.g., cystitis, allergic rhinitis, simple sprain)	MRI/CT, PFTs Superficial needle biopsies Clinical lab test requiring arterial puncture Skin biopsies	OTC drugs Minor surgery with no identified risk factors PT/OT IV fluids without additives
Moderate	One or more chronic illnesses with mild exacerbation, progression, or side effect of treatment Acute illness systemic symptoms (e.g., pyelonephritis, pneumonitis) Two or more stable chronic illnesses Acute complicated injury (e.g., vertebral compression fracture, head injury with brief LOC) Undiagnosed new problem with uncertain prognosis (e.g., lump in breast)	Diagnostic endoscopies with no identified risk factors Cardiovascular imaging studies with contrast, no risk factors (e.g., arteriogram) Arthrocentesis, LP Physiologic tests under stress test (e.g., cardiac stress test) Deep needle or incisional biopsy	Prescription drug management Minor surgery with identified risk factors IV fluids with additives Therapeutic nuclear medicine Elective major surgery (open, percutaneous, or endoscopic) with no identified risk factors Closed treatment of fracture or dislocation without manipulation

(continues)

Table 17-3 Risks Associated with Complexity Level of Visit *(continued)*

Level of Risk	Presenting Problem	Diagnostic Procedures Ordered	Management Options Selected
High	One or more chronic illnesses with severe exacerbation, progression, or side effects of treatment Acute or chronic illness that may pose a threat to life or bodily function (e.g., progressive severe RA, multiple trauma, acute myeloid leukemia, PE, severe respiratory distress, psych illness with threat to self or others, acute renal failure) An abrupt change in neurological status (e.g., seizure, TIA, weakness, or sensory loss)	Cardiac EP tests Cardiovascular imaging studies with contrast, with identified risk factors Diagnostic endoscopies with identified risk factors Discography	Elective major surgery with risk factors Emergency major surgery Administration of parenteral controlled substances Drug therapy requiring intensive monitoring for toxicity Decision not to resuscitate or to de-escalate care because of poor prognosis

Complexity of MDM Services Not Office or Outpatient

Number of Diagnoses or Management Options	Amount and/or Complexity of Data to Be Reviewed	Risks of Complications and/or Morbidity or Mortality	Type of MDM
Minimal	Minimal or None	Minimal	Straightforward
Limited	Limited	Low	Low Complexity
Multiple	Moderate	Moderate	Moderate Complexity
Extensive	Extensive	High	High Complexity
Number of Diagnoses or Management Options	Amount and/or Complexity of Data to Be Reviewed	Risks of Complications and/or Morbidity or Mortality	Type of MDM

BPN = benign prostatic hyperplasia; CT = computed tomography; EKG/ECG = electrocardiography; EP = electrophysiology; HTN = hypertension; IV = intravenous; LOC = loss of consciousness; LP = lumbar puncture; MRI = magnetic resonance imaging; NIDDM = noninsulin-dependent diabetes mellitus; OT = occupational therapy; OTC = over the counter; PE = pulmonary embolism; PFT = pulmonary function test; PT = physical therapy; RA = rheumatoid arthritis; TIA = transient ischemic attack; UA = urinalysis

Key Components of Reimbursement **421**

Table 17-4 Documentation Grid for Patients

Code	Level of MDM (Based on 2 of 3 of the Elements of MDM)	PROBLEMS Number and Complexity of Problems Addressed	Number	Level
99202 99212	Straightforward	**Minimal** ■ 1 self-limiting or minor problem		
99203 99213	Low	**Low** ■ 2 or more self-limiting or minor problems or ■ 1 stable chronic illness or ■ 1 acute, uncomplicated illness or injury		
99204 99214	Moderate	**Moderate** ■ 1 or more chronic illnesses with exacerbation, progression, or side effects of treatment or ■ 2 or more stable chronic illnesses or ■ 1 undiagnosed new problem with uncertain prognosis or ■ 1 acute illness with systematic symptoms or ■ 1 acute complicated injury		
99205 99215	High	**High** ■ 1 or more chronic illnesses with severe exacerbation, progression or side effects of treatment or ■ 1 acute or chronic illness or injury that poses a threat to life or bodily injury		

(continues)

Table 17-4 Documentation Grid for Patients *(continued)*

Code	Level of MDM (Based upon 2 out of 3 Elements)	DATA		
		Amount and Complexity of Data to Be Reviewed and Analyzed	Patient Results	Level
99202 99212	Straightforward	Minimal or none		
99203 99213	Low	**Limited (must meet the requirement of at least 1 of the 2 categories)** **Category 1: Tests and documents (any combination of 2 of the following)** ■ Review of prior external note(s) for each unique source ■ Review of the result(s) of each unique source ■ Ordering of each unique test or **Category 2: Assessment requiring an independent historian(s)** (For the categories of independent interpretations of tests and discussion of management or test interpretation, see moderate or high)		
99204 99214	Moderate	**Moderate** (must meet the requirements of at least 1 out of 3 categories) **Category 1: Tests, documents, or independent historian(s)** Any combination of 3 from the following: ■ Review of prior external note(s) from a unique source ■ Review of the result(s) of each unique test* ■ Ordering a unique test* ■ Assessment requiring an independent historian(s) or		

99205 99215	High	**Category 2: Independent interpretation of tests**
- Independent interpretation of a test performed by another physician/other qualified HC professional (not separately reported) or

Category 3: Discussion of management or test interpretation
Discussion of management or test interpretation with external physician/other qualified HC professional/appropriate source (not separately reported)

Extensive (Must meet the requirements of at least 2 out of 3 categories)

Category 1: Tests, documents, or independent historian(s)
Any combination of 3 from the following:
- Review of prior external note(s) from each unique source*
- Review of the result(s) of each unique test*
- Ordering of each unique test*
- Assessment requiring an independent historian(s) or

Category 2: Independent interpretations of tests
- Independent interpretation of a test performed by other physicians/other qualified healthcare professional (not separately reported) or

Category 3: Discussion of management or test interpretation
Discussion of management or test interpretation with external physician/other qualified healthcare professional/appropriate source (not separately reported) |

(continues)

Table 17-4 Documentation Grid for Patients *(continued)*

Code	Level of MDM (Based on 2 of 3 of the Elements of MDM)	RISK — Risk of Complications and/or Morbidity or Mortality of Patient Management
99202 99212	Straightforward	Minimal risk of morbidity from additional diagnostic testing or treatment
99203 99213	Low	Low risk of morbidity from additional diagnostic testing or treatment
99204 99214	Moderate	Moderate risk of morbidity from additional diagnostic testing or treatment *Examples only:* ■ Prescription drug management ■ Decision regarding minor surgery with identified patient or procedure risk factors ■ Decision regarding elective major surgery without identified patient or procedure risk factors ■ Diagnosis or treatment significantly limited by social determinants of health
99205 99215	High	High risk of morbidity from additional diagnostic testing or treatment *Examples only:* ■ Drug therapy requiring intensive monitoring for toxicity ■ Decision regarding elective major surgery with identified patient or procedure risk factors ■ Decision regarding emergency major surgery ■ Decision regarding hospitalizations ■ Decision not to resuscitate or to de-escalate care because of poor prognosis

*Each unique test, order, or document contributes to the combination of 2 or combination of 3 in Category 1.
Data from 2019 American Medical Association. All rights reserved.

Coding by Time vs. MDM

The NP can opt to select coding by time instead of MDM. Time includes the total time for the patient visit on the date of service (DOS). This includes face to face and work before or after the visit. This is the time spent by the NP and does not include any work done by ancillary staff.

Activities include:

- Preparing to see the patient (review of tests, notes)
- Obtaining and/or reviewing separately obtained history
- Performing a medically necessary examination and/or evaluation
- Counseling and educating the patient/family/caregiver
- Ordering medication(s), tests(s), or procedure(s)
- Referring and communicating with other HCP (when not separately reported)
- Documenting clinical information in the EHR
- Independently interpreting results (not separately reported) and communicating results to the patient/family/caregiver
- Care coordination (not separately reported)

There are specific time elements associated with coding by time. **Table 17-5** details the codes and time associated with each.

How to Bill for a Visit

To bill for a visit, you must know what ICD-10 and CPT codes to use. In review, know where your feet are planted, and use the specific location codes for where the care is provided. Decide if the patient is a new or established patient. Perform a level of history, physical examination appropriate for the patient encounter. Then decide if you are using MDM or Time for Office and Outpatient visits. All other visits use the levels of history, physical examination, and MDM for the level of service provided.

Coding Conundrums

Some coding situations can be a challenge or a benefit if you know what they are and how to use them effectively. Evaluation and management plus procedure, modifiers, shared evaluation and management, and "incident to" are examples described

Table 17-5 Patient Codes and Associated Timeframes

New Patient Code	Time	Established Patient Code	Time
99202	15–29 minutes	99212	10–19 minutes
99203	30–44 minutes	99213	20–29 minutes
99204	45–59 minutes	99214	30–39 minutes
99205	60–75 minutes	99215	40–54 minutes

in greater detail. Understanding these situations can make a difference in revenue for the practice and help avoid legal pitfalls.

Evaluation and management plus a procedure occur when the same provider performs the evaluation and management plus the procedure on the same patient on the same day. For example, a diabetic patient comes into the office for a follow-up visit (evaluation and management) and asks about a warty growth on his or her shoulder. It is a seborrheic keratosis, and the NP performs cryosurgery (procedure) on the lesion. The nurse practitioner bills a 99214 for the diabetic visit and codes for the cryosurgery one lesion (17000). Because there is a duplication in work effort, there will be a modifier (25) placed on the office visit, and the value will be decreased but the procedure will be reimbursed at the highest rate. There needs to be separate documentation for each service provided. Be aware that a preventative visit and a same-day evaluation and management pose a problem. The patient has no copay associated with a preventative visit and will need to pay a copay for the evaluation and management part of the visit. This should be disclosed to the patient prior to the preventative visit.

Modifiers are a way to show the evaluation and management code has changed. The service or procedure is altered. Modifiers can increase or decrease a value. It can indicate bilateral or multiple procedures. It can also indicate additional work was performed in rendering the service. The two-digit modifier is always attached to the evaluation and management code. Most modifiers are used in the surgical arena.

Shared evaluation and management occur when the nurse practitioner sees a patient in the hospital and documents the visit in the medical record. Later, the physician sees the patient and further documents in the medical record. The visit from both providers can be billed as a shared visit and billed under the physician's national provider number. There must be clear, separate documentation in the patient medical record. It does not mean the physician has to cosign the nurse practitioner's note. This is used for hospital billing and reimbursement purposes. This is different than "incident to" billing.

"Incident to" billing has been used in the care of Medicare patients. The term "incident to" has been used by physicians to bill for various services provided in the office by healthcare personnel that are performed in "relation to" or "incident to" the care the physician provides (Rapsilber, 2019). In this situation, the nurse practitioner bills for her services with the physician's national provider number. The visit is reimbursed at 100%. This is problematic in that the NP is not visible in this method of billing and cannot show the income he or she is generating for the practice.

There are three major criteria that must be met by the practice before "incident to" billing can occur. The first criterion is that the nurse practitioner must be employed and directly supervised by the physician. This is problematic, for in most states, nurse practitioners either practice autonomously or in collaboration with a physician. This stipulation means the physician must be available onsite to provide consultation to the NP. The physician cannot be in the hospital, on vacation, or out of the office. It does not mean the physician has to see the patient, but the physician must be available for questions if the need arises. The second criterion for "incident to" billing to occur is that the physician must see the patient for the initial visit and develop the treatment plan. The nurse practitioner cannot see any new Medicare patients under the current guidelines. The last criterion is that the physician must

> **Box 17-3** Basic Components of a Compliance Plan
>
> Internal auditing system
> Policies and procedures specific to the practice
> Compliance officer in the practice to oversee and enforce the plan
> Education of all employees about the plan
> Prompt responses to any errors or offenses with corrective action
> Open communication
>
> Used with author permission.

have ongoing participation in the patient's care. The patient cannot have a new problem when they see the nurse practitioner. The physician cannot simply cosign the nurse practitioner's documentation in this situation but must actually see the patient and modify the treatment plan, or otherwise bill the service under the nurse practitioner's NPI number.

There are numerous problems with this type of billing for a nurse practitioner. The Office of Inspector General is looking at the use of "incident to" billing and checking to see the rules are being followed. Significant monetary penalties may be levied and there is the chance of potential removal as a Medicare provider for violation of the rules. In addition, there are considerations subjecting the practice to an audit. Audit triggers include billing noncovered services as covered, double billing, coding all visits at the same level, coding that does not meet medical necessity, "incident to" billing when the physician is not present in the office, waiving of copays, and documentation not supportive of the level billed. NPs should check their state nurse practice acts for reasons for loss of professional licensure such as false reports, willful misrepresentation, submitting false statements, or other unprofessional conduct (Phillipsen, 2008). **Box 17-3** shows basic components of a compliance plan that should be instituted in each practice setting.

Value-Based Reimbursement

There is a significant change to reimbursement with attention to quality (outcomes) versus quality (procedures). The Quality Payment Program (QPP) established by Medicare as part of the 2015 Medicare Access and CHIP Reauthorization Act (MACRA) seeks to improve quality of care to keep patients healthier. Federal Register (2015). Nurse practitioner participation is imperative. There are two ways one can enter this program: through MIPS (Merit-based Incentive Payment System) or APM (Advanced Alternative Payment Model). Both programs offer participants incentives for providing quality care. Failure to participate will result in a reduction in payments or penalty. Nurse practitioners who see greater than 200 Medicare patients and provide more than 200 Part B services and bill more than $90,000 in Part B services should participate. Participation can be checked by entering a National Provider Number (NPI) into the QPP data base. (Centers for Medicare and Medicaid. (2021). There is a timeline for participation. Participation occurs on a three-year cycle. Data is submitted in year one, and reviewed and analyzed in year two. In year three, payment adjustments in the form of an incentive (positive payment adjustment) or penalty (negative payment adjustment) will be rendered yielding. As the programs progresses, the adjustments will be more significant.

The nurse practitioner is responsible for what is billed during the patient encounter. The practice, physician, and billing staff is not. It is imperative the nurse practitioner understand the method to code and bill for a patient visit properly to avoid an audit and avoid fraudulent activity. With the changes to reimbursement under MACRA, reimbursement will be affected. Nurse practitioner care allows the opportunity for success in this program. Education and participation are crucial. It is fiscally prudent to have an understanding of this process.

Seminar Discussion Questions

Two case studies are presented. Read the following case studies and answer the questions that follow.

♀ CASE STUDY ONE

Jenna Ward is a 19-year-old female who presents to the clinic with a chief complaint of 2-day history of burning with urination and vaginal discharge. The discharge is foul smelling. She has tried OTC vaginal treatment without improvement. She has been sexually active with several partners. She is G1, P0, A1. She takes oral contraceptives and menses are regular. She denies any cramping, abdominal pain, or unusual vaginal bleeding. No fever or chills. No routine medications. NKDA.

Past Medical History: Appendectomy age 16
Family History: M 32 A&W F 33 IDDM, B 22 asthma
Smokes ½ PPD, denies alcohol or drug use
She is 5'4" in height and weighs 137 lbs. Her blood pressure is 120/62, P 76. NAD, afebrile, abdomen soft, +BS, tender in suprapubic area. GU: external genitalia WNL with thick white vaginal discharge noted. No bleeding noted, Cervix pink, no CMT, GC & Chlamydia cultures taken, wet mount obtained, PAP smear performed, bimanual examination WNL no adnexal masses or tenderness.
Labs: UA 20-30 WBCs per HPF/C&S sent, wet mount: + whiff test, + clue cells

1. What are the potential ICD-10 codes in this case?
2. How can the NP determine if this patient is a new patient versus an established patient at the clinic?
3. What components of care will be used for reimbursement decisions for Ms. Ward?
4. What type of physical examination level best fits what was performed on Ms. Ward?
5. If you were coding the visit for Ms. Ward, how would you determine what decision-making level you would choose? Provide your rationale, and be specific.

♀ CASE STUDY TWO

Robert Jones is a 45-year-old male who presents for diabetes. He has been struggling with blood sugar control. He travels for his job and eats out most days. He walks or goes to the gym when he can at least once a week. Takes metformin but forgets to take the second dose. AM BS 200-300, PM BS 300-400. Did not go to diabetic education classes. "I could not fit them into my busy schedule."

Past Medical History:
Back surgery for "protruding lumbar disc" 5 years ago
Depression
Allergies:
Codeine; rash
Medications:
Zoloft 100 mg QD
Metformin BID
Family History:
Osteoarthritis, DM, HTN; mother 75 y.o. Cerebral vascular accident; father deceased age 60 y.o.
Social History:
Happily married to an attorney for 15 years, works in sales
Nonsmoker
No children
< 3 alcoholic drinks weekly
Review of Systems:
General: Denies fever, weight loss, actually gained 10 lbs, night sweats
Respiratory: Denies difficulties
Cardiac: No CP or palpitations
Gastrointestinal: Appetite good, denies problems
GU: Denies urinary frequency, no nocturia
Musculoskeletal: Denies numbness, weakness, or sensation of pain in the upper extremities.
Physical Examination:
General: NAD. HT 5'9", WT 285 lbs, BP 130/80, P-76, R-18.
Cardiac RRR, S1,S2 no S3,S4, 3/6 SEM throughout precordium (new finding), Lungs CTA, Abd: soft, +BS no HSM, extremities no edema noted

1. What are the potential ICD-10 codes in this case?
2. How can the NP determine if this patient is a new patient versus an established patient at the clinic?
3. What components of care will be used for reimbursement decisions for Mr. Jones?
4. What type of physical examination best fits what was performed on Mr. Jones?
5. If you were coding the visit for Mr. Jones, how would you determine what decision-making level you would choose? Provide your rationale, and be specific.

References

Aalseth, P. (2006). *Medical coding: What it is and how it works*. Sudbury, MA: Jones & Bartlett.
American Association of Professional Coders. (2021). *What is HCPCS?* Retrieved from https://www.aapc.com/resources/medical-coding/hcpcs.aspx
American Medical Association. (2021). *CPT changes 2021: An insider's view*. American Medical Association.
Centers for Disease Control and Prevention (2021). *Classification of Diseases, Functioning, and Disability*. Retrieved from: https://www.cdc.gov/nchs/icd/index.htm
Centers for Medicare and Medicaid. (2020). *Final policy payment*. Retrieved from https://www.cms.gov/newsroom/fact-sheets/final-policy-payment-and-quality-provisions-changes-medicare-physician-fee-schedule-calendar-year-1
Centers for Medicare and Medicaid. (2021). *Quality payment program*. Retrieved from https://qpp.cms.gov/
Contexo Media. (2015). Procedural coding expert ultimate guide to CPT coding. *Contexo Media*, 1–33.
Department of Health and Human Services. (2007). *Direct billing and payment for non-physician practitioner services*. Baltimore, MD: Centers for Medicare & Medicaid Service. Retrieved from https://www.cms.gov/Outreach-and-Education/Medicare-Learning-Network-MLN/MLNMattersArticles/downloads/MM5221.pdf
Federal Register. (2015). *Public Law 114-10: Medicare Access and CHIP Reauthorization Act*. Retrieved from https://www.congress.gov/114/plaws/publ10/PLAW-114publ10.pdf
Goodson, J. (2007). Unintended consequences of resource-based relative value scale reimbursement. *Journal of American Medical Association*, 298(19), 2308–2310.
Medicare Learning Network. (2010). *Evaluation and management services guide*. CMS. Retrieved from https://www.cms.gov/Outreach-and-Education/Medicare-Learning-Network-MLN/MLNProducts/Downloads/eval-mgmt-serv-guide-ICN006764.pdf
National Center for Health Statistics. (2012). *Classification of diseases, functioning, and disability: International classification of diseases* (10th rev. ed., Clinical Modification [ICD-10-CM]). Retrieved from http://www.cdc.gov/nchs/icd/icd10cm.htm
National Plan and Provider Enumeration System. (2021). *National provider identifier*. Retrieved from https://nppes.cms.hhs.gov/#/
Phillipsen, P. S. (2008). The most costly billing practices ever. *Journal for Nurse Practitioners*, 4(10), 761–765.
Rapsilber, L. M. (2019). Incident to and NP value in value reimbursement. *The Nurse Practitioner Journal*, 44(2), 15–17.
Rapsilber, L. M., & Anderson, E. H. (2000). Understanding the reimbursement process. *Nurse Practitioner*, 25(5), 36–56.
Stanley, J. (2010). *Advanced practice nursing: Emphasizing common roles* (3rd ed.). Philadelphia, PA: F.A. Davis.

CHAPTER 18

Professional Employment: Preparing for Licensure, Certification, and Credentialing

Susan M. DeNisco

Nurse Practitioner Certification

National board certification in your specialty area is a mark of excellence and establishes that a new graduate NP has met the educational criteria and clinical competencies to work as a safe and prudent clinician. This chapter will help the new graduate understand the steps needed to prepare them for certification and state licensure. There is much confusion among healthcare providers, insurance companies, and consumers regarding the role of the NP and the rigorous practice requirements needed to attain and maintain certification and licensure.

Preparing for Graduation

It is an exciting time for the NP student when getting ready to graduate and start in a new professional role. The process of certification and advanced practice licensure can be quite confusing, and the student needs to develop a timeline for this at least 3 months prior to graduation. It is very easy to procrastinate as one is busy completing didactic and clinical requirements, but there is paperwork that the NP graduate and the academic institution need to complete prior to the NP taking the national certification examination.

A signature from the NP academic program director may be needed for verification of the advanced pharmacology requirements and certain national certification examination applications. Official academic institution transcripts need to be sent to the state department for advanced practice licensure, as well as the national certification body the graduate will be applying to. Staying organized is key to completing the appropriate paperwork on a timely basis to ensure early certification and licensure. Employers typically require that the NP be legally ready to practice and have the ability to go through the credentialing process required by many institutions and insurance companies.

National Certification

Upon completion of the graduation requirements, the NP should apply for national board certification from either the American Academy of Nurse Practitioners (AANP) or the American Nurses Credentialing Center (ANCC). Graduates of women's health or neonatal NP programs should apply to the National Certification Corporation for the obstetric, gynecologic, and neonatal nursing specialties. Candidates for the pediatric NP examination should apply to the Pediatric Nursing Certification Board.

The candidate should check with the board of nursing for the state in which he or she plans to practice to see which certifications are acceptable for licensure application. All states require an NP to be board certified in order to practice, except for California. New York does not require it if the graduate attended the NP program in NYS. In recent years, there have been efforts to allow multistate compacts so NPs can legally practice in more than one state with one license.

What to Expect on the Certification Examination

Most certification examinations allot at least 3 hours, except for the ANCC, which allows 3.5 hours for the examination. The candidate must go to the website of the chosen organization to review the domains that will be covered in the examination. The ANCC Family Nurse Practitioner Examination covers the following content domains:

- Assessment
- Diagnosis
- Clinical Management
- Professional Role

Detailed test content information can be found on the ANCC website that outlines specific topics for each domain. The examination contains 200 questions, of which 175 questions will be scored. Once the eligibility requirements to take the certification examination are completed and the NP has successfully passed the exam, the credential is awarded: family nurse practitioner–board certified (FNP-BC) by the National Commission for Certifying Agencies. The Accreditation Board for Specialty Nursing Certification accredits this ANCC certification. Certification is awarded for a 5-year time period.

AANP National Certification Examinations are entry-level, competency-based examinations for nurse practitioners reflective of nurse practitioner knowledge and expertise for each of the following specialties: adult-gerontology, family nurse practitioner, and a new emergency nurse practitioner specialty for family nurse practitioners. The AANP examinations have four knowledge areas:

- Assessment
- Diagnosis
- Plan
- Evaluation

The examination contains 150 questions, of which 135 will be scored. Go to the website to review the updated domains for testing to familiarize yourself with them and to choose which examination may be best suited for you as well as acceptable to your state and potential practice site(s).

Practice, practice, practice before taking the board certification examination. Since all the certification examinations are multiple choice, the applicant should practice taking test questions answering one per minute. Both the AANP and ANCC offer a multiple-choice practice examination for the FNP certification candidates to identify areas in which further study may be needed in anticipation of taking an official competency-based examination. This is highly recommended—practice makes perfect. It is wise to study with a partner or in small groups. Preparation for taking the certification examination should start months before graduation; attending a review course or purchasing review CDs is a wise way to become familiar with the material covered in the certification examinations. Many successful certified NPs listened to the review CDs to and from class and work for weeks or even months preparing for the examination. Remember that the exams are developed for entry-level NPs, and extremely complex questions will not be on the test.

Nurse Practitioner Licensure for Prescription Privileges

Currently, nurse practitioners must be licensed in the state where they plan to practice, in order to have prescriptive authority. They prescribe medications, including controlled medication with varying levels of restriction, and should be checked in the state practice act. Variation exists among states in the area of authorization to prescribe controlled medications, as well as the relationship, if any, that must be maintained with a physician. Nurse practitioners should refer to the Drug Enforcement Administration website to clarify what the controlled substances prescriptive authority is in each state.

Advanced Practice State Licensure

Once the certification exam has been passed successfully, the graduate sends required documentation to the state in which she or he is applying to practice in for advanced practice nurse licensure. Most states require successfully completing 30 hours of education in pharmacology for advanced nursing practice, as well as holding a master's degree in nursing or in a related field recognized for certification as a nurse practitioner, such as a clinical nurse specialist or a nurse anesthetist recognized by one of the certifying bodies. Most states will want the application to be notarized and have photo identification.

The American Association of Nurse Practitioners has detailed, updated information on state practice acts, as well as prescriptive authority. In addition, the *Pearson Report* is an excellent reference for all nurse practitioners; it provides an annual state-by-state national overview of nurse practitioner legislation and healthcare issues. It is very important that the NP understand the specific functions included in his or her state's definition of NP scope of practice related to diagnosing, treatment, prescribing practices, hospital admission privileges, referrals, education, and ordering diagnosis tests (Buppert, 2021). Each state's scope of practice delineates what the legal role and requirements are of physician involvement in the NP practice. Language such as *collaboration*, *supervision*, *independent practice*, and *consultation* are examples of varying forms of physician involvement with the NP.

Drug Enforcement Administration (DEA) Licensure

In addition, the NP must apply for the state-controlled substances licensure and the DEA (U.S. Drug Enforcement Administration) licensure. Through the Department of Justice and DEA, the NP must apply for a DEA number pursuant to Title 21, Code of Federal Regulations, Section 1300.01(b28), which states

> The term *mid-level practitioner* means an individual practitioner, other than a physician, dentist, veterinarian, or podiatrist, who is licensed, registered, or otherwise permitted by the United States or the jurisdiction in which he/she practices, to dispense a controlled substance in the course of professional practice. (U.S. Drug Enforcement Administration, 2021)

Examples of midlevel practitioners include, but are not limited to, healthcare providers such as nurse practitioners, nurse midwives, nurse anesthetists, clinical nurse specialists, and physician assistants, who are authorized to dispense controlled substances by the state in which they practice.

National Provider Identification (NPI)

The Health Insurance Portability and Accountability Act of 1996 (HIPAA) mandated the adoption of a standard unique identifier for healthcare providers. This is particularly important for reimbursement of healthcare services that the NP provides. In 2004, the Centers for Medicare and Medicaid Services (CMS) adopted the National Provider Identifier (NPI) as the standard unique identifier number for all healthcare providers to use when filing and processing healthcare claims (Stanley, 2010). All NPs are required to apply for a national provider number and are assigned only one number that will follow the NP wherever she or he practices. The application must be completed by the nurse practitioner to avoid any potential error that could delay billing and reimbursement (National Plan and Provider Enumeration System, 2021).

Malpractice Insurance

Professional liability is a recognized risk for nurse practitioners and advanced practice clinicians. With increased autonomy and responsibility at the point of care comes an increased risk for errors and omissions that can result in harm to the patient. It is your professional responsibility to understand the current care practice environment and the methods of risk reduction. It is important to remember to change the malpractice insurance policy from student NP and RN to NP malpractice insurance, even if the workplace offers to put the NP under its umbrella. While you may be an employee of a hospital, physician office, or other healthcare organization and are considered to be covered under the employer's malpractice program, it behooves the NP to carry individual malpractice insurance to avoid conflicted interests of the employer (Joel, 2018). Check with state and federal regulations to see what may affect malpractice insurance and what the advisable amounts of coverage are. Additionally, it is the NP's responsibility to minimize the risk of being sued by maintaining current clinical skills and knowledge, clearly documenting all ordered or refused diagnostic testing and treatments, and carefully evaluating the patient's response to treatment.

Résumé vs. Curriculum Vitae Development for Nurse Practitioners

The current job market for nurse practitioners is highly competitive. Some experts recommend that nurse practitioners use curricula vitae as opposed to résumés (Beauvais, 2021). Although the two documents are similar, there are some significant differences. A résumé is typically an abbreviated document that gives an overview of education, employment history, and achievements in one to two pages. Curricula vitae, on the other hand, are typically longer and more detailed. Curricula vitae are used when seeking positions in an academic setting, but often nursing professionals will use them if seeking a leadership role in the healthcare field.

As a new graduate, you will want to highlight your clinical education and the hours spent in each specialty area because you have no formal work experience as an NP (Dahring, 2012). Whether you use a résumé or a curriculum vitae, the NP must have a well-organized and coherent document that highlights the individual's abilities, skills, and accomplishments to promote his or her career. **Box 18-1** provides an outline of a résumé for a new graduate nurse practitioner.

Do's and Don'ts of Résumé Writing

The résumé is the nurse practitioner's first introduction to a potential employer, making it imperative that the NP use this opportunity to make a positive impression with the goal of being invited to a first interview. However, a résumé can quickly leave a negative connotation if it contains errors such as misspellings, typos, and poor grammar. If the employer receives a document that is poorly constructed, this will likely give the impression that the NP is inattentive to detail and perhaps is unprofessional. It has been stated that over 75% of organization leaders interviewed indicated that only one or two typos in a curriculum vitae would eliminate the candidate from consideration for the position (Hosking, 2010).

Print your résumé on high-quality paper using a professional font such as 10- to 12-point Times New Roman, because it is easy to read (Beauvais, 2021). Be sure your email address is professional sounding, and avoid using your current employer's email address or telephone number. Account for all gaps in your employment

> **Box 18-1** Graduate Nurse Practitioner Résumé Outline
>
> - Summary of Qualifications
> - Education
> - Clinical Rotations:
>   - Name and type of clinical facility
>   - Population focus of the rotation
>   - Number of clinical hours
>   - Number of patients seen daily
>   - Level of autonomy
>   - Procedures mastered
> - Work History
> - Certifications and Licensure
> - Awards and Honors
> - Activities
> - Languages
> - References Available on Request

history, and do not list nonmedical employment history. Include a cover letter explaining how your skills and talents can provide immediate benefits to the organization (Beauvais, 2021).

Job Satisfaction

As the NP student prepares for graduation, or for the NP considering workplace change, it is imperative to consider factors that enhance the work environment to be able to choose a successful practice option. The initial transitional year of professional practice is thought to provide the critical foundation on which new professionals build their knowledge and expertise. Having a supportive workplace environment has been shown to improve work effectiveness, enhance the ability to provide high-quality patient care, contribute to cost effectiveness, and promote the retention of NPs in successful collaborative practices in a variety of healthcare settings (DeNisco, 2021).

Job satisfaction has proven to decrease absenteeism, improve employee retention, improve productivity, and enhance job performance (Kacel et al., 2005). In a study looking at factors leading to job satisfaction and dissatisfaction in NPs from the Midwest, the Misener Nurse Practitioner Job Satisfaction Scale (MNPJSS) was used. The MNPJSS consists of 44 items grouped into six categories: intrapractice partnership/collegiality; challenge/autonomy; professional, social, and community interaction; professional growth; time; and benefits. The factors that received the highest ratings for satisfaction were sense of accomplishment, challenge in work, and level of autonomy.

Job satisfaction has been linked to autonomy and is important in attracting and retaining NPs in the workplace, in addition to greater outpatient clinical productivity (Chumbler et al., 2000; Schiestel, 2007). Clearly, autonomy is an important factor to consider when selecting a practice site.

Nurse practitioners working in nurse-managed health centers (NMHCs) have been shown to be accessible to their clients and provide health care that is at the least equitable to, and has been shown to be better than, in some cases, other providers (Pron, 2012). Nurse practitioners who work in this type of setting are the main healthcare providers but frequently have to deal with the numerous barriers to practice related to recognition by insurers and adequate resources. In a study published by Pron (2012), the majority of NPs working in NMHCs were found to perceive themselves as autonomous and had good job satisfaction as it related to the concept of autonomy. A sense of accomplishment was noted to be very high in this group of NPs, with the suggestion that this is related to the ability to provide improvement in the health care of the vulnerable patients that use NMHCs.

Successful practice for NPs has been linked to intrinsic factors such as challenge, sense of accomplishment, ability to deliver quality care, and level of autonomy (Kacel et al., 2005; Pron, 2012). The NP/DNP has much to offer in providing health care to the vulnerable and underserved populations needing improved health. In any case, the graduating NP/DNP should consider the various options and the pros and cons of the various practice settings that will provide job satisfaction.

Collaboration

Although the topic of collaboration has been discussed earlier in this book, the relationship between collaboration and job satisfaction, as well as success, will be reviewed here. Relational theory suggests that fostering collaborative relationships within the workplace can enhance empowerment and increase job effectiveness. Collaboration is an important component for NP practice, and one that is inherent to nursing in general. Collaborative care may be defined as "an arrangement whereby an NP and a physician provide primary health care to a group of patients, with the professionals sharing authority for providing care within their scope of practice" (Bellini & Shea, 2006, p. 233). Resnick and Bonner (2003) defined collaboration as "a joint and cooperative enterprise that integrates the individual perspectives and expertise of various team members" (p. 344), and they identified collaboration as a foundation for successful practice.

Collaboration has been associated with improvements in patient outcomes, healthcare costs, decision making, and as part of a response to the current nursing shortage (Hojat et al., 2003).

Nurse practitioners perceive that they collaborate well with physicians (Maylone et al., 2011), but some physicians may not understand what NPs' roles are. Bellini and Shea (2006) assessed medical residents' perceptions of nurse practitioners who worked in a collaborative model with assessments before and 1 year after implementation of the model. The majority of medical residents had a positive view of NPs prior to the collaborative model implementation; yet 1 year after the implementation, results indicated that more medical residents viewed NPs as colleagues and appreciated NPs' clinical judgment.

Successful collaborative practices need an orientation to the process of collaboration, education to the NP role and scope of practice to prevent underutilization of NPs, and promotion of effective collaborative care (Bailey et al., 2006). Trust, mutual respect, and open communication are critical components of a collaborative practice (Hallas et al., 2004).

Empowerment

Empowerment… It sounds important, but what exactly is it? Power has been defined as "the ability to get things done, to mobilize resources, to get and use whatever it is that a person needs for the goals he or she is attempting to meet" (Kanter, 1993, p. 166). Empowerment has been said to be a central component of advanced practice nursing (Ackerman et al., 1996). There are two perspectives of empowerment within the work environment: structural and psychological. Laschinger's (Almost & Laschinger, 2002; Laschinger et al., 2004) and Spreitzer's (1995, 2007) studies suggest that there are at least two components of empowerment—structural and psychological—that are separate from each other, although a positive relationship appears to exist between them.

Structural empowerment occurs when nurse practitioners have access to "information, support, resources, and opportunities to learn and grow" (Laschinger et al., 2004, p. 528). Psychological empowerment is a process that occurs when one has a sense of motivation in relation to the workplace environment (Manojlovich, 2007; Manojlovich & Laschinger, 2007).

When NPs' values, beliefs, and behaviors are congruent with their workplace's requirements, the NPs find meaning in professional practice (Stewart, 2008). Findings from these studies suggest that workplace environments that foster collegiality, provide support and access to resources, afford opportunities for professional growth, and permit visibility can enhance job satisfaction.

Psychological empowerment is felt to be a motivator for people and has been associated with an increased sense of self-efficacy and increased self-determination, which can encourage involvement and commitment by these individuals (Knol & Van Linge, 2009; Laschinger et al., 2007; MacPhee et al., 2011; Spreitzer & Doneson, 2005).

Interviewing Skills

Going on a job interview may seem intimidating to the newly minted nurse practitioner, but honing interview skills can help transform the experience into a steppingstone to a new career. The interview process is competitive given the influx of primary care providers, so the NP needs to set him or herself above the rest. According to the Keiser Family Foundation, there are approximately 250,000 practicing nurse practitioners and 112,000 practicing physician assistants in 2020. This estimate represents approximately over 50% more nurse practitioners that report having NP in their title in a 2008 national survey (Agency for Health Care Research & Quality, 2011).

The Interview Process

For many candidates, the first step in the interview process may be a telephone interview. The telephone interview is used as a mechanism to screen candidates in order to decide if they warrant a face-to-face interview or video interview. The NP should not take a casual approach to the telephone interview, and should be prepared with questions as if he or she were in an in-person interview; some experts

Box 18-2 Potential Discussion Items for the Interview

What key tasks do you see yourself doing as a nurse practitioner?
What are the most important knowledge and skills that you bring to the NP role?
What do you know about this organization?
Describe two major trends in your profession.
What nonclinical qualifications do you bring to your role as a NP?
What are your strengths and weaknesses?
Where do you see yourself in 5 years?
When will you receive certification and licensure?

---

believe that standing while being interviewed will make you stronger and increase your confidence. NPs that make it past the initial telephone interview should not assume they have the position (Kess, 2011).

If called in for a face-to-face interview or video-based interview, the NP must prepare by dressing professionally, having several copies of his or her résumé in hand, and have a list of questions for the employer. Doing research on the company's mission and goals shows interest and initiative on the part of the NP. **Box 18-2** shows discussion items that the NP should be prepared to answer during an interview for a clinical position.

Questions for the Employer

Too often, nurse practitioners will ask about salary and benefits on the first interview. While compensation packages are important, this should be reserved for the second interview, as finding a position that is a "good fit" for your skills, talents, and personal needs should be of upmost importance. The NP should be prepared to ask myriad questions regarding practice issues, the employer contract, and credentialing, which will be discussed later in this chapter. Other important questions will pertain to the patient population, practice hours, and facility setup, such as exam rooms and equipment. Very often, job satisfaction is dependent on the availability of a strong support team that helps make the practice as efficiently productive as possible. Ask about the number of patients you will be expected to see per day.

New graduate NPs often start out at between 8 and 12 patients a day, while experienced NPs usually see between 18 and 22 patients a day (Tumolo, 2005). Higher patient numbers may increase job pressure, but again, if your salary is productivity-based, it could increase your bottom line (Tumolo, 2005). **Box 18-3** lists important questions the NP should ask a potential employer.

Negotiating an Employment Contract

Every employment agreement or contract is unique, and various factors should be addressed before negotiation. The NP must determine his or her needs while assessing the potential employer's needs. Reflecting on and balancing your needs and your family's needs is paramount before accepting a position and negotiating your contract. Understand what aspects of the position are desired, negotiable, and

> **Box 18-3 Questions to Ask a Potential Employer**
>
> What is the expected patient volume?
> Expected hours/day/week?
> Weekend hours?
> "On-call" expectations?
> "Moonlighting" allowed?
> Number of days/hours for orientation?
> Peer review process and timeline?
> Orientation to policies and procedures?
> Offsite facilities?
> Physician support?
> Nursing support staff?
> Community education program attendance?
> Provider mix: NPs, PAs, MDs?
> Billing for services?

non-negotiable. In the previous section, compensation package, job obligations, and practice issues were areas of negotiable elements. The process of negotiating a contract should include preparation, bargaining, and finalizing (Chien, 2002).

Preparation

Do your research ahead of time and be able to clearly articulate what you know about local and national compensation patterns. According to the U.S. Bureau of Labor Statistics, the mean annual salary was $112,000 in 2019. The NP should have a reference range for both annual and hourly wages for similar positions and write down what the bottom line is for both earnings and benefits. The NP should also be prepared to understand the potential offers in regard to the reimbursement system for the office or organization. In addition, the NP should research and find out if it is a fee-for-service practice or a capitated practice. Ask the employer if there are bonus opportunities as well as rewards for productivity and effort.

Bargaining

The NP must market him or herself as a high-quality, cost-effective healthcare provider. Highlight your previous contributions to nursing and as an NP. Familiarize yourself with the business of medicine. Savvy negotiators will calculate the NP's potential revenue for the practice. Be flexible and listen to the employer's perspective; gaining the trust of the employer will facilitate the negotiating process.

Finalizing

Once an agreement is reached, it is important for the NP to finalize the contract with a written agreement. There are varying opinions on whether or not a formal contract is needed for a NP and the employer. There are many advantages of a written employment contract:

- Increased job security and control over professional practice
- Legal protection in relation to finances and job responsibilities

- Up-front agreement on potential problems and professional issues
- Protection from termination

NPs should secure an attorney familiar with NP law and business contracts. If any employer has a well-established, profitable practice, the NP should expect to be rewarded well under the employment agreement. If the practice is losing money, the NP will find it difficult under the best circumstances to negotiate an acceptable agreement, no matter what the skill set and experience the NP has (Buppert, 2021).

Credentialing

The public has the right to safe, quality health care delivered by healthcare professionals with the appropriate education, training, and experience. The Joint Commission, the Accreditation Association for Ambulatory Healthcare, and managed care organizations take this commitment very seriously (Magdic et al., 2005). One mechanism required by these agencies to ensure patient safety is the process of credentialing and delineation of clinical privileges for medical staff, including nurse practitioners. Obtaining clinical privileges was once reserved for physicians, but as nurse practitioners have integrated themselves as equal partners in the healthcare delivery system, credentialing and obtaining clinical privileges to practice is now commonplace. Nurse practitioners must become familiar with the regulations that impact and guide the process of credentialing and obtaining clinical privileges.

Credentialing and clinical privileging follows licensure and is the process through which a provider obtains authorization to practice in a select healthcare or hospital setting. Typically the credentialing process involves verification of education, licensure, certification, health requirements, and reference checks. Ongoing clinical privileges are contingent on maintaining skills and board certification. Clinical privileges are a specifically delineated list or description of the privileges granted within your scope of practice. For example, standard clinical privileges for a nurse practitioner would include obtaining a history and physical examination and ordering and interpreting diagnostic tests. A peer review process is a usual part of maintaining the privileges, which are reviewed by your employer periodically.

Collaborative Agreements

The nurse practitioner must be familiar with the legal scope of practice in the state she or he wishes to practice in. Each state has regulations that define the scope of practice; some statutes are governed by state legislature and other states give the board of nursing the authority to enforce the scope of practice law (Buppert, 2021). Each state must define the legal requirement for physician involvement in the nurse practitioner's practice. This involvement, if any, is depicted as "supervision" or "collaboration" and further explains the details of the terms of the involvement. Some state laws give tremendous detail in regard to the specifics of the level of involvement, ranging from prescribing controlled substances to establishing a referral and consultation arrangement between the physician and NP. When entering an employment contract in a state where the scope of practice statute mandates a "collaborative" agreement between an advanced practice nurse and a physician, it is important to draft a mutually agreeable collaborative practice agreement that will support the scope of practice law in your state. **Table 18-1** is a sample collaborative practice agreement that details prescriptive authority, systems for peer review, coverage in the absence of the clinician, and referral and consultation arrangements.

Table 18-1 Collaborative Practice Agreement for Advanced Practice Nurses Requesting Prescriptive Authority

1. Complete names, home and business addresses, zip codes, and telephone numbers of the licensed practitioner and the advanced practice nurse:

Licensed Practitioner:	*Advanced Practice Nurse:*
Licensed practitioner name and license number	Advanced practice nurse name and license number
Street address of home	Street address of home
City, state, & zip of home	City, state, & zip of home
Home phone number	Home phone number
Business street address	Business street address
City, state, & zip of business	City, state, & zip of business
Business phone number	Business phone number

2. List of all locations where prescriptive authority is authorized by this agreement.

Business street address	Business street address
City, state, & zip of business	City, state, & zip of business
Business phone number	Business phone number

3. List all specialty or board certifications of the licensed practitioner and the advanced practice nurse.
   Licensed practitioner is board certified in a medical practice specialty. The advanced practice nurse is a nurse practitioner, clinical nurse specialist, certified nurse midwife, etc., with a specialized certification as a family nurse practitioner, etc.

4. Briefly describe the specific manner of collaboration between the licensed practitioner and advance practice nurse. *Specifically, how they will work together, how they will share practice trends and responsibilities, how they will maintain geographic proximity, and how they will provide coverage during an absence, incapacity, infirmity, or emergency by the licensed practitioner.*

   How they will work together:
   The licensed practitioner and advanced practice nurse shall collaborate on a continual basis, etc.

   How they will share practice trends and responsibilities:
   The advanced practice nurse shall make rounds at the request of the licensed practitioner and consult with the license practitioner as needed, etc.

   How they will maintain geographic proximity:
   The licensed practitioner will maintain a physical presence within a reasonable geographic proximity to the advanced practice nurse's practice location.

   How they will provide coverage during absence, incapacity, infirmity, or emergency by the license practitioner:
   In the case of the absence, incapacity, or unavailability of the licensed practitioner, coverage and consultation will be coordinated and maintained by another licensed practitioner as arranged in advance by the licensed practitioner and the advanced practice nurse.

(continues)

Table 18-1 Collaborative Practice Agreement for Advanced Practice Nurses Requesting Prescriptive Authority *(continued)*

5. Provide a description of limitations, if any, that the licensed practitioner has placed on the advanced practice nurse's prescriptive authority.
There are no additional limitations on the advanced practice nurse or there are the following limitations on the advanced practice nurse, etc.

6. Provide a description of the time and manner of the licensed practitioner's review of the advanced practice nurse's prescribing practices. Specifically, the description should include provisions that the advanced practice nurse must submit documentation of prescribing practices to the licensed practitioner within 7 days. Documentation of prescribing practices shall include, but not be limited to, at least a 5% random sampling of the charts and medications prescribed for patients.
The advanced practice nurse must submit documentation of the advanced practice nurse's prescribing practices within 7 days to the licensed practitioner for review. The documentation of prescribing practices shall include at least a 5% random sampling of the charts and medications prescribed for patients.

7. Provide a list of all other written practice agreements of the licensed practitioner and advanced practice nurse.
There are no other practice agreements, or list all other practice agreements, etc.

8. Provide the duration of the written practice agreement between the licensed practitioner and advanced practice nurse.
Either party may terminate this practice agreement without cause at any time, effective immediately upon notice to the other party, etc.

| *Signature of licensed practitioner:* | *Signature of advanced practice nurse:* |
| Date: | Date: |

The Consensus Model—Stay Tuned!

Licensure, accreditation, certification, and education is the collaborative work of the APRN Consensus Work Group and National Council of State Boards of Nursing (NCSBN) APRN Advisory Committee. The Consensus Model was intended to ease the confusion surrounding advanced practice nursing. It clarifies the population foci for APNs to include certified registered nurse anesthetists, certified nurse midwives, clinical nurse specialists, and certified nurse practitioners (NCSBN, 2009). After receiving critical input from NP educators and practicing APNs, some changes related to the overlap that occurs between acute care and primary care APNs were suggested. The goal remains for all NPs to have a DNP as entry level into practice; however, due to the myriad state licensing regulations, it is difficult to expect that will be mandated anytime soon. As shown in many research studies, NPs have been providing high-quality, cost-effective health care with master's level education for years.

The addition of doctoral education is a goal to have parity with our colleagues, such as physicians, physical therapists, psychologists, and pharmacists. Having additional preparation to improve the NP's ability to expand leadership initiatives in individual, community, and global health is the direction we need to be heading in these tumultuous times in our current healthcare system. Kudos to those of you who are reaching that goal, and we encourage those obtaining MSNs to seriously consider continuing on with your education to obtain a DNP. Either way, we know you will connect with your patients and make a difference in their lives.

Seminar Discussion Questions

1. Discuss the elements important to you when seeking a place of employment. What is negotiable and what is non-negotiable?
2. Share your résumé with a peer. Discuss the strengths and weaknesses of your peer's current résumé and offer suggestions for improvement.
3. Discuss the process of certification and licensure, and list what steps need to be taken to become gainfully employed after graduation.
4. What resources are available to the NP in understanding the state-by-state NP scope-of-practice laws?
5. Identify the benefits of formal employment.

References

Ackerman, M. H., Norsen, L., Martin, B., Wiedrich, J., & Kitzman, H. J. (1996). Development of a model of advanced practice. *American Journal of Critical Care, 5*(1), 68–73.

Agency for Health Care Research & Quality. (2011). *Primary care workforce: Facts and stats No. 2: The number of nurse practitioners and physician assistants practicing primary care in the United States.* Retrieved from https://www.ahrq.gov/sites/default/files/publications/files/pcwork2.pdf

Almost, J., & Laschinger, H. S. (2002). Workplace empowerment, collaborative work relationships, and job strain in nurse practitioners. *Journal of the American Academy of Nurse Practitioners, 14*(9), 408–420.

Bailey, P., Jones, L., & Way, D. (2006). Family physician/nurse practitioner: Stories of collaboration. *Journal of Advanced Nursing, 53*(4), 381–391.

Beauvais, A. (2021). Entering the jobmarket and promoting future success. In S. DeNisco (Ed.), *Advanced practice nursing: Essential knowledge for the profession* (pp. 901–923). Burlington, MA: Jones & Bartlett Learning.

Bellini, L. M., & Shea, J. A. (2006). Improvement of resident perceptions of nurse practitioners after the introduction of a collaborative care model: A benefit of work hour reform? *Teaching and Learning in Medicine, 18*(3), 233–236.

Buppert, C. (2021). *Nurse practitioners' business practice and legal guide* (7th ed.). Sudbury, MA: Jones & Bartlett Learning.

Chien, A. (2002). Negotiating a contract. In M. Goolsby, *Nurse practitioner secrets: Questions and answers to reveal the secrets to successful NP practice* (pp. 1–4). Philadelphia, PA: Hanley & Belfus.

Chumbler, N. R., Geller, J. M., & Weier, A. W. (2000). The effects of clinical decision making on nurse practitioners' clinical productivity. *Evaluation & the Health Professions, 23*(3), 284–304.

Dahring, R. (2012). *Nurse practitioner job search*. Retrieved from http://www.nursepractitionerjobsearch.com/nurse-practitioner-resume.html

DeNisco, S. (2021). *Advanced practice nursing: Essential knowledge for the profession* (4th ed.). Burlington, MA: Jones & Bartlett Learning.

Hallas, D. M., Butz, A., & Gitterman, B. (2004). Attitudes and beliefs for effective pediatric nurse practitioner and physician collaboration. *Journal of Pediatric Health Care, 18*(2), 77–86.

Hojat, M., Gonnella, J. S., Nasac, T. J., Fields, S. K., Cicchetti, A., Lo Scalzo, A., Torres-Ruiz, A., et al. (2003). Comparisons of American, Israeli, Italian, and Mexican physicians and nurses on the total and factor scores of the Jefferson scale of attitudes toward physician-nurse collaborative relationships. *International Journal of Nursing Studies, 40,* 427–435.

Hosking, R. (2010). Top 10 tips for job seekers. *OfficePro, 70*(2), 5.

Joel, L. A. (2018). *Advanced practice nursing: Essentials for role development* (4th ed.). Philadelphia, PA: F.A. Davis.

Kacel, B., Miller, M., & Norris, D. (2005). Measurement of nurse practitioner job satisfaction in a midwestern state. *Journal of the American Academy of Nurse Practitioners, 17*(1), 27–32.

Kaiser Family Foundation. (2020). Total number of nurse practitioners. Retrieved from https://www.kff.org/other/state-indicator/total-number-of-nurse-practitioners/?currentTimeframe=0&sortModel=%7B%22colId%22:%22Location%22,%22sort%22:%22asc%22%7D

Kaiser Family Foundation. (2020). Total number of physician assistants. Retrieved from https://www.kff.org/other/state-indicator/total-number-of-physician-assistants/?currentTimeframe=0&sortModel=%7B%22colId%22:%22Location%22,%22sort%22:%22asc%22%7D

Kanter, R. M. (1993). *Men and women of the corporation* (2nd ed.). New York, NY: Basic Books.

Kess, S. (2011). *Clinical advisor*. Retrieved from http://www.clinicaladvisor.com/job-interview-tips-for-physician-assistants-and-nurse-practitioners/article/197218

Knol, J., & Van Linge, R. (2009). Innovative behavior: The effect of structural and psychological empowerment on nurses. *Journal of Advanced Nursing, 65*(2), 359–370.

Laschinger, H. K., Finegan, J. E., Shamian, J., & Wilk, P. (2004). A longitudinal analysis of the impact of workplace empowerment on work satisfaction. *Journal of Organizational Behavior, 25,* 527–545.

Laschinger, H. K., Purdy, N., & Almost, J. (2007). The impact of leader-member exchange quality, empowerment, and core self-evaluation on nurse manager's job satisfaction. *Journal of Nursing Administration, 37*(5), 221–229.

MacPhee, M., Skelton-Green, J., Bouthillette, F., & Suryaprakash, N. (2011). An empowerment framework for nursing leadership in development: Supporting evidence. *Journal of Advanced Nursing, 68*(1), 159–169.

Magdic, K. S., Hravnak, M., & McCartney, S. (2005). Credentialing for nurse practitioners: An update. *American Association of Critical Care Nurses Clinical Issues, 16*(1), 16–22.

Manojlovich, M. (2007). Power and empowerment in nursing: Looking backward to inform the future. *Online Journal Issues of Nursing, 12*(1). Retrieved from http://www.medscape.com/viewarticle/553403

Manojlovich, M., & Laschinger, H. (2007). The nursing worklife model: Extending and refining a new theory. *Journal of Nursing Management, 15,* 256–263.

Maylone, M., Ranieri, L., Quinn Griffin, M., McNulty, R., & Fitzpatrick, J. (2011). Collaboration and autonomy: Perceptions among nurse practitioners. *Journal of the American Academy of Nurse Practitioners, 23*(1), 51–57.

National Council of State Boards of Nursing. (2009). *Consensus model for APRN regulation: Licensure, accreditation, certification & education*. Retrieved from https://www.ncsbn.org/Consensus_Model_for_APRN_Regulation_July_2008.pdf

National Plan and Provider Enumeration System. (2021). *National provider identifier*. Retrieved from https://nppes.cms.hhs.gov/NPPES/StaticForward.do?forward=static.npistart

Pron, L. (2012). Job satisfaction and perceived autonomy for nurse practitioners working in nurse-managed health centers. *Journal of the American Academy of Nurse Practitioners, 25*(4), 213–221.

Resnick, B., & Bonner, A. (2003). Collaboration: Foundation for a successful practice. *Journal of the American Medical Directors Association,* 344–349.

Schiestel, C. (2007). Job satisfaction among Arizona adult nurse practitioners. *Journal of the American Academy of Nurse Practitioners, 19,* 30–34.

Spreitzer, G. (1995). Psychological empowerment in the workplace: Dimensions, measurement, and validation. *Academy of Management Journal, 38*(5), 1442–1465.

Spreitzer, G. (2007). Toward the integration of two perspectives: A review of social-structural and psychological empowerment at work. In C. Cooper & J. Barling (Eds.), *The handbook of organizational behavior*. Thousand Oaks, CA: Sage.

Spreitzer, G., & Doneson, D. (2005). Musings on the past and future of employee empowerment. Forthcoming in T. Cummings (Ed.), *Handbook of organizational development*. Thousand Oaks, CA: Sage.

Stanley, J. (2010). *Advanced practice nursing: Emphasizing common roles* (2nd ed.). Philadelphia, PA: F.A. Davis.

Stewart, J. (2008). Psychological empowerment, structural empowerment, and collaboration among nurse practitioners (doctoral dissertation). Cleveland, OH: Case Western Reserve University.

Tumolo, J. (2005). *Advance for NPs & PAs*. Retrieved from http://nurse-practitioners-and-physician-assistants.advanceweb.com/Article/Question-Authority-2.aspx

U.S. Bureau of Labor Statistics. (2019). Occupational Employment and Wages, 29-1171 Nurse Practitioners. Retrieved from https://www.bls.gov/oes/current/oes291171.htm

U.S. Drug Enforcement Administration. (2021). *Mid-level practitioners authorization by state*. Retrieved from https://www.deadiversion.usdoj.gov/drugreg/practioners/index.html

CHAPTER 19

Nurse Practitioner as a Business Owner: Entrepreneurship and Practice Management

Kimberly Testo and Tiffany Teixeira

Introduction

As access to health care grows in demand, the NP has answered the ever-important call to heal those in need at every corner of the healthcare system. As nurses, our approach is more holistic in nature, and this lends great synergy to creating a business from concept to operational status. Entrepreneurship is often viewed as a function that involves the exploitation of opportunities existing within a market. Such exploitation is most commonly associated with the direction and/or combination of productive inputs.

The role of the nurse practitioner entrepreneur is continuing to evolve across the world with the need for more highly skilled medical professionals to help handle the shortages across all medical fields. Physician availability to patients has been recognized as one of the top barriers to meeting the medical needs of patients. It is estimated there will be a shortage of up to 139,000 physicians by 2033 (Heiser, 2020). Additionally, the numbers of medical students and residents specializing in primary care have continued to decline in recent years (Naylor & Kurtzman, 2010; Daly, 2009). This primary care physician deficit, coupled with our aging population and the implementation of the Affordable Care Act in 2010, has resulted in a strained healthcare delivery system starved for innovation. The World Health Organization (WHO) explains that "health innovation" improves the efficiency, effectiveness, quality, and affordability of health care. Health innovation responds to unmet public health needs by creating new ways of thinking and working. Nurses have been healthcare innovators for centuries. From the revolutionary hygiene practices of Florence Nightingale into the 21st century where nurse practitioners themselves are serving as disruptive innovators, we are now on the brink of a fundamental shift in health care and nurse practitioners are positioned to be its pioneers. Conley & Judge-Ellis (2021).

Nurses are an integral part of the healthcare delivery system and make up the largest section of the health profession. It is reported there are approximately 29 million nurses and midwives globally, with 3.9 million of those individuals in the United States. Nurse practitioner jobs are set to grow exponentially over the next 10 years at a rate of 35%, five times the overall employment rate in the United States (Haddad et al., 2020). Additionally, evidence has shown that nurse practitioners provide an equal level of care when compared to physicians and are well-positioned to provide high-quality and affordable health care. A 2018 Cochrane review of 18 randomized controlled trials suggested that nurses provide care equivalent to physicians and achieve similar patient outcomes (Laurant et al., 2018). Nurse practitioners are ready and willing to meet the increasing healthcare demand for quality care, but to do so they must first be seen as equal partners in health service provision. Nurses are being encouraged to practice to the full extent of their skills and take on significant leadership roles in health policy and planning (Wilson et al., 2013). However, regulations limiting their scope of practice vary greatly by state. As of 2021 in the United States, 23 states and the District of Columbia have full practice authority. Nurse practitioners continue to actively work with legislators in the hope of removing the barriers to practice and patient care so as to meet the growing healthcare demands nationwide.

The ability to provide high-quality and affordable care makes nurse practitioners well-suited for business ownership. Nurse practitioners are taking a healthcare problem and reframing it into an opportunity for innovation. A combination of social, economic, and political reasons have driven more nurse practitioners to become entrepreneurs and advance the profession through entrepreneurial endeavors.

Nurses have been starting businesses for over a century, dating back to the 1800s. The most widely recognized nurse entrepreneur and the founder of modern nursing, Florence Nightingale, established St. Thomas' Hospital and the Nightingale Training School for Nurses in 1860 (Karimi & Masoudi Alavi, 2015). Mary Seacole, a British-Jamaican nurse, established the British Hotel where she cared for wounded officers during the Crimean War, and Clara Barton established the Bureau of Records of Missing Army Men and founded the American Red Cross in 1881 (Phillips, 2021).

In the 1900s, many nurses were self-employed, providing care as private-duty nurses. However, following the Great Depression, private-duty nursing made a shift toward institutional nursing because private-duty nursing was no longer affordable for many families. Despite this, the work that private-duty nurses did may arguably have laid the foundation for future nurse entrepreneurs.

Practice Start-up

Are you ready to take the leap and open your own practice? If so, the first question most people ask is where to start. To do this, you need to first determine your passion. A wise person once told me that you will never work a day in your life if you love what you do. Look at your community. Where are there deficits for patient access? What area are you licensed in (geriatric, pediatrics, family, midwife, etc.)? And what do you want to achieve by creating your own business? These questions will help you fine-tune your area of interest so you can do a deep dive into the next step: creating a business plan (US, SBA, n.d.).

Steps to completing a business plan:

- Executive Summary
- Business Description
- Marketing Analysis
- Organization and Management
- Service or Product Line
- Marketing and Sales
- Funding Request
- Financial Projections

Every business starts with a plan. You first need to develop your executive summary. This summary is created to tell your reader about your company and why it will be successful. This section should include your mission statement, products and services, a brief overview of your company's leadership team, employees, and location. You also want to make sure you include financial information and growth plans if you plan to ask for financial assistance. For most of us, this may sound foreign, but the role of your growth plan is to clearly state your objectives and the steps and activities you plan on implementing to achieve these objectives. This can include things like the financial and operating standards, along with policies and procedures that must be in place for your business to grow. You should also create plans for rollout and expansion, as well as the staffing needs required to support your projected growth.

The next part of your business plan is your company description. In this section, you want to clearly define the problem your business will solve. For most, the major problem will be the lack of medical providers available for the patient population. But it could be the fact that there is no one certified or qualified to offer a service/treatment in your area. The purpose in this section is for the reader to understand the competitive advantages your business will offer.

Once you have described your business, it is time to complete the market analysis. Determine your target group of clients and investigate your competition. Delve into what makes them successful and what you can do better. Do your research, because this will help you be as successful as you can be in the early stages of your business, which will then help you in the long run. Arm yourself with all the knowledge you can to make your business succeed. Organization and management is the next area to be tackled in your business plan. Will you be operating as a LLC, S, or C Corp? You may want to seek assistance from an accountant to determine which avenue will be the most beneficial for your business, because there are benefits to each structure. You also want to state who will be running the business. Create an organizational chart to help the reader understand the chain of command within the business, and also attach the résumés of those who will be part of the team. They want to know who will be taking the lead and what support you will have in your endeavor.

Our next category to complete is the explanation of your services and/or product lines. This is where you show the reader how your practice will shine in comparison to competitors. What can you offer your patients and what services will make you stick out from your competitors?

Now that we have written our summary, defined our business, evaluated the market, discussed the team that will make the business happen and what services you have to set yourself apart from your competitors, it is time to plan your marketing strategy. How are you going to reach your patients? Who is going to be your referral base? Will you be using word of mouth, social media, or business to business? When marketing your business, you need to remember that it is a contact sport. The one who stays in the minds of the community (i.e., consumers) will get the referral. We all know that when someone drops off information at the front desk, it will only get to the providers if there is a benefit to their patients. So, come up with a strategy to get in front of your local community and use your professional and social contacts to spread the word about your new business. Consider using forms of social media to gain access to your target market, because around 7 out of 10 Americans currently use social media applications (Pew Research, 2021).

The last task required to complete your business plan is to determine if you will be asking for funding. If you need funding, be sure to specify how much money you will require, what it will be used toward, and how it will be distributed over the next 5 years. Backers need to clearly understand the breakdown of the financial obligations of the business, from start-up costs to maintenance and expansion opportunities. Financial projections are also required to convince the reader that the business is stable and worth giving the financial investment requested. Lenders will evaluate the risk associated with their investment and if the business will be successful over a 5-year period. Support your request for financial funding with clear explanations of your projections. There are many resources available to you as a small business owner. Also be aware that there can be benefits to those businesses that are more than 50% owned by women and veterans. So, talk to your lenders to see if you qualify for any of these benefits. Also. do not give up if you are not given funding on the first attempt. Take their recommendations, modify your plan, and go to another lender, because where there's a will, there's a way.

Target markets:

- Primary Care
- Mental Health
- Visiting Nurse Practitioners
- Assisted Living and Long-Term Care Facilities
- Specialty Care: Endocrinology, Urology, Dermatology, Pain Management
- Aesthetics
- Alternative: Holistic-Integrative Care
- Opioid Treatment Programs
- Concierge Practice
- Mobile Units

The Legal Aspects of Owning a Practice

Now that your business plan is complete and you have gotten funding to begin your practice, you need to think about the legal aspects. You must register your business with the state. This will give you a Tax ID number, which will be used to open up bank accounts and credit cards for your business. Then you will want to seek legal counsel and create an operating agreement. Depending upon if you are a sole proprietorship, LLC, S-, or C-Corp will determine the language required to protect all parties within the business. If you are not a sole proprietorship, this is one of the most important documents in your practice. Make sure you and any partners have reviewed the document and understand all its aspects in its entirety, because this document will be used if there are ever any issues within the business organization that can't be resolved. Then you want to set up your bank account so payments can be directed to this account once credentialing is complete and services are being rendered.

As nurse practitioners, we understand the importance of having malpractice insurance, but that is not the only insurance you will require when operating a practice. You need to consider general liability insurance for your practice location, whether you are renting or you own the building your practice is located in. This will cover you for any possible slip-and-fall injuries that might occur on the premises. If you will employ staff, you will also need workers, compensation insurance. Workers, compensation insurance provides benefits to employees who become sick or injured on the job. Be aware that most states require businesses to carry workers, compensation insurance, so be sure to check your state's regulations. Also know that without coverage, your employees can sue you for a work-related injury or illness to help pay for their medical costs or lost wages. Employees have the right to sue their employer for the tort of negligence (The Hartford, 2021). In addition to insurance as a medical practice owner, you need to go back to basics and remember that HIPAA is of the utmost importance. What form of EHR system will you be using? Do you have a secure fax and or email? Have your patients signed a HIPAA consent form? And do you have a release of information form for when medication records are requested or need to be obtained? These are all things you will need before you open your doors to patients. Also, you want to create an employee handbook, because it gives employees information about the organization's history, mission, values, policies, procedures, and benefits in a written format. This can be used to support a reason for termination of an employee if they fail to follow the values and policies of the practice. It is there to keep the communication open and transparent between the employee and employer.

Collaborative Agreements vs. Independent Practice

The next question you need to ask yourself is: Are you able to practice independently? Your state of practice will determine what types of agreements you must have in place to operate your business. As of 2021 in the United States, 23 states and the District of Columbia have full practice authority (**Figure 19-1**).

Please be aware, however, that just because a state has full practice authority, it doesn't mean you will be able to prescribe all controlled substances. Certain states still have limitations on what schedule of narcotics the NP can prescribe. So be sure to review your state's prescribing practices, because you would not want to open a pain management clinic in a state where you can't prescribe narcotics.

When it comes to being an independently practicing NP, also educate yourself about your state's requirements to maintain your independence, whether it concerns a specific number of clinic practice hours per year, completing a certain number of CEUs and/or the specific training you need to maintain (such as

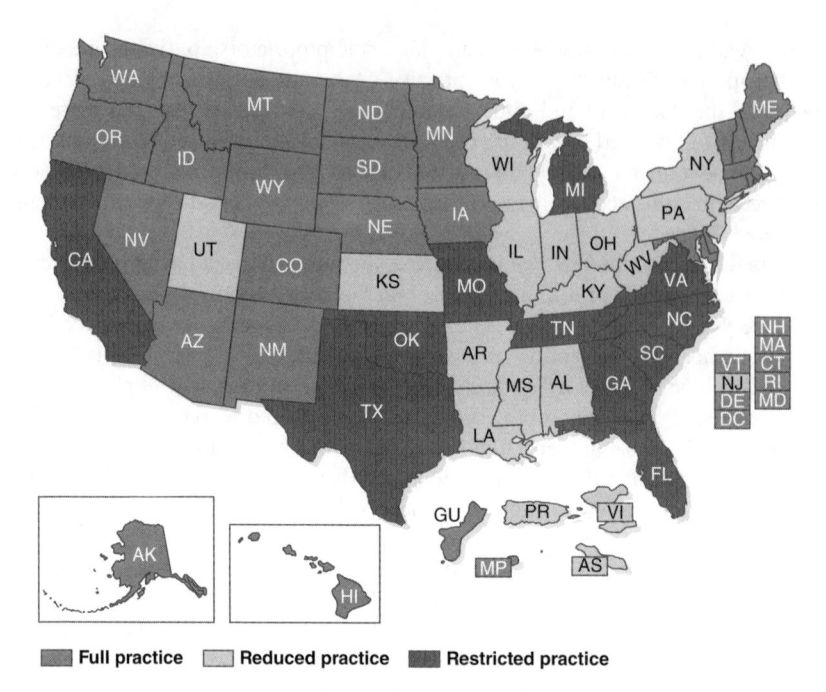

Figure 19-1 Practice Authority for Nurse Practitioners by State

Reproduced from State practice environment. (n.d.). Retrieved April 01, 2021, from https://www.aanp.org/advocacy/state/state-practice-environment

harassment in the workplace), HIPAA training, and/or emergency response preparedness, etc. State regulatory agencies have the right to audit NPs at any time, so be proactive and be sure to keep all required education, hours, and training up to date so you aren't sited for not following the state's guidelines for practicing independently.

For those nurse practitioners who can practice with collaboration, be sure to educate yourself on state guidelines of your approved scope of practice. Knowing what is allowed and what requires referral to a higher level of care for your patients is important for liability and the maintenance of state licensure. When collaborating, determine if your state allows you to collaborate with another NP or if you are required to use an MD. Many states are working to pass legislation to allow fellow nurse practitioners to collaborate with each other to help meet the growing shortage of healthcare providers in our community. In states where an MD is required for supervision, determine what is needed as part of the collaboration agreement. In regard to how long you require collaboration, find out if there will be a fee associated with the MD's service, how often they expect you to meet, and what will be discussed during meetings. Also have a clear start and stop date for the agreement, as well as an exit clause that allows either party to leave the agreement with a specific amount of time and written notice. The collaboration should be fair and beneficial to both parties.

Credentialing for Insurance Panels

First, you need to create a practice National Provider Identifier (NPI) number. This is required in addition to your individual provider NPI number. Once this number is created, you will be able to start the application process with the insurances of your choice. You again must have a bank account set up for the business where electronic payments will be deposited, along with proof of malpractice insurance, and copies of the board certifications for all practicing providers in the practice. Be aware that not all insurances are always accepting new providers. When it comes to credentialing as a medical practice, you need to first determine which insurance companies you would like to work with. Certain companies work easily with independently run nurse practitioner practices, while others can make it more challenging, asking for collaborating MDs despite state law saying they are not required (AANP, 2021). It is also important you get the fee schedule for the insurance company, to determine the financial reimbursement that will be received for each service. Remember, too, that there will be differences in reimbursement between different insurance companies, as some will pay more while others will pay significantly less for the same billing code. You need to determine if joining a specific insurance is financially beneficial for the practice. For instance, do you have to see more patients to be paid the same reimbursement from a higher-paying company? We want to be able to assist all patients no matter their insurance; however, we must keep in mind that we are running a business, not a charity. Financial considerations need to be made when it comes to credentialing with lower-paying insurance companies. When credentialing, you also need to keep in mind the length of time it takes from application submission to approval. Depending on the insurance, it can take anywhere from 30 to 90 days. The sooner you complete the application and submit all the requested supporting documents, the faster you will be able to open your doors, begin treating patients, and working toward turning a profit.

For those NPs who will be doing cash businesses, there is no need to credential; however, in the aesthetics world there are still treatments like Botox for migraines which can be processed under insurance. So, do the research on reimbursements to determine if it would be beneficial to credential with those companies that cover the treatments you offer. The process of credentialing can be very overwhelming in the beginning. It is important to keep track of when the application was submitted and to have a contact person so you can follow up on the status of the application throughout the process. They may need more documents signed or CVs may be needed. The sooner you can produce the information, the faster your approval will come. Your approvals from the insurance companies will come through at different times. By keeping track of this information, you can begin to schedule patients with the insurances you are currently credentialed with to prevent any further delays in providing treatment to the patients in your local community. And as you are approved with more companies, you can continue to expand your market.

There are services available for NPs who are overwhelmed or not willing to complete the leg work of credentialing. They will complete all of the applications, submit the supporting documentation, and manage the renewals of the contracts with the insurance company. They can even negotiate the terms of the agreement on your behalf to enhance reimbursement, which is something a new entrepreneur may not be that confident in immediately. Be sure to look at multiple options and their costs to determine who will provide the best services for the most appropriate cost. Remember, cheaper is not always better.

Selecting an EHR

When choosing the best electronic health records (EHR) for your practice, you want to determine your needs, likes, and wants. EHR systems can become very costly very quickly. Defining what you require to do your job will take priority over the added bells and whistles some EHR systems offer. Take a look at your business and review how much was designated for your EHR, then based on how many licenses you need, you can determine your budgeted amount for EHR. The estimated costs for a five-person practice to implement an EHR system are approximately $162,000 in the first year and $85,000 a year in maintenance costs (Tucker, 2019; Milliman, J 2019). Keep in mind that the right EHR does not have to break the bank. For a new practice, choosing a web-based system that has the availability of e-prescribing is a great place to start. Determine how many support staff licenses you are allowed for every prescriber you have in your practice to make sure there is enough access for everyone on your team. On average, you are allowed three support staff licenses for every prescriber. Those added licenses are assigned to your support team (e.g., medical assistants, registered nurses, administrative staff). The support staff licenses will have designated limitations on access for safety purposes to prevent unlicensed medical staff from being able to send prescriptions. Palabindala, Pamarthy & Jonnalagadda (2016).

When it comes to e-prescribing, you also want to determine if there is an extra cost for prescribing controlled substances, because there will need to be a two-step verification process in order for you to prescribe controlled substances through an EHR. You will want to know if this is part of the cost of the EHR or if there is an additional cost and whether or not it is through a third party. To improve your patient workflow, also investigate what the EHR offers in regard to ordering and receiving lab and radiology information. Most EHR systems have agreements in place with national chains to allow blood work and radiological exams to be ordered directly through the her, after which results will be sent directly to the patient's chart. This is extremely helpful for ease of access and in saving time for support staff. These systems cut down on unnecessary legwork. The goal is to use every aspect of your EHR to improve the work processes for your business to improve efficiency, which in turn will help to improve revenue.

The next thing to consider when choosing the best EHR for your practice is to look at which devices are able to utilize the system. In this day and age of working parents, many providers have other responsibilities when the workday ends. However, we know the job of the NP is never done. Investigate if staff are able to access the EHR from the IOS or android platforms, or if they can utilize a tablet. Some EHRs limit access to using specific web browsers. Know the limitations and benefits of using each system so you can make an educated decision in choosing the best system to support your business and its expected growth. But, have no fear. If after a fair trial of the system it is not able to support the needs of your practice, you can always change. There is no shortage of EHR systems on the market, so do not feel like you are stuck. As the saying goes, if at first you don't succeed, try try again.

Planning for Practice Growth

The time will come when your new business is growing faster than you can keep up. This is a good thing but can become overwhelming in the moment. Being proactive in planning for your expected growth will save you stress in the long run.

Part of your business plan was to make projections for your business. We hope to beat these goals, and when we do, we need to be able to support the expansion of the practice to meet the needs of the community. Recruitment is an integral part of preparing for expansion and meeting the demands of your population. There are many ways to recruit for your practice; the easiest being a recruitment solution such as Indeed, Monster.com, and Zip Recruiter. These avenues will give you access to thousands of résumés and eligible candidates, but know that it comes with a cost. As a new business, extra financial spending may not be readily available. So, do not feel there are no other options. Utilize your company website to post an ad for available positions in your practice. Create social media accounts for your businesses, if you have not already done so, and post the ad there and ask family, friends, and colleges to share it. We live in the day and age of the worldwide web and information travels fast. By utilizing social media, you are able to reach many people without any financial cost. Yes, there are ways to pay to boost the number of people who can see your posts, but it is not necessary if you utilize your connections. Your family, friends, and colleges want to see you succeed, so most people will share the post or tag a friend who might be interested in the position. This removes a lot of the legwork because it sends potential candidates to you. Recruitment is not limited to the use of services. Many have found employees through collaborations with local schools. As you know, nurse practitioners are required to complete clinical hours in order to graduate, so consider precepting students from surrounding schools, as this will introduce students to your practice for a future referral base, but they may also be your next hire.

When you train a student and they are a great fit to the practice, hiring this individual is extremely beneficial for both parties. When they are fully licensed, there is no delay in their revenue production, because they are already trained in the policies and procedures of your practice, and can deal with one of the biggest challenges: familiarizing themselves with the use of EHR. Recruitment of staff is not limited to NPs. Many schools are looking for clinical sites for the certified nursing assistant and medical assistant students. Again, training and hiring these individuals upon completion of their program means they are ready to take on all aspects of the role on their first day of hire, thus leading to improved workflow and greater productivity for the business.

Practice Management

Medical practice management is an important aspect of your business. This is usually a software solution, which is either part of your electronic health record system or a separate system altogether. The practice management system is the "headquarters" of the practice. This is where your day-to-day operations are tracked. A practice management system encompasses your schedules for all staff at all of their locations, phone/text/email reminders for appointments, insurance verification, and billing and administrative tasks. Depending on which EHR system you choose, this will determine if the practice management system is included or separate. I highly recommend when starting your business that you utilize a system where both the EHR and practice management system are included in the same platform. This is beneficial usually from a financial standpoint, but also for accessibility and ease of use. The appointment schedule is like a calculator for success. In the beginning it may be slow to start, but through your efforts of marketing and being registered with insurance companies, the referral base will increase. The schedule will help you to project your financial capability and determine if and when you need to bring on new staff to support the needs of the practice. It is always best to be proactive instead of reactive. If you know that your weekly appointments are low, you have to expect your financial reimbursements will be low in the 2 weeks following, potentially making covering the cost to do business more challenging. The schedule is a key performance indicator for the financial stability and growth of the practice. In order to help keep patients accountable for their appointments, I recommend looking for a system that does email, call, and text reminders. Mehra et al (2018) found no-show rates in outpatient settings ranging between 23.1% and 33.6%, resulting in decreased efficiency, lost time, and higher use of resources. Moore et al. (n.d.) found that no-shows adversely affected approximately 25% of scheduled time in a family medicine clinic and cost 14% of anticipated daily revenue. The lesson here is to follow your schedules closely and determine where there can be gaps that need to be filled. Also, do everything to support the compliance of your patients in regard to them showing up for their scheduled visits.

The financial management aspect of your practice is necessary for success. When an office visit is completed, the billing code and diagnosis are sent to the insurance company for review and payment. However, it is not always that easy. There are special codes and modifiers that can lead to payment for your visit being denied. In medical practices, medical billing denial rates range from 5–10%, with better performers averaging 4%. Some organizations even see denial rates on first billing as high as 15–20%. For those providers, one out of every five medical claims has to be reworked or appealed. Rework costs average $25 per claim, and success rates vary from 55–98%, depending on the medical denial management team's capabilities. When all else fails, write-offs can range from 1–5% of net patient revenue (Lachney, 2017). It is recommended to use a billing system that can "scrub" your claims to make sure there are no issues before forwarding them to the insurance company. This is process can save you time in having to resubmit the claim and prevent delays in payment. Most practice management systems or EHRs have built-in programs that are either managed by the suppliers or a third party. Either way, it is important to have someone like a certified biller/coder on staff or use an outside source to complete your practices billing. The price of billing services may seem costly, but know that having a designated person or system to do this task will lead to increased revenue in the long run. It may also be financially beneficial to see if your billing company or employee would be able to do your credentialing, as they go hand in hand. This can be an avenue to receive multiple benefits for service with a lower cost for using the same company. Again, bundling all your services together—like your EHR, practice management system, billing company, and credentialer—can save you time and money.

When it comes to treating patients, we as nurse practitioners are above board. We evaluate all aspects of the patients to ensure we are addressing their physical, social, and emotional needs. Nurse practitioners use evidence-based practice to improve clinical outcomes. We have been taught to implement the best practices into every daily care to improve patient outcomes. We can also track the improvement of our patient populations over time by tracking the data through our EHR systems. Creating standard work in a new practice is imperative to allow for highly consistent quality of care. This does not mean you will be told which drugs to use and how much. Instead, you will be given guidelines that have been proven to have successful results. This will allow providers to use the most up-to-date information. With that being said, guidelines should be reviewed and updated annually to make sure the latest evidence is implemented into the practice.

Resources and Support for NP Entrepreneurship

Toolkit:

- Epocrates
- Doximity
- GoodRx
- Hopkins Guides
- https://www.practicalpainmanagement.com/treatments/pharmacological/opioids/evaluation-comparison-online-equianalgesic-opioid-dose-conversion
- IBM Drug Reference
- https://www.nnpen.org

⚲ CASE STUDY: A SUCCESSFUL NP ENTREPRENEUR

In 2013, I was working as a nurse practitioner in a long-term care facility. I was finding it extremely challenging to find providers to manage my patients who were on opiates upon discharge. This was a time when primary care providers were gravitating away from prescribing controlled substances. When looking at the need in my community, along with the number of patients who have complaints of pain on a daily basis, I determined there was a large market that had significant gaps in care. I created a business plan, even though I did not require financial funding. I wanted to be able to look at my projections over the next 5 years and meet my yearly milestone. I independently began the credentialing process. I did the research and filed all the applications. I have to admit that I had some denials at first. I had to learn the hard way, as I was on a tight budget. At the time of opening, the HR that I incorporated into my practice was a free web-based service; however, since that time it has turned into a pay-per-provider system. I initially taught myself how to do billing and coding through the insurance websites and filed paper claims when necessary. But as the practice grew, we became more financially independent and were able to hire a company to complete the billing for all our providers. Also, as we grew we began to take on students to help with different roles in the practice. We collaborated with local technical schools for medical assistance and with local colleges for APRN students. We use these avenues to help with recruitment and retention for our practice. Since 2013, we have grown into the only fully-run nurse practitioner pain management clinic in the state of Connecticut, and currently provide services in two locations with local long-term care facilities and have a total of six nurse practitioners. We continue to set goals of national expansion and hope to make our evidence-based practices the industry's standards.

References

American Association of Nurse Practitioners. (2021). *State practice environment*. Retrieved April 1, 2021, from https://www.aanp.org/advocacy/state/state-practice-environment

Conley, V. M., & Judge-Ellis, T. (2021). Disrupting the system: An innovative model of comprehensive care. *The Journal for Nurse Practitioners, 17*(1), 32–36. doi:10.1016/j.nurpra.2020.09.012

Daly, R. (2009). AAMC issues alert about looming physician shortage. *Psychiatric News, 44*(2), 4-4. doi:10.1176/pn.44.2.0004a

Haddad, L., Toney-Butler, T., & Annamaraju, P. (2020). *Nursing shortage*. Retrieved March 30, 2021, from https://www.ncbi.nlm.nih.gov/books/NBK493175/

The Hartford. (2021). Workers' compensation insurance. Retrieved March 1, 2021, from https://www.thehartford.com/workers-compensation

Heiser, S. (2020). New AAMC report Confirms Growing Physician Shortage. Retrieved March 30, 2021, from https://www.aamc.org/news-insights/press-releases/new-aamc-report-confirms-growing-physician-shortage

Karimi, H., & Masoudi Alavi, N. (2015). Florence Nightingale: The mother of nursing. *Nursing and Midwifery Studies, 4*(2). doi:10.17795/nmsjournal29475

Lachney, K. (2017). *Medical billing denials are avoidable: How to help prevent the top 10*. Retrieved April 1, 2021, from http://promos.hcpro.com/pdf/MedicalBillingDenialsAreAvoidable_McKessonW.pdf

Laurant, M., Van der Biezen, M., Wijers, N., Watananirun, K., Kontopantelis, E., & Van Vught, A. J. (2018). Nurses as substitutes for doctors in primary care. *Cochrane Database of Systematic Reviews*. doi:10.1002/14651858.cd001271.pub3

Mehra, A., Hoogendoorn, C. J., Haggerty, G., Engelthaler, J., Gooden, S., Joseph, M., Guiney, P. A., et al. (2018). Reducing patient no-shows: An initiative at an integrated care teaching health center. *The Journal of the American Osteopathic Association, 118*(2), 77. doi:10.7556/jaoa.2018.022

Millman, J. (2019). *Electronic health records were supposed to be everywhere this YEAR. They're not—but it's okay*. Retrieved April 1, 2021, from https://www.washingtonpost.com/news/wonk/wp/2014/08/07/electronic-health-records-were-supposed-to-be-everywhere-this-year-theyre-not-but-its-okay/

Moore, C. D., Wilson-Witherspoon, P., & Probst, J. C. (n.d.). *Time and money: Effects of no-shows at a family practice residency clinic*. Retrieved April 1, 2021, from https://pubmed.ncbi.nlm.nih.gov/11456244/

Naylor, M. D., & Kurtzman, E. T. (2010). The role of nurse practitioners in reinventing primary care. Health affairs (Project Hope), 29(5), 893–899. https://doi.org/10.1377/hlthaff.2010.0440

Palabindala, V., Pamarthy, A., & Jonnalagadda, N. R. (2016). Adoption of electronic health records and barriers. *Journal of Community Hospital Internal Medicine Perspectives, 6*(5), 32643. doi:10.3402/jchimp.v6.32643

Pew Research Center. (2021). Social Media Fact Sheet. Retrieved March 1, 2021, from https://www.pewresearch.org/internet/fact-sheet/social-media/

Phillips, L. (2021). *Nurse Practitioner Entrepreneurship* [PowerPoint slides]. https://cdn.ymaws.com/www.pacnp.org/resource/resmgr/2017_Handouts/Phillips_Lynn_-_Nurse_Practi.pdf

Tucker, M.E., 2019) Physician Burnout Tied to Automated EHR Messages, American Psychiatric Association: Psychiatric News. Retrieved from:https://psychnews.psychiatryonline.org/doi/10.1176/appi.pn.2019.8b33

U.S. Small Business Association. (n.d.). *Write your business plan*. Retrieved March 1, 2021, from https://www.sba.gov/business-guide/plan-your-business/write-your-business-plan

Wilson, A., Whitaker, N., & Whitford, D. (2013). Rising to the challenge of health care reform with entrepreneurial and intrapreneurial nursing initiatives. *Creative Nursing, 19*(3), 166–168. doi:10.1891/1078-4535.19.3.166

Index

Note: Page numbers followed by *b*, *f*, *t* indicate boxes, figures and tables respectively.

A

AACN. *See* American Association of Colleges of Nursing; American Association of Critical Care Nurses
AAMC. *See* Association of American Medical Colleges
AANP. *See* American Academy of Nurse Practitioners; *See* American Association of Nurse Practitioners
AAP. *See* American Academy of Pediatrics
access to care
  enhancing through telehealth/telemedicine, 378–379
  telehealth, 334–335
Accreditation Association for Ambulatory Healthcare, 441
Accreditation Board for Specialty Nursing Certification, 432
ACE-Q screener, 145
ACE Star model, 38, 39*t*
ACEs. *See* adverse childhood experiences (ACEs)
acetaminophen, 199
ACP PIER. *See* American College of Physicians—Physicians Information & Education Resource
acute pain, 198
addiction, substance use disorders and. *See* substance use disorders
Advanced Alternative Payment Model (APM), 427
advanced practice nurses(APNs), 4, 13–16
  in telehealth, 332–333
    access to care, 334–335, 335*b*
    healthcare provider shortages, 333–334, 333–334*t*
    preventive education, management of complex and chronic diseases, and improving outcomes, 335–336
  competencies for, evidence-based practice, 37–38
  and palliative care, 193
  educational foundation for, 6–8
  The Essentials: Core Competencies for Professional Nursing Education, 6–8
    competencies, 8, 8–13*t*
    core nursing concepts, 8, 8*t*
    major domains, 8, 8–13*t*
  nurse anesthetists, 15–16
  nurse-midwives, 13–15, 15*f*
  professional identity, 352, 354–355
advanced practice registered nurses (APRNs), 4, 6
  Consensus Work Group, 375
  Joint Dialogue Group Report, 375
  legal scope of practice, 376
  prescriptive authority for, 229–231
  Regulatory Model, 376*f*
advancing nurse practitioner practice
  healthcare legislation, 371–372, 373*f*
  healthcare regulation, 372–373, 374*f*
adverse childhood experiences (ACEs), 103–105
  ACE Pyramid, 145, 145*f*
  BRFSS module prologue, 104–105*b*
  pyramid, 104*f*
  management, treatment, and referrals considerations, 144–146, 145*f*
  transgenerational trauma, 105–106
advocacy, 101
Affordable Care Act (ACA). *See* Patient Protection and Affordable Care Act of 2010
AFP. *See* American Academy of Family Physicians
Agency for Health Care Quality and Research (AHCQR), 107
Agency for Healthcare Research and Quality (AHRQ), 140, 42*t*
  national healthcare quality and disparities report, 217
  patient-centered outcomes research interventions, 62
  patient safety and medication errors, 232
  questions to guide for health care, 217
AGREE II tool, 50*t*, 55, 55*t*
AHCQR. *See* Agency for Health Care Quality and Research
AHRQ. *See* Agency for Healthcare Research and Quality
AIDS. *See* HIV/AIDS
"all-hands-on-deck" effort, 384
altruism, 359–361
American Academy of Family Physicians (AFP), 131
American Association of Nurse Practitioners (AANP), 249, 432
  National Certification Examinations, 432–433
American Academy of Pediatrics (AAP), 131

462 Index

American Association of Colleges of Nursing
(AACN), 157, 158, 277
Formal Health Policy Education, 369
American Association of Critical Care Nurses
(AACN), 46, 46t
American Association of Nurse Practitioners
(AANP), 131, 361, 434
American College of Physicians—Physicians
Information & Education Resource (ACP
PIER), 42t
American Nurses Association (ANA), 158
Culturally Congruent Standard, 158, 159b
American Nurses Credentialing Center (ANCC),
249, 432
Family Nurse Practitioner Examination, 432
American Recovery and Reinvestment Act (ARRA),
307–308
American Society of Addiction
Medicine (ASAM), 111
ANA. *See* American Nurses Association
ANCC. *See* American Nurses Credentialing Center
anorexia, 200
anticonvulsions, for pain management, 199
antidepressants, for pain management, 199
anxiety, 202
disorders, 139
anxiolytic agents, for dyspnea, 201
APM. *See* Advanced Alternative Payment Model
APNs. *See* advanced practice nurses
APRNs. *See* advanced practice registered nurses
ARCC model, 38, 39t
architecture, 319
ARRA. *See* American Recovery and Reinvestment Act
ASAM. *See* American Society of Addiction Medicine
Association of American Medical
Colleges (AAMC), 367
AstraZeneca, 279, 291t
authentic listening, 23
autonomy, 355–358
awareness, 149

B

balance, 149
Balanced Budget Act, 403
bamlanivimab, 292
bandwidth/broadband, 339–340
bargaining, employment contract, 440
baricitinib, 292
Barker-Sullivan Model of Mentor Partnerships, 395
Beck Depression Inventory (BDI), 203
B.E.L.T. framework, 339, 340f
best-of-breed *vs.* integrated systems, 319–320
billing resources, coding and. *See* coding, and billing resources
bills
drafted, 372
for visit, 425
organization to work, 371
biological racial differences, 163
biological variations, 162–163

biomedical practitioners, 22
bipolar and related disorders, 138
bipolar I disorder, 138
bipolar II disorder, 138
bouncing back process, 74. *See also* resilience
broadband, 339–340
bronchodilators, for dyspnea, 201
buprenorphine, 380
business owner, nurse practitioner as
entrepreneurship, 449
resources and support for, 459
owning practice, legal aspects of
collaborative agreements *vs.* independent
practice, 453–454, 454f
credentialing for insurance panels, 454–455
electronic health records, selecting, 456
practice growth, planning for, 456–457
practice management, 457–459
practice start-up, 450–452

C

cachexia, 200
CAGE-AID, 112
CAGE questionnaire, 112
Calgary Family Assessment Model (CFAM),
80, 82
Campbell Collaboration, 43t
cancer
anorexia and cachexia in, 200
fatigue in, 202
CAPC. *See* Center to Advance Palliative Care
CARA. *See* Comprehensive Addiction
and Recovery Act
care coordination
electronic health records and, 311
communication and, 224–225
increased, 306
care depletion, 148
care transitions, 189
CARES Act. *See* Coronavirus Aid, Relief and
Economic Security (CARES) Act
caring, defined, 20
CAS. *See* cultural awareness and sensitivity
case presentation, 255–256. *See also* oral case
presentation
casirivimab, 292
CASP critical appraisal checklists, 49t
CBT. *See* cognitive behavioral therapy
CCA tool, 168
CCB. *See* cultural competence behaviors
CCNE. *See* Commission on Collegiate Nursing
Education
CDC. *See* Centers for Disease Control and
Prevention
CDS. *See* clinical decision support
Center for Evidence-Based Medicine
(Oxford), 43t
Center for Transdisciplinary Evidence-based Practice
(CTEP), 36
Center to Advance Palliative Care (CAPC), 192

Centers for Disease Control and Prevention
        (CDC), 132
    chronic diseases, 193
    Telehealth/Telemedicine, 379
Centers for Medicare and Medicaid Services (CMS),
        140, 434
    national provider number, 404
certification
    distribution, top practice setting, and clinical
        focus area by area of, 7t
    examination, 432–433
certified midwives (CMs), 14, 15f
certified nurse-midwife (CNM), 4,
        14–15, 15f
certified registered nurse anesthetist (CRNA),
        4, 15–16
CFAM. See Calgary Family Assessment Model
chain of infection, 281, 281f
change theory, 74
chief complaint, 257, 260, 416
children, living in poverty, 102
CHMM. See Collaborative Health Management
        Model
chronic diseases (CD), 193–194
    management of complex and, 335–336
    nurse practitioner, role of
        community health workers, 195
        self-management programs, 194–195
    palliative care and. See palliative care
    symptom management, 196, 197–198b
        anorexia/cachexia, 200
        anxiety, 202
        depression, 202
        dyspnea, 200–201
        fatigue, 201–202
        pain, 196, 198–200
chronic pain, 198
CHWs. See community health workers
CINAHL. See Cumulative Index to Nursing Allied
        Health Literature
CINAHL Plus with Full Text, 43t
CLAS standards. See Culturally and Linguistically
        Appropriate Services in Health Care
clinical decision support (CDS), 318
clinical education, 237–239
    current trends in, 249
    daily reflective questions, 239
    Doctorate of Nursing Practice
        community health and population
            focus, 248
        leadership and management, 248
        postmaster's NP clinical education in,
            247–248
        teaching/learning, 248
    evaluation and clinical time documentation,
        246–247
    faculty, role of, 239–241
    final project, 248–249
    future of, 249–250
    pandemic's impact on, 250
    preceptor, role of, 244–246
    student, role of, 241–244

clinical education, cultural competency and,
        157–160, 159b
clinical evidence, 43t
clinical nurse specialist (CNS), 4
clinical practice, integration of telehealth
        into, 337
Clinical Prevention and Population Health (CPPH)
        Curriculum Framework, 293
clinical prevention, defined, 278
clinical privileging, 441
clinical time documentation, 246–247
clinician burnout, electronic health records and,
        320–321
clinician, cultural competence and
    cultural competence, determining, 168–169,
        168f, 169–170b
    culture awareness and cultural sensitivity, 167
"cloud"-based systems, 319
CMs. See certified midwives
CMS. See Centers for Medicare and Medicaid
        Services
CNM. See certified nurse-midwife
CNS. See clinical nurse specialist
coach, 391, 392t
Cochrane Collaboration, 43t
Cochrane Database of Systematic
        Reviews, 41, 44
Cochrane Library, 41, 44
Code of Ethics, 332
coding
    and billing resources
        CPT and ICD-10 books, 405–406
        medical coding, defined, 405
        medical necessity, 406, 407–411
    by time vs. medical decision making,
        425, 425t
    conundrums, 425–427, 427b
    general guidelines, 413–414
        CPT procedure codes, 414
        ICD-10 diagnoses codes, 414
        outpatient and office visits, significant changes
            to, 415
        patient encounter, levels of, 415
        patient encounter, location of, 414, 415b
cognitive behavioral therapy (CBT), 142–143
collaboration, 263–264, 361, 437
    defining, 264
    by state statute, 264
    interprofessional. See interprofessional
        collaboration
collaborative agreements
    employment contract, 441–442
    for advanced practice nurses requesting
        prescriptive authority, 442–444t
    independent practice vs., 453–454, 454f
collaborative care, defined, 437
Collaborative Health Management Model (CHMM),
        271–273
Columbia Suicide Severity Rating Scale
        (C-SSRS), 140
Commission on Collegiate Nursing Education
        (CCNE), 249, 270

464　Index

communication
  and care coordination, 224–225
  cultural awareness, 160–161
  electronic health records and, 311
  interprofessional, 270
  language and, 174–175, 174f
    community partnerships, 177–178
    evaluation, 180
    listening, 175, 176b
    pulling it all together, 178–180, 179b
    trust, 175–177
  style, misinterpretation of, 165–166
community health and population, 248
community health workers (CHWs), 195
community partnerships, 177–178
compassion fatigue, 148
compassion satisfaction, 148
competencies. *See also* core competencies; cultural competence
  based education, 7
  enhancement/development, process for, 165–166, 166b
  for advanced practice nurses, evidence-based practice, 37–38
compliance plan, 427, 427b
Comprehensive Addiction and Recovery Act (CARA), 380
computerized provider order entry (CPOE), 318
connection, 149
consultant's responsibilities, 267–268
consultation, 263–264
  consultant's responsibilities, 267–268
  defining, 264–265
  formal, 267b
  mechanisms for, 265b
  process, 266–267
  reasons for, 265–266, 266b
continuous quality improvement (CQI), 215–216
contract tracing, 291
Controlled Substances Act (CSA), 380
convalescent plasma, 292
conversion, electronic health record
  go-live, 317
  implementation
    configuration, 316
    paper chart migration, 317
    testing, 316–317
    training, 316
  post-go-live, 317–318
  preparation
    available resources, 314
    communication plan, 315
    readiness assessment, 314
    request for proposal, 315
    setting goal and vision, 314
    workflow documentation, 314
  system/product selection
    contracting, 316
    vendor demonstration, 315
core competencies, 13, 13b
  advanced practice nursing foci, 13–16
  for effective mentoring, 394

nurse anesthetists, 15–16
nurse-midwives, 13–15, 15f
Coronavirus Aid, Relief and Economic Security (CARES) Act, 384
coronavirus disease 2019. *See* COVID-19
Coronavirus Preparedness and Response Supplemental Appropriation Act, 328
corticosteroids, for COVID-19, 292
cost savings, electronic health records and, 311–312
countertransference, 148
COVID-19, 278, 284
  affiliated with severe infection, 288
  and prevention levels, 288–293
    primary prevention, 289–291
    secondary prevention, 291–292
    tertiary prevention, 292–293
  impact on clinical education, 250
  in older adults, 288–289
  telehealth, 328–329, 344
  transmission of, 289
  transmission-based precautions, 292
  traumatic impacts from, 131
  vaccine, 278–279, 290–291t
CPOE. *See* computerized provider order entry
CPT. *See* Current Procedural Terminology
CQI. *See* continuous quality improvement
CRAFFT test, 112
credentialing
  employment contract, 441
  for insurance panels, 454–455
  form, 404
  third-party, 404
critical appraisal
  clinical practice guidelines, 54–59
  of evidence, 48–50, 49–50t, 51–52t
  of single intervention study, 54
  tools, 49–50, 49–50t, 51–52t
Critical Appraisal Sheets, 49t
CRNA. *See* certified registered nurse anesthetist
CSA. *See* Controlled Substances Act
CTEP. *See* Center for Transdisciplinary Evidence-based Practice
cultural approach, 165
cultural awareness
  communication, 160–161
  social organization, 161
  space, 161
  time, 161
cultural awareness and sensitivity (CAS), 168
cultural competence
  and clinical education, 157–160, 159b
  and clinician, 165–167, 166b
    culture awareness and cultural sensitivity, 167
  determining, 168–169
  promoting in primary health care, 169–170b
  puzzle, demystifying, 171–174
  Pyramid Model of Intercultural Competence, 168f
cultural competence behaviors (CCB), 168
cultural dimensions theory, 163

Index

cultural humility, 163–164, 165b
cultural immersion experiences, 170–171
cultural sensitivity and global health, 155–156
    cultural awareness
        communication, 160–161
        social organization, 161
        space, 161
        time, 161
    cultural competence and clinician, 165–167, 166b
        culture awareness and cultural sensitivity, 167
        determining, 168–169, 168f, 169–170b
    cultural competence puzzle, demystifying, 171–174
    cultural competency and clinical education, 157–160, 159b
    cultural humility, 163–164, 165b
    cultural immersion experiences, 170–171
    environmental control, 161–162
        biological variations, 162–163
        Hofstede's cultural dimensions theory, 163
    global diversity, 156–157
    language and communication, 174–175, 174f
        community partnerships, 177–178
        evaluation, 180
        listening, 175, 176b
        pulling it all together, 178–180, 179b
        trust, 175–177
cultural variations, 165
Culturally and Linguistically Appropriate Services in Health Care (CLAS standards), 164, 175
culture awareness and cultural sensitivity, 167
culture of safety, 219
Cumulative Index to Nursing Allied Health Literature (CINAHL), 41, 44
Current Procedural Terminology (CPT), 379, 405–406
    structure of procedure codes, 414
curriculum vitae, résumé vs., 435, 436b
    résumé writing, do's and don'ts of, 435–436

D

DA. *See* decision aids
DCVMRC. *See* Division of the Civilian Volunteer Medical Reserve Corps
DEA. *See* Drug Enforcement Administration
decision aids (DA), 59
Dempster Practice Behavior Scale (DPBS), 357
depression, 202
depressive disorders, 138
developmental approach, 73
dexamethasone, 292
Diagnostic and Statistical Manual of Mental Disorders, fifth edition (DSM-V), 132
    mental illness, 137
    substance-related and addictive disorders, 139
    trauma- and stressor-related disorders, 143
diagnostic studies, 261
differential diagnosis, 261

"dimensions of diversity" model, 160
disparities, vulnerabilities and, 99
    advocacy, 101
    literacy, 100–101
    poverty. *See* poverty
    social determinants of health, 99–100, 100t
    vulnerability and resilience, 103
dissemination, evidence-based practice, 62
Division of the Civilian Volunteer Medical Reserve Corps (DCVMRC), 300
divorced families, 82
DNP. *See* Doctorate of Nursing Practice
DNP Essentials, 216, 370
Doctor of Nursing Practice (DNP) Roadmap, 62
doctoral education, quality in, 216
Doctorate of Nursing Practice (DNP), 16–18, 37, 237
    community health and population focus, 248
    leadership and management, 248
    postmaster's NP clinical education in, 247–248
    teaching/learning, 248
DPBS. *See* Dempster Practice Behavior Scale
Drug Enforcement Administration (DEA), 434
dual-diagnoses, 139
dyspnea, 200–201

E

Early and Periodic Screening, Diagnosis, and Treatment (EPSDT), 140
EBM. *See* evidence-based medicine
EBP. *See* evidence-based practice
ecomap, 91–92
economic stability, 135
education access and quality, 135
educational programs, 5–6
education/environment, 340
efficiency, electronic health records and, 306–307, 311–312
ehealth, 330t, 331
EHRs. *See* electronic health records
elderly. *See* older adults
older adults
    and poverty, 102
    COVID-19 in, 288–289
    trauma-informed care, 147–148
    substance abuse, 148
electronic documentation. *See* electronic health records
electronic health records (EHRs), 229
    and clinician burnout, 320–321
    barriers and challenges to adoption, 313
    benefits of using, 310–312
        enhanced patient safety, 311
        improved care coordination and communication, 311
        improved quality of patient care, 310–311
        increased efficiencies and cost savings, 311–312
        increased population health, 312
        reduction in medical errors, 311

466 Index

electronic health records (EHRs) (*Continued*)
  conversion
    go-live, 317
    implementation, 316–317
    post-go-live, 317–318
    preparation, 314–315
    system/product selection, 315–316
  core functionalities of, 306
  features and functionality
    administrative processes, 318
    decision support, 318
    electronic communication and connectivity, 318
    health information and data, 318
    order management, 318
    patient support, 318
    reporting and population health, 319
    result management, 318
  health information exchange, 312
  influencing forces, 307–308
  meaningful use, 308f
    stage 1, 308–309
    stage 2, 309
    stage 3, 309
  reasons for
    complete and accurate patient information, 305–306
    greater efficiency, 306–307
    increased care coordination, 306
    patient participation and empowerment, 307
  technical considerations
    architecture, 319
    best-of-breed versus integrated systems, 319–320
    hardware options, 320–321
  selecting, 456
electronic medical records (EMRs), 229, 310
electronic prescribing (E-prescribing), 231
elevator speech, 371
ELNEC. *See* End of Life Nursing Education Consortium
emergency
  defined, 297
  preparedness, 297–301
empathy, 24
employer provider number, 404
employer, questions for, 439, 440b
employment contract negotiation, 439–440, 440b
  bargaining, 440
  collaborative agreements, 441–442, 442–444t
  Consensus Model, 445
  credentialing, 441
  finalizing, 440–441
  preparation, 440
empowerment, 361, 438
  patient participation and, 307
EMRs. *See* electronic medical records
End of Life Nursing Education Consortium (ELNEC), 192
endemic, 282
Enhanced Calgary Cambridge Guide, 224

entrepreneurship, 449
  resources and support for, 459
entry-level primary provider, guidelines for, 331–332
environmental control, 161–162
  biological variations, 162–163
  Hofstede's cultural dimensions theory, 163
e-prescribing, 456
epidemic, 282
epidemiological triangle, 281, 281f
epidemiology, 277–279
  defined, 278
  population health, 282–283
  terminology in, 279–282, 280b, 281f
EPQA. *See* Evidence-Based Practice Process Quality
EPSDT. *See* Early and Periodic Screening, Diagnosis, and Treatment
equipment and platform finding, 342
eradication, 282
The Essentials: Core Competencies for Professional Nursing Education, 6–8
  competencies, 8, 8–13t
  core nursing concepts, 8, 8t
  major domains, 8, 8–13t
The Essentials of Doctoral Education for Advanced Nursing Practice, 216, 369–370
ethics
  Code of Ethics, 332
  professional nurse practitioner, 358–359
  values and ethics for interprofessional practice, 270
ethnic groups, and poverty, 102
ETHNIC mnemonic, 175, 176b
evaluation, 180
  and clinical time documentation, 246–247
  and management documentation guidelines, 413
  and management plus procedure, 425–426
evidence
  critical appraisal of, 48–50, 49–50t, 51–52t
  searching databases for current, 40–45, 42–44t
  searching for, 38, 40, 41f, 42f
  sources of, 42–44t
  synthesis and recommendations. *See* evidence synthesis
  thing counts as evidence, 45–48, 46–47t, 48t
evidence-based medicine (EBM), 33
evidence-based practice (EBP)
  barriers to, 62–63
  competencies for advanced practice nurses, 37–38
  defined, 34–35
  disseminating, 62
  evidence
    critical appraisal of, 48–50, 49–50t, 51–52t
    hierarchies, 45–48, 46–47t, 48t
    searching databases for current, 40–45, 42–44t
    searching for, 38, 40, 41f, 42f
    synthesis and recommendations. *See* evidence synthesis
  history of, 33–34
  key assumptions of, 35
  nursing and, 34–36
  reason for nurse practitioner using, 36–37

Index 467

outcomes of, 59, 60–61t
shared decision making, 59, 62
translating into practice, 38, 39–40t
preceptor, 246
Evidence-Based Practice Process Quality (EPQA), 62
evidence synthesis
    and recommendations, 53–54, 53t
        AGREE II instrument, 55t
        critical appraisal of clinical practice guidelines, 54–59
        critical appraisal of single intervention study, 54
        grading system for clinical practice recommendations, 57–58t
        USPSTF recommendation grades and suggestions, 56t

F

face-to-face interview, 438–439
facilitators, integrative review of, 357
faculty, role of, 239–241
Faculty/Student Healthcare Mission, 359–361
Family Assessment and Intervention Model, 80
family capacity, 79–80, 79f
family development theory, 73, 81–82
family-focused clinical practice
    divorced families, 82
    family capacity, 79–80, 79f
    family development, 81–82
    family function, 81
    family structure, 80–81
    family theory, 71–72
        macrosystem, application to clinical practice, 72–73
        microsystem, application to clinical practice, 73–74
    nontraditional families
        foster families, 83–84
        grandparents raising grandchildren, 84–85
        same-sex couple families, 83
        single-parent families, 82–83
    resilience, 74–75
        family resilience, 74–79
        theoretical model, 76f
    structural assessment and family interviews
        ecomap, 91–92
        family pedigree, 88–91, 90–91f, 90b
        family problem list, 92–93
        family problem list/case study exercises, 94–95
        family risk assessment tools, 91, 92b
        genograms. See genograms
family function, 81
family interviews, structural assessment and
    ecomap, 91–92
    family pedigree, 88–91, 90–91f, 90b
    family problem list, 92–93
    family problem list/case study exercises, 94

family risk assessment tools, 91, 92b
    genograms. See genograms
family pedigree, 88–91, 90–91f, 90b
    drawing, 90f
    key questions for a family history warranting, 90b
    symbols, 91f
family problem list, 92–93
    case study exercises, 94–95
family resilience, 74–79, 76f
family risk assessment tools, 91, 92b
family stress theory, 74
family structure, 80–81
family systems approach, 73
family theory, 71–72
    macrosystem, application to clinical practice
        developmental approach, 73
        interactional approach, 73
        structural approach, 72–73
    microsystem, application to clinical practice
        change theory, 74
        family stress theory, 74
        family systems approach, 73
family tree, 88
fatigue, 201–202
Federal Bureau of Primary Health Care, 106
Federal Bureau of Prisons, 117
federally qualified health centers (FQHCs), 117–118
fellowship program, 397
finalizing, employment contract, 440–441
financial management of practice, 458
"5 As" approach, 21
The Flexner Report, 351
FNS. *See* Frontier Nursing Service
formal health policy education for nurse practitioner, 369–370
foster families, 83–84
FQHCs. *See* federally qualified health centers
Framingham Heart Study, 280
Friedman Family Assessment Model, 80
Frontier Nursing Service (FNS), 13–14

G

GAD. *See* generalized anxiety disorder
GAF. *See* Global Assessment of Functioning
Gamaleya (Sputnik-V), 290t
gap analysis, 125
gender dysphoria, 120
gender expression, 120–122
gender identity, 120–122, 121t
generalized anxiety disorder (GAD), 139
genetics, 162
genograms, 85–86
    interview data
        expanded events, 87b
        factual events, 87b
        relationships, 88b
    key indicators to develop, 86b
    process of developing, 86–87
    themes, 88b
    understanding and interpreting, 87–88

Index

genomics, 162
Geographic Practice Cost Index (GPCI), 412
geriatrics. *See* older adults
gifting, 394
Global Assessment of Functioning (GAF), 136
global diversity, 156–157
global health, cultural sensitivity and. *See* cultural sensitivity and global health
Golden Rule, 155
GPCI. *See* Geographic Practice Cost Index
Grading of Recommendations, Assessment, Development and Evaluations (GRADE) approach, 55–56
grading system for clinical practice recommendations, 57–58t
graduation, preparing for, 431–432
grandchildren, grandparents raising, 84–85
grandparents raising grandchildren, 84–85
grounded theory, 243

H

HADS. *See* Hospital Anxiety and Depression Scale
Hamric's Model of Advanced Practice Nursing competencies, 244
hardware options, 320–321
HCPCS. *See* Healthcare Common Procedure Coding System
health disparities, 132–134
  social determinants of health, 134–135, 134f
health information exchange (HIE), 312
Health Information Technology for Economic and Clinical Health Act (HITECH), 308
health innovation, 449
Health Insurance Portability and Accountability Act of 1996 (HIPAA), 341, 404, 434, 453
health literacy. *See* literacy
health policy, 367–368
  advancing nurse practitioner practice through
    healthcare legislation, 371–372, 373f
    healthcare regulation, 372–373, 374f
  current issues
    access to care through telehealth/telemedicine, 378–379
    opioid crisis, 379–380
    Patient Protection and Affordable Care Act, 378
    scope of practice. *See* scope of practice
  formal health policy education for nurse practitioner, 369–370
  getting involved, 380–382
  history of nurse practitioner and related, 368–369
  nurse practitioner health policy exemplars
    exemplar 1, 382–383
    exemplar 2, 383–385
health-related outcomes, 280
healthcare access and quality, 135
Healthcare Common Procedure Coding System (HCPCS), 406
healthcare disparities. *See also* disparities, vulnerabilities and

chronic diseases and, 194
healthcare legislation, 371–372, 373f
healthcare provider shortages, 333–334, 333–334t
healthcare regulation, 372–373, 374f
Healthy People 2030, 166, 293–297, 294–295b, 298f
Healthy People Curriculum Task Force, 293
Helene Fuld Health Trust National Institute for Evidence-based Practice in Nursing and Healthcare Center, 36
herd immunity, 282
HIE. *See* health information exchange
HIPAA. *See* Health Insurance Portability and Accountability Act of 1996
history
  and reimbursement decisions, 416
  of nurse practitioner and related health policy, 368–369
history of present illness (HPI), 260, 416
HITECH. *See* Health Information Technology for Economic and Clinical Health Act
HIV/AIDS, 123–114, 285
  and prevention levels, 286–288
    primary prevention of, 287
    secondary prevention, 287–288
    tertiary prevention, 288
  CDC recommendation for testing, 287
  community partnerships, 178
  related discrimination, 123
  related stigma, 123
  transmission of, 286
Hofstede's cultural dimensions theory, 163
holistic care, nurse practitioners role in, 132
homeless health care
  assessing for homelessness at point of care, 107b
  barriers to, 109–110
  clinical practice guidelines, 107, 107b, 108–109t
  defining, 106–107
Hospice and Palliative Nurses Foundation (HPNF), 191
hospice care, 188, 188f
Hospital Anxiety and Depression Scale (HADS), 203
HPI. *See* history of present illness
HPNF. *See* Hospice and Palliative Nurses Foundation
Human Genome Project, 89, 163
Human immunodeficiency virus (HIV)/acquired immunodeficiency syndrome (AIDS). *See* HIV/AIDS
human trafficking, 118–119, 119f
  sex trafficking on victims, 120t
  telephone numbers for victims and healthcare providers, 120b

I

IAT. *See* Implicit Association Test
ICN. *See* International Council of Nurses
identifying individuals/team to lead, 342
IHI. *See* Institute for Healthcare Improvement
illness and disease, 281
imdevimag, 292
immigrant health, refugee and. *See* refugee and immigrant health

immunization. *See* vaccination
Implicit Association Test (IAT), 167
implicit bias, 156, 167
imposter syndrome, 242–243
in-house computer system, 319
in-person provider visits *vs.* telehealth, 331
"incident to" billing, 425–427
independent practice
    autonomy and, 357
    collaborative agreements *vs.*, 453–454, 454*f*
individual life span theory, 73
informatics, 229
    and healthcare technologies, 12*t*
Institute for Healthcare Improvement (IHI), 224
Institute of Medicine (IOM), 174
    interprofessional collaboration, 268
    quality reports, 218–219
insurance panels, credentialing for, 454–455
integrated systems, best-of-breed *vs.*, 319–320
integrating with electronic medical record, 342
interactional approach, 73
International Classification of Diseases, Tenth Edition (ICD-10), 136, 405–406
    structure of diagnoses codes, 414
International Council of Nurses (ICN), 358
interprofessional collaboration (IPC), 268–270, 270*b*
    barriers and benefits to effective, 273
    competency domains
        interprofessional communication, 270
        roles and responsibilities, 270
        teams and teamwork, 271
        values and ethics for, 270
interprofessional education (IPE), 268
Interprofessional Education Collaborative (IPEC), 269–270
interprofessional partnerships, 11*t*
interprofessionality, defined, 269
interview data. *See* family interviews, structural assessment and
    collection, 80
    expanded events, 87*b*
    factual events, 87*b*
    relationships, 88*b*
interviewing skills
    employer, questions for, 439, 440*b*
    interview process, 438–439, 439*b*
intra-professional tensions, impact of, 362–363
introduction/chief complaint, 257, 260
IOM. *See* Institute of Medicine (IOM)
Iowa Model of Evidence-Based Practice to Promote Quality Care, 38, 39*t*
IPC. *See* interprofessional collaboration
IPE. *See* interprofessional education
IPEC. *See* Interprofessional Education Collaborative

J

JHNEBP Model, 53–54
Joanna Briggs Institute, 43*t*, 45
job satisfaction, 436–437
Johns Hopkins Nursing EBP Model, 38, 39*t*

Johnson & Johnson, 279, 290*t*
The Joint Commission, 227, 441
just culture, 219

K

King's framework, 20
knowledge for nursing practice, 9*t*

L

lack of role clarity, 362
lack of uniformity, 362
language and communication, 174–175, 174*f*
    community partnerships, 177–178
    evaluation, 180
    listening, 175, 176*b*
    pulling it all together, 178–180, 179*b*
    trust, 175–177
leadership, 307
    and management, 248
    interprofessional collaboration, 271
    professional nurse practitioner, 361–362
    quality principles, 219
    telehealth, 340
Leading Health Indicators (LHI), 294–295*b*
Leininger's theory on diversity, 157
lesbian, gay, bisexual, and transgender (LGBT), 122, 122*t*
lesbian, gay, bisexual, transgender, queer, questioning, and intersex (LGBTQ/QI), 120
levels of evidence hierarchy, 45–48
LGBT. *See* lesbian, gay, bisexual, and transgender
LGBTQ/QI. *See* lesbian, gay, bisexual, transgender, queer, questioning, and intersex
LHI. *See* Leading Health Indicators
LIAASE tool, 178–179, 179*b*
    for culturally sensitive care, 179–180
licensure for prescription privileges
    advanced practice state licensure, 433–434
    Drug Enforcement Administration licensure, 434
    national provider identification, 434
life course theory, 73
lifelong learning, 397–398
    benefits of, 398*b*
    for professional nurse practitioner, 398*b*
    personal growth activities, 398*b*
listening, 175, 176*b*
literacy, 100–101
live videoconferencing, 329, 330*t*

M

MACRA. *See* Medicare Access and CHIP Reauthorization Act
macrosystem
    application of family theory to clinical practice
        developmental approach, 73
        interactional approach, 73
        structural approach, 72–73

470 Index

malpractice insurance, 434–435, 453, 455
management plan, 261–262
MDM. *See* medical decision making
Meaningful Use (MU), 307
   advanced clinical processes, 309
   conceptual approach to, 308f
   data capture and sharing, 309
   improved outcomes, 309
   stage 1, 308–309
   stage 2, 309
   stage 3, 309
MEASUREevaluation. *See* monitoring and evaluation to assess and use results (MEASURE) evaluation
medical coding, defined, 405
medical decision making (MDM)
   and reimbursement, 417–418, 419–420t
   coding by time *vs.*, 425, 425t
   for office and outpatient, 418, 421–424t
medical errors, reduction in, 311
Medical Literature Online (MEDLINE), 41, 44t, 45
medical necessity, 406, 407–411
medical practice management, 457–458
medical record documentation, 406, 412, 412f
medical reserve corps (MRC), 300
Medicare Access and CHIP Reauthorization Act (MACRA), 427
medication errors, 232, 233t
MEDLINE. *See* Medical Literature Online
mental health and primary care, 131
   health disparities, 132–134
      social determinants of health, 134–135, 134f
   importance of self-care, 148–149
      scope of practice, 149–150
   management, treatment, and referrals
      considerations, 142–143
      adverse childhood experiences, 144–146, 145f
      trauma, 143–144
   mental health
      defined, 135–136
      mental illness. *See* mental illness
      mental status exam, 141–142
      screening, 140–141
   nurse practitioners role in holistic care, 132
   trauma-informed care
      geriatric considerations, 147–148
      pediatric considerations, 146–147
mental illness, 136–137
   anxiety disorders, 139
   bipolar and related disorders, 138
   depressive disorders, 138
   substance-related and addictive disorders, 139
   suicide, 140
mental status exam (MSE), 141–142
mentor, 391–396
   nurse practitioner residency and fellowship programs, 397
   nurse practitioners as lifelong learners, 397–398, 398b
   preceptor, coach *vs.*, 392t
   sample mentor and mentee agreement, 395f
   stages of mentor relationship, 394b

mentoring and lifelong learning
   coach, 391, 392t
   mentor, 391–396
      nurse practitioner residency and fellowship programs, 397
      nurse practitioners as lifelong learners, 397–398, 398b
      preceptor, coach *vs.*, 392t
      sample mentor and mentee agreement, 395f
      stages of mentor relationship, 394b
   preceptor, 389–390, 392t
   role model, 390–391
mentoring, defined, 392
mentor–mentee relationship, 392–396
   stages of, 394b
mentorship program, 393
Merit-based Incentive Payment System (MIPS), 427
mHealth. *See* mobile health
MI. *See* motivational interviewing
microsystem
   application of family theory to clinical practice
      change theory, 74
      family stress theory, 74
      family systems approach, 73
mid-level practitioner, 434
middle range theory, 20
military's "mission first" approach, 383
Mini-CEX, 240
MIPS. *See* Merit-based Incentive Payment System
Misener Nurse Practitioner Job Satisfaction Scale (MNPJSS), 436
mistrust, 175–177
MNPJSS. *See* Misener Nurse Practitioner Job Satisfaction Scale
mobile health (mHealth), 330t, 331, 339
Model for EBP Change, 38, 40t
model of practice, 27f
Moderna, 279, 290t
modifiers, 425–426
monitoring and evaluation to assess and use results (MEASURE) evaluation, 296–297
morbidity, 280
mortality, 280, 280b
motivational interviewing (MI), 142–143
MRC. *See* medical reserve corps
MSE. *See* mental status exam
MU. *See* Meaningful Use
My AGREE PLUSSoftware, 50t, 55

N

NAMI. *See* National Association of Mental Illness
NAPNAP. *See* National Association of Pediatric Nurse Practitioners (NAPNAP)
NARA. *See* National Archives and Records Administration
National Alliance to End Homelessness, 106
National Archives and Records Administration (NARA), 372
National Association of Mental Illness (NAMI), 140

Index

National Association of Pediatric Nurse Practitioners (NAPNAP), 131, 369, 381
National Cancer Institute (NCI), 192, 199
National Center for Children in Poverty (NCCP), 102
national certification, 432
National Coalition for Hospice and Palliative Care (The Coalition), 191
National Commission for Certifying Agencies, 432
National Consensus Project (NCP), 191–192
National Council of State Boards of Nursing (NCSBN), 336, 377
    APRN Advisory Committee, 5, 375, 445
National Diabetes Prevention Program (NDPP), 194
National Health Care for the Homeless Council (NHCHC), 106, 107, 107t
National Institutes of Health and Clinical Excellence, 43t
National Organization for Nurse Practitioner Faculties (NONPF), 13, 18, 255, 331, 370, 390
national organizations, 191–192
National Patient Safety Goals (NPSGs), 227
National Provider Identification (NPI), 434, 454–455
national provider number, 404
National Quality Forum (NQF), 191
National Quality Strategy (NQS), 217
NCCP. *See* National Center for Children in Poverty
NCI. *See* National Cancer Institute
NCP. *See* National Consensus Project
NCSBN. *See* National Council of State Boards of Nursing
NDPP. *See* National Diabetes Prevention Program
needs assessment, 124
    framework and plan, 124–125
    gap analysis and results, 125
    process measures, 125
negotiation, 24–25
    employment contract, 439–440
neighborhood and built environment, 135
network bandwidth, 339–340
neurological procedures, for pain management, 199
new patient, defined, 413
NHCHC. *See* National Health Care for the Homeless Council
Nightingale, Florence, 19, 215, 368, 449
NLM database, 44t
NMHCs. *See* nurse-managed health centers
non-research evidence, 35
non-steroidal anti-inflammatory drugs (NSAIDs), 199
NONPF. *See* National Organization for Nurse Practitioner Faculties
nontraditional families
    foster families, 83–84
    grandparents raising grandchildren, 84–85
    same-sex couple families, 83
    single-parent families, 82–83
Novavax, 279, 290t
NP. *See* nurse practitioner
NPI. *See* National Provider Identification
NPs. *See* nurse practitioners
NPSGs. *See* National Patient Safety Goals
NQF. *See* National Quality Forum
NQS. *See* National Quality Strategy
NSAIDs. *See* non-steroidal anti-inflammatory drugs
nurse anesthetists, 15–16
nurse-managed health centers (NMHCs), 436–437
nurse-midwives, 13–15, 15f
Nurse Practice Act, 336
nurse practitioners (NPs)
    approach to patient care, 18–19
    as business owner. *See* business owner, nurse practitioner as
    as lifelong learners, 397–398, 398b
    beyond, 13–16
    biomedical practitioners *vs.*, 22
    certification, 431
        certification examination, 432–433
        graduation, preparing for, 431–432
        national certification, 432
    core competencies, 13, 13b
        advanced practice nursing foci, 13–16
        nurse anesthetists, 15–16
        nurse-midwives, 13–15, 15f
    education and title clarification, 5–6
    emergency preparedness and, 297–301
    entrepreneurship, resources and support for, 459
    ethnographical study of student, 243–244
    formal health policy education for, 369–370
    health policy. *See* health policy
    history and related health policy, 368–369
    in chronic diseases
        community health workers, 195
        self-management programs, 194–195
    in holistic care, 132
    licensure for prescription privileges
        advanced practice state licensure, 433–434
        Drug Enforcement Administration licensure, 434
        national provider identification, 434
    model of practice, 27f
    nursing theories for, 20–21
    objectives for educational program, 164
    reason for using evidence-based practice, 36–37
    reimbursement for. *See* reimbursement
    residency and fellowship programs, 397
    résumé *vs.* curriculum vitae development for, 435, 436b
    résumé writing, do's and don'ts of, 435–436
    role of, 21–23, 23t
        authentic listening, 23
        empathy, 24
        going above and beyond expectation, 25–28
        historical perspective, 3–4
        negotiating, 24–25
        today, 6, 7t
    role transition, 241–242
    Stewart Model of, 28f
    work of, 19–20
Nurse Practitioner Preceptorship Tax Credit Fund, 249
nurses, and palliative care, 192–193
nursing and evidence-based practice, 34–36
    reason for nurse practitioner using, 36–37
nursing theories, 20–21. *See also specific theories*

O

Objective Structured Clinical Examination (OSCE), 240
OCP. *See* oral case presentation
OCR. *See* Office for Civil Rights
ODPHP. *See* Office of Disease Prevention and Health promotion
office and outpatient
  medical decision making for, 418, 421–424*t*
  visits
    changes to, 415
    services provided other than, 416, 417*t*
Office for Civil Rights (OCR), 336
Office of Administration of Children and Families, 118
Office of Disease Prevention and Health promotion (ODPHP), 293
Office of Minority Health (OMH), 174–175
Office of the National Coordinator for Health Information Technology (ONCHIT), 307
OMH. *See* Office of Minority Health
ONCHIT. *See* Office of the National Coordinator for Health Information Technology
opioids
  crisis, 379–380
  for dyspnea, 201
  for pain management, 198–199
oral case presentation (OCP), 256–257, 262–263*b*
  components of, 258–259*b*
    diagnostic studies, 261
    differential diagnosis, 261
    history of present illness, 260
    introduction or chief complaint, 257, 260
    management plan, 261–262
    physical examination, 260
  tips for effective, 257*b*
OSCE. *See* Objective Structured Clinical Examination
outpatient visits. *See* office and outpatient, visits
owning practice, legal aspects of, 452–453
  collaborative agreements *vs.* independent practice, 453–454, 454*f*
  credentialing for insurance panels, 454–455
  electronic health records, selecting, 456
  practice growth, planning for, 456–457
  practice management, 457–459
Oxford Centre for Evidence-Based Medicine 2011 Levels of Evidence, 46–47, 47*t*

P

pain
  assessment, 198–199
  management, 196, 198–200
palliative care
  background, 187–188, 188*f*
  defined, 187–188, 188*f*
  goals of, 189
  hospice care *vs.*, 188
  national organizations, 191–192
  nurses and, 192–193
  quality of life, 189–191, 190*f*
  symptom management, 196, 197–198*b*
    anorexia/cachexia, 200
    anxiety, 202
    depression, 202
    dyspnea, 200–201
    fatigue, 201–202
    pain, 196, 198–200
  transitions, 189
pandemic, 282
panic attack specifier, 139
paraphernalia, 287
PARIHS framework, 38, 39*t*
partnership, defined, 177–178
passive immunization, 292
past family and social history (PFSH), 416
patient care, approach to, 18–19
patient-centered care, 223–224
Patient Centered Medical Home (PCMH), 271
patient-centered outcomes research interventions (PCORI), 62
patient-centered telehealth practices, 343
patient encounter
  levels of, 415
  location of, 414, 415*b*
Patient History Questionnaire (PHQ-9), 140
patient information, complete and accurate, 305–306
patient-nurse relationship, 20
patient participation and empowerment, 307
Patient Protection and Affordable Care Act of 2010, 3, 217, 256, 269, 378
patient safety and medication errors, 232, 233*t*
patients education, 343
payment for services, 412–413, 413*b*
PCMH. *See* Patient Centered Medical Home
PCORI. *See* patient-centered outcomes research interventions
PDMPs. *See* Prescription Drug Monitoring Programs
PDSAframework. *See* Plan-Do-Study-Act (PDSA) framework
PEARLS. *See* Related Life-events Screener
Pearson Report, 434
Pediatric ACEs Screening, 145
Pediatric Nursing Certification Board, 432
Pediatric Symptom Checklist (PSC), 147
pediatrics, trauma-informed care, 146–147
pedigree. *See* family pedigree
peer mentoring, 396
peer review process, 441
person-centered care, 9*t*
personal attributes of autonomy, 356
personal, professional, and leadership development, 13*t*
personal space, 161
Pfizer-BioNTech, 279, 291*t*
PFSH. *See* past family and social history
phenomenological community, 283
physical examination, 260
  and reimbursement decisions, 416–417, 418*t*
physicians, objectives for educational program, 164
Physicians Health Questionnaire 9 (PHQ-9), 203

Index 473

PICOT questions, 38, 40–41, 41–42f
PIT. *See* professional identity theory
Plan-Do-Study-Act (PDSA) framework, 226
Planetree Model, 223
Platinum Rule, 155, 158
POMR. *See* problem oriented medical record
population-based programs, 124–125
    needs assessment for
        gap analysis and results, 125
        needs assessment framework and plan, 124–125
        process measures, 125
population health, 9–10t, 278, 282–283
    and *Healthy People 2030*, 293–297, 294–295b, 298f
    electronic health records and, 312
post-traumatic stress disorder (PTSD), 147
postmaster's NP clinical education, 247–248
poverty
    definition, 101–102
    elderly and, 102
    ethnic groups and, 102
    women and children living in, 102
power, defined, 438
practice authority, 405
practice-focused doctoral programs, 369
practice growth, planning for, 456–457
practice management, 457–459
practice of medicine, 336
pre-exposure prophylaxis (PrEP), 287
PRECEDE-PROCEED model, 297, 298f
preceptor, 389–390, 392t
    role of, 244–246
PrEP. *See* pre-exposure prophylaxis
prescription
    electronic prescribing, 231
    writing, 232–234, 233f
Prescription Drug Monitoring Programs (PDMPs), 230
prescriptive authority, 229–231
    electronic prescribing, 231
    patient safety and medication errors, 232, 233t
    writing prescription, 232–234, 233f
prevention levels, 283
    COVID-19 and, 288–293, 290–291t
    HIV and, 286–288
    primary prevention, 284–285, 284b
    secondary prevention, 285–286
    tertiary prevention, 286
preventive education, 335–336
primary care, mental health and. *See* primary care, mental health and
primary healthcare providers, 165b
primary prevention, 284–285, 284b
    of COVID-19, 289–291
    of HIV, 287
priority setting, in disaster, 300
prison health
    clinical practice guidelines for, 117
    healthcare needs of prisoners, 116–117
    incarceration timeline risk factors, 117t
    interventions for reintegration post-incarceration, 117–118, 118b

privacy and protective health information requirements relevant to, 336, 337b
problem list
    family problem list, 92–93
        case study exercises, 94–95
problem oriented medical record (POMR), 92
professional accountability, 219
professional attributes of autonomy, 356
professional employment
    collaboration, 437
    collaborative agreements, 441–442, 442–444t
    Consensus Model, 445
    credentialing, 441
    employment contract negotiation, 439–440, 440b
        bargaining, 440
        finalizing, 440–441
        preparation, 440
    empowerment, 438
    interviewing skills
        interview process, 438–439, 439b
        questions for employer, 439, 440b
    job satisfaction, 436–437
    malpractice insurance, 434–435
    nurse practitioner certification, 431
        certification examination, 432–433
        graduation, preparing for, 431–432
        national certification, 432
    nurse practitioner licensure for prescription privileges
        advanced practice state licensure, 433–434
        Drug Enforcement Administration licensure, 434
        national provider identification, 434
    résumé *vs.* curriculum vitae development for nurse practitioners, 435, 436b
    résumé writing, do's and don'ts of, 435–436
professional identity theory (PIT), 352
professional liability, 434–435
professional nurse practitioner
    characteristics of, 355
    concepts and challenges of
        autonomy, 355–358
        barriers, 362–363
        ethics, 358–359
        leadership, 361–362
        professionalism, 351–355
        service/altruism, 359–361
professionalism, 12t, 351–355
program evaluation, 60–61t
Prospero, 44t
providers education, for telehealth, 342–343
PSC. *See* Pediatric Symptom Checklist
psychological empowerment, 438
PTSD. *See* post-traumatic stress disorder
public health
    nursing, 277
    emergency, scope of practice expanding during, 377–378
PubMed, 41, 44t, 45
pursed lip breathing, 201
Pyramid Model of Intercultural Competence, 168, 168f

Q

QA. *See* quality assurance
QI. *See* quality improvement (QI)
QOL. *See* quality of life
QPP. *See* Quality Payment Program
QSENinitiative. *See* Quality and Safety Education for Nurses (QSEN) initiative
quality, 215–216
   and safety education for nurses, 220, 220–223*t*
   attributes of, 218–219
   communication and care coordination, 224–225
   dimensions of, 218
   electronic health records and, 310–311
   in doctoral education, 216
   informatics, 229
   Institute of Medicine reports, 218–219
   patient-centered care, 223–224
   professional accountability and teamwork, 219
   quality improvement planning, 225–227
   safety, 10–11*t*
   TeamSTEPPS, 229
   U.S. healthcare system, 216–218
Quality and Safety Education for Nurses (QSEN) initiative, 220
   knowledge, skills, and attitudes for quality improvement, 221–223*t*
   knowledge, skills, and attitudes for safety, 220–221*t*
quality assurance (QA), 216
quality improvement (QI), 60–61*t*, 215
   planning, 225–227
   QSEN knowledge, skills, and attitudes for, 221–223*t*
quality of life (QOL), 189–191, 190*f*
Quality Payment Program (QPP), 427

R

race-based medical mistrust, 177
radiation therapy, for pain management, 199
rapid critical appraisal checklists, 49*t*, 55
RBRVS. *See* resource-based relative value scale
RC. *See* relational coordination
RCA for Evidence-Based Guidelines, 49*t*
Re-Aim Framework, 343
realize, defined, 146
recognize, defined, 146
Recovery and Reinvestment Act of 2009, 269
referral
   defining, 265
   process, 266–267
   reasons for, 265–266, 266*b*
   tracking, 267
refugee and immigrant health
   common healthcare issues and torture, 114–115, 115*t*
   major host countries, 113–114, 114*f*
   refugee health profiles, 115–116, 116*t*
   resettlement issues, 114
   top countries of origin, 113
refugee health profiles information, 115–116, 116*t*
regionalism, transmission of information and, 161
registered nurses (RNs)
   prescriptive authority for, 229
   to advanced practice nurse, 244
   to nurse practitioner, 241–242
reimbursement
   bill for visit, 425
   coding and billing resources
      CPT and ICD-10 books, 405–406
      medical coding, defined, 405
      medical necessity, 406, 407–411
   coding conundrums, 425–427, 427*b*
   eligibility, important steps in, 403–404
      employer provider number, 404
      national provider number, 404
      practice authority, 405
      third-party credentialing, 404
   evaluation and management documentation guidelines, 413
   general coding guidelines, 413–414
      CPT procedure codes, 414
      ICD-10 diagnoses codes, 414
      outpatient and office visits, significant changes to, 415
      patient encounter, levels of, 415
      patient encounter, location of, 414, 415*b*
   key components of, 415
      coding by time *vs.* MDM, 425, 425*t*
      history and reimbursement decisions, 416
      medical decision making and reimbursement, 417–418, 419–420*t*
      medical decision making for office and outpatient, 418, 421–424*t*
      physical examination and reimbursement decisions, 416–417, 418*t*
      services provided, 416, 417*t*
   medical record documentation, 406, 412, 412*f*
   payment for services, 412–413, 413*b*
   value-based reimbursement, 427–428
reintegration post-incarceration, interventions for, 117–118, 118*b*
Related Life-events Screener (PEARLS), 145
relational coordination (RC), 306
relational resilience, 78
remdesivir, 292
remote management/monitoring/coaching, 338
remote patient monitoring (RPM), 330*t*, 331
RePort, 44*t*
request for proposal (RFP), 315
research, 60–61*t*
   appraisal questions, 49*t*
resettlement issues, refugee and immigrant health, 114
residency program, 397
resilience
   defined, 74–75
   family resilience, 74–79

theoretical model, 76f
   vulnerability and, 103
resisting re-traumatization, 146
resource-based relative value scale (RBRVS), 412, 412b
responding, defined, 146
résumé vs. curriculum vitae for nurse practitioners, 435, 436b
   résumé writing, do's and don'ts of, 435–436
résumé writing, do's and don'ts of, 435–436
review of systems (ROS), 416
Revised Standards for QUality Improvement Reporting Excellence (SQUIRE) 2.0, 62
Wolf's Caring Behaviors Inventory instrument, revised, 21
RFP. *See* request for proposal
RNs. *See* registered nurses
Robert Wood Johnson Foundation (RWJF), 375
role model, defined, 390–391
ROS. *See* review of systems
RPM. *See* remote patient monitoring
RWJF. *See* Robert Wood Johnson Foundation

S

SaaS. *See* software as a service
safety, 227–228
   electronic health records and, 311
   informatics, 229
   patient safety and medication errors, 232, 233t
   QSEN knowledge, skills, and attitudes for, 220–221t
   quality and safety education for nurses, 220, 220–223t
   TeamSTEPPS, 229
SAGE acronym, 394
same-sex couple families, 83
SAMHSA. *See* Substance Abuse and Mental Health Services Administration
SARS. *See* severe acute respiratory syndrome
scholarship, 361
   for nursing discipline, 10t
scope of practice, 149–150, 441–442
   defining, 375–377, 376f
   expanding during public health emergency, 377–378
screening, mental health, 140–141
SDM. *See* shared decision making
SDOH. *See* social determinants of health
secondary prevention, 285–286
   of COVID-19, 291–292
   of HIV, 287–288
self-care, importance of, 148–149
   scope of practice, 149–150
self-efficacy, 393
self-management programs (SMP), 194–195
self-medication, 139
seroconversion period, 286
services
   payment for, 412–413, 413b
   professional nurse practitioner, 359–361

severe acute respiratory syndrome (SARS), 289
sex trafficking, impact of, 119, 120t
sexual preference, 120–122, 121t
SHARE Approach, 59
shared decision making (SDM), 59, 62
shared evaluation and management, 425–426
simulation, 240
single database, 320
single-parent families, 82–83
Sinopharm, 291t
SIT. *See* social identity theory
site visits, supervising students by, 240–241
smallpox vaccination, 278
smoking cessation, intervention in, 21
SMP. *See* self-management programs
SNL. *See* standardized nursing language
social and community context, 135
social determinants of health (SDOH), 217, 283, 295–296
   domains of, 134f
   mental health and primary care, 134–135
   vulnerabilities and, 99–100, 100t
social identity theory (SIT), 352
social organization, 161
Social Security Act, 369
software as a service (SaaS), 319
sound bite, 371
source of data, 320
space, 161
staff education, for telehealth, 342–343
standardized nursing language (SNL), 21–22
state regulations, for telehealth, 341
steroids
   for dyspnea, 201
   for pain management, 199
Stewart Model of Nurse Practitionering, 27, 28f
The Stimulus Act. *See* American Recovery and Reinvestment Act
store-and-forward technology, 329, 330t, 331
stressor-related disorders, 143
Strong model, 361
structural approach, 72–73
structural empowerment, 438
student, role of, 241–244
substance abuse, geriatrics, 148
Substance Abuse and Mental Health Services Administration (SAMHSA), 110, 146, 380
substance-related and addictive disorders, 139
Substance Use-Disorder Prevention that Promotes Opioid Recovery and Treatment (SUPPORT) Act, 380
substance use disorders (SUDs)
   and addiction, 110
      characteristics of, 111f
      evaluation of, 112, 112b
      impact on patients, 111
      screening, 112
   management and treatment of, 113
   trends in, 110f
   vulnerable populations and, 111–112

476 Index

suicide, 140
SUPPORTAct. *See* Substance Use-Disorder Prevention that Promotes Opioid Recovery and Treatment (SUPPORT) Act
symptom management, 196, 197–198*b*
syndromic surveillance, 299
system-based resilience model, 75
systems-based practice, 11*t*

T

talk therapy, 142
TB. *See* tuberculosis
teaching/learning theory, 248
teams, interprofessional collaboration, 271
TeamSTEPPS, 229
teamwork, 219
  interprofessional collaboration, 271
technology, telehealth, 340
telehealth, 250, 327
  advanced practice nurse practitioner in, 332–333
    access to care, 334–335, 335*b*
    healthcare provider shortages, 333–334, 333–334*t*
    preventive education, management of complex and chronic diseases, and improving outcomes, 335–336
  clinical practice, integration into, 337
  enhancing access to care through, 378–379
  evaluation of systems, 343
  frameworks
    bandwidth/broadband, 339–340
    B.E.L.T. framework, 339, 340*f*
    education/environment, 340
    leadership, 340
    mobile health, 339
    remote management/monitoring/coaching, 338
    technology, 340
    Telehealth Service Implementation Model, 338, 339*f*
    telemedicine, 338
    Tietze Telehealth Framework, 338, 340*f*
    videoconferencing, 339
  future of, 344
  guidelines for entry-level primary provider, 331–332
  history of, 328–329
  in-person provider visits *vs.*, 331
  modalities, 330*t*
    live videoconferencing, 329
    mobile health/ehealth, 331
    remote patient monitoring, 331
    store-and-forward, 329, 331
  privacy and protective health information requirements relevant to, 336, 337*b*
  regulations, 336
  services under bad faith provision, 337*b*
  steps for implementing, 341
    equipment and platform finding, 342
    HIPAA and state regulations, 341
    identifying individuals/team to lead, 342

integrating with electronic medical record, 342
patient-centered telehealth practices, 343
patients education, 343
staff and providers education, 342–343
use in practice, 341
telemedicine *vs.*, 327–328
Telehealth Service Implementation Model, 338, 339*f*
telemedicine, 338
  enhancing access to care through, 378–379
  telehealth *vs.*, 327–328
  uses, 335*b*
telephone interview, 438–439
tertiary prevention, 286
  of COVID-19, 292–293
  of HIV, 288
third-party credentialing, 404
Tietze Telehealth Framework, 338, 340*f*
time, concept of, 161
transcultural nursing theory, 20
Transdisciplinary Model of EBP, 38, 40*t*
transgenerational/intergenerational trauma, 105–106
  based precautions, 292
  COVID-19, 289
  HIV/AIDS, 286
  of family patterns, 86
transmission, 281
trauma
  from adverse childhood experiences, 145
  management, treatment, and referrals considerations, 143–144
  transgenerational/intergenerational, 105–106
trauma-informed care
  geriatric considerations, 147–148
  pediatric considerations, 146–147
Trinity EBP model, 38, 40*t*
TRIP. *See* Turning Research into Practice Database
trust, 175–177
Truvada (tenofovir/emtricitabine), 287
tuberculosis (TB), 279
Turning Research into Practice Database (TRIP), 44*t*

U

United Nations High Commission for Refugees (UNHCR), 113
United States Preventive Services Task Force (USPSTF), 112, 285
  grading system, 55, 56*t*
  recommendation grades and suggestions, 56*t*
"universal precautions" approach, 146
UpToDate, 44*t*, 56, 57–58*t*
U.S. Department of Health and Human Services (USDHHS), 134, 372–373
  Organizational Chart, 374*f*
USDHHS. *See* U.S. Department of Health and Human Services
U.S. healthcare system, 216–218
USPSTF. *See* United States Preventive Services Task Force
U.S. Surgeon General's Family History Initiative, 89

Index

V

vaccination
  COVID-19, 278–279, 290, 290–291t
  primary prevention, 284–285
  smallpox, 278
value-based reimbursement, 427–428
values and ethics for interprofessional practice, 270
vendor demonstration, 315
Vendor Rating Tool, 315
vicarious traumatization, 148
video interview, 438–439
videoconferencing, 339
visits
  bill for, 425
  office and outpatient
    changes to, 415
    services provided other than, 416, 417t
  risks associated with complexity level of, 419–420t
volunteering, 299–300
vulnerability, 283
vulnerable populations
  adverse childhood events, 103–105
    BRFSS module prologue, 104–105b
    pyramid, 104f
    transgenerational trauma, 105–106
  gender identity, expression, and sexual preference, 120–122, 121t, 122t
  HIV/AIDS, 123–114
  homeless health care
    assessing for homelessness at point of care, 107b
    barriers to, 109–110
    clinical practice guidelines, 107, 107b, 108–109t
    defining, 106–107
  human trafficking, 118–119, 119f
    sex trafficking on victims, 120t
    telephone numbers for victims and healthcare providers, 120b
  needs assessment for
    gap analysis and results, 125
    needs assessment framework and plan, 124–125
    process measures, 125
  population-based programs, 124–125
  prison health
    clinical practice guidelines for, 117
    healthcare needs of prisoners, 116–117, 117t
    interventions for reintegration post-incarceration, 117–118, 118b
  refugee and immigrant health
    common healthcare issues and torture, 114–115, 115t
    major host countries, 113–114, 114f
    refugee health profiles, 115–116, 116t
    resettlement issues, 114
    top countries of origin, 113
  special populations, direct care, and access. *See* specific populations
  substance use disorders and addiction. *See* substance use disorders
  vulnerabilities and disparities, 99
    advocacy, 101
    literacy, 100–101
    poverty. *See* poverty
    social determinants of health, 99–100, 100t
    vulnerability and resilience, 103

W

Watson's Theory of Human Caring, 20
WHO. *See* World Health Organization (WHO)
women, living in poverty, 102
World Health Organization (WHO)
  health innovation, 449
  International Classification of Diseases, 136–137
  interprofessional collaboration, 269
  social determinants of health, 134
World Health Organization Disability Assessment Schedule 2.0 (WHODAS 2.0), 136